A CLINICAL GUIDE TO
PEDIATRIC NURSING

Second Edition

A CLINICAL GUIDE TO PEDIATRIC NURSING

Marilyn Lang Evans, R.N., M.Ed.
Associate Professor
School of Nursing
The University of North Carolina at Greensboro
Greensboro, North Carolina

Beverly Desmond Hansen, R.N., M.N.
Assistant Director of
Hospital Operations
Children's Hospital
New Orleans, Louisiana

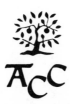

APPLETON-CENTURY-CROFTS/Norwalk, Connecticut

0-8385-1129-5

Notice: The author(s) and publisher of this volume have taken care that the information and recommendations contained herein are accurate and compatible with the standards generally accepted at the time of publication.

Copyright © 1985 by Appleton-Century-Crofts
A Publishing Division of Prentice-Hall, Inc.

85 86 87 88 89 / 10 9 8 7 6 5 4 3 2

Prentice-Hall International, Inc., London
Prentice-Hall of Australia, Pty. Ltd., Sydney
Prentice-Hall Canada, Inc.
Prentice-Hall of India Private Limited, New Delhi
Prentice-Hall of Japan, Inc., Tokyo
Prentice-Hall of Southeast Asia (Pte.) Ltd., Singapore
Whitehall Books Ltd., Wellington, New Zealand
Editora Prentice-Hall do Brasil Ltda., Rio de Janeiro

Library of Congress Cataloging in Publication Data

Evans, Marilyn Lang, 1939-
  A clinical guide to pediatric nursing.

  Rev. ed. of: Guide to pediatric nursing, c1980.
  Bibliography: p.
  Includes index.
  1. Pediatric nursing. I. Hansen, Beverly Desmond,
1940-   . II. Evans, Marilyn Lang, 1939-
Guide to pediatric nursing. III. Title. [DNLM: 1. Pedia-
tric Nursing—outlines. WY 18 E93g]
RJ245.E828 1984   610.73'62   84-16944
ISBN 0-8385-1129-5

Design: Jean M. Sabato-Morley

In honor of my parents, Margaret and Charles E. Lang,
and in loving memory of Eileen and Robert G. Evans, Sr.,
for all they have given me.

M. L. E.

To my son Scott
for taking the book in stride

B. D. H.

CONTENTS

PREFACE

As demonstrated in the first edition, we strongly believe that holistic nursing care of the pediatric patient necessitates including the family in all aspects of hospital and well child care. Preparing the child and family for what to expect during and following a contact with the health care system is essential. Taking time to accomplish the teaching of the child and family, and to arrange community follow-up are important parts of quality nursing care. Recognition of the psychosocial needs of the child and parents and implementing nursing measures to support them are integral to our philosophy of pediatric nursing.

We recognize that continuing to provide comprehensive care which incorporates these beliefs will become more challenging to the pediatric nurse as economic resources for health care diminish.

The delivery of health care to children has continued to change since the first edition of this book. Changes in treatment approaches and greater involvement of parents in the care of their children, as well as increasing pressure to make health care more cost effective and efficient, have resulted in shorter hospitalizations, greater outpatient treatment of conditions which formerly required hospitalization, and more children being seen in ambulatory settings in shorter time periods.

Nursing students, and practicing clinicians, are experiencing limited contact with children and their families in both hospital and ambulatory settings while being expected to deliver quality care. In many situations, nursing students no longer have the opportunity to prepare in advance for the care they will provide. These conditions demand that nurses make maximal use of their contact time and that there be an up-to-date, readily available source of information that can be used as the basis for providing health care to children and their families.

The goal of this edition, like that of the first, is to present a clear, direct, concise approach to the nursing care of children in a variety of settings. The General Considerations section, which precedes Nursing Management for each topic, provides the knowledge base essential for safe care. The Nursing Management sections, which consistently include instructions for care of the child in the home, present a plan of care which meets standards of quality assurance and are easily individualized for a particular child. Alphabetical arrangement of topics permits immediate access to information and extensive cross referencing eliminates repetition. Prospective payment systems require initiation of discharge planning on admission and the format of this book reinforces that concept.

Every topic from the first edition has been updated to reflect current accepted practice and new topics have been added. The expanded appendices contribute to the nurse's ability to perform a rapid assessment of the child. Health care of the adolescent has been given particular emphasis in order to make the book applicable to the full range of the pediatric population.

PREFACE
FROM THE FIRST EDITION

The health care of children is changing as health professionals increase their focus on promotion of the child's physical and emotional well-being. Parents are assuming more responsibility for the health care of their children. Hospitalizations are less frequent and are shorter in length. As a result, those who provide nursing care for children and their families must use the limited contact time wisely and efficiently.

This book provides a clear, direct, and concise approach to nursing management. In order to help the reader find essential information immediately, the topics have been arranged alphabetically in an outline format. A reference system has been used to minimize repetition. The book's scope includes selected aspects of both ambulatory and acute pediatric nursing.

The consistent inclusion of instructions for home management will assist the nurse in meeting the standards for quality assurance. The book also provides nursing students with basic information in those clinical situations where preparation in advance is impossible.

We wish to acknowledge the contribution of Rebecca Smoak Parrish, B.S.N., M.S.N., P.N.P., Assistant Professor at The University of North Carolina at Greensboro School of Nursing for content and suggestions related to ambulatory care in the early portion of the book. We are deeply indebted to Becky Patterson, B.S.N., M.S.N., Instructor at The University of North Carolina at Greensboro School of Nursing for her diligent review of material, her suggestions for organization of content, and her constant, enthusiastic support.

We also wish to thank Leslie Boyer, our nursing editor, for her understanding of the need for this book, and for her constant support during the past year. Our special thanks go to Gayle Mandigo who typed the major portion of the text, and to Linda Allen, Connie Prater, and Patricia Rockwood for their assistance. Additional typing help was offered by Judy Allen, Janet Poole, and Beverly Bradshaw. We also appreciate the assistance of Margie Kent and her faith in us while we worked. We are grateful for the encouragement of our families, colleagues, and students.

ACKNOWLEDGMENTS

We are deely indebted to Becky Patterson, B.S.N., M.S.N. and Becky Knight, B.S.N., M.S.N., for their diligent reviewing of material and suggestions for organization of content. We also wish to thank our nursing editor, Marion Kalstein-Welch, for her assistance in completing this edition.

Our thanks also go to Ila Falgout for typing the revisions. We are also appreciative of the gracious assistance of our medical librarians, Nancy Keller, Leslie Mackler, and Kristi Marshall.

The book has no senior author. Either name could come first since it represents the equal work of two persons committed to a single goal.

INSTRUCTIONS FOR USE

The topics in this text are listed alphabetically. Each topic is divided into two sections. General Considerations includes information about the topic. Nursing Management includes nursing procedures for the child and family.

The reader will be referred to additional topics by the use of either *italics* or SMALL CAPITALS. Topics in *italics* contain material essential to the topic being reviewed. This material should be read immediately so the information can be used in patient/family care.

Topics in SMALL CAPITALS contain material supplemental to the topic being reviewed. This material will expand the reader's knowledge, but need not be read immediately.

Example: You want to read about Admission to the Hospital, Elective (Page 10).

1. Read General Considerations.
2. Read Nursing Management.
3. Read *Hospitalization, Support During* (Page 148) and *Preparation for Procedures* (Page 225).
4. Read DISCHARGE PLANNING AND HOSPITALIZATION, RESPONSE TO as soon as time permits.

INTRODUCTION

Framework of Reference
for Pediatric Nurses

The authors have presented their introduction in an outline format similar to that used throughout the text. We hope this will familiarize the reader with the unique structure of A Clinical Guide to Pediatric Nursing; 2nd Edition.

Introduction to the care of children—Selected aspects of child development which are basic to quality nursing care.

A. General Considerations.
   1. Children are competent.
      a. Infants are born with protective reflexes.
      b. Infants can summon help by crying.
      c. Competency and responsibility for personal actions increase with age in normal children.
   2. Although the rate varies with each child, the sequence of development is the same. See *Appendix 5.*
   3. Children also exhibit individuality in their growth and development.
      a. Acquisition of skills may be early, average, or late.
      b. Cultural patterns influence learning (e.g., speech development).
      c. Family social environment may determine emphasis on accomplishment of certain tasks.
   4. Growth and development are directional.
      a. Cephalocaudal (e.g., arm control before hand control, newborn more advanced near the head).
      b. General to specific (e.g., vocalization precedes speech; gross motor coordination precedes fine motor coordination).
      c. Proximodistal (e.g., shoulder control before head control).
   5. There is a time span called the critical period when accomplishment of a developmental task is most favorable (e.g., learning to walk around 13–14 months of age).
   6. Children demonstrate a compulsion to master a new task through repetition (e.g., standing or walking).
   7. A child can master only one new task at a time.
   8. The environment may dictate focus on a certain task. (e.g., The immobilized child experiences his environment primarily through vision.)
   9. Developmental aspects are interrelated and the child must be assessed as a whole.

B. Nursing Management.
   1. Assess factors which affect the child's behavior.
      a. Parent-child relationship.
      b. Genetic endowment.
      c. Modified family life experiences:
         1. Single parent. See *Single Parent Families.*

2. Adopted Child. See *Adoption*.
3. Family crisis.
4. Poverty.
5. Chronic illness of family members.
d. Parents' child-rearing practices. See *Parenting*.
e. Sibling and peer relationships.
2. Identify and support the child's usual coping patterns. See *Coping*.
a. How does he usually deal with new experiences?
b. How does he usually express his feelings when he is troubled?
3. Support the child in using his own resources of energy, intelligence, and coordination to help him accomplish developmental tasks.
4. Encourage the child's support system (parents, teacher, nurse) to participate actively in the child's contact with the health care system.

A CLINICAL GUIDE TO PEDIATRIC NURSING

TOPICS

Abandonment, fear of. See *Fears.*

Abscess. A localized collection of pus.

Abscess, epidermal. Bacterial infection between skin layers.

A. General Considerations.
1. Incision and drainage may be necessary.
2. Heat application may be ordered before and/or after incision and drainage.

B. Nursing Management.
1. Support the child and parents during hospitalization. See *Hospitalization, Support During.*
2. Initiate discharge planning. See *Discharge Planning.*
3. Apply restraints when necessary to prevent the young child from disturbing the site, particularly during afternoon naps and nighttime sleep. See *Restraints.*
4. Observe, record, and report the child's response to antibiotic therapy.
5. Enlist the child's cooperation. See *Preparation for Procedures.*
   a. Let him make choices about the time of the procedure within reasonable limits.
   b. Teach him the steps in the application of compresses and soaks using terminology appropriate to his age and ability to understand.
   c. Have him hold unopened gauze dressings until you need them.
6. Check temperature of compresses or soaks to prevent injury to the child's sensitive skin.
7. Apply dressings securely so that the child can engage in active play.
8. Explain to parents the importance of handwashing to prevent secondary infection.

Abscess, retropharyngeal. Infection of lymph nodes located behind the posterior wall; usually caused by group A beta-hemolytic streptococcus.

A. General Considerations.
1. Symptoms follow an upper respiratory infection.
   a. High fever.
   b. Anorexia.
   c. Refusal to swallow.
   d. Drooling.
2. If I.V. antibiotic therapy is begun immediately, surgery may not be required.
3. If the mass is fluctuant, surgical incision will be performed.

B. Nursing Management.
1. Support the child and parents during hospitalization. See *Hospitalization, Support During.*
2. Initiate discharge planning. See *Discharge Planning.*
3. Use the mummy restraint to restrain the child securely during physical examination.
4. Place the child in Trendelenburg position.
5. Have suction equipment available.
6. Observe, record, and report the child's response to antibiotic therapy.
7. Institute measures to reduce fever as ordered. See *Fever Reduction.*
8. Perform gentle, oral suction if absolutely necessary without touching mass.
9. Prepare the child and parents if surgery must be done. See *Preoperative Care* and *Preparation for Surgery.*
10. Meet the postoperative needs of the child. See *Postoperative Care.*
    a. Elevate the foot of the bed and position the child on the abdomen or side after incision and drainage.
    b. Apply restraints if the child becomes restless.
    c. Give mouth care frequently.
    d. Observe, record, and report the following:
       1. Increased respiratory rate.
       2. Nasal flaring.
       3. Cyanosis.
       4. Frequent swallowing.
       5. Bright, bloody drainage.

A

Abused child. A child who has been injured by non-accidental means or who has received improper care from his parent(s) or caregiver(s).

A. **General Considerations.**
1. Maltreatment of the child can be classified as: (Miller, 1982)
   a. Physical abuse—infliction of physical injuries.
   b. Sexual abuse—sexual exploitation.
   c. Psychologic abuse—maladapted parent-child interactions.
   d. Physical neglect—failure to provide food, shelter, clothing.
   e. Medical care neglect—parental refusal to adhere to medical recommendations.
   f. Intentional drugging—sedating a child to control behavior.
   g. Education deprivation—intentional parental induced truancy.
   h. Abandonment or lack of supervision—intermittent or permanent nonsupervision of the child by an adult.
2. Factors which are associated with high risk for child abuse and neglect include:
   a. Parents who were abused as children.
   b. Parents who lack knowledge of normal growth and development and lack parenting skills.
   c. Parents with aggressive tendencies (Altermeier et al., 1982).
   d. Unplanned or unwanted pregnancy.
   e. Major birth defect or prematurity which interferes with bonding.
   f. Multiple births.
   g. Chronic family stress, e.g., marital discord, poverty, unemployment, drug or alcohol addiction.
   h. Acute parent/family crisis.
3. Diagnosis is based on:
   a. Physical examination of the child.
   b. Comprehensive past history and history of present illness.
   c. Radiographic or bone scintigraphy for infant with physical abuse.
4. High quality color photographs should be obtained when there are observable physical manifestations of abuse.
5. It is common for parents to provide an explanation of the child's condition which is inconsistent with the objective symptoms or inconsistent with the child's developmental level.
6. Parents may be inappropriately overconcerned or underconcerned with the child's condition.
7. Health professionals are required by law to report suspected child abuse and neglect to proper authorities.
8. Successful treatment of the abused child and his caretakers requires a team approach.
9. The goal of intervention is safe return of the child to his family.
10. A therapeutic nursing approach emphasizes parental strengths and shared concern of the parents and nurse for the child.
11. The nurse must resolve personal attitudes and feelings about abusive parents in order to be a positive influence on modifying parental behavior.
12. The nurse should initiate activities with high risk families to prevent abuse. See *Crisis Intervention.*
    a. See that basic needs of parents are met so they can then consider the child's needs (Hall, DeLaCruz, and Russell, 1982).
    b. Promote parental attachment to the child.
    c. Assist the parents in identifying positive child-rearing practices, particularly discipline.
    d. Identify support systems for the parents and encourage parents to use them.
    e. Improve the parents' self-esteem by reinforcing positive parent–child interactions.
    f. Refer to community agencies or health professionals for classes on parenting skills.
13. Individualized assistance to families can be provided through child protective services which encourage voluntary self-referral (DePanfilis, 1982).

B. **Nursing Management.** See *Crisis Intervention.*
1. Reduce the parents' anxiety level before obtaining the nursing history.
2. Remember that the parents may have already been interviewed by police, social worker, etc.
3. Observe, record, and report the following characteristics of parents:
   a. Reactions to the child.
   b. Questions about the child.
   c. Comforting behaviors.
   d. Knowledge about the child.
   e. Expectations of the child.
   f. Perceptions of the child.
4. Support the child and parents during hospitalization. See *Hospitalization, Support During.*
5. Initiate discharge planning. See *Discharge Planning.*
6. Observe and record selected aspects of the child's behavior without stating judgments or conclusions, e.g., record a description of how and with whom the child played rather than "enjoyed the playroom."
   a. Developmental level and abilities.
   b. Coping mechanisms. See *Coping.*
   c. Response to treatment.

d. Participation in unit activities.

e. Interactions with parents, other adults, and peers.

7. Offer additional preparation for and support during traumatic procedures that may remind the child of abusive actions of parents. See *Preparation for Procedures*.

8. Use a consistent approach to the child, particularly if consistent staff assignments are not possible.

a. Remember that first and foremost this is a "child" not an "abused child."

b. Set limits and tell the child what they are. See *Discipline*.

c. Provide anticipatory affection so the child does not seek this indiscriminately from personnel or other parents, e.g., plan cuddle or rocking chair time after morning care and at bedtime.

d. Provide anticipatory attention so the child does not provoke attention through negative behavior.

e. Provide positive experiences through play and informal nurse-child interactions.

f. Encourage the child to verbalize his feelings, but avoid forcing discussion.

g. Comment on disliked behavior, but not dislike of the child.

9. Protect the rights of the child and parents to privacy and confidentiality.

a. Refrain from discussion with peers or co-workers.

b. Decrease the hostility of other parents toward the abusing parents.

c. Prevent other parents from discussing the events with the abused child.

10. Observe and record the following selected aspects of the parents' behavior without stating judgments or conclusions:

a. Interactions with the child and with each other.

b. Interactions with other parents and with authority figures.

c. Knowledge of normal growth and development.

d. Response to stressful situations.

e. Use of supportive individuals and/or agencies.

11. Identify and implement a consistent approach to working with the parents.

a. Keep them informed of the child's progress.

b. Encourage them to participate in the child's care.

c. Serve as a role model for alternate methods of managing the child's behavior.

d. Give information on normal growth and development if needed.

e. Demonstrate acceptance of the parent's guilty feelings, but do not deny the need for these feelings.

12. Make discharge plans based on the court's decision for care of the child.

a. Placement.

1. Assess parental needs and communicate this data to the health professionals providing follow-up.

2. Prepare the child for placement by sharing information about his new caregivers, if possible.

3. Encourage the new caregivers to visit the hospital and learn about the child.

4. Support the parents in accepting placement by having them meet the new caregivers to share information about the child's individual needs.

5. Allow the parents to ventilate their feelings about having the child removed from their care.

b. Return home.

1. Prepare the parents for posthospital behavior.

2. Inform parents of agencies and support groups within the community.

3. Establish communication with public health nurse and/or psychiatric nurse specialist.

Accidents. Unplanned event which results in injury to the child. See *Poisoning*.

A. **General Considerations.**

1. Caregivers must assume responsibility for accident prevention for the very young child.

2. The focus should move toward education of the child as he matures.

3. Product modification of manufactured items is the most direct means of decreasing accidents, e.g., changes in child car seats.

4. Multiple factors, including the child's behavior, are involved in causing most accidents.

5. The concept of "accident proneness" has not been substantiated.

6. Any disruption in family routine increases the likelihood of an accident occurring, e.g., parental illness, marital discord, babysitters, etc.

7. Parents need information on normal growth and development in order to anticipate safety precautions for the child.

8. The child who is impulsive or immature is more likely to have accidents.

B. **Infants.**

1. General Considerations.

a. The caregiver must anticipate developmental tasks to be accomplished next and take appropriate preventive measures.

b. Black infants frequently attain motor skills earlier than textbook norms.

c. Mothers often over- or underestimate the infant's abilities.

2. Types of accidents and specific precautions for the caregiver.

a. Falls.

1. Keep crib sides all the way up all the time and fasten securely.

2. Discard hand-me-down cribs manufactured prior to 1974, as they may have a distance greater than $2\frac{3}{8}$ inches between the bars or an unsafe distance between the mattress and crib ends.

3. Do not place infant on adult bed or sofa unattended; today may be the day the baby learns to roll over.

4. Position the baby perpendicular to the crib sides when diapering so the infant will roll toward the crib end, not over the side.

5. Place baby care items within reach.

6. Place hand on baby's abdomen if caregiver must turn away to reach diaper, soap, etc.

7. Place infant seat on firm surface, away from edge.

8. Keep floors free of hazards to prevent tripping while carrying infant.

9. Place gates on stairs before child begins to creep.

10. Restrain infant in infant seat, high chair, feeding table, etc.

b. Aspiration or suffocation.

1. Keep baby pillows out of crib.

2. Do not drape blanket, diaper, etc., over crib side.

3. Use a firm mattress.

4. Remove plastic bags from environment.

5. Do not prop bottles.

6. Position baby on side or abdomen after feeding, or upright in infant seat.

7. Do not place infant in adult's bed for sleep as adult may roll over and suffocate child.

8. Do not attach pacifier to string around infant's neck.

9. Use pacifier of one-piece construction with loop handle.

10. Attach cradle gym or mobile high enough to prevent child from strangling on string.

11. Place crib away from venetian blind cords or shorten cords.

12. Remove inflated balloons from crib or playpen if infant is unsupervised.

13. Check environment frequently for small objects such as beads, pins, coins, etc.

14. Do not feed nuts or popcorn to an infant.

15. Do not use styrofoam cups for feeding, since child can bite them.

16. Use a modified Heimlich maneuver or turn child's head down if choking, but do not slap the child on the back, as this will cause the child to gasp and inhale the object.

c. Burns

1. Test bath water with elbow before placing baby in tub.

2. Keep crib and playpen away from windows, as sun rays are also potent through the window panes.

3. Keep electrical cords out of reach so infant does not bite them.

4. Use cool mist vaporizers only.

d. Drownings.

1. Supervise the baby when bathing; ignore the telephone and doorbell.

2. Maintain firm control of infant while bathing; leave at least one extremity unlathered.

3. Place towel or diaper at the bottom of tub to prevent slipping.

4. Do not overestimate the infant's swimming ability after an infant swim program.

e. Miscellaneous.

1. Keep diaper pins closed and out of reach.

2. Select toys appropriate to the infant's developmental level.

3. Control rodent population to prevent rat bites.

4. Remove lead-based paint from crib, playpen, window sills, etc.

5. Use an infant car bed or seat which meets the Federal Motor Vehicle Safety Standards.

6. Keep tablecloths or other items from dangling and tempting infant.

7. Shake baby powder on hand and apply to diaper area; inhaling the powder may result in aspiration pneumonia.

C. Toddlers.

1. General Considerations.

a. Toddlers are very curious, mobile, and increasingly independent.

b. Toddlers learn by trial and error.

c. Caregivers must constantly supervise the toddler.

2. Types of accidents and specific precautions for the caregiver.

a. Falls.
1. Keep all windows screened securely and avoid placing furniture near windows.
2. Open windows only from the top if the toddler is unattended or sleeping.
3. Teach the toddler how to climb stairs safely.
4. Keep gates at the top and bottom of stairs.
5. Keep the child in an enclosed space when outdoors and unsupervised.
6. Provide safe objects on which child can practice climbing.
7. Keep floor clear of scatter rugs, toys, spilled liquids, excess wax, etc.
8. Equip stairs with additional handrails at proper height to keep child from falling under existing rail.
9. Put safety strips in bottom of bathtub.
10. Keep crib rails fully raised and mattress at lowest level.
11. Shorten pant legs to prevent tripping.

b. Drownings.
1. Supervise child during bathing.
2. Empty backyard wading pools and turn over so they cannot be filled by rainwater when not in use.
3. Supervise child near pools, ditches, lakes, ponds, etc.
4. Teach the child to swim.
5. Cover open wells.

c. Motor vehicles.
1. Purchase a car seat that meets federal safety standards and install as directed.
2. Lock car doors.
3. Teach the child not to play in driveways, streets, or near curbs in pile of leaves, snow, or in large, empty boxes.

d. Burns.
1. Supervise bathing so child will not turn on hot water faucet.
2. Keep water heater temperature at a maximum of 140°F.
3. Keep handles of cooking utensils turned toward back of stove.
4. Remove stove burner knobs if they are located at front of stove.
5. Place hot food containers away from edge of table.
6. Keep hot irons out of reach.
7. Screen fireplaces and space heaters.
8. Cover radiators.
9. Shorten electrical appliance cords to prevent dangling.
10. Keep matches, lighters, and burning candles out of reach.

e. Miscellaneous.
1. Cover unused electrical outlets.
2. Keep sharp objects locked out of reach.
3. Supervise the toddler when fans are used.
4. Select safe toys.
5. Close safety pins.
6. Remove doors from unused refrigerators.
7. Supervise child if wringer washer is used.
8. Make a safety check of the home periodically.
9. Evaluate potential environmental hazards when visiting other homes, particularly if there are no young children in the household.
10. Use a toddler seat with foot braces and straps if the child rides behind the parent on a bicycle.
11. Teach the child not to approach strange animals.
12. Forbid child to carry sharp or pointed objects, lollipops, popsicles, etc. while walking or running.

D. Preschoolers.
1. General Considerations.
a. Preschoolers are usually receptive to safety teaching.
b. Safe behavior of adult role models will be imitated by young children.
c. Preschooler can be given specific safety responsibilities to satisfy his initiative.
2. Types of accidents and specific precautions for the parent.
a. Falls.
1. Keep doors locked where there is danger of falls, e.g., in the basement.
2. Put guards or bars across windows.
3. Do not allow child to play on fire escapes.
b. Drowning.
1. Supervise bathing.
2. Teach child to empty water after bath.
3. Introduce swimming rules.
c. Motor vehicles.
1. Use approved car seat placed in rear seat.
2. Give child responsibility for seeing that all doors are locked and passengers are wearing seat belts.
3. Do not leave child unattended in parked car.
4. Do not allow child to pretend to drive parked car.
5. Teach safety rules for crossing streets and review frequently; children do not

always remember colors of traffic signals.

6. Teach child not to chase balls into street.

d. Burns
1. Keep matches, lighters, and burning candles out of reach.
2. Do not allow preschooler to cook on stove, barbecue, fireplace, etc.
3. Keep child away from rubbish or other outdoor burning.
4. Teach the child to roll on the floor or ground, not run, if clothes catch on fire.
5. Teach child not to hide in closet or under the bed if there is a fire.

e. Miscellaneous.
1. Keep firearms unloaded and locked in a safe place.
2. Teach the child safe places to play hide and seek.
3. Teach proper use of scissors.
4. Teach the child not to talk to strangers or to accept rides, candy, etc.
5. Have child learn how to make emergency calls.
6. Do not allow child near a lawn mower while in operation.
7. Teach risks of throwing sharp objects.
8. Dress the child in light clothing with long pants and long-sleeved shirt for walks in woods. Check for ticks, particularly in hair.

E. Schoolchildren.
1. General Considerations.
a. Increased cognitive ability makes them receptive to safety information.
b. Their background of experience improves their judgment in coping with hazards.
2. Types of accidents and specific precautions for the parent.
a. Motor vehicles.
1. Use seat belts. Lap belts should be used for a child weighing over 50 pounds; shoulder harness should never be used for a child less than 55 inches in height.
2. Keep doors locked.
3. Teach child to walk facing traffic and to wear light-colored clothing.
b. Drowning.
1. Teach the child to swim.
2. Enforce the following water safety rules:
a. Call for help only if really needed.
b. Swim with a buddy.
c. Explore unfamiliar lake, pond, etc., before diving.
d. Walk into water and swim back to

shore to prevent tiring while in deep water.
e. Do not dunk others.
3. Keep rope, stick, or buoyant object available to throw to a swimmer in difficulty.
c. Bicycles and minibikes.
1. Choose the right size bike.
2. Teach safety rules for bicycles.
a. Follow automobile driving rules.
b. Wear light-colored clothing.
c. Equip bicycle with reflectors, lights, and bell or horn.
d. Do not hitch rides on motor vehicles.
e. Do not dart from behind parked vehicles.
f. Do not carry passengers.
g. Never stunt ride.
3. Check brakes, tires, nuts, screws, etc., frequently.
4. Ride defensively.
5. Teach safety rules for minibikes.
a. Wear a helmet and shatterproof goggles or face shield.
b. Ride only on a safe, dry surface.
c. Do not ride in streets.
d. Do not carry passengers.
e. Never stunt ride.
d. Firearms.
1. Keep firearms unloaded and locked in a safe place.
2. Enforce safety rules.
a. Treat every gun as if it were loaded.
b. Point the gun in a safe direction.
c. Keep the safety on until ready to shoot.
e. Falls.
1. Teach the child to avoid dead or small limbs when tree climbing and to wear nonslippery shoes.
2. Supervise construction of tree houses.
3. Forbid climbing on electrical poles, water towers, etc.
4. Enforce safety rules for skateboarding.
a. Wear long pants, long-sleeved shirt, helmet, and knee and elbow pads.
b. Have the child learn techniques of rolling and somersault to reduce injury.
c. Use skateboards in a safe location, preferably a graded track with earthen shoulders.

F. Adolescents.
1. General Considerations.
a. The desire to meet peer expectations greatly influences risk-taking behavior.

b. Adolescent rebellion and/or a need for independence may lead to ignoring safety rules.
c. Rapid physical changes may increase "clumsiness" and result in accidents, particularly in sports.
d. Safety habits taught throughout childhood will reduce serious accidents.
2. Types of accidents and specific precautions for the caregiver.
   a. Motor vehicles.
      1. Enroll teenager in driver education program.
      2. Parent should demonstrate safe driving practices.
      3. Discuss the relationship of alcohol and drugs in causing accidents.

Acidosis. *See Fluid and Electrolyte Imbalance.*

Acne. Chronic inflammatory disease of the sebaceous glands and hair follicles of the skin.

A. **General Conditions.**
   1. The sebaceous glands become active at puberty and trapped sebum becomes darkened from accumulated dirt forming blackheads and comedones.
   2. There are two basic types of lesions.
      a. Noninflamed lesions (comedones).
         1. Whiteheads.
         2. Blackheads.
      b. Inflamed lesions.
         1. Papules.
         2. Pustules.
         3. Nodules.
         4. Cysts.
   3. Sites usually involved are the scalp, neck, face, back, upper arms, and external ear.
   4. The inflammatory response is caused by the normally harmless bacteria, *Propionibacterium acnes,* or by secondary invasion by *Staphylococcus albus.*
   5. Treatment of noninflammatory acne includes:
      a. Oral sebostatics.
      b. Comedone removal.
      c. Peeling agents.
         1. Cleansing agents.
         2. Astringents.
         3. Topical preparations.
         4. Cryoslush therapy (freezing skin with carbon dioxide).
         5. Ultraviolet light.
         6. Topical application of vitamin A.
   6. Treatment for inflammatory acne includes:

a. Acne surgery (incision and drainage of cystic and pustular lesions).
b. Chemotherapy.
   1. Broad-spectrum antibiotics (e.g., tetracycline, erythromycin).
   2. Corticosteroids.
   3. Estrogen-progestins.
c. X-ray therapy.
d. Dermabrasion.
7. Irreparable physical scarring can occur with inflammatory acne.
8. The adolescent's concern about appearance of the skin may lead to an undue self-consciousness that affects school performance and social relationships.

B. **Nursing Management.**
   1. Obtain a history of exposure to possible causative factors.
      a. Cosmetics.
      b. Hair pomades.
      c. Medication, prescription or non-prescription.
      d. Occupational products such as cooking grease, paints, varnishes, oils.
      e. Clothing irritation.
      f. Emotional stress.
      g. Past acne treatments, self-administered or prescribed (Stone, 1982).
   2. Facilitate compliance with treatment by discussing the pathogenesis of the disease and realistic expectations of management.
   3. Teach the adolescent and parents about home management.
      a. Review instructions for the use of benzoyl peroxide.
         1. Begin use once daily with a 5 percent solution and adjust frequency and strength to individual response.
         2. Some redness and peeling is expected, but excessive response should dictate decreasing the frequency of application or reducing the strength.
         3. Avoid application to sensitive skin and areas around eyes and mouth.
      b. Review instructions for the use of retinoic acid.
         1. Explain that the therapeutic response to the medication is an acne exacerbation 2 to 4 weeks after treatment begins.
         2. Increase frequency of application only as directed.
         3. Apply at bedtime, at least 15 minutes after washing.
         4. Stinging or warmth on application, followed by slight drying or redness is the expected response.
         5. Avoid exposure to sunlight unless a sunscreen is used.

A

c. Teach the use of the comedone extractor.
   1. Wash the face with soap and water before and after the extraction.
   2. Place the hole directly over the blackhead.
   3. Apply gentle pressure against the skin with a slight sliding movement.
   4. Clean the instrument with soap and water and store in alcohol or clean with alcohol and store in a clean container.
d. Discuss antibiotic therapy. See *Administration of Medications, Parental.*
   1. Tell the female that monilial vaginitis may be a side effect of tetracycline therapy. See *Candida albicans.*
   2. Tell the teenager that it may take 2 to 3 weeks for the antibiotics to become effective.
4. Discuss with the adolescent and parents that food restrictions are unnecessary unless a specific food is known to be irritating.
   a. Support the adolescent so he can accept the food restrictions without feeling his popularity is jeopardized.
5. Discuss with the female adolescent the probable exacerbation of acne 7 to 10 days prior to the onset of menstruation.
6. Tell the child and parents that temporary sensitivity to sunlight occurs when tetracycline or vitamin A therapy are prescribed.
7. Explore what the condition means to the adolescent. *See Body Image.*
   a. Discuss activities in which the teenager does well and which will increase self-esteem.
   b. Provide opportunities for the adolescent to verbalize frustrations and feelings.
   c. Reassure the adolescent that the acne is not related to veneral disease, masturbation, or sexual activity.

Acyanotic Heart Disease. See *Congenital Heart Disease.*

Adenoidectomy. See *Tonsillectomy and Adenoidectomy.*

Administration of medications.

A. **General Considerations.**
   1. Medication dosages must be individualized for each child.
   2. No child should ever receive a dose higher than the adult dose.
   3. Child's body surface area or weight should be used to calculate safe drug dosage. See *Appendix iii.*

4. Child's age should be used to calculate drug dosage only when pediatric dose not specified by manufacturer (Howry, Bindler, Tso, 1981).
B. **Nursing Management. See** *Appendix iii.*
   1. General.
      a. Be kind and positive in your approach to the child.
      b. Expect that the child will try to cooperate.
      c. Praise the child for taking medications.
      d. Allow for expression of fears.
      e. Tell the child the truth, e.g., If a medication is sour, say so.
      f. Do not threaten, punish, or use force.
      g. Administer medications according to developmental level.
      h. Restrain the child only for safety.
      i. Offer choices where possible, e.g., Do you want coke or juice with your pill?
      j. Do not offer the child a choice about a medication if there is no choice.
      k. Use medication administration times to teach the older child and adolescent about the medication and to answer questions.
   2. Oral medication administration. See *Appendix iii.*
      a. Use appropriate technique.
      b. Use dropper, nipple, syringe or cup to administer medications depending on the child's age.
      c. Taste a small amount of the medication so that you can tell child what to expect about its taste.
      d. Place syringe or dropper on center back portion of tongue in child under 6 months due to extrusion reflex.
      e. Give medication at rate the child can swallow without difficulty.
      f. Support infant's head.
      g. Let the child hold own cup if possible.
      h. Do not mix medications with essential foods.
      i. Use the smallest amount of food or fluid possible when mixing it with medicine to promote taking of total dose.
      j. Use gelatin capsules to administer bitter pills; place pill in capsule and have child swallow.
      k. Involve parents or significant caregiver in administering oral medications to young child to gain child's cooperation.
      l. Prevent development of dental caries from use of sweetened medications (Babington, Spandaro, 1982).
         1. Have physician prescribe sugar-free or reduced sugar form, if possible, or prescribe pill/tablet form, if available.
         2. Teach parents to prevent caries formation. See *Dental Care Administration.*
   3. Intramuscular medications.

a. Give clear, concise explanations to the child.
b. Prepare all injections out of the child's sight.
c. Use one of the following sites based on the child's age and development.
   1. Vastus lateralis: all ages.
   2. Ventro gluteal: over age 1.
   3. Upper outer quadrant of gluteal muscle: over age 2.
   4. Deltoid: over age 1.
d. Restrain the child as needed for safe care.
e. Take someone with you if you will need assistance in restraining child.
f. Inject slowly into relaxed muscle to promote absorption.
g. Massage the area following the injection to promote absorption unless contraindicated.
4. Intravenous medication Administration.
   a. Dilute intravenous drugs that may irritate vein.
   b. Add all medications to intravenous out of the child's sight, since he may react to seeing the needle.
   c. Explain why a particular infusion is needed.
5. Eye medication administration.
   a. Do not administer eye drops if the child is crying.
   b. Keep eye drops at room temperature.
   c. Use appropriate technique.
      1. Use sterile technique.
      2. Hyperextend child's head over your arm or pillow.
      3. Stabilize hand holding dropper by resting it on child's forehead.
      4. Tell older child to close eyes; gently retract lower lid and place medication in sac-like area formed by this action (Bindler, Howry, Tso, 1981).
      5. Hold bottle tip/dropper parallel to the eye.
      6. Have child keep eyes closed and head hyperextended for several minutes, if possible.
6. Ear medication administration.
   a. Use sterile technique if eardrum is ruptured.
   b. Administer drops at room temperature to prevent pain, nausea, or vertigo.
   c. Use appropriate technique.
      1. Place child on side with affected ear up.
      2. Pull auricle down and back in child under 3 years of age.
      3. Pull auricle up and back in child over 3 years of age.
      4. Direct drops toward the side of the ear canal.
      5. Have child remain on side a few minutes to ensure contact with tympanic membrane.
      6. Insert cotton pledgets if ordered. See *Otitis Media*.

7. Nasal medication administration.
   a. Use clean technique.
   b. Do not use oil-based drops since they may be aspirated.
   c. Use medications at room temperature.
   d. Use appropriate technique for administration.
      1. Position infant with head tilted back.
      2. Position older child with head extended over pillow.
      3. Tell older child to breathe through mouth during administration to avoid sniffing medication into sinuses.
      4. Tell older children they will taste the medication.
      5. Direct drops toward superior turbinate by having child tilt head at a 30 degree angle.
      6. Keep head tilted back for 1 minute to maximize contact with turbinate.
      7. Observe for signs of aspiration.
8. Rectal medication administration.
   a. Do not split suppositories since dose cannot be measured accurately.
   b. Be aware that the intrusive nature of this procedure is upsetting to the child.
   c. Use appropriate technique.
      1. Provide privacy.
      2. Insert suppository gently past internal anal sphincter.
      3. Use fifth finger to insert suppository in child under 3 years, use index finger in child over 3 years (Howry, Bindler, Tso, 1981).
      4. Show older child how to pant or breathe deeply to avoid reflex bearing down.
      5. Hold buttocks together firmly for 5 to 10 minutes after insertion.
      6. Examine any stool expelled within 30 minutes of administration for undissolved suppository.
9. Vaginal medication administration.
   a. Be aware that the intrusive nature of this procedure is upsetting to the young child.
   b. Assess and support the older child's and adolescent's response because the vagina is a sexual organ.
   c. Support parents responding to use of this route of administration because of its relation to sexuality.
   d. Use appropriate technique for administration.
      1. Provide privacy.
      2. Place child supine with legs flexed.
      3. Use good light to visualize opening.
      4. Insert medication gently with gloved finger.
      5. Teach adolescent to insert own medication.

Administration of medication, parental.

A. General Considerations.

1. Support parents' compliance in giving medications to child so response can be assessed accurately.
2. The following factors are known to contribute to noncompliance.
   a. Illness not perceived as being serious.
   b. Failure to understand directions.
   c. High cost of medication.
   d. Side effects associated with medication.
   e. Duration of time medication must be given.
   f. Complexity of medication regimen.
   g. Cultural and religious beliefs/practices.
   h. Inconsistencies in teaching parents/caregivers about medication.

B. Nursing Management.

1. Consult with the physician about prescribing the most economical form of the drug.
2. Ask the physician to order the drug in the form the child takes most easily.
3. Teach the parents what they need to know about the drug(s):
   a. Name of drug.
   b. Why child is getting the drug.
   c. How to administer the drug.
   d. Amount of drug to be given in each dose.
   e. Number of doses per day and whether schedule can be altered.
   f. How many days the drug should be given.
   g. Expected results of the drug and when they can be expected.
   h. Side effects and toxicity of the drug(s).
   i. What the consequences may be if drug regimen is not followed.
   j. Indications for calling physician.
4. Coordinate teaching efforts with other health care providers to support compliance with drug regimen.
5. Assist the parents.
   a. Write out directions in language the parent(s) understands.
   b. Adjust drug schedule to life-style, e.g., hospital schedule: 10:00, 2:00, 6:00, 10:00. Home schedule: 8:00 (breakfast), 12:00 (school lunch), 4:00 (home from school), 8:00 (before bed).
   c. Give them a standard measuring device.
   d. Suggest they have a dosage chart and mark off doses given.
6. Teach parents to keep a medication history for each child including:
   a. Name of drug.
   b. Date(s) given.
   c. Illness for which drug was given.
   d. Drug dose.
   e. Child's response to the drug.
7. Make a community health nurse referral if needed to assess parents' ability to handle drug administration at home.
8. Review safty precautions related to drug administration.
   a. Check the label each time the drug is given; do not rely on memory.
   b. Do not put drug in another container.
   c. Pour liquid medications on side away from label so label stays clean and can be read.
   d. Do not alter the dose.
   e. Do not chew enteric coated medications.
   f. Chew chewable medication before swallowing.
   g. Give drug before or after meals as instructed.
   h. Do not give drug to anyone else.
   i. Do not store drugs in sunlight or areas with high humidity.
   j. Do not give the drug past expiration date.

Admission to hospital, elective. Planned entry into the hospital for tests and/or specific treatment.

A. General Considerations.

1. Admission procedures set the tone of the hospital experience for parent and child.
2. The child's responses are influenced by the level of preparation for hospitalization.
3. Parental behaviors reflect a response to the child's illness and hospitalization.
4. The adolescent may find hospital admission procedures very stressful because they threaten the need for privacy, independence and peer contact.
5. Consistency in people and practices promotes security.
6. Nurse's role should complement, not replace, parental role.
7. The nursing care plan should be begun when the child is admitted.
8. Discharge planning is an essential component of quality care and should be initiated upon admission.
9. Involve both parents in the admission procedure.
10. The nurse should serve as an advocate for the child/adolescent and parents. See *Advocate*.

B. Nursing Management. See DISCHARGE PLANNING and HOSPITALIZATION, RESPONSE TO.

1. Support the child and parents. See *Hospitalization, Support During*.
   a. Introduce yourself and others caring for the child.
   b. Call the parents by name, and the child by name or nickname.
   c. Communicate at eye level.
   d. Use anticipatory guidance for each step of the admission.

e. Explain what you are going to do.
f. Keep explanations brief to promote understanding.
g. Reinforce information.
h. Be nonjudgmental of behavior.
i. Postpone painful intrusive procedures until some trust is developed with the child.
j. Do all intrusive procedures in the treatment room if appropriate. *See Preparation for Procedures.*
k. Allow as much mobility as possible.
l. Encourage the child in play activities. See *Play.*
m. Orient child and parents to hospital room and unit/hospital policies.

2. Promote continuity of care.
   a. Assign one nurse to complete the admission.
   b. Encourage parental involvement in the admission.
   c. Obtain nursing history as a basis for individualized care. See *History Taking* and *Appendix iv.*
   d. Familiarize parent and child with the physical environment and hospital routines and services.
   e. Promote wearing of own clothing and bringing of familiar articles from home, e.g., pillow, stuffed toys, etc.

3. Use developmental guidelines during admission.
   a. Infant.
      1. Encourage parent to hold the child.
      2. Approach infant slowly.
   b. Toddler.
      1. Encourage parent to hold.
      2. Promote handling of unfamiliar equipment.
      3. Let the child hold security object, e.g., blanket, doll.
      4. Give simple explanations.
      5. Let parent change the child into hospital gown.
   c. Preschooler.
      1. Have parents present.
      2. Promote trust prior to intrusive procedures.
      3. Encourage handling of unfamiliar equipment.
      4. Explain all actions.
      5. Let parent help by undressing the child and putting on hospital gown.
      6. Permit child to keep on own underpants.
      7. Provide privacy and respect modesty.
   d. Schoolchild.
      1. Encourage participation in admission.
      2. Promote handling of equipment.
      3. Explain all actions and procedures.
      4. Reward the child's cooperation with a smile or a pat.
      5. Encourage independence.
      6. Permit child to keep on own clothing.
      7. Provide privacy and respect modesty.
   e. Adolescent (Klein and Showalter, 1974).
      1. Admit in room as an adult.
      2. Obtain nursing history separate from parents, since adolescent may be uncomfortable discussing some topics in their presence.
      3. Place with similar age group.
      4. Permit wearing of own clothes when possible.
      5. Orient to surroundings in order of importance to adolescent: phone, television, visiting hours, hospital routines.
      6. Keep restrictions to a minimum, but make sure they are clearly stated.

4. Orient parents to the pediatric unit and hospital.
   a. Explain what they may do for the child and what the nurse will do.
   b. Encourage their participation in care.
   c. Introduce them to other parents.
   d. Provide information about eating and sleeping arrangements and location of phones and bathrooms.

Admission to hospital, emergency. Unplanned entry into the hospital as a result of worsening of preexisting condition, sudden illness or accident.

A. **General Considerations.**
   1. Emergency admission is more stressful because of the following (Roskies, 1977):
      a. Child often more acutely ill.
      b. Painful and intrusive procedures are often greater in number.
      c. Preparation for hospitalization has been brief or nonexistent.
      d. Medical tasks take precedence over emotional support.
      e. Parental stress levels often render them unable to support the child.
   2. Many emergency admissions are in the under 5 years of age group.
   3. Coping mechanisms may be inadequate to meet the stresses imposed by emergency. See *Coping.*
   4. The child and the parents may be very frightened.
   5. Nurse should act as an advocate for the child and parents.

B. **Nursing Management.** See DISCHARGE, PLANNING, and HOSPITALIZATION, RESPONSE TO.
   1. Support the child during an emergency admission.

a. Assign a nurse to remain with the child at all times during the emergency admission if parents are unavailable.

b. Tell the child where parents are waiting, if parents not in room with child.

c. Introduce yourself, and establish some relationship with the child, if possible, before starting procedures.

d. Explain all procedures as they are done; keep them brief to promote understanding.

e. Encourage the child to verbalize feelings.

f. Support coping mechanisms. See *Coping*.

g. Recognize that the fears specific to each age group will influence the child's response. See *Fears*.

2. Support parents. See *Hospitalization, Support during*.

a. Focus your attention on the child.

b. Answer questions as quickly and honestly as possible.

c. Inform parents of what you are doing or where you are taking the child.

d. Encourage parents participation in care, if possible.

e. Be aware of parental needs/concerns, e.g., location of phone, concern about other children at home.

3. Employ crisis intervention techniques in working with parent and child. See *Crisis Intervention*.

4. Start a nursing history as situation permits.

5. Accompany child to unit to promote continuity of care and provide support.

Adolescent. Child in the developmental period between puberty and the time physical growth is complete and/or emotional maturity is attained.

A. **General Considerations.**

1. The adolescent is faced with accomplishing multiple tasks:

   a. Achieving independence.

   b. Developing peer relationships.

   c. Deciding on a career.

   d. Making heterosexual adjustments.

   e. Developing a set of personal and social values.

   f. Accepting physical development.

   g. Achieving emotional control.

2. The sequence of development will be the same but the time at which tasks are accomplished varies.

3. Adolescence qualifies as a developmental crisis period because of the following:

   a. New situations are presented.

   b. New behaviors are called into use.

   c. Old behavior patterns no longer meet the child's needs.

4. Adolescent behavior often exhibits the following sequence in a cyclic form (Denyes and Altshuler, 1979).

   a. Self-assertion in a particular situation, e.g., staying out past curfew.

   b. Involvement in situation beyond the adolescent's ability to cope.

   c. Emotional response to the inability to cope characterized by fear and anxiety.

   d. Regression to a more comfortable level.

   e. Inability to accept regression.

   f. Renewed self-assertion.

5. Conflict with parents may develop if the parents:

   a. Cannot allow the adolesent to develop independence.

   b. Do not agree with the adolescent about areas in which independence should be allowed.

   c. Are experiencing life crises themselves, e.g., accepting an "empty nest" as children leave home.

   d. Are not aware of the developmental tasks the adolescent must achieve.

6. Rapid growth and physical changes make adolescents very conscious of their bodies.

7. The peer group is the most important social group for the adolescent.

8. The reaction of an adolescent to illness will be affected by:

   a. The nature of the illness.

   b. The time the illness occurs in the developmental sequence.

   c. How many adjustments in behavior will be required.

   d. Whether it will affect body image or capabilities.

   e. How it may affect the future.

9. Hospitalization may be especially difficult for the adolescent because of the:

   a. Confinement which threatens independence.

   b. Presence of younger children which may cause concerns about regression.

   c. Separation from peers and school.

   d. Pressure to adopt the patient role which is passive and depersonalized and conflicts with the drive toward independence and identity.

   e. Similarity between the nurturing role of the nurse and mothering which the adolescent may wish to avoid (Klein and Showalter, 1974).

10. The concept of death is on an adult level.

B. **Nursing Management.**

1. Observe dress, verbal and nonverbal behavior, and interpersonal relations, since these

provide important information about the adolescent.

2. Employ a warm, friendly approach.
3. Encourage questions and give honest answers.
4. Involve the adolescent in planning care to meet individualized needs.
5. Promote self-care as much as possible.
6. Provide privacy for care and visiting.
7. Allow reasonable noise, e.g., radio, television, record player.
8. Promote continuation of social activities, e.g., plan group get-togethers in the playroom after younger children are gone.
9. Provide for diet preferences.
   a. Talk with dietician.
   b. Let friends and parents bring in favorite foods.
   c. Allow kitchen privileges or permit keeping of snacks in room.
10. Permit wearing of clothes rather than pajamas if possible.
11. Obtain permission for adolescent to go to lobby, snack-bar, gift shop, and outside for walk as condition permits.
12. Intervene on basis of where adolescent is in behavior cycle as appropriate.
   a. Support self-assertion.
   b. Accept regression in nonjudgmental manner.
   c. Recognize that anxiety may prevent adolescent from participating in care.
13. Provide information to the adolescent as needed/requested in relation to the following:
   a. Growth and development norms. See *Appendix v.*
   b. Nutrition. See *Nutrition, Obesity, Appendix vii.*
   c. Dental care. See *Dental Care.*
   d. Safety. See *Accidents.*
   e. Health promotion and maintenance. See *Appendix vi.*
   f. Substance abuse. See *Alcoholism, Drug Abuse, Smoking.*
   g. Sexuality. See *Menstruation, Nocturnal Emissions, Sex Education.*
   h. Sexually transmitted diseases. See *Sexually Transmitted Diseases.*
   i. Management of chronic illnesses. See *Chronic Illness.*
   j. Management of minor illnesses. See *Home Management of Minor Illnesses.*
14. Teach parents to:
   a. Expect that adolescent behavior will be erratic.
   b. Recognize that adolescent needs parents' support, reassurance, and guidance.
   c. Continue to set appropriate limits but begin to let go of adolescent.
   d. Accept fact that life goals of adolescent may differ markedly from theirs.
   e. Feel comfortable in expressing concerns and frustrations associated with rearing adolescents.

Adoption. A socially constructed parent–child relationship in which, by a legal act, a child is taken as one's own (Watson, 1978).

A. **General Considerations.**
   1. Developmental tasks of adoptive families (Watson, 1978).
      a. Accepting that family is different.
      b. Explaining adoption to the child.
      c. Recognizing the child's biological family.
      d. Accepting appropriate parenting role.
      e. Recognizing expectations of the child.
   2. There is no traditional societal support system for the adoptive family.
   3. How the child copes with his adopted status is influenced by how the family meets his needs.
   4. The developmental level of the child influences his reaction to knowledge of his adoptive status.
   5. Children over age 7 have more cognitive ability to deal with the concept of adoption.
   6. Lack of information about the biological family may place the adopted child at greater risk for health problems.
   7. Girls seem to have more difficulty accepting/dealing with adoption than do boys (Clore, Newberry, 1981).

B. **Nursing Management.**
   1. Assess coping mechanisms of the family.
   2. Support family in developmental tasks. See *Parenting.*
      a. Accept their **difference** from other families.
      b. Provide informat.. n on explaining adoption.
      c. Recognize biological family's impact on the child.
      d. Help parents recognize that they have the same rights as biological parents in establishing their own methods of child rearing.
      e. Refer for appropriate counseling, if indicated.
   3. Use Freud and Piaget as a guide in helping parents cope with telling the child about his adoption. See *Appendix v.*
   4. Assist the parents in helping the child master Erickson's developmental tasks (Clore, Newberry, 1981).
      a. Trust vs. Mistrust: The older infant may experience feelings of abandonment and need extra contact with parents.
      b. Autonomy vs. Shame and Doubt: Avoid overprotectiveness, accept child's level of ability to perform.

c. Initiative vs. Guilt: Accept child's questioning, begin to introduce concept of adoption as child indicates readiness, support child in dealing with comments/attitudes of relatives and friends.

d. Industry vs. Inferiority: Accept child's level of performance realistically, encourage child's expression of concerns/feelings about adoption.

e. Indentity vs. Role Confusion: Accept adolescent's need to question about/make contact with birth parent(s), recognize that the adolescent may use adoption as a "weapon" in conflicts, expect that feelings related to having been "given up" may recur.

5. Involve family in planning an acceptable schedule for health assessment.

Advocate. Primary role of the nurse in which commitment is made to serving the patient–client within the system.

A. **General Considerations.**
1. The nurse develops the ability to assume this role by:
   a. Continuing professional education.
   b. Involvement in local, state, and national issues affecting health care delivery.
   c. Membership in professional organizations.
2. The nurse is prepared to assume this role when care is provided using:
   a. The nursing process.
   b. Theories of child and family development, e.g., Freud, Piaget, Erikson, and Maslow's hierarchy of human needs.
   c. Knowledge of cultural and religious beliefs and practices that influence health.
   d. Knowledge of the disease process, when applicable.
   e. Community resources and referrals to meet continuing health care needs.

B. **Nursing Management.**
1. Be willing to assume the role of child and family advocate.
2. Accept the fact that assumption of this role may place you in conflict with the system.
3. Work with the child and family to establish priorities for change if there is more than one area of conflict between the child's and family's needs and the policies of the system.
4. Use appropriate channels to achieve change, e.g., nursing care conference with the head nurse.
5. Employ an appropriate manner.
   a. Approach the situation with the belief that you can help the child and family.
   b. Identify people and/or resources that can be

of assistance, e.g., dietician, public health nurse, Child Protective Services.
   c. State the facts clearly and concisely.
6. Implement changes.
   a. Discuss the changes that will be made with the child and family.
   b. Record all changes on the Kardex or chart to promote consistency in care.
7. Deal with unresolved conflicts.
   a. Discuss with the child and family alternative, acceptable approaches that might be used.
   b. Maintain the attitude that change is possible.

Aganglionosis. See *Hirschsprung's Disease*.

Aggression, child. Anger displayed as biting, kicking, uncooperativeness, yelling, or destroying property.

A. **General Considerations.**
1. Aggressive feelings should be expected when the child must cope with:
   a. Major physical hurt.
   b. Loss of close relationships.
   c. Immobilization.
   d. Intrusive procedures, e.g., rectal temperatures, injection.
2. Tightly controlled environments cause the child to repress aggressive feelings.
3. Counteraggressive responses from adults are frightening for the child, e.g., yelling at the child who yells at you.
4. Hospital staff are frequently the objects of displaced anger the child feels for himself or others.

B. **Nursing Management.**
1. Encourage verbalization of the older child's aggressive impulses by expressing sympathy for his feelings, e.g., "I would be angry, too, if I had to stay in bed for 3 weeks."
2. Establish a consistent plan of approach to aggressiveness.
   a. Use firmness, not hostility, to control behavior.
   b. Provide a permissive, secure environment that allows the child to express negative feelings.
   c. Allow the child to displace his anger verbally to staff members until he can deal with his feelings cognitively.
3. Help the toddler or preschooler name his angry feelings, e.g., "You feel mad when I hurt you by changing your bandage."
4. Provide young children with toys such as pounding boards, bean bags, soft sponge balls,

balloons, etc., which allow physical release of aggression.

5. Provide the child, preschool age and older, with therapeutic play equipment. See *Play, Therapeutic.*
6. Provide motor activities such as walks outside the hospital, physical therapy, and isometric exercises for the older child as physical condition permits.
7. Reinforce positive behavior and ignore negative behavior that can be tolerated.

Aggression, parental.
Verbal, angry response to personnel with minimal or no provocation.

A. General Considerations.
1. Guilt for not meeting societal expectations of keeping a child well may cause anger at staff.
2. Demands of the ill child toward the parent may lead to parents' demanding of the staff.
3. Anger with the child may be manifest as anger with the staff.
4. Lack of trust in the staff's competency and caring may result in aggression.
5. The parents may need the child to fill a "sick" role and become angry with staff who make him well.

B. Nursing Management.
1. Ensure that accurate, consistent communication is maintained about the etiology of the child's illness.
   a. Accompany the physician when explanation is given to parents.
   b. Clarify any misunderstanding the parents have about the physician's explanations.
   c. Record information on the Kardex so it is available to all personnel to read.
2. Help the parents to understand how illness alters the child's normal behavior. See *Hospitalization, Response to.*
3. Recognize that being able to express anger is important to the parents' psychological health.
4. Maintain interaction with parents and praise their abilities to cope with this crisis.
5. Initiate interdisciplinary conferences if parents are receiving or perceiving inconsistencies in nursing or medical management.
6. Initiate referrals to community mental health agencies if negative family dynamics cannot be altered during brief hospitalizations.

Alcoholism.
Excessive use of or dependence on alcohol (ethanol).

A. General Considerations.
See ADOLESCENT, DRUG ABUSE, and SUICIDE.
1. Alcohol is the most frequently used, and abused, drug and acts as a central nervous system depressant.
2. Alcohol is unique among the major drugs abused in that it can be legally purchased without a prescription by anyone 18 to 21 years of age depending on state laws (Schonberg, Litt, Cohen, 1982).
3. The child may drink because of powerful drives toward emancipation, experimentation, and acquisition of adult status.
4. The child may find it impossible to avoid peer pressure to drink.
5. Characteristics of the child who abuses alcohol include:
   a. Isolation.
   b. Negative self-image.
   c. Disturbed relationships.
   d. Dependence on alcohol for psychological support.
6. Alcohol is often combined with other drugs which potentiate its effects, e.g., barbiturates, tranquilizers.
7. Severe alcohol withdrawal symptoms are less common in children than adults and withdrawal usually is over in 48 hours.
8. Complications of alcohol abuse include:
   a. Safety hazards related to poor judgment, e.g., auto accidents.
   b. Nutritional deficiencies.
   c. Gastritis, possibly hemorrhagic.
   d. Pancreatitis.
   e. Overdose (alcohol level = 500 mg/dl blood) resulting in coma and death.
9. Long-term use of alcohol leads to eventual destruction of liver and brain cells.
10. Treatment modalities include:
    a. Short-term symptomatic treatment.
    b. Long-term rehabilitation based on individual needs, e.g., counseling, the use of Antabuse in conjunction with counseling, etc.

B. Nursing Management.
1. Support the child hospitalized for alcohol abuse. See *Hospitalization, Support During.*
2. Initiate discharge planning. See *Discharge Planning.*
3. Observe, record, and report the following signs and symptoms associated with alcohol abuse:
   a. Lethargy, stupor.
   b. Incoordination.
   c. Impaired judgment and perception.
   d. Loss of inhibitions.
   e. Labile emotions.
4. Observe, record, and report the following signs and symptoms associated with withdrawal:
   a. Tremors.
   b. Restlessness.
   c. Mild diaphoresis.
   d. Mild disorientation.

7A

e. Hallucinations.

f. Short convulsions (rare).

5. Observe, record, and report signs and symptoms associated with:

a. Gastritis.

1. Epigastric pain.

2. Anorexia.

3. Vomiting.

4. Gastrointestinal bleeding.

b. Pancreatitis.

1. Severe abdominal pain.

2. Profuse vomiting.

6. Meet the physical needs of the child during withdrawal.

a. Promote a quiet environment.

1. Keep lights dim.

2. Avoid loud talking, television, radio, etc.

b. Prevent injury.

1. Keep bed in low position.

2. Keep side rails up. (Pad if necessary.)

3. Assist with ambulation if incoordination is present.

c. Administer tranquilizing drugs as ordered.

d. Promote fluid intake and observe for signs of fluid and electrolyte imbalance. See *Fluid and Electrolyte Imbalance.*

e. Promote adequate nutrition. See *Nutrition.*

7. Meet the psychological needs of the child during withdrawal.

a. Use a nonjudgmental approach in your care.

b. Permit the child to make choices as the situation allows and his condition improves, e.g., select menu, times for hygienic care.

c. Involve the child in setting appropriate limits and adhere to them. See *Discipline.*

d. Reinforce positive behaviors and ignore negative behaviors.

8. Support the child in accepting long-term therapy if this is required.

a. Encourage verbalization about feelings about alcohol dependence.

b. Make sure that the adolescent is aware of treatment options and participates in the selection of a treatment modality suited to individual needs, e.g., residential treatment in a drug abuse center, joining a Young People's Alcoholics Anonymous group, etc.

9. Work with the family.

a. Encourage other family members who are dependent on alcohol to join Alcoholics Anonymous.

b. Support the family in restructuring their lives to find satisfaction in life without the use of alcohol.

c. Stress the need for parents to be role models.

d. Identify resources for counseling as indicated, e.g., Crisis Control, Hot Line, family service agency.

10. Meet the needs of the child who will be on disulfram (Antabuse) as an adjunct to therapy.

a. Explain that the drug prevents the body from handling alcohol.

b. Tell the child that the ingestion of even small amounts of alcohol will produce:

1. Flushing.

2. Headache.

3. Tachycardia.

4. Hypotension.

5. Profuse vomiting.

6. Vertigo.

c. Explain the need to avoid preparations that contain alcohol, e.g., vanilla extract, cough syrups.

d. Explain that reactions to disulfram may occur up to 5 days after last dose.

Alkalosis. See *Fluid and Electrolyte Imbalance.*

Allergic rhinitis. Allergic manifestation involving the upper respiratory tract.

A. **General Considerations.**

1. Allergens are usually foods in the young child and inhalants in the older child.

2. Seasonal allergic rhinitis (hay fever) is caused by sensitivity to molds, pollens, and house dust.

3. Perennial allergic rhinitis is caused by sensitivity to house dust, wool, feathers, molds, and animal dander.

4. Signs and symptoms include:

a. Sneezing.

b. Rubbing the nose to relieve itching.

1. Allergic salute; movement of the hand to push the nose up and back.

2. Mouth wrinkling.

3. Nose wrinkling.

c. Nasal stuffiness.

d. Red and itching conjunctiva.

e. Pale and swollen mucous membranes of the nose.

f. Nasal discharge.

1. Clear and profuse initially.

2. Purulent as secondary infection occurs.

g. Sore throat due to mouth breathing and drainage of nasal secretions.

h. "Allergic shiners"; dark areas around the eye orbit due to back pressure of the blood circulation.

5. The clinical course may be milder than that of other allergic diseases.

6. The child may have a history of frequent colds, recurrent epistaxis, or recurrent otitis media.

7. Serous otitis media can occur as a consequence of perennial allergic rhinitis.
8. Treatment includes:
   a. Removal of antigens.
   b. Desensitization.
   c. Control of infections.
   d. Relief of symptoms.
      1. Antihistamines.
      2. Oral decongestants.
      3. Nasal sprays.

B. **Nursing Management.**
1. Refer the child who comes in for well child evaluation, but manifests allergic symptoms.
2. Document any history of respiratory infections.
3. Teach the child and parents how to control the environment. See *Allergy*.
4. Discuss the use of antihistamines and/or nasal mucous membrane constricting agents. See *Administration of Medications, Parental.*
   a. Give antihistamines at bedtime to relieve symptoms and induce sleep.
   b. Contact the physician for adjustment in the dosage if the drug causes drowsiness during the day.
   c. Use nasal decongestants for a maximum of 5 days to prevent the rebound phenomenon.
5. Use a vaporizer or humidifier to relieve nasal stuffiness.
6. Teach the child and the parents how to prevent infections.
   a. Good hygiene.
   b. Adequate sleep. See *Sleep*.
   c. Adequate nutrition. See *Nutrition*.
   d. Limit exposure to crowds.

Allergy. An altered tissue reactivity to one or more substances.

A. **General Considerations.**
1. Allergic reactions result from the interaction of antigens and antibodies.
2. Clinical manifestations include:
   a. Allergic rhinitis.
   b. Asthma.
   c. Atopic dermatitis.
   d. Serum sickness.
3. Sensitization may result from:
   a. Contactants such as wool or poison ivy.
   b. Inhalants such as pollen or dust.
   c. Ingestants such as chocolate or orange juice.
   d. Injectables such as serum used in immunizations.
4. The development of allergic manifestations is influenced by heredity, susceptibility, and psychological factors involved in stress.
5. Skin and serum radioallergosorbent tests (RAST) can help identify allergens such as animal dander and mold.
6. A home visit by a nurse may be the most effective way to identify allergens when the symptoms cannot be linked to obvious allergens or when the child is not responding to treatment (Jennings, 1982).
7. Treatment includes:
   a. Removing the offending allergens.
   b. Decreasing the sensitivity to specific known allergens.
   c. Altering the response to offending allergens.

B. **Nursing Management.**
1. Obtain a detailed history of the allergic responses of the child and his family.
2. Assist the parents to assess the home environment as well as school, day care center, baby sitter's home, etc. for offending allergens:
   a. Molds.
   b. Dust.
   c. Dust mites and other insects.
3. Teach the child and parents general preventive measures.
   a. Good hygiene.
   b. Adequate nutrition. See *Nutrition*.
   c. Adequate rest. See *Sleep*.
   d. Limit exposure to crowds.
   e. Prompt treatment of respiratory infections.
4. Teach the child and parents about the elimination diet.
   a. Discuss which food products contain the allergens.
   b. Add one new food to the diet at a time.
   c. Use a scrapbook, food models, or magazine with pictures to test food knowledge.
   d. Place the allergen on the child's plate and offer positive reinforcement if the child notices and refuses to eat it.
5. Prepare the child and parents for a desensitization program.
   a. Discuss the rationale and the procedure.
   b. Provide "needle play" if the child is fearful of injections.
   c. Have adrenaline available to treat a reaction.
   d. Teach the child and parents to administer the allergen extract according to protocol.
6. Discuss environmental control of allergens.
   a. Foam pillows.
   b. Plastic covered mattress and pillow.
   c. Washable, cotton curtains and rugs.
   d. Washable window shades.

e. Metal, plastic, or wooden toys.

f. Washable, cotton or synthetic blankets and spread.

g. Plain, simply designed furniture.

h. Remove all carpeting from child's room.

i. Change heating and air conditioning filters frequently.

j. Vacuum and damp dust the child's room daily.

k. Avoid contact with the family pet.

l. Avoid exposure to smoke, strong odors, perfumes, etc.

m. Keep humidity level at 30 to 50 percent.

n. Avoid spray insecticides; use other types with caution.

o. Use an air cleaner only if it has proved effective when rented on a trial basis.

7. Explore ways in which family stress can be reduced if this is a contributing factor.

8. Teach the child and parents about medications and discourage self-prescribed drugs which may lead to intractability. See *Administration of Medications, Parental*.

9. Encourage the parents to initiate contact with the school nurse.

10. Discuss with the child and parents the long-term implications of the disease. See *Chronic Illness*.

Amblyopia. Loss of central vision in one eye from lack of use.

A. **General Considerations.**

1. Amblyopia may result from:

a. Anisometropia (Anisometropic amblyopia): unequal refractive power of the eyes.

b. Strabismus (strabismic amblyopia): imbalance of the extraocular muscles resulting in diplopia.

2. Amblyopia in anisometropia occurs in the eye with the greatest refractive error.

3. Amblyopia in strabismus occurs in the deviating eye when the brain suppresses the confusing image from that eye in order to avoid diplopia (double vision).

4. Diagnosis of amblyopia:

a. Is made on the basis of two line difference between eyes on a Snellen test (Pollard, 1977).

b. Requires that each eye be tested while the other one is covered.

5. Loss of visual acuity may range from slight loss of acuity to just being able to perceive light and is not related to the amount of deviation in strabismus.

6. The condition may be arrested or reversed if treatment is instituted before age 6.

7. The earlier treatment is begun the more likely the child is to retain vision.

8. Treatment consists of:

a. Patching the good eye to promote central vision in the affected eye.

b. Use of corrective lenses with anisometropia.

9. Schoolage children may have difficulty adjusting to wearing a patch because:

a. It makes them different from classmates.

b. Being forced to use the weak eye interferes with schoolwork.

10. Frequent evaluation of both eyes will be necessary during treatment to:

a. Evaluate response of the amblyopic eye.

b. Prevent occlusion amblyopia in the patched eye.

B. **Nursing Management.** See STRABISMUS

1. Assess the child and parents' understanding of the reason for wearing a patch.

2. Facilitate expressions of concern regarding outcome of treatment.

3. Support the child and parents in acceptance of altered body image. See *Body Image*.

4. Praise the child for cooperation in treatment program.

5. Explain rationale for periodic reevaluation of condition. See *Vision Screening*.

6. Teach child and parents activities which foster visual focusing, e.g., stringing beads, tracing designs.

Ambulatory care. Health care provided on an outpatient basis.

A. **General Considerations.**

1. Research supports the benefits to the child and family if care can be managed at home.

2. Emphasis in pediatric nursing care has shifted from the care of hospitalized children to the equally important role of caring for ambulatory children.

3. Parents, with support, are becoming more capable and desirous of caring for their children at home.

4. Children should be actively involved in their own health care, beginning with the preschooler.

5. Achieving optimal results requires compliance with the plan of care.

6. Parents may bring a child to an ambulatory care setting, or an adolescent may come alone, with a stated chief complaint but an unstated concern may be the real reason for the visit.

7. An initial nursing history should be obtained and updated at subsequent visits.

8. The cost of health care is less if the child can be treated at home.

9. Hospitalization should be reserved for those instances in which the child's condition or treatment warrant it and/or the parents are unable to manage it at home.

B. **Nursing Management.** See ADVOCATE and WELL-CHILD CARE.
1. Facilitate the use of ambulatory health care services.
   a. Give specific appointments and adhere to the schedule.
   b. Address the child and parents by name.
   c. Conduct all interviews in a manner that indicates the child and parents are important. See *History Taking*.
   d. Provide enough interview time to permit additional concerns to be expressed.
   e. Provide services at times when the parents can bring the child for care.
   f. Encourage the adolescent to use ambulatory health care services.
      1. Set aside specific hours for adolescent visits.
      2. Provide a teen atmosphere, e.g., remove toys, turn on popular radio station, subscribe to magazines which appeal to the adolescent.
2. Discuss the results of the physical exam, developmental evaluation, nutritional assessment, any lab or screening tests.
   a. See younger child and parents together.
   b. See adolescent separate from parents, then together if necessary.
3. Provide health teaching tailored to the specific needs and circumstances of the child and parents.
4. Promote open discussion of the child's condition to decrease anxiety and allay any guilt.
   a. Provide privacy for talking with parents.
   b. Provide play activities for the younger child so parent can be free to talk.
5. Encourage compliance with the health care plan. Use the nursing history as a basis for planning care.
   a. Include the child, adolescent and parents in making decisions about health care.
   b. Develop a plan consistent with the family's life style, culture, religious beliefs, finances, etc. See *Cultural Aspects of Health Care* and *Religious Aspects of Health Care*.
   c. Provide information as needed about medications, diet, activity, procedures, etc. See *Administration of Medications, Parental*.
   d. Answer questions honestly.
   e. Give the parents a phone number where a physician or nurse practitioner can be reached.
   f. Make an appointment for a return visit.

6. Make appropriate referrals as needed, e.g., nutritionist, dentist.
7. Assess whether a home visit would be of benefit to the child and parents before the next visit.

Amenorrhea. See *Menstruation*.

Amputation. See *Ewing's Sarcoma and Osteosarcoma*.

Anemia, iron deficiency Iron supply inadequate to meet requirements for optimal red blood cell formation. Red blood cells are pale and small.

A. **General Considerations.**
1. Mild iron deficiency anemia is usually asymptomatic and is detected by decreased hemoglobin values.
2. Signs and symptoms associated with moderate to severe anemia include:
   a. Irritability.
   b. Weakness.
   c. Anorexia.
   d. Decreased exercise tolerance.
   e. Shortened attention span.
   f. Pale mucous membranes.
   g. Decreased resistance to infection.
   h. Tachycardia and cardiomegaly when hemoglobin concentration level is below 6Gm/dl.
3. Fatigue due to anemia may manifest itself in hyperactive behavior.
4. Gastrointestinal irritation may occur with normal or toxic doses of iron supplements.
5. Iron is retained in the body when intake is excessive causing toxicity.
6. Iron-fortified formula is recommended for the first year of life.
7. Treatment may involve:
   a. Improvement of dietary iron intake. See *Appendix vii*.
   b. Use of oral iron preparations.

B. **Nursing Management.**
1. Assess.
   a. Foods usually eaten.
   b. Feeding methods used with the child.
   c. Child's reaction to feeding situation.
2. Promote improved nutrition.
   a. Feed slowly.
   b. Offer small, frequent feedings.
   c. Feed solids before offering liquids.
   d. Introduce iron rich foods when child is hungry.
   e. Limit milk intake. See *Appendix vii*.
3. Prevent constipation due to iron therapy.

a. Include roughage in diet.
b. Offer fluids frequently, include orange and prune juices.
4. Promote absorption of iron supplement.
   a. Give iron with orange juice as it promotes absorption.
   b. Avoid giving with milk which impedes absorption.
   c. Give between meals since bulk decreases absorption.
5. Prevent tooth discoloration from liquid iron preparations.
   a. Use dropper for infant.
   b. Use straw for older child.
   c. Have older child rinse mouth and brush teeth after taking iron supplement.
6. Observe, record, and report the following:
   a. Signs of infection.
   b. Vomiting and/or diarrhea which may signal gastric irritation.
7. Teach the child and parents home management.
   a. Base teaching on:
      1. Child's age.
      2. Sources of iron rich foods appropriate for income.
      3. Availability of iron rich foods in store(s) used for shopping.
      4. Cultural food patterns.
   b. Teach administration of iron preparation if ordered. See *Administration of Medications, Parental.*
   c. Tell parents that stools will be black when the child takes iron.
   d. Protect the child from infection.
   e. Encourage rest periods and quiet activity time during day to reduce fatigue.
   f. Reduce milk intake.

Anemia, sickle cell. Autosomal recessive disorder, found predominantly in blacks in which an abnormal hemoglobin (Hgb SS) causes sickling of red blood cells in the presence of decreased oxygen tension, acidosis, stress, dehydration, or cold.

A. General Considerations.
   1. Rigid, sickled cells increase blood viscosity, decrease blood flow, and may become sequestered in areas wherever blood flow is slow.
   2. Two major types of crisis characterize sickle cell anemia.
      a. Vaso-occlusive (pain) crises are common, result from infarction and necrosis, and are accompanied by:
         1. Episodic pain.
         2. Soft tissue swelling.
         3. Warmth over affected joints.
         4. Jaundice.
         5. Anorexia.
         6. Weakness.
         7. Low grade fever.
      b. Anemic crises, which are less common, include:
         1. Aplastic: resulting from decreased red blood cell production and increased red blood cell destruction; child is pale and lethargic.
         2. Splenic sequestration: occur spontaneously or follow a viral infection, and may cause death from profound anemia and cardiovascular collapse; child is pale, lethargic, and appears shocky.
         3. Hyperhemolytic: resulting from increased rate of red blood cell destruction (rare); child exhibits increasing jaundice.
   3. Hand-foot syndrome (dactylitis) is a vaso-occlusive crisis of the short tubular bones in children between 6 months and 2 years of age accompanied by fever, leukocytosis, and painful swelling over the affected areas which resolves in approximately 2 weeks.
   4. No specific measures can prevent a crisis.
   5. All vital organs are eventually involved and clinical manifestations include:
      a. Spleen: increasing fibrosis which reduces the ability to filter bacteria and release phagocytes.
      b. Liver: progressive focal necrosis leading to cirrhosis.
      c. Bones: development of skeletal deformities and aseptic necrosis of the femoral head.
      d. Central nervous system: visual impairment and strokes.
      e. Blood: marked hemolysis resulting in increased iron storage (hemosiderosis).
      f. Heart: heart failure.
      g. Musculoskeletal: infarction, infection, and necrosis.
      h. Endocrine: delayed sexual maturation.
      i. Skin: ulcerations.
      j. Genitourinary: hematuria, decreased urine concentration, enuresis, priapism.
   6. Children with sickle cell anemia:
      a. Adjust to low hemoglobin values. See *Appendix ii.*
      b. Have a decreased resistance to infection, especially pneumococcal and salmonella.
      c. May have delayed growth but usually reach normal adult height.
      d. Have a shortened life span.
   7. Adolescents with sickle cell anemia are prone to cardiac and gallbladder complications, leg ulcers, and aseptic necrosis of the femoral head.

8. Pregnancy is hazardous to both mother and fetus and requires intensive supervision.
9. Treatment measures for sickle cell crisis include:
   a. Bedrest to decrease oxygen demands.
   b. Hydration to promote hemodilution.
   c. Restoration of electrolyte balance since hypoxia leads to metabolic acidosis.
   d. Pain reduction.
10. Additional treatment measures may include:
    a. Antibiotic therapy for infection.
    b. Splenectomy or recurrent splenic sequestration.
    c. Administration of bicarbonate for acidemia.
    d. Blood transfusions for treatment of aplastic crises, prevention of recurrent strokes, promotion of healing of leg ulcers, management of the pregnant patient, and prophylactically prior to surgery.
    e. Use of experimental antisickling drugs.
11. Oxygen therapy is indicated only for the child who is hypoxemic; it has no effect on vaso-occlusive crises.
12. Parents may express or exhibit guilt over having passed the disease to their child.

B. **Nursing Management.** See CHRONIC ILLNESS and LIFE-THREATENING ILLNESS.
   1. Support the child and parents during hospitalization. See *Hospitalization, Support During.*
   2. Initiate discharge planning. See *Discharge Planning.*
   3. Handle pain crisis with:
      a. Hydration. See *Forcing Fluids.*
      b. Relief of pain. See *Pain.*
      c. Reduction of fever if present. See *Fever Reduction.*
      d. Rest periods.
      e. Warmth.
      f. Optimal nutrition. See *Nutrition.*
      g. Emotional support.
   4. Avoid those factors that predispose to sickling.
      a. Chilling.
      b. Tight clothing.
      c. Tight restraints.
      d. Positions that impede blood flow.
      e. Giving analgesic before assessing temperature.
      f. Stressful situations when possible.
   5. Observe, record, and report the following:
      a. Pain episodes and severe pain.
      b. Signs of infection.
      c. Increasing pallor.
      d. Jaundice.
      e. Lethargy.
      f. Difficulty waking child.
      g. Irritability.
      h. Fever.
      i. Signs of acidosis in the child receiving aspirin. See *Poisoning.*
   6. Observe, record, and report signs of less common but more severe crises:
      a. Aplastic: child is pale and lethargic.
      b. Hyperhemolytic: child exhibits increased jaundice.
      c. Acute sequestration: child is pale, lethargic, and may be in shock.
   7. Support parents in management of the child's condition.
   8. Administer packed red blood cell transfusions as ordered.
   9. Teach the child and parents to:
      a. Provide for health promotion.
         1. Keep immunizations up to date.
         2. Care for all breaks in skin as they occur.
         3. Dress the child appropriately for weather.
         4. Avoid excessively stressful situations if possible.
         5. See a dentist twice a year.
         6. Prepare well-balanced, iron-rich meals.
         7. Inform school about the child's health status.
      b. Call the physician for (McFarlane, 1977):
         1. Complaints of pain.
         2. Increasing pallor.
         3. Lethargy.
         4. Increasing jaundice.
         5. Difficulty waking the child.
         6. Soft tissue swelling.
         7. Temperature of 100°F for more than 2 days or initial elevation of 104°F.
      c. Schedule periodic blood value evaluation (McFarlane, 1977):
         1. Under age 2 years: every 1 to 2 months.
         2. Over age 2 years: every 3 to 6 months.
      d. Carry identification card with the child's:
         1. Diagnosis.
         2. Usual lab values.
         3. Allergies.
         4. Current medications.
   10. Refer family for sickle cell screening by hemoglobin electrophoresis to determine presence of sickle cell trait or anemia.
   11. Explain that sickle cell trait:
       1. Is a genetic carrier state of sickle cell anemia.
       2. Does not become sickle cell anemia.
       3. Does not produce symptoms under normal conditions.
       4. Requires no treatment.
   12. Provide genetic counseling referrals for family members with sickle cell trait if desired. See *Genetic Counseling.*

Anomalies, parents' reaction to. See *Exceptional Child.*

Anorectal malformation. An anomaly of the anorectal structures which occurs during fetal life.

A. **General Considerations.**
1. Anomalies may be classified as follows:
   a. Anal stenosis: corrected by digital dilatation.
   b. Imperforate anal membrane: corrected by surgical perforation in the newborn period.
   c. Anal agenesis: corrected by anoplasty in the newborn period.
   d. Rectal agenesis: colostomy is performed in the newborn period followed by a pull-through procedure at 6 to 12 months.
   e. Rectal atresia: colostomy is performed in the newborn period followed by a pull-through procedure at 6 to 12 months.
2. Signs and symptoms include:
   a. No anal opening observed during newborn examination.
   b. A finger or thermometer cannot be inserted into the rectum.
   c. Absence of stools.
   d. Abdominal distention after 2 to 3 days of life.
   e. Vomiting.
3. Female infants frequently have rectovaginal fistulas which allow surgery to be deferred since stool passage occurs.
4. Associated genitourinary, gastrointestinal (particularly tracheoesophageal fistula), and cardiac anomalies increase the mortality rate.
5. Abdominal x-rays and excretory urography are performed to diagnose the defect and to rule out associated anomalies.
6. Continence is achieved more slowly and is strongly influenced by social motivation in the older child.

B. **Nursing Management.**
1. Support the child and parent during hospitalization. See *Hospitalization, Support During.*
2. Initiate discharge planning. See *Discharge Planning.*
3. Meet the needs of the infant preoperatively. See *Preoperative Care* and *Preparation for Surgery.*
   a. Observe, record, and report meconium flecks in the urine which indicate rectourinary fistula.
   b. Assist with the insertion of a nasogastric tube which is used to decompress the stomach.
   c. Irrigate the nasogastric tube as ordered to insure patency.
   d. Monitor I.V. accurately.
   e. Position the baby on the abdomen or side to prevent aspiration if the infant vomits.
   f. Take axillary temperatures.
4. Meet the needs of the infant after colostomy. See *Postoperative Care.*
   a. Provide good skin care around the stoma.
      1. Wash around the stoma with soap and water.
      2. Apply zinc oxide, silicone ointment, or a Karaya preparation around the stoma.
      3. Apply gauze or tissue dressings and secure with a cloth diaper folded lengthwise.
      4. Fit the infant with a colostomy bag when possible.
   b. Take axillary temperatures.
   c. Teach parents home management of the colostomy.
      1. Remember the parents are learning to care for the new infant and the colostomy care. See *Neonate* and *Infant.*
      2. Demonstrate the care and have parents perform the demonstration.
      3. Explain that changes of the dressing or bag will need to be frequent, since the baby eliminates frequently and there is increased likelihood of skin breakdown.
5. Meet the needs of the infant after anoplasty or pull-through procedure. See *Postoperative Care.*
   a. Take axillary temperatures.
   b. Clean the suture line after each bowel movement with hydrogen peroxide or other solution as ordered.
   c. Position in a side-lying prone position with the hips elevated or in a supine position with the legs suspended at a 90 degree angle to decrease tension on perineal sutures.
   d. Teach parents home management.
      1. Teach dilatation procedure if ordered.
      2. Review administration of stool softener if ordered. See *Administration of Medications, Parental.*
      3. Anticipate that toilet training will cause greater anxiety in these parents and identify resources for the family to use when teaching is appropriate.

Anorexia in hospitalized child. See *Hospitalization, Support During.*

Anorexia nervosa. Severe weight loss in preadolescent or adolescent not attributed to a physical cause.

A. **General Considerations.**
1. Signs and symptoms include:
   a. Weight loss of 25 to 30 percent.
   b. Aversion to food.
   c. Low body temperature.

d. Increased, lanugo type body hair.
e. Decreased pulse.
f. Low blood pressure.
g. Dry skin and brittle nails.
h. Amenorrhea or delayed menses.
i. Constipation.
j. Vomiting after eating.
k. Distorted body image.
l. Hyperactivity.
2. Laboratory studies show anemia, lowered serum potassium and albumin, and increased cholesterol.
3. Fluid and electrolyte imbalance may develop. See *Fluid and Electrolyte Imbalance.*
4. The etiology is unclear but factors believed to contribute to the development of anorexia nervosa include:
   a. Dieting that has been carried to the extreme.
   b. Disturbed interpersonal relationships within the family, especially with the mother.
   c. Difficulty accepting the physical changes of puberty and sexual development.
   d. The development of a personality characterized by overconformity and overcompliance in the presence of feelings of being unable to control one's own life.
   e. Hypothalamic dysfunction.
5. Contributing factors to the weight loss are self-induced starvation, induced vomiting, and use and abuse of laxatives, enemas, and diuretics. See *Bulimia.*
6. The adolescent may engage in strenuous physical exercise to attain or maintain an unrealistic weight goal.
7. Obsession with food may lead the adolescent to assume responsibility for family food preparation.
8. Some adolescents may have been overweight originally, and parents may experience guilt if they nagged the child to lose.
9. Death from circulatory collapse or starvation is possible, and hospitalization is necessary for initial treatment.
10. Treatment includes:
    a. Behavior modification techniques:
       1. A firm, consistent, supportive approach.
       2. Reinforcement of appropriate behavior.
       3. Ignoring inappropriate behavior.
    b. Deemphasizing eating.
    c. Use of I.V. nasogastric tubes or total parenteral nutrition as required. See *Total Parenteral Nutrition.*
    d. Psychotherapy and/or counseling for the adolescent and the family.
    e. Hormonal treatment of amenorrhea.

B. Nursing Management. See ADOLESCENT.
1. Support the adolescent and parents during hospitalization. See *Hospitalization, Support During.*
   a. Develop a specific care plan and record it on the Kardex.
   b. Discuss the plan in conference so all staff understand how care is to be handled and the use of behavioral modification techniques.
   c. Limit the number of staff working with the adolescent to decrease the need for developing new relationships.
   d. Explain the treatment plan to the adolescent and parents and involve them in setting goals since knowing exactly what is expected decreases anxiety and limits manipulative behavior.
   e. Involve the adolescent in the planning as the condition permits in order to provide some sense of control.
   f. Help the family accept the need for professional counseling.
2. Initiate discharge planning. See *Discharge Planning.*
3. Encourage compliance with the dietary regimen ordered.
   a. Use a friendly, firm, consistent approach with feedings.
   b. Act as if you expect the adolescent will cooperate.
   c. Do not force, threaten, or punish the adolescent who refuses food.
   d. Reinforce positive eating behaviors.
   e. Explain why I.V. or nasogastric tube feeding is necessary (if used).
4. Observe, record, and report the following:
   a. Parent–child interactions.
   b. Response to counseling sessions.
   c. Intake and output (urine, stool, vomitus).
   d. Eating behaviors.
   e. Alterations in temperature, pulse, and blood pressure.
   f. Weight.
   g. Condition of skin.
5. Explore the adolescent's body image perception.
6. Decrease activity level by selecting and supervising exercise.
7. Observe for behaviors which interfere with treatment plan (Misik, 1981).
   a. Self-induced vomiting of food or vitamin/mineral supplements.
   b. Food hoarding.
   c. Disposal of food.
   d. Secret exercising.
   e. Adding weighted items to clothing before daily weighings.

8. Support the adolescent's level of development.
   a. Allow increasing control as condition improves.
   b. Provide peer contact.
   c. Encourage recreational activities.
   d. Provide appropriate sex role models.
9. Teach child and parents.
   a. Need for following dietary regimen that has been established.
   b. Positive behaviors should be reinforced and negative behaviors ignored.
   c. The adolescent should be allowed to assume increasing responsibility as the condition improves.
   d. Counseling may be required for the child and family for an extended period to relieve the underlying cause.
   e. The adolescent should be encouraged to become involved in peer group and school activities.

Anus, imperforate. See *Anorectal Malformations*.

Anxiety. A reaction to real or anticipated danger.

Anxiety in the Child.
A. General Considerations.
   1. Sources of anxiety include:
      a. Separation from parents.
      b. Separation from familiar environment and routine.
      c. Intrusive procedures, e.g., rectal temperature, injections.
      d. Loss of control over situations.
      e. Dependency.
      f. Absence from school.
      g. Lack of knowledge about his illness.
      h. Change in body image.
      i. Death fears.
      j. Fear of mutilation.
   2. Manifestations of anxiety include:
      a. Use of specific coping mechanisms.
      b. Aggression.
      c. Crying.
      d. Fearful facial expressions.
      e. Frequent questioning or no questioning.
      f. Clinging.
      g. Sleep disturbance.
      h. Refusal to eat.
      i. Inability to play.
      j. Hyperactivity.
B. Nursing Management.
   1. Observe and record behavior that may help identify the source of anxiety, e.g., response to parents, response to procedures.

2. Provide consistency in assignment of caregivers and in implementation of nursing care.
3. Follow home routines and rituals as much as possible.
4. Prepare the child for all procedures. See *Preparation for Procedures*.
5. Allow the child to make choices about his care whenever possible.
6. Encourage the child to assume responsibility for aspects of his own care when appropriate.
7. Meet educational needs by arranging for homebound teacher, having parents bring in homework assignments and establishing quiet, uninterrupted time for study.
8. Provide the child with information about his illness by using textbook pictures, drawings, and audio-visual materials.
9. Help the child cope with body image changes. See *Body Image* and *Coping*.
10. Allow the child to express feelings about death or mutilation directly through verbalization or indirectly through drawings or fantasy. See *Death, Concept Development of* and *Play, Therapeutic*.
11. Describe specifically how surgery, suture removal, cast application, etc., will affect the child's body integrity.

Parental Anxiety.
A. General Considerations.
   1. Sources of parental anxiety include:
      a. Uncertainty about diagnosis and treatment.
      b. Concern for the child's recovery.
      c. Unfamiliar hospital environment.
      d. Loss of the parental role and responsibility for child care.
      e. Guilt for "allowing the child to become ill."
      f. Concern for siblings.
      g. Financial concerns.
   2. High anxiety levels interfere with the ability to take in new information.

B. Nursing Management.
   1. Anticipate some degree of communication difficulty because of parental anxiety.
      a. Write down specific instructions and information.
      b. Record what parents have been told by the physician in order to prevent misunderstandings.
      c. Use lay terms rather than medical jargon.
      d. Give small amounts of information when the parent is able to listen.
      e. Use the same words and explanations used by other personnel.
      f. Answer questions calmly and honestly

even if the parent has asked the same question before.

2. Orient the parents to hospital routine and environment.
3. Encourage parents to participate in the child's care.
4. Give and/or reinforce information on how the child will be affected by diagnostic tests and treatment.
5. Allow parents to voice concerns about the child's recovery.
6. Interpret the child's behavioral response to hospitalization and treatment. See *Hospitalization, Response to.*
7. Allow parents to make appropriate decisions about child care, e.g., choice of fluids to be offered, how to explain procedures.
8. Identify and support positive aspects of parents' care of the child and teach alternative methods tactfully. See *Parenting.*
9. Discuss responsibility for care of other family members and make suggestions appropriately.
   a. Help mother identify who needs her the most; the sibling or the hospitalized child.
   b. Encourage telephone contact with the hospital when the parent is at home.
   c. Explore family and community resources for relief either at the hospital or at home.
10. Make appropriate referrals to social service, crippled children's services, etc., if finances are a problem.

Aorta, coarctation. See *Congenital Heart Disease.*

Aortic Stenosis. See *Congenital Heart Disease.*

Appendicitis. Inflammation of the appendix, usually secondary to obstruction by fecal matter.

A. **General Considerations.**
1. Early signs and symptoms are anorexia, behavioral changes, and diffuse, cramping abdominal pain, irritability, and "just not acting right."
2. Later signs and symptoms include sharp pain localized in the right lower quadrant, vomiting and nausea, fever, and elevated white blood count.
3. Young children are irritable and unable to report pain sites accurately.
4. The child may lie on the side with knees flexed and refuse to move.
5. Admission for observation may be necessary if the symptoms are inconclusive.
6. I.V. therapy may be necessary preoperatively if the child is dehydrated from frequent vomiting.
7. Cathartics and heat to the abdomen may cause rupture.
8. Barium enema may be used to establish the diagnosis.
9. Surgery is performed on an emergency basis.

B. **Nursing Management.**
1. Support the child and parents during hospitalization. See *Hospitalization, Support During.*
2. Initiate discharge planning. See *Discharge Planning.*
3. Give concise and specific explanations to the child and parents, since emergency admission and surgery causes high anxiety levels.
4. Meet the needs of the child preoperatively. See *Preoperative Care* and *Preparation for Surgery.*
   a. Tell the child what to expect during the physical examination.
      1. Warn the child before abdominal palpation that this maneuver will be painful. Palpation should be performed only by the nurse practitioner or physician because of the discomfort.
      2. Tell the child what you are listening for when you do auscultation for bowel sounds.
      3. Explain the rectal exam procedure.
   b. Prepare the child for routine complete blood count, chest x-ray, and urine specimen collection.
   c. Apply ice packs to abdomen as ordered.
   d. Position in semi-Fowler's or side-lying position for comfort.
   e. Explain why he is NPO and the rationale for I.V. or nasogastric therapy if used preoperatively.
   f. Provide general information as time and the child's condition permit.
   g. Prepare the abdomen of the older child as ordered.
5. Meet the needs of the child postoperatively. See *Postoperative Care.*
   a. Offer opportunities for the child to explore fears and concerns related to emergency surgery and limited preparation. See *Play, Therapeutic.*
   b. Record and report signs and symptoms of abscess.
      1. Irritability.
      2. Reluctance to move.
      3. Prolonged complaints of pain.
      4. Anorexia.
      5. Rigid abdomen.
      6. Shallow respirations.
      7. Fever.
   c. Prepare the child for discharge in 5 to 7 days and return to school in another week.

7A

d. Caution the child about restrictions of strenuous activity and sports and bicycle riding for several more weeks.

Appendix, ruptured. Bursting of the appendiceal wall.

A. **General Considerations.**
1. Bacteria escaping through the appendiceal wall may result in peritonitis or abscess.
2. The child will appear more ill at diagnosis, and the course of recovery will be longer.
   a. Rapid temperature elevation.
   b. Progressive abdominal distention.
   c. Tachycardia.
   d. Rapid, shallow respirations.
   e. Pallor.
   f. Chills.
   g. Restlessness and irritability.
3. Pain decreases after rupture and before peritonitis begins.
4. Conservative treatment with I.V. antibiotics followed by interval appendectomy 4 to 6 weeks later may be attempted (Powers et al., 1981).
5. If conservative treatment is ineffective after 12 to 24 hours, surgery will be performed.

B. **Nursing Management.**
1. Meets the needs of the child preoperatively. See *Preoperative Care* and *Preparation for Surgery.*
   a. Place the child in semi-Fowler's position so infected drainage will drain into pelvis.
   b. Administer oxygen, I.V. fluids, blood replacement, and I.V. antibiotics as ordered.
2. Meet the needs of the child postoperatively. See *Postoperative Care.*
   a. Apply warm soaks three to four times a day as ordered.
   b. Change and/or reinforce dressings carefully so penrose drains are not dislodged.
   c. Use Montgomery straps to prevent skin breakdown, since dressing changes are frequent.
   d. Keep the child in semi-Fowler's position.
   e. Turn to right side frequently to facilitate drainage through penrose drains.
   f. Prevent abdominal distention by ensuring functioning of nasogastric tube and by inserting rectal tube as ordered.
   g. Implement appropriate isolation techniques to prevent spread of infection.
   h. Explain to the child how drains will be "advanced" and then removed in 1 to 2 weeks.
   i. Help parents and child understand the reason for I.V. antibiotic therapy.
   j. Begin ambulation as ordered.
   k. Encourage the child and parents to express feelings about the complications and result-

ant disappointment over a longer hospitalization.

Arthritis, juvenile rheumatoid. A chronic, idiopathic, inflammatory disease which involves the joints and may cause connective tissue and visceral lesions.

A. **General Considerations.**
1. The disease has three distinct courses:
   a. Systemic onset—any joint may be involved.
   b. Pauciarticular—usually affects joints of lower extremities.
   c. Polyarticular—any joint, hip or spine frequently involved, usually asymmetric involvement of small joints.
2. The affected joint(s) are stiff (particularly in the morning), swollen, warm to the touch, and limited in motion.
3. Fever, malaise, lymphadenopathy, organomegaly, and rash may occur with systemic onset.
4. Diagnosis is often made when other diseases are eliminated as the cause of symptomatology.
5. Growth may be affected by the disease.
   a. Growth may be retarded during exacerbation, and a growth spurt may occur during remission.
   b. Growth is significantly retarded in children with chronic disease.
   c. Corticosteroid therapy contributes to growth retardation.
6. A milder disease course is associated with:
   a. An acute and painful onset.
   b. Involvement of only a few joints.
7. A longer, more disabling course is associated with:
   a. A gradual onset.
   b. Involvement of many joints.
8. Chronic disability occurs in approximately one-third of the children.
9. Treatment is aimed toward preservation of joint function, prevention of deformities, and relief of symptoms.
   a. Drugs.
      1. Salicylates.
      2. Corticosteroids.
      3. Gold salts.
      4. Antimalarial drugs.
   b. Physical therapy.
   c. Synovectomy in the older child may be recommended occasionally.
10. Drug levels must be monitored regularly, since the margin between therapeutic and toxic levels is narrow.

11. Infections, injuries, or surgery may precipitate an exacerbation of the disease.
12. Compliance with treatment is improved when the adolescent has a high self-esteem and is allowed more autonomy (Litt, Cresky, and Rosenberg, 1982).

B. **Nursing Management.** See CHRONIC ILLNESS.
   1. Support the child and parents during hospitalization. See *Hospitalization, Support During*.
   2. Initiate discharge planning. See *Discharge Planning*.
   3. Observe, record, and report the following:
      a. Joint pain, stiffness, or swelling.
      b. Fever, particularly during evening.
      c. Presence of salmon pink rash during febrile episodes.
   4. Prepare the child for diagnostic tests. See *Preparation for Procedures*.
      a. Serum immunoglobulins, sedimentation rate, and agglutination tests for the rheumatoid factor.
      b. X-rays of extremities.
      c. Joint aspiration.
   5. Obtain thin pillow for bed, since a fat pillow pushes the head forward and interferes with cervical alignment.
   6. Do not place pillows under involved joints.
   7. Meet hygiene needs of the acutely ill child, then gradually give the child responsibility for selfcare.
   8. Place a pillow at the back to shorten the depth of the chair seat and provide a stool to prevent feet dangling from the chair.
   9. Initiate teaching for the child and parent(s).
      a. Involve the child and parent in planning a home routine which fits in with family life style, e.g., hot bath, limbering-up exercises, school, intense physical therapy in afternoon or evenings.
      b. Assist the parents in learning physical therapy measures to be used at home.
      c. Give a warm tub bath for morning stiffness.
      d. Use warm compresses to facilitate joint motion.
      e. Help the family identify appropriate activities such as swimming for total exercise.
      f. Encourage the child to lie flat on a firm mattress for sleep.
      g. Have the child watch television lying face-down with hips in full extension and abduction.
      h. Apply half-shell night splints to prevent foot drop during sleep.
      i. Explain that splints are not to be used during waking hours.
      j. Discuss adjustment of home and school furniture to meet physical needs.
      k. Assist the parents to plan well balanced meals which do not result in excessive weight gain.
      l. Encourage parents to seek medical assistance promptly if the child develops symptoms of an infection.
      m. Discuss with parents the need to evaluate the effectiveness of unorthodox treatments which may harm the child.
      n. Teach the child and parents about medications. See *Administration of Medications, Parental*.
         1. Give aspirin at mealtime and parent's bedtime.
         2. Give aspirin with milk or an antacid or use an enteric-coated pill with the older child.
         3. Give corticosteroids every other day as instructed to minimize side effects.
      o. Review the need for frequent eye examinations, since eye inflammation (iridocyclitis) may occur asymptomatically as a complication.
      p. Explore with the child and parents how body image concerns and peer relationships may be affected by the disease. See *Body Image*.
      q. Discuss the need for the child to participate in normal, developmentally appropriate activities even if the activities are somewhat inappropriate to the medical problem.
      r. Establish and maintain communication with the public health nurse for follow-up.

Arthritis, septic. Joint inflammation usually caused by *Staphylococcus, Streptococcus,* or *Hemophilus influenzae.*

A. **General Considerations.**
   1. The joint infection is secondary to an acute infectious disease, otitis media, or penetrating wound.
   2. A history of trauma to the involved joint is common.
   3. One or more joints may be involved.
   4. Signs and symptoms include:
      a. Guarding of the joint.
      b. Fever.
      c. Muscle spasm around the joint.
      d. Edema of the joint.
      e. Positioning the joint in slight flexion.
      f. Malaise.
      g. Vomiting.
   5. Treatment may include:
      a. Joint aspiration.

A

b. Surgical drainage.
c. I.V. antibiotics.
d. Intra-articular antibiotics.
e. Immobilization by splints, cast, or traction.
f. Physical therapy during recuperative phase.

6. Complications include:
   a. Osteomyelitis.
   b. Necrosis, fragmentation, or pathologic dislocation of the femoral or humeral head.
   c. Fibrous ankylosis of the affected joint.

7. Prompt, adequate treatment usually results in full recovery of joint function.

B. **Nursing Management.** See IMMOBILIZED CHILD.
1. Support the child and parents during hospitalization. See *Hospitalization, Support During*.
2. Initiate discharge planning. See *Discharge Planning*.
3. Observe, record, and report symptoms that could aid in diagnosis.
4. Prepare the child and parents for procedures. See *Preparation for Procedures*.
   a. Blood and/or wound cultures.
   b. Surgical aspiration for fluid for culture.
   c. I.V. therapy.
   d. X-rays.
   e. Bone scan.
   f. Application of splints, traction, or cast, See *Cast Care*.
   g. Surgical drainage.
5. Observe, record, and report the child's response to medication and treatment.
6. Assess the neurovascular status of the limb.
   a. Sensation.
   b. Circulation.
   c. Pain.
   d. Color.
   e. Swelling.
   f. Heat.
   g. Tenderness.
7. Move and turn the child gently to minimize discomfort.
8. Assess the child's need for pain medication. See *Pain*.
9. Monitor the administration of wound irrigation solution if ordered.
10. Provide age-appropriate diversion and stimulation. See *Stimulation*.
11. Provide or reinforce physical therapy during recuperative phase as ordered.
12. Teach the child and parents home management.
    a. Review the administration of oral antibiotics. See *Administraton of Medications, Parental*.

b. Have parents demonstrate dressing change technique if needed.
c. Evaluate the older child's ability to use crutches.
d. Have the child and parents demonstrate physical therapy exercises.
e. Initiate contact with community resources if indicated.
f. Discuss the need for medical follow-up on a consistent basis.

Asthma. Reversible, obstructive disease of the lower respiratory tract usually caused by allergic hypersensitivity to foreign substances.

A. **General Considerations.**
1. Increased production of tenacious mucus, mucosal edema, and bronchospasm result in airway obstruction and lung hyperinflation.
2. Allergies are common in children with asthma.
   a. Food allergies are common in infants.
   b. Inhalant allergies are more common in older children.
   c. Infants and older children may be allergic to dust.
3. Other associated factors are:
   a. Rapid changes in environmental stress, especially cold.
   b. Physical stress of fatigue and exertion.
   c. Psychological stress, e.g., tension, fear, anxiety.
   d. Infections of the respiratory tract, ears, sinuses, etc.
4. The onset of an attack may be:
   a. Gradual, with sneezing, nasal congestion, and slight cough usually caused by an infection.
   b. Sudden, with wheezing, coughing spasms, and cyanosis usually caused by allergen exposure.
5. Infants may present with failure to thrive, vomiting, diarrhea, excessive mucus or bronchiolitis.
6. Diagnostic tests include:
   a. Chest x-ray.
   b. Examination of sputum, nasal secretions, and peripheral blood for eosinophils.
   c. Skin testing.
   d. Pulmonary function tests.
7. When a child with severe asthma fails to respond to drug therapy, the child is considered to be in status asthmaticus.
8. Treatment includes:
   a. Preventive measures.
      1. Hyposensitization.
      2. Removal of antigens.
      3. Bronchodilators, e.g., ephedrine, aminophylline, theophylline.

b. Management of acute attacks.
1. Bronchodilators, e.g., sympathomimetics (administered by IPPB or orally) and methylxanthines (administered by I.V., I.M., orally, or rectally). See *Administration of Medications.*
2. Corticosteroids.
3. Expectorants.
4. Antibiotics.
5. Sedatives. (Morphine is contraindicated.)
6. Combination drugs.
c. Management of status asthmaticus.
1. I.V. fluids to correct acidosis, liquefy secretions, and provide means of medication administration. See *Fluid and Electrolyte Imbalance.*
2. Humidified oxygen.
3. Intermittent positive pressure breathing (IPPB).
4. Antibiotics for infection.
5. Chest physiotherapy.
6. Monitoring of vital signs and central venous pressure (CVP), if necessary.
7. Determination of arterial blood gas and electrolyte levels.
8. Correction of acidosis with sodium bicarbonate or tromethamine.
9. Assisted ventilation with a volume-type respirator.
d. Long-term management.
1. Medications.
2. Allergen control.
3. Physical therapy.
4. Exercise program.
5. Hyposensitization.
9. Asthma attacks and hospitalizations are fewer when the child and parents participate in programs which teach self-management skills (Fireman et al., 1981).
10. Long-term hospitalization in a specialized hospital may be necessary if the home is not conducive to recovery.

B. **Nursing Management.** See LIFE-THREATENING ILLNESS.
1. Support the child and parents during hospitalization. See *Hospitalization, Support During.*
2. Initiate discharge planning. See *Discharge Planning.*
3. Observe, record, and report the following:
a. Characteristics of respiration, particularly during bath, feeding, or if child out of mist tent and oxygen.
1. Wheezing: an expiratory sound which may be audible with or without a stethoscope.
2. Dyspnea (difficulty breathing).
b. Color.
4. Keep child well hydrated to decrease sputum viscosity.
a. Maintain I.V. rate accurately.
b. Encourage oral fluids. See *Forcing Fluids.*
c. Offer fluids at room temperature, since cold fluids may cause coughing spasms.
d. Monitor urine specific gravity.
e. Measure intake and output.
f. Assess signs of hydration. See *Fluid and Electrolyte Imbalance.*
5. Observe, record, and report child's response to medications.
a. Monitor pulse, respirations, and blood pressure before, during, and after aminophylline administration.
b. Observe for signs of drug toxicity since child may have received medication at home or in the physician's office.
6. Assist with administration of mist and oxygen. See *Preparation for Procedures.*
a. Mist tent. See *Mist Tent.*
b. Vaporized inhalations (IPPB).
1. Allow the child to become familiar with equipment.
2. Let the child participate as much as possible in responsibility for procedure.
c. Oxygen.
1. Maintain ordered low flow rate, since a high flow rate will increase alveolar CO_2 tension and cause hypoxia.
2. Provide the child with a safe mechanisms to call for the nurse, e.g., small bell.
7. Provide or assist with chest physiotherapy.
a. Schedule postural drainage at times which are before meals and after medications.
b. Do not administer postural drainage if there is significant wheezing, cyanosis, or shortness of breath.
8. Promote comfort.
a. Position the child upright with arms supported, e.g., leaning over padded overbed table, to provide greater chest expansion.
b. Offer fluids and foods frequently, but in small amounts.
c. Organize nursing care to allow the child adequate rest periods.
d. Provide age-appropriate diversion. See *Stimulation.*
e. Prevent emotional conflicts that could result in respiratory difficulty by using a consistent nursing approach.
f. Reassure parents and keep them informed of the child's treatment and progress.
9. Teach the child and parents home management of an asthmatic attack.
a. Teach the child to begin breathing exer-

cises and to drink warm water when symptoms begin.

b. Teach the child to seek help if above measures are ineffective.

c. Teach parents how to administer subcutaneous injections.

d. Review protocol for medications as ordered.

1. Aqueous epinephrine is usually given and repeated in 20 minutes if needed.

2. Sus-Phrine may then be given for long-term effectiveness.

3. Bronchodilators by nebulizer may be used.

e. Review proper use of nebulizer or aerosol devices since incorrect use or abuse is common (Kirilloff and Tibbals, 1983).

1. The young child is unable to coordinate breathing with administration.

2. Children may become "spray happy."

f. Administration of disodium cromoglycate (cromolyn), particularly before exercise.

10. Teach the parents and child the importance of control of allergens. See *Allergy.*

11. Help parents to understand variations in appetite, growth rate decelerations, and chest circumference changes.

12. Encourage exercise such as swimming, calisthentics, baseball, and skiing if medically approved.

13. Teach parents to use play techniques which improve the child's respiratory capacity, e.g., blowing cotton balls, pinwheels, feathers, ping-pong balls, etc.

14. Assist the child and parents to understand long-term effects of the diagnosis. See *Chronic Illness.*

15. Refer to a parent support group, if available (Walsh, 1981; Pituch and Bruggeman, 1982).

Athlete's foot. See *Tinea.*

Atrial septal defect. See *Congenital Heart Disease.*

Autism. A severe psychosis beginning in infancy characterized by an inability to relate interpersonally.

A. **General Considerations.**

1. There are four major criteria for infantile autism (Rutter, 1971).

a. Onset before the age of 3 months.

b. The appearance of aloofness and distance with a general lack of interest in others.

c. Ritualistic and compulsive behavior, particularly with mechanical objects.

d. Speech and language delays.

2. The etiology is unknown although central nervous system abnormalities may be a factor.

3. The lack of known etiology and limited success of psychotherapy, drug intervention, and behavior modification techniques cause severe stress to parents of autistic children.

4. Most autistic children score less than 50 on standard IQ tests.

5. Behavioral characteristics of the autistic child include:

a. Lack of involvement with others.

1. No eye contact.

2. No response to verbal communication.

3. Resist touching and other signs of affection.

4. Perceptual dysfunction leads the child to operate only from his own reality.

b. Lack of verbal communication.

1. Echoing or parrot speech.

2. No use of personal pronouns.

3. No self-image development.

c. Intense preoccupation with inanimate objects and own body.

1. Odd, repetitive behaviors.

2. Frequent, self-stimulating activities.

d. Frequent temper tantrums.

1. Destructive rages toward himself or others.

2. Fear of harmless things.

3. Extreme response to changes in routine.

6. The differential diagnosis between autism and mental retardation, childhood schizophrenia, or deafness is often difficult.

7. The goals of therapy are to help the child to:

a. Identify own body as separate from those of other people.

b. Integrate the concept of self.

c. Develop relations with other human beings.

B. **Nursing Management.**

1. Support the child and parents during hospitalization. See *Hospitalization, Support During.*

2. Initiate discharge planning. See *Discharge Planning.*

3. Obtain a nursing history which includes the following specific information (Killion and McCarthy, 1980):

a. Type of therapy used at home/school.

b. General level of understanding.

c. Specific communication words, phrases, or signals.

d. Specific routines or rituals, e.g., meal time, bed time, etc.

e. Food preferences.

f. Methods of managing problem behaviors.

g. Need for supervision.

4. Communicate the plan for managing the child's behavior via nursing staff conferences and the Kardex.
   a. Anticipate that the child may become enraged if health care requires a change in routine.
   b. Recognize that the treatments must be implemented despite the child's objections.
   c. Allow the child to engage in nonharmful self-stimulating behavior if this serves as a comfort measure.
   d. Respond to temper tantrums by isolating the child from interpersonal events, but maintain his safety.
5. Inspect the child's room frequently to assure that there are no hazards to the child's safety.
6. Facilitate effective communication (Killion and McCarthy, 1980).
   a. Identify the goal of your interaction.
   b. Establish eye contact.

c. Break the desired behavior into small, attainable goals.
d. Give precise, concise instruction; repeat as necessary.
e. Reward correct response to question or instruction, but do not reward attempts which are unsuccessful.
7. Meet nutritional needs by providing familiar, preferred foods since the autistic child resists change.
8. Promote rest and sleep by following home routines.
9. Promote appropriate behavior by setting firm, consistent limits.
10. Provide support for the family and initiate referrals for financial, social, or mental assistance as needed.

Automobile Safety. See *Accident Prevention.*

Battered child. See *Abused Child.*

Bedwetting. See *Enuresis.*

Bee stings. See *Home Management of Minor Emergencies.*

Behavior problems. Forms of behavior which occur in response to stress and are inappropriate to the child's developmental level, the setting in which they occur, and/or are maladaptive.

A. **General Considerations.**
   1. Knowledge of normal development is a prerequisite to management of behavior problems. See *Appendix v.*
   2. Behavior problems may develop when:
      a. Parents misinterpret normal, adaptive coping responses as a problem, e.g., the toddler who hangs onto a favorite toy or blanket when stressed.
      b. Age appropriate stimulation is not provided, e.g., infants not provided with adequate stimulation may resort to excessive body rocking and head banging.
      c. Expectations of the adults in the child's en-

vironment are inappropriate to the child's level of development, e.g., expecting too high a level of performance in school may lead to cheating.
      d. The approach to the child is inconsistent, e.g., a parent first ignores then responds to a child's temper tantrums.
      e. There is minimal brain dysfunction, e.g., the child who cannot keep up with his peers may become disruptive.
   3. Treatment of behavior problems is based on:
      a. Identification and eradication of the underlying stress, if possible.
      b. Support of the development of age appropriate coping. See *Coping.*
      c. Understanding that reinforced behaviors continue whereas nonreinforced behaviors become extinguished.
      d. Recognition that parent(s) and child must be treated together.
   4. Learning age appropriate, adaptive behaviors requires time and both parent(s) and child will need consistent support.
   5. The greater the number of functional areas affected by a behavior problem, the more severe the problem.
   6. The child's developmental level, not his chronological age, should be used as a basis for expectation of behaviors.

B. Nursing Management. See DISCIPLINE and TEMPER TANTRUMS.

1. Obtain a nursing history to assess:
   a. Parents' knowledge and comprehension of normal developmental behaviors.
   b. Parents' perception of their child, e.g., a "difficult" baby.
   c. Duration of symptom(s).
   d. Number of functional areas with which problem interferes, e.g., problem interferes with child's home, school, and peer relationships.
2. Do not seek to blame anyone for the child's behavior.
3. Observe parent and child interaction as a basis for intervention.
   a. Tone of voice used with the child.
   b. Amount and type of physical contact.
   c. Ratio of positive statements about the child to negative ones.
4. Intervene.
   a. Assist parents in identifying stressors in the child's environment which can be modified or eliminated.
   b. Teach parents general management of behavior problems.
      1. Teach growth and development norms to be used as a basis for expectations of the child.
      2. Teach parents age-appropriate activities for the child.
      3. Teach techniques to promote appropriate, adaptive behavior.
      4. Use a consistent method in your approach to avoid manipulation by the child.
      5. Ecourage parents to work with the school in maintaining a consistent approach.
   c. Teach promotion of appropriate, adaptive behavior through behavior modification.
      1. Do not use threats, bribes, or sarcasm in response to a child's misbehavior.
      2. Ignore negative behaviors that are exhibited unless they are unsafe.
      3. Reinforce positive behaviors, e.g., "you played so well with the other children."
      4. Agree among staff on a consistent approach to the child and record it on the chart or Kardex.
      5. Provide age-appropriate activities for the child. See *Play*.
   d. Role model appropriate responses to the child's behavior.
5. Support parents in their use of behavior modification techniques.
6. Remember that illness and hospitalization may cause regression in behavior. See *Regression*.
7. Care for the hospitalized child with a behavior problem.
   a. Assess how parents are handling problem at home.
   b. Work with parents to develop a plan of care.
   c. Record plan on Kardex to promote consistency in nursing approach.
   d. Use the time child is hospitalized to teach parents management of behavior problems when parents indicate an interest and child's condition permits.

Bicycle safety. See *Accident Prevention.*

Birth defects, parent's reactions to. See *Exceptional Child.*

Bites. See *Home Management of Minor Emergencies.*

Blindness. Absence of vision. See *Exceptional Child* and *Stimulation.*

A. General Considerations.
1. Blind children have the same basic needs as children who have sight.
2. The age at which blindness occurs, the cause, and the presence of other handicaps will affect how both parents and child will cope with blindness.
3. Parents will require ongoing support in order to help their blind child achieve his potential.
4. Blind children require assistance in learning in the following areas where vision plays a central role (Fraiberg, 1977).
   a. Human attachment, since the child will not receive visual cues given by human behavior, e.g., smiles.
   b. Prehension, since the child will not be focused to the midline by seeing his hands come together.
   c. Locomotion, since the child will not be stimulated to explore his world by what he sees.
   d. Language, since the child does not have a visual representation of what he is told.
5. Midline organization is a prerequisite for the development of the ability to reach out and experience the environment.
6. Behavior problems may be more intense in the child who is blind (Friedman and Hoekelman, 1980).
7. Public Law 94-142 effective September, 1977 mandates free and appropriate education for all handicapped children.

B. Nursing Management.
1. Focus your care on the "child" not on his "handicap" to promote optimal development.
2. Meet the special needs of the blind child in the hospital or clinic setting.

a. Find out home routines and record on Kardex to promote consistency.
   1. Daily routines.
   2. Self care capabilities, e.g., dressing, toileting.
   3. Feeding techniques.
   4. Food preferences.
   5. Sleep patterns.
b. Assist child in adapting to new environment.
   1. Explain new sounds, e.g., "the bell you hear tells the nurse to come."
   2. Let child handle all materials and equipment that will be used in his care.
   3. Place items child will use in the same place and record on Kardex, e.g., table always on left side of bed.
   4. Walk the child around his room and orient him to where things are located.
   5. Do not move the furniture without reorienting the child.
   6. Place your arm through the child's when walking him somewhere rather than pushing the child by the elbow.
   7. Assess the environment for safety hazards and remove so the child may be mobile, e.g., keep cords from equipment out of the traffic path.
c. Facilitate meal times.
   1. Allow enough time for the child to finish his meal.
   2. Select foods with distinct smells in order to stimulate the child's appetite.
   3. Name the foods on the child's plate so he learns to identify specific tastes with names of foods.
   4. Do not feed the child if he can feed himself.
   5. Give preschoolers finger foods.
   6. Place food in small bowls for the child using a spoon.
   7. Tell the child which foods are hot and which are cold.
   8. Tell the child who can identify time on a clock face that different foods are at different times, e.g., ham is at 6 o'clock.
d. Provide verbal cues where visual ones would normally be used by the child.
   1. Identify yourself when you enter the room and tell the child when you are leaving.
   2. Speak to the child before you touch him.
   3. Tell the child what you are doing in the room as you work.
   4. Introduce the child to other people in the unit.
e. Encourage the child to do everything for himself that he is able to do.
f. Foster peer group relationships.

   1. Introduce the child to other children.
   2. Place in a room with children of the same age.
   3. Take to the playroom and involve the child in group activities.
3. Support development of the blind infant. (Scott, 1977). See *Handicapped Child.*
   a. Promote human attachment.
      1. Hold, cuddle, and rock.
      2. Carry child with you when you can.
      3. Place infant in a room with auditory stimuli.
   b. Promote bringing of hands together in a midline position in order to develop midline organization.
      1. Place infant's hands on the bottle during feeding.
      2. Hang a mobile, which makes a noise when touched, in the middle over the crib.
      3. Play pat-a-cake.
   c. Encourage the infant to explore his environment by use of auditory stimuli placed in front of him, e.g., musical toys, wind-up clock.
   d. Facilitate language development by reading, talking, and singing to the infant.
   e. Encourage development of body movement and hand control by tactile stimulation.
      1. Stroke infant under chin to promote holding head up.
      2. Permit exploration of the house.
      3. Promote increasing experience with the outside world.
   f. Encourage child to do all he can for himself.

Body image. A constantly changing mental picture of one's own body.

A. **General Considerations.**
   1. Factors that affect body image development include:
      a. Physical experiences, such as sensation and mobility.
      b. Physiological functioning.
      c. Developmental maturation.
      d. Attitudes of others.
   2. Most children less than 10 or 11 years of age have a poor understanding of what is inside their body.
   3. Young children believe all body parts are essential for survival.
   4. Concern about changing body image is characteristic of the adolescent.
   5. Body image distortion occurs as a result of illness and/or surgery.
   6. Pain and large bandages magnify body image distortion.

B

B. **Nursing Management.**
1. Help the child understand what he is experiencing.
   a. Find out what the child believes has happened or will happen to his body.
   b. Consider the body concerns specific to the age group when giving explanations. See *Fears*.
   c. Tell the child how he will feel during and after a procedure.
   d. Tell the young child that his body part(s) will be "fixed" not removed.
   e. Remember that the toddler and preschooler believe that bandages and sutures keep body insides intact.
   f. Provide information on the technical aspects of a procedure for the older child who indicates a need for this knowledge.
   g. Allow the child to see and touch bandages and body parts when he is ready.
      1. Offer a mirror so that the child can inspect his body.
      2. Give him sterile gloves, if needed, and let him participate in care of the affected part.
   h. Describe what he is now experiencing in relation to his past experiences, e.g., growth of new skin after a blister, abrasion, etc.
   i. Provide experiences that provide feedback about his body.
      1. Play games such as "pat-a-cake," "this little piggy," and naming body parts during bath.
      2. Tell the young child his body part is still under the bandage, cast, etc.
      3. Encourage all caregivers to hold, stroke, and touch the child.
      4. Reposition the child frequently using minimal restraints.
   j. Remember that constant focus on an affected body part by health professionals will increase the child's concern.
2. Demonstrate respect for and acceptance of the child.
   a. Promote cleanliness, comfort, and a pleasant appearance.
   b. Provide privacy.
   c. Protect from undue exposure.
   d. Initiate physical contact frequently to reinforce acceptance.
   e. Support coping behaviors such as control and avoidance.
3. Help parents to cope with the child's body image changes. See *Coping*.
   a. Encourage them to verbalize their expectations about how the child will look as a result of illness and/or surgery.
   b. Provide accurate information about the child's appearance.
   c. Explain how a positive approach by the parents will help the child.
      1. Visits and gifts are interpreted as acceptance by the child.
      2. Abandonment, pity, and aversion are interpreted as rejection.
   d. Support their attempts to talk with the child about his appearance.
      1. Discuss alternative explanations based on their knowledge of the child and your knowledge of growth and development.
      2. Remain in the room during explanations if the parents wish.
   e. Help them plan what to tell relatives, neighbors, school teacher, etc., about the child's appearance if necessary.
4. Maintain the child's positive body image.
   a. Make the hospital experience as normal as possible.
      1. Follow home routines.
      2. Encourage peer interactions.
      3. Let the child wear his own clothes.
      4. Provide diversion.
      5. Help him keep up with school work.
   b. Encourage the child to express his feelings and concerns.
      1. Self-drawings may give clues to the child's self image.
      2. Anger and grief are frequent responses to loss of a body part.

Bottle mouth syndrome. See *Nursing Bottle Syndrome*.

Braces. See *Legg-Perthes Disease*.

Brain, minimal dysfunction. See *Minimal Brain Dysfunction*.

Brain tumor. Abnormal growth of cells located in the brain or metastasized from neoplasm of another body part.

A. **General Considerations.**
1. Most brain tumors in children occur in the posterior third of the brain resulting in symptoms of increased intracranial pressure.
2. Early diagnosis is difficult because of the tumor's insidious nature.
3. The prognosis for infants is poor because the tumor grows to a large size before being diagnosed.
4. Surgery is the treatment of choice, but most tumors cannot be totally removed.
5. Surgical complications include infection, hematoma formation, and neurological deficits (Damon and Taylor, 1980).
6. Shunting procedures may be utilized to relieve

obstructive hydrocephalus. See *Hydrocephalus.*

7. Radiation therapy and/or chemotherapy are usually used postoperatively.
8. Irritation of the temperature control area of the brain will result in fever postoperatively.

B. Nursing Management. See LIFE-THREATENING ILLNESS.

1. Support the child and parents during hospitalization.
2. Initiate discharge planning. See *Discharge Planning.*
3. Meet the needs of the child preoperatively. See *Preoperative Care* and *Preparation for Surgery.*
   a. Observe, record, and report signs of increased intracranial pressure. See *Increased Intracranial Pressure.*
   b. Observe, record, and report signs and symptoms that would help localize the tumor.
      1. Decreased rate or change in nature of pulse and respiration.
      2. Hypothermia or hyperthermia.
      3. Change in blood pressure, especially rise in systolic pressure with widening pulse pressure.
      4. Behavior changes, e.g., irritability, lethargy, coma.
      5. Quality of speech.
      6. Level of consciousness.
      7. Visual defects, e.g., nystagmus, diplopia, strabismus, decreased visual acuity, visual field defects.
      8. Head tilt.
      9. Seizures.
      10. Ataxia.
      11. Vomiting, with or without nausea.
      12. Headache, particularly those which wake the child from sleep, occur when arising, are prolonged or incapacitating, or altered in quality, frequency, or pattern (Honig and Charney, 1982).
      13. Cranial enlargement in child under 18 months.
      14. Papilledema.
   c. Prepare the child and parent(s) for diagnostic procedures.
      1. Computerized tomography.
      2. Radionucleide imaging.
      3. Brain scan.
      4. Echoencephalography.
      5. Roentgenography.
      6. Cerebral angiography.
   d. Keep side rails up since the child may be confused or drowsy.
   e. Assure adequate hydration. See *Fluid and Electrolyte Imbalance.*
      1. Refeed after vomiting since nausea is usually absent.
      2. Measure intake and output.
      3. Test urine specific gravity.
      4. Observe for signs of dehydration.
   f. Tell the child and parents what to expect the child to look like after surgery.
      1. Bulky head dressing.
      3. Edema, particularly of orbital area.
      3. Head will be shaved.
   g. Introduce child and parents to Intensive Care Unit staff if appropriate.
4. Meet the needs of the child postoperatively. See *Postoperative Care.*
   a. Position child with the bed flat or slightly elevated as ordered.
      1. Change position hourly with slow, careful movements.
      2. Move the head and neck as a single unit if surgery was performed in the low occipital area.
      3. Position on side that was not operated on unless ordered otherwise.
      4. Do not lower the head of the bed or elevate the foot of the bed.
   b. Monitor I.V. accurately to prevent increased intracranial pressure.
   c. Observe, record, and report the following:
      1. Significant variation in vital signs.
      2. Rapid increase in drainage or bright red blood on head dressing.
      3. Changes in pupil response.
      4. Abnormal reflexes, handgrip, or function of the cranial nerve.
      5. Regression in level of consciousness.
      6. Increase in facial or neck edema.
      7. Urinary incontinence or retention.
   d. Initiate fever reduction measures as ordered. See *Fever Reduction.*
      1. Help parents understand that the fever is not unexpected.
      2. Explain the purpose and operation of the hypothermia equipment.
      3. Administer antipyretics as ordered.
   e. Reinforce the head dressing with sterile towel or pads.
      1. Use a ballpoint pen to outline drainage since fluid from a felt tip pen may penetrate the dressing.
      2. Clarify with the surgeon how much drainage should be expected.
   f. Avoid upsetting conversation in the child's presence even if he appears to be unconscious.
   g. Promote comfort.
      1. Provide irrigations, eye drops, or eye dressings as ordered.
      2. Use cool compresses to reduce edema if ordered.
      3. Provide mouth care.
      4. Provide meticulous skin care.

B

5. Provide a quiet, safely lit environment.
6. Avoid jarring movements such as banging against the bed.
   h. Restrain the child only if absolutely necessary. See *Restraints*.
      1. Restraints may increase the child's frustration and result in increased intracranial pressure.
      2. Use elbow restraints or mitts if restraints are required.
   i. Anticipate that parents will need help in adjusting to diagnosis, particularly if the tumor was not removed totally.
5. Meet the needs of the child during the recovery period.
   a. Encourage the child's return to independence when his condition improves.
      1. Explain that edema and surgical trauma make return to normal functioning a slow process.
      2. Support the parents so they do not overprotect the child.
   b. Help the child adjust to changes in body image when the dressing is removed. See *Body Image*.
      1. Obtain a cap, scarf, or ruffled sleeping bonnet.
      2. Have the child wear a wig until hair grows.
   c. Help the child and parents cope with chemotherapy and/or radiation therapy. See *Chemotherapy* and *Radiation Therapy*.
      1. Reinforce physician's explanation of treatment goals.
      2. Review action and side effects of therapy.
   d. Refer the family to the community health nurse for teaching, reinforcement, and family support.
   e. Initiate contact with the child's teacher and school nurse.
      1. Classmates need to expect change in child's appearance and behavior.
      2. Activity restrictions must be explained.
      3. Rest periods should be planned initially.

Breast feeding. See *Nutrition*.

Bronchiolitis. Viral infection of lower respiratory tract accompanied by inflammatory obstruction of the small bronchioles due to cellular debris from tissue necrosis, edema, and mucus.

A. **General Considerations.**
1. Signs and symptoms usually occur during the course of an upper respiratory infection and include:

   a. Low grade to moderate fever.
   b. Paroxysmal cough.
   c. Dyspnea.
   d. Tachypnea.
   e. Nasal flaring.
   f. Wheezing.
   g. Rales.
   h. Intercostal and subcostal retractions at rest.
   i. Barrel-shaped chest in severely ill child due to hyperinflation.
2. Cyanosis and right heart failure may develop in severe cases.
3. A decrease in wheezing may represent worsening of the condition as plugging increases and airflow is diminished.
4. Chest x-rays reflect evidence of air trapping.
5. Treatment is supportive and includes:
   a. Humidified oxygen; percent based on results of arterial blood gas studies.
   b. Hydration.
   c. Positioning for maximum air exchange.
   d. Pulmonary hygiene as condition permits.
   e. Rest.
   f. Antibiotics for any secondary infection.
6. Mild cases are managed at home but severely ill or young infants are hospitalized.
7. Bronchiolitis may be difficult to differentiate from asthma.
8. Sedatives should not be used, since they would mask the signs of increased respiratory distress.
9. A trial dose of epinephrine may be given to rule out reactive airway disease.

B. **Nursing Management.**
1. Support the child and parents during hospitalization. See *Hospitalization, Support During*.
2. Initiate discharge planning. See *Discharge Planning*.
3. Observe, record, and report the following:
   a. Sudden temperature elevation which may indicate secondary infection.
   b. Changes in retraction, rales, and/or wheezing which may indicate improvement or further deterioration of child's condition.
   c. Signs and symptoms of heart failure.
      1. Easy fatigability.
      2. Weak, rapid pulse.
      3. Dyspnea.
      4. Tachycardia.
      5. Diaphoresis.
4. Position child in semi-Fowler's position or on abdomen to facilitate breathing since weight of chest helps expiration.
5. Place in oxygen hood as ordered. See *Mist Tent*.
6. Prevent fatigue.
   a. Schedule care in blocks of time to provide rest periods.
   b. Feed slowly.

c. Do not permit infant to cry for long periods.
7. Promote hydration.
   a. Offer fluids frequently. See *Forcing Fluids.*
   b. Monitor I.V. accurately if receiving I.V. fluids.
8. Observe, record, and report infant's response to medications, if ordered.
9. Teach the parents home management of milder cases.
   a. Promote hydration.
   b. Facilitate breathing by use of cool steam vaporizer.
   c. Provide adequate rest periods.
   d. Administer medications as instructed. See *Administration of Medications, Parental.*
   e. Call physician if signs of secondary infection or respiratory distress occur.

Bronchitis. Inflammation of the mucous membranes of the bronchi.

A. **General Considerations.**
1. Usually accompanies or follows a viral upper respiratory infection.
2. Signs and symptoms include:
   a. Cough which progresses from nonproductive to loose, gurgly productive state.
   b. Low grade fever.
   c. Coarse rales and rhonchi, which clear when the child coughs.
   d. Wheezing in some cases.
3. Treatment includes:
   a. Increased air humidification.
   b. Expectorants.
   c. Antibiotics for secondary bacterial infection.
4. Bronchodilators may be used when wheezing is present because asthma is often present in such cases (Loughlin, 1983).
5. Cough suppressants and antihistamines should not be used, since the aim of therapy is to liquify and loosen secretions.
6. Untreated bronchitis may lead to pneumonia.
7. Home treatment is usually possible.

B. **Nursing Management.**
1. Explain the condition to the child and parents.
2. Teach parents how to:
   a. Promote hydration. See *Forcing Fluids.*
   b. Use nasal aspirator to remove secretions.
   c. Increase air humidity. See *Home Management of Minor Illnesses.*
3. Tell parents that child under 4 cannot usually cough up secretions.
4. Explain why antihistamines and cough suppressants are not used.
5. Tell parents to observe for signs of secondary bacterial infection and call physician if the child develops:

a. Sudden high fever.
b. Increased cough.
c. Purulent sputum.

Bronchopulmonary dysplasia. Diffuse pulmonary fibrosis following long-term treatment of idiopathic respiratory distress syndrome (hyaline membrane disease) with endotracheal intubation, mechanical ventilation, and high inspired oxygen concentration.

A. **General Considerations.**
1. The disease progresses through four overlapping stages with the following symptoms (Voyales, 1981):
   a. Stage I, actually idiopathic respiratory distress syndrome, days 1 to 3: tachypnea, cyanosis in room air, grunting, and retractions.
   b. Stage II, days 4 through 10: difficulty with ventilation due to obstruction caused by tissue regeneration; pulmonary edema may develop in this period as a result of a patent ductus arteriosus.
   c. Stage III, days 10 through 30: transition to chronic state of bronchopulmonary dysplasia with increased mucus production and alternating atelectic and emphysematous lung areas.
   d. Stage IV, 1 month to 2 to 3 years of age: chronic state with hypoxemia, emphysema, and perivascular fibrosis.
2. Complications which may develop during the long healing process include: pulmonary hypertension, congestive heart failure, growth retardation, poor nutrition, and exercise intolerance.
3. Treatment is directed at:
   a. Slow withdrawal of ventilation and oxygen to prevent hypoxemia and pulmonary hypertension.
   b. Providing adequate nutrition.
   c. Reduction of stress.
   d. Prompt treatment of respiratory infections.
   e. Use of bronchodilators and mild sedation for wheezing which may develop.
   f. Use of diuretics to treat fluid overload (digitalis is not helpful) (Bland, Tooley, 1982).
4. The majority of children are symptom free by 2 to 3 years of age, although residual symptoms may persist up to 5 to 7 years.
5. Many children can be cared for at home with the use of supplemental oxygen.

B. **Nursing Management.**
1. Support the child and parents during hospitalization. See *Hospitalization, Support During.*
2. Initiate discharge planning as the child's condition permits. See *Discharge Planning.*
3. Observe, record, and report signs and symp-

B

toms of congestive heart failure. See *Congestive Heart Failure*.

4. Provide respiratory support.
   a. Administer cool humidified oxygen as ordered.
   b. Position for maximum lung expansion.
   c. Promote mucus removal by postural drainage, percussion, and/or suctioning as ordered.
5. Administer medications as ordered and observe, record, and report the child's response.
6. Promote adequate nutrition. See *Nutrition*.
   a. Meet additional caloric needs due to increased respiratory rate.
   b. Restrict fluid and salt intake as ordered if child has cardiac involvement.
   c. Offer smaller, more frequent feedings.
   d. Provide oxygen as needed during feedings.
   e. Feed older infant with a spoon and offer high caloric foods.
7. Stimulate age-appropriate development within the child's activity tolerance. See *Stimulation*.
8. Teach parents home management.
   a. Assist parents in developing procedures for administration of supplemental oxygen.
   b. Teach parents how to carry out postural drainage, percussion, and suctioning.
   c. Teach parents to administer medications. See *Administration of Medications, Parental*.
   d. Provide nutrition guidance.
   e. Teach parents ways in which they can stimulate growth and development.
   f. Help parents develop sources of support.
      1. Refer to home health care agency or public health nurse.
      2. Tell them to notify their local emergency service of child's special needs.
      3. Support them in locating and teaching a competent baby sitter how to care for their child so that they can have some time for themselves.

Bulemia Psychiatric disorder characterized by binge-eating episodes followed by vomiting.

A. General Considerations.
1. The adolescent may gorge herself with food (up to 55,000 calories), then induce vomiting or take laxatives or diuretics to avoid weight gain.
2. This binge–purge syndrome may also be a symptom of anoxeria nervosa, but bulemia victims usually have normal or near-normal weight. See *Anorexia Nervosa*.
3. Symptoms include:
   a. Tooth decay caused by destruction of tooth enamel by acidic vomitus.
   b. Persistent sore throat.

c. Liver damage.
d. Nutritional deficiencies.
e. Stomach rupture.
f. Fluid and electrolyte imbalance. See *Fluid and Electrolyte Imbalance*.

4. The adolescent is frequently depressed and there may be family history of depression.
5. The adolescent is aware of her abnormal eating pattern and may voluntarily seek help with her problem.

B. Nursing Management.
1. Be alert to clues that an adolescent may be controlling her weight by binging and purging episodes.
   a. Ask how the adolescent controls her weight while you are performing a nursing history. See *Nursing History*.
   b. Listen for statements by parents that it is impossible to keep food in the house.
2. Support the adolescent who admits to bulemic practices and encourage her to seek treatment.
   a. Group therapy.
   b. Individual psychotherapy.
   c. Family therapy.
   d. Antidepressants or other pharmacotherapy.

Burns, chemical. Tissue damage of the oropharynx, esophagus, stomach due to ingestion of a corrosive substance.

A. General Considerations.
1. Household cleaners containing the strong alkalis potassium or sodium hydroxide (lye) are the most commonly ingested corrosive substances.
2. Concentrated acids produce coagulative necrosis and severe burns due to lack of buffering by gastric secretions.
3. Concentrated alkalis produce liquefaction of tissue, especially the esophagus, since gastric acid acts as a buffer in the stomach.
4. Weak acid or alkali solutions produce erythema and edema but not tissue necrosis.
5. Signs and symptoms produced by the ingestion of a concentrated solution include:
   a. Pallor.
   b. Excessive salivation.
   c. Hoarseness.
   d. Dysphagia.
   e. Edema; may be severe enough to require tracheostomy.
6. Acute symptoms resolve within several days.
7. Treatment includes:
   a. Maintenance of a patent airway.
   b. Antibiotics.
   c. Adequate nutrition and hydration to promote healing.

d. Repeated esophageal dilatation for strictures requiring hospitalization.

e. Corticosteroids, begun when diagnosis of esophageal burn is made, to decrease edema, and continued during healing process to decrease or prevent strictures (controversial).

8. Vomiting is never induced.

9. Milk or water may be given at the time of ingestion to dilute corrosive substances but severe burns can occur within seconds of contact.

10. Complications include:
   a. Stricture formation.
   b. Perforation of the esophagus during the acute stage or later during dilatations.
   c. Erosion into the mediastinum and/or peritoneum.
   d. Tracheoesophageal fistula.

11. A gastrostomy tube may be needed to maintain nutrition if the child is unable to swallow.

12. Surgical reconstruction of the esophagus using a segment of the colon may be needed.

13. Hospitalization occurs under emergency circumstances and both child and parents may be very frightened.

14. Severe burns of the mouth may require extensive oral plastic surgery and dental care.

B. Nursing Management. See *Poisoning.*

1. Support the child and parents during hospitalization. See *Hospitalization, Support During.*

2. Initiate discharge planning. See *Discharge Planning.*

3. Observe, record, and report signs of increasing airway obstruction due to edema.
   a. Restlessness and/or anxiety.
   b. Rapid breathing.
   c. Increased pulse rate.
   d. Flaring of the nares.
   e. Retractions.
   f. Dysphagia and drooling.

4. Observe, record, and report signs that a tracheoesophageal fistual has developed.
   a. Coughing.
   b. Choking.
   c. Circumoral cyanosis.

5. Observe, record, and report signs and symptoms of peritonitis.
   a. Severe abdominal pain.
   b. Fever.
   c. Nausea.
   d. Vomiting.
   e. Abdominal rigidity and distention.

6. Observe, record, and report signs and symptoms of mediastinitis.
   a. Dyspnea.
   b. Fever.
   c. Chest pain.

7. Observe, record, and report the child's response to medications.

8. Administer analgesics for pain as ordered and observe, record, and report the child's response.

9. Maintain hydration by oral or I.V. route as ordered.

10. Meet the nutritional needs of the child on oral feedings.
   a. Offer liquid or soft high protein foods.
   b. Serve small amounts frequently if child has difficulty swallowing.
   c. Use a tube feeder like those used with cleft lip if child has difficulty opening his mouth.

11. Support the child and parents during repeated admissions for dilatations.
   a. Assign the same nurse to care for the child.
   b. Admit the child to the same room if possible.
   c. Support coping mechanisms since the child and parents may be stressed by reminders of initial trauma. See *Coping.*
   d. Assess how the family has been managing at home and provide assistance/referral as needed.
   e. Prepare the child for each procedure; never assume that details of prior preparation are remembered.
   f. Assess the child after dilatation for airway obstruction.
      1. Noisy respirations.
      2. Grunting.
      3. Elevated respiratory rate.
      4. Restlessness.
   g. Assess the child after dilatation for perforation of the esophagus.
      1. Fever.
      2. Tachycardia.
      3. Tachpnea.

12. Observe, record, and report the child's response to the dilatation procedure.

13. Prepare the child and parents for the insertion of a gastrostomy tube if this is required for feeding.

14. Meet the needs of the child after insertion of a gastrostomy tube.
   a. Provide gravity drainage for the first day.
   b. Aspirate before feeding and subtract amount returned from quantity ordered to be given.
   c. Progress the position of the tube as ordered.
      1. Leave open to gravity drainage between feedings.
      2. Elevate the tube between feedings.
      3. Clamp the tube between feedings.

B

d. Feed slowly and at a consistent rate.

e. Do not force the feeding into the tube.

f. Protect the skin around the tube with karaya powder, zinc oxide ointment, etc.

g. Keep the area around the tube clean and dry.

h. Anchor the tube so there is no pull on it.

15. Teach the child and parents home management.

a. Tell parents signs and symptoms that should be reported to the physician.

b. Review medications ordered and method of administration. See *Administration of Medications, Parental.*

c. Discuss the importance of following the schedule of esophageal dilatations if this is planned.

d. Have parents return a demonstration of tube feeding if the child has a gastrostomy.

e. Provide anticipatory guidance in the area of accident prevention.

f. Make a referral to a community health nurse if parents indicate need for assistance at home.

Burns, electrical of mouth. Tissue damage caused by contact with an electrical current.

A. **General Considerations.**

1. Signs and symptoms include:

a. Pale gray areas where the current entered and left the body.

b. Edema.

c. Tissue necrosis; progressive after 24 to 36 hours.

d. Eschar formation; separation occurs in about 12 to 14 days.

2. Minor burns can usually be managed at home after initial evaluation and treatment.

3. Severe burns require hospitalization and treatment, which includes antibiotics, wound care, and the use of tetanus toxoid depending on the child's immunization status.

4. Complications include infection and hemorrhage due to erosion of blood vessels in a highly vascular area.

5. Scar tissue may develop and interfere with the child's speech.

6. Surgical repair of a lip or cheek burn can be done in a two-stage procedure, approximately 2 weeks after the burn, in which the defect is filled with a flap made from the tongue (Ortiz-Monasterio and Foster, 1980).

7. Severe wounds should not be permitted to heal by secondary intention in order to prevent: narrowing of the mouth due to scar tissue formation; dental deviation; and persistent drooling.

B. **Nursing Management.**

1. Support the child and parents during hospitalization. See *Hospitalization, Support During.*

2. Initiate discharge planning. See *Discharge Planning.*

3. Observe, record, and report the child's response to medications.

4. Care for the wound.

a. Rinse the mouth with water after feeding.

b. Clean the wound as ordered.

c. Restrain the child as needed to prevent further injury to the area.

5. Promote increased protein intake to enhance healing.

6. Administer analgesics as ordered.

7. Observe, record, and report signs of infection or bleeding.

8. Teach the parents home care of the burn.

9. Prepare the child and parents for reconstructive therapy if this is planned. See *Preoperative Care* and *Preparation for Surgery.*

10. Care for the child after pedicle flap construction (Isler, 1976). See *Postoperative Care.*

a. Prevent injury to the surgical site.

1. Restrain infants and toddlers if needed. See *Restraints.*

2. Keep small objects out of child's reach.

3. Feed infant with soft rubber tube.

4. Do not use forks, spoons, or straws.

5. Do not give infant a pacifier.

6. Feed older child from side of spoon or cup.

b. Prevent wound breakdown and infection.

1. Give only clear liquids until diet order is progressed by physician.

2. Remove milk and/or remaining food with sterile water.

3. Use antiseptic mouthwash with older child as ordered.

4. Keep wound as dry as possible.

5. Administer antibiotics as ordered.

c. Provide substitute comfort measures for infant deprived of sucking, e.g., cuddle, rock, walk, etc.

d. Provide age-appropriate, quiet play activities for older child.

e. Observe, record, and report any signs of wound breakdown or infection.

11. Teach parents home care of the child after a pedicle flap construction.

12. Meet the needs of the child after release of pedicle flap and wound reconstruction using care plan from pedicle flap construction.

13. Teach parents home care after plastic repair is completed.

14. Provide anticipatory guidance in relation to accident prevention. See *Accident Prevention.*

15. Initiate referral for speech therapy if required.

Burn, thermal. Tissue injury that results from excessive exposure to thermal or electrical agents.

A. **General Considerations.**
1. Burns are classified according to depth of tissue destruction.
   a. Superficial (first degree).
      1. Appear red (due to vasodilation) and dry.
      2. Do not blister or scar.
      3. Are painful.
      4. Blanch readily on pressure and refill quickly.
      5. Peel after approximately 1 week.
   b. Partial thickness (second degree) are further classified as:
      1. Superficial: appear blistered, mottled, pink or red; are painful and sensitive to air exposure; blanch readily on pressure and refill quickly; and heal within 3 weeks with minimal scarring.
      2. Deep: appear mottled, red, dull, blistered; may be moist or dry; require 4 to 8 weeks to heal, and have more extensive scarring.
   c. Full thickness (third degree).
      1. Destroy entire dermis and may extend to underlying subcutaneous tissue.
      2. Are painless.
      3. May appear black and charred, yellow-brown, or translucent.
      4. Do not blister.
      5. Require grafting.
2. Deep superficial burns are susceptible to conversion to full thickness burns in the presence of poor perfusion and/or infection.
3. The "Rule of Nines," used in determining the percentage of body surface burned in the adult, cannot be used with children, because the head is proportionately larger and the legs are proportionately smaller.
4. Hospitalization for burn care is needed when (Stein, 1979):
   a. The face, hands, feet and/or perineum have been burned:
   b. Partial or full thickness burns cover:
      1. 20 percent or more of body surface in older child.
      2. 12 to 15 percent of body surface in infants.
      3. 10 percent of body surface in neonates.
   c. Full thickness burns cover 0.5 percent or more of body surface and require immediate excision and grafting.
   d. Child abuse is suspected.
   e. Electrical burns are present.
5. Transfer to a burn treatment center is advisable when:
   a. Partial thickness burns cover more than 20 percent of body surface area.
   b. Full thickness burns cover more than 10 percent of body surface area.
   c. There are complicating factors, e.g., additional trauma such as fractures, intercurrent or chronic illness, inhalation burns.
6. Hospital treatment will be based on accurate assessment of the depth and percent of the burns and is developed to:
   a. Prevent shock during the emergent period 24 to 48 hours following the burn.
   b. Prevent infection.
   c. Promote healing.
   d. Maintain or restore maximal function.
   e. Minimize psychological problems resulting from the burns.
7. Burn care for the hospitalized child may include:
   a. Intravenous fluids to replace fluid losses.
   b. Insertion of an indwelling catheter to measure output.
   c. Insertion of an nasogastric tube to prevent gastric distention.
   d. Pain medication.
   e. Tetanus prophylaxis.
   f. Prophylactic antibiotics.
   g. Frequent monitoring of vital signs.
   h. Wound care, which may include:
      1. Debridement of nonviable tissue.
      2. Hydrotherapy to loosen dead tissue.
      3. Application of topical antibacterial agents.
      4. Covering or leaving burn sites exposed.
      5. Early excision of burn followed by autografting.
      6. Use of biological (human amniotic membrane, cadaver allograft, porcine xenograft) and/or synthetic (polyethylglycol with methylcryate) skin coverings until autografting can be done, i.e., granulation bed is clean and well vascularized.
      7. Protective isolation.
   i. Positioning and/or splinting and use of pressure garments.
   j. Administration of an antacid to prevent stress ulcers (Curling ulcer).
   k. Avoidance of hypothermia.
   l. High caloric, high protein diet.
   m. Psychological counseling.
8. Optimal care for the burned child may require a team effort of physician, nurse, physical therapist, occupational therapist, recreational therapist, dietician, social worker, respiratory therapist, surgeon, teacher, parent, and child.
9. Itching is a major problem with healing burns.
10. Loss of zinc in the urine contributes to loss of taste and anorexia.

B

11. Burn scars (Surveyer and Cloughedly, 1983):
    a. Change from pink to deeper red as healing occurs.
    b. Become hard and raised (hypertrophic) due to whorl-like pattern of collagen fibers in tissue.
    c. Will be less hypertrophic when pressure garments are used.
    d. Vary in color when they are fully healed:
       1. Superficial, superficial partial thickness, and donor sites are usually normal or near normal skin color.
       2. Deep-partial and full-thickness burns show changes in color.
12. Anticipate that the child with major burns will require repeated hospitalizations for release of contractures and cosmetic surgery.

B. **Nursing Management.** See ADMISSION TO HOSPITAL, EMERGENCY, and LIFE-THREATENING ILLNESS.
1. Support the child and parents during hospitalization. See *Hospitalization, Support During*.
2. Initiate discharge planning as soon as condition permits See *Discharge Planning*.
3. Meet the needs of the child during the emergent period.
   a. Give concise, specific explanations to the child and parents, since emergency admission and burns cause high anxiety levels.
   b. Obtain baseline physiological data, e.g., weigh, participate in assessment of wounds, obtain laboratory studies as ordered.
   c. Obtain nursing history of the injury.
   d. Observe, record, and report.
      1. Signs and symptoms of shock: altered level of consciousness, thirst, poor peripheral circulation, decreased urinary output, decreased blood pressure, weak, thready pulses.
      2. Symptoms of respiratory distress: wheezing, air-hunger, wet rales, and sooty secretions.
      3. Signs and symptoms of fluid and electrolyte imbalance. See *Fluid and Electrolyte Imbalance*.
   e. Observe, record, and report the child's response to medications.
      1. Check before using I.M. route, since poor peripheral circulation may hinder absorption.
      2. Check immunization record before giving tetanus prophylaxis.
   f. Monitor intake and output accurately.
   g. Explain why child may be kept NPO, since he may be very thirsty due to fluid shift.

   h. Give frequent mouth care while child is NPO.
   i. Use sterile equipment and aseptic technique.
4. Meet the needs of the child during the convalescent period.
   a. Prevent infection.
      1. Follow isolation technique as ordered.
      2. Wash hands before giving any care.
      3. Administer antibiotics as ordered.
      4. Do not assign staff members with infections to care for child.
      5. Carry out good hygienic care to reduce the bacterial count of the skin.
      6. Do not allow visitors who have any infections.
   b. Observe, record, and report signs of wound infection.
      1. Offensive odor.
      2. Temperature elevation.
      3. Gray green color indicative of *Pseudomonas*.
      4. Blue black color indicative of sepsis.
      5. Redness at wound edge indicative of cellulitis.
   c. Assess for signs of sepsis:
      1. Tachypnea.
      2. Tachycardia.
      3. Hypothermia or hyperthermia.
      4. Paralytic ileus.
   d. Promote adequate hydration. See *Forcing Fluids*.
   e. Administer medications as ordered and observe for side effects.
   f. Assist with or carry out wound care as ordered.
      1. Prepare child for procedure. See *Preparation for Procedures*.
      2. Use aseptic technique at all times.
      3. Permit child to express his feelings about care.
      4. Promote child's ability to cope by giving him a task he can do, e.g., hand you supplies. See *Coping*.
   g. Observe, record, and report coffee grounds vomitus or aspirant from a nasogastric tube which may indicate development of a Curling's ulcer.
   h. Stimulate deep breathing exercises, e.g., have child blow pin wheels or Kleenex held in front of mouth.
   i. Prevent contractures and pressure areas.
      1. Maintain joints in neutral position or extension.
      2. Put shoes on child to prevent footdrop, but remove periodically to prevent pressure areas.
      3. Apply splints as ordered.

4. Carry out active and passive range of motion exercises at each dressing change.
5. Turn the child from side to side frequently.
6. Carry out skin care to avoid breakdown, e.g., use Nivea cream.

j. Promote nutrition intake needed for healing.
1. Provide a high caloric, high protein diet.
2. Allow the child to choose what appeals to him, since anorexia is a common problem.
3. Offer small frequent feedings rather than large meals.
4. Do not threaten the child or use food as a weapon.
5. Encourage red meats and/or seafood which are high in zinc.

k. Assist the child in coping with immobilization, pain, and isolation that may accompany therapy. See *Immobilization, Isolated Child*, and *Pain*.
1. Visit child at times other than when you are giving care.
2. Provide rest periods by scheduling care in blocks of time.
3. Provide age-appropriate play activities. See *Play*.
4. Encourage therapeutic use of play. See *Play, Therapeutic*.
5. Place bed where child can see activity around him.
6. Avoid personalizing outbursts of anger which child may express.
7. Be consistent in your approach and record it on the Kardex.
8. Promote peer contact if appropriate.

l. Care for the child undergoing grafting. See *Postoperative Care, Preoperative Care*, and *Preparation for Surgery*.
1. Explain types of grafts used, e.g., homograft, heterograft are temporary whereas autograft is permanent.
2. Explain procedures to be used.
3. Follow principles involved in autografting: keep graft in contact with recipient bed, immobilize the grafted site as ordered, avoid unnecessary manipulation, observe for vascularity, adherence, and infection.

m. Help minimize itching which accompanies healing.

1. Administer antihistamines as ordered.
2. Apply lotion with high lanolin content.

n. Prepare the child and parents for discharge.
1. Recognize that the child may have concerns about going home due to altered body image. See *Body Image*.
2. Discuss exposing the child gradually to activities of daily living.
3. Suggest clothes that would cover scars.
4. Teach parents how to prepare teacher and classmates of severely burned child for child's return to school: visit classroom and talk to teacher and children, take current picture of child to show (with child's permission only), show pictures of, or actual, pressure garments or splints.
5. Teach administration of any medications. See *Administration of Medications, Parental*.
6. Teach how to do dressing changes at home.
7. Teach any exercises which may be ordered.
8. Teach child and parents use and care of pressure garment(s) (Surveyer and Cloughedly, 1983).
   a. Wear garment(s) 24 hours a day; remove only for hygienic care.
   b. Assess garment(s) for proper fit.
   c. Wash garment(s) by hand in mild soap and water, rinse completely, and air dry.
   d. Use water base skin creams under garment(s) since oil base destroys elastic thread.
9. Suggest the use of nonperfumed alcohol free makeup to cover healed burns.

5. Meet the needs of the child during the rehabilitative period.
a. Anticipate that readmission of the child for release of contractures or cosmetic surgery may reactivate fears related to initial hospitalization.
b. Prepare the child for all procedures.
c. Teach the child and parents proper use of any correctional orthopedic appliances.
d. Explain types of clothing that can be worn over appliances which may be large and bulky.

Caloric needs See *Nutrition.*

Candida albicans (monilia). Infection caused by the fungus *Candida albicans.*

A. **General Considerations.**
1. The fungus prefers warm, moist areas and is normally present in skin folds and in the mucous membranes of the mouth and vagina.
2. Infections may occur:
   a. When the infant passes through the mother's vagina at birth.
   b. As a secondary invader in diaper dermatitis. See *Dermatitis, Diaper.*
   c. Following antibiotic treatment that alters normal alimentary flora.
   d. In the presence of immunosuppression.
   e. When skin disorders, poor nutrition, or other diseases lower resistance.
   f. Following sexual intercourse.
   g. In the adolescent taking birth control pills.
3. Candida infection of the mouth called "thrush":
   a. Produces a white, flaky coating or patches which appear on the buccal mucosa, tongue, gingiva, and, sometimes, the lips.
   b. May be accompanied by bleeding if the white patches are removed.
   c. Frequently interferes with feeding.
4. Candida infection of the diaper area:
   a. Produces raised salmon-colored, confluent lesions with smaller satellite lesions.
   b. May be followed by secondary bacterial infection which produces pustules.
5. Candida infection of the vulva and vagina (vulvovaginitis) produces:
   a. Intense itching.
   b. A thick, yellow-white, curdy discharge.
   c. Severe burning sensation when urine touches the affected areas.
   d. Red, swollen, painful labia.
   e. Excoriation of the perianal area.
   f. Satellite lesions similar to those seen in monial diaper rash (less common).
6. Treatment measures include:
   a. Antifungal medications applied to the lesions.
   b. Good hygienic practices.
   c. Comfort measures.
7. Treatment of vulvovaginitis should continue during the menstrual period since blood is an excellent growth medium.

8. The use of douches and antiseptic vaginal suppositories may increase symptoms.
9. The adolescent with diabetes and/or taking birth control pills may have difficulty eradicating a candida infection.
10. Systemic infection may occur.

B. **Nursing Management.**
1. Use meticulous handwashing technique, since the infection may be spread by hands.
2. Teach application of antifungal medication.
   a. Oral preparations are to be swabbed around the mouth after feeding.
   b. Creams are to be applied in a thin layer that covers the area.
   c. Vaginal suppositories or creams are to be placed deep in the vaginal canal by use of a clean applicator.
3. Explain to the parents that the infant with thrush may feed poorly and be irritable.
4. Teach parents to:
   a. Feed yogurt to a child on antibiotics since it helps restore normal intestinal flora.
   b. Prevent reinfection of the mouth by:
      1. Boiling rubber nipples for bottle-fed infant.
      2. Applying antifungal cream to nipples of breastfeeding mother.
5. Teach comfort measures.
   a. Thrush: rinse mouth with clear water after feeding and offer clear, cool liquids to older child.
   b. Candida diaper dermatitis: wash with cool water and thoroughly pat dry the area, avoid rubber pants, and change wet diapers promptly.
   c. Candida vulvovaginitis: use tepid water sitz baths as needed, wear absorbent cotton underpants, and avoid nylon panty hose and tight slacks.
6. Encourage adolescent with vulvovaginitis to have any sexual partner(s) seek treatment.

Cardiac catheterization Diagnostic procedure in which there is placement of a radiopaque catheter within the chambers of the heart in order to trace anatomic defects, measure pressure in the heart chambers, sample oxygen content of the blood and assess changes in cardiac output.

A. **General Considerations.**
1. An arterial or venous approach may be used for left heart catheterization.

2. A venous approach is used for right heart catheterization.
3. The groin or antecubital space is used most frequently for the introduction of the catheter.
4. Cardiac catheterization is often combined with angiocardiography: the injection of radiopaque dye through the catheter followed by films of its dilution and circulation.
5. Pain is not generally associated with the procedure once the catheter is inserted; pressure may be felt at the insertion site as the catheter is advanced.
6. Local anesthesia and sedation are usually employed; general anesthesia may be used.
7. The child must remain immobile while the procedure is done.
8. The room temperature in the cardiac catheterization lab may be cool and serve as a stressor.
9. A cardiac monitor may be used following the procedure.
10. Digitalis dose may be withheld prior to the procedure.

B. Nursing Management.
  1. Meet the needs of the child before the procedure.
     a. Prepare the child and parents for the procedure. See *Preparation for Procedures.*
     b. Tell the child what he will feel before and during the insertion of the catheter and what he can do to help himself, e.g., lie still.
     c. Tell the child he may feel a warm flush when the medicine is injected.
  2. Meet the needs of the child after the procedure.
     a. Find out if an arterial or venous approach was used.
     b. Move the child gently.
     c. Instruct the child not to sit up suddenly, since postural hypotension may occur.
     d. Observe, record, and report the following:
        1. Heart rate; count pulse for a full minute.
        2. Blood pressure.
        3. Pulses distal to the catheter insertion site. (Pulse may be weaker initially but should gradually increase.)
        4. Skin temperature, color, and sensation in the extremity distal to the site used for catheterization.
     e. Observe, record, and immediately report signs of complications.
        1. Slow or irregular pulse due to disturbance of cardiac electrical conduction system.
        2. Absence of pulse distal to catheter insertion site, coolness, and cyanosis of the extremity that may indicate vessel obstruction.
        3. Bleeding at insertion site.
        4. Drop in blood pressure that may result from internal bleeding or reaction to dye.
        5. Dyspnea that may signal a pulmonary embolus or pneumothorax.
        6. Increased temperature that may indicate infection or an allergic reaction to the dye.
        7. Vomiting from premedication or the dye.
     f. Initiate emergency management of any bleeding.
        1. Apply pressure to the site.
        2. Elevate the extremity if venous oozing occurs.
        3. Do not release the pressure on an arterial dressing site.
     g. Provide fluids when fully awake since the child has been NPO for several hours.
     h. Keep the child flat for several hours after the procedure.
     i. Keep the child warm.
     j. Help the child work through the experience.
        1. Provide therapeutic play opportunities.
        2. Facilitate verbalization of feelings.
  3. Teach parents to call the physician if they observe impaired circulation.

Carditis in rheumatic fever. See *Rheumatic Fever.*

Cast care Nursing measures taken to meet the needs of the child immobilized in a cast.

  A. General Considerations.
     1. Cast materials used to immobilize body parts vary with the need.
        a. Gauze tapes impregnated with plaster of Paris are used for casting severely displaced bones, unstable fractures or extremities after a surgical procedure.
        b. Synthetic cast tapes of polyester and cotton, fiberglass, or thermoplastic polyester are used for simple fractures.
     2. Synthetic casts can usually be immersed in water, plaster casts cannot.
     3. Synthetic casts are:
        a. Less likely to be indented during the short drying period.
        b. Less restrictive because they are lightweight.
        c. Less bulky so that regular clothing can be worn over them.

d. Immersible in water, if approved by the physician.

e. More expensive and require special equipment for removal.

f. Rougher in finish so they snag clothing, scratch furniture, and abrade the skin.

g. More difficult to mold which decreases their utilization in difficult fractures.

4. The water temperature for preparing the synthetic cast varies with the fabric as does the drying time and procedure.

B. Nursing Management.

1. Prepare the child and parents for application of a synthetic cast. See *Preparation for Procedures.*

   a. Explain how the specific cast fabric being used will be prepared and how long it will take to dry.

   b. Inspect the child's skin for redness, abrasions, etc. before the cast is applied.

   c. Tell the child and parents there will be a change in the child's body image. See *Body Image.*

2. Perform a neurovascular assessment as ordered and observe, record, and report the following:

   a. Blueness, paleness, or coldness of the distal part.

   b. Lack of peripheral pulse.

   c. Numbness or tingling in any toe or finger.

   d. Pain.

   e. Edema which does not improve if the part is elevated.

   f. Loss of motion.

3. Teach patient/parent home management of the synthetic cast (Lane and Lee, 1983).

   a. Avoid too vigorous activity which could disturb fracture alignment.

   b. Use a mild soap when bathing and apply only a small amount near the cast.

   c. Assure tub or bath safety by using a hand rail and/or by applying rubber decals to the bottom of the tub.

   d. Flush the cast with water after swimming or bathing to prevent skin irritation and maceration.

   e. Rinse the cast thoroughly if sand, dirt, or other foreign particles get under the cast.

   f. Dry a wet cast as follows:

      1. Blot with a towel to remove the excess water.

      2. Set a blow dryer on cool or warm and use sweeping motions over the entire cast.

   g. Avoid getting the cast wet if the child/parent is unwilling to spend approximately 1 hour's time to dry the cast.

h. Tell the child/parent which observations must be reported to the physician.

   1. Foul odor or drainage.

   2. Pain in casted part.

   3. Fever.

   4. Skin breakdown or sores.

   5. "Hot spots" on cast.

   6. Cast that is too loose or too tight.

4. Prepare the child and parents for application of a plaster cast. See *Preparation for Procedures.*

   a. Wet strips of plaster of Paris feel cool when first applied.

   b. As evaporation begins, the child will feel warm.

   c. The feeling of warmth will not be permanent.

   d. The extremity and/or body will feel very heavy after the cast is applied.

   e. The child will experience a change in body image. See *Body Image.*

   f. Inspect the child's skin for redness, abrasions, etc. before the cast is applied.

5. Perform a neurovascular assessment as ordered and observe, record, and report:

   a. Blueness, paleness, or coldness of the distal part.

   b. Lack of a peripheral pulse.

   c. Numbness or tingling in any toe or finger.

   d. Pain.

   e. Edema which does not improve if the part is elevated.

   f. Loss of motion.

6. Care for the wet plaster cast.

   a. Use the open palms to move the cast since finger indentions cause pressure points.

   b. Support the cast on cloth covered pillows.

   c. Avoid fans and heaters since these may cause uneven drying.

   d. Mark outline of drainage from a surgical incision with a ball point pen, since fluid from a felt tip marker may penetrate through the cast.

7. Care for the dry plaster cast.

   a. Cover edges with petals of waterproof adhesive.

   b. Tape plastic wrap around cast at the genital area.

   c. Clean soiled areas of the cast with a damp cloth and a nonchlorine bleach such as Bon Ami.

   d. Rub pressure areas and areas around and under cast edges with alcohol T.I.D. to toughen skin.

   e. Avoid oils or powders that soften the skin and may cause irritation.

   f. Give a sponge bath daily and avoid getting the cast wet since this weakens the cast.

g. Turn the child every 2 hours when in bed.

h. Use a stroller, wagon, cart, etc. to change position and provide stimulation.

i. Explain to the child and parents that use of coat hangers or knitting needles to scratch under the cast will injure the skin and cause infection.

8. Meet the special needs of the child in a spica cast.

a. Use a Bradford frame for positioning, if available, or keep child in semi-Fowler's position.

b. Turn the child every 2 hours.

c. Prop partially filled ice bags to sides, but not on top of cast for 24 to 48 hours.

d. Do not use the abduction bar on a spica cast to aid in turning.

e. Use folded diaper or sanitary pads to keep young child dry.

f. Avoid using 24-hour urine collecting bags which irritate the skin.

g. Pin diapers so they do not cover cast.

h. Avoid use of plastic pants.

i. Use a bib or napkin to cover the top edge of a body or spica cast during feeding.

j. Obtain overhead traction bar for the older, hospitalized child.

9. Teach parents home management of spica cast.

a. Review observations, protection of the dry cast, and skin care as stated above.

b. Discuss safety measures.

1. Keep small objects out of reach so they cannot be put down into cast.

2. Use proper body mechanics for moving child.

3. Elevate the child's head during eating and drinking.

4. Arrange for downstairs room for the child.

5. Obtain a small bell for child to use when he needs assistance.

c. Teach dietary modifications.

1. Provide an adequate fluid intake for age. See *Forcing Fluids*.

2. Increase intake of whole grain cereals, fresh fruits and vegetables.

d. Review observations to be reported to the physician.

1. Foul odor or drainage.

2. Pain in casted part.

3. Fever.

4. Skin breakdown or sores.

5. "Hot spots" on cast.

6. Cast that is too loose or too tight.

10. Give parents information on what to expect when the cast is removed so they can prepare the child.

a. Cast cutters are noisy and frightening to the child.

b. Tell parents to ask person who will remove cast to demonstrate that it will not cut skin.

c. The yellow, flaky skin under the cast should be removed by soaking the area with oil for several hours, then washing.

Cellulitis. Infection of skin, underlying subcutaneous tissue, and regional lymph nodes.

A. **General Considerations.**

1. Local signs and symptoms include:

a. Warmth.

b. Tenderness.

c. Swelling.

d. Redness.

e. Induration.

2. General signs and symptoms include:

a. Fever.

b. Malaise.

c. Swelling of regional lymph nodes.

d. Lymphangitis, "streaking," on an extremity.

3. Treatment includes:

a. Culturing to identify the causative organism.

b. Antibiotic therapy appropriate to the organism.

c. Warm soaks if the area is nonsuppurative.

4. Hospitalization may be necessary for the child with systemic symptoms or cellulitis of the face.

B. **Nursing Management.**

1. Support the child and parents during hospitalization. See *Hospitalization, Support During.*

2. Initiate discharge planning. See *Discharge Planning.*

3. Observe and record signs of localized infection.

a. Warmth.

b. Redness

c. Induration.

d. Tenderness.

4. Observe, record, and report the following signs and symptoms of systemic spread of infection:

a. Red streaking along lymphatic drainage path.

b. Enlarged, tender regional lymph nodes.

c. Elevation of temperature.

d. Malaise.

5. Administer antibiotics as ordered and observe for side effects.

6. Apply warm soaks as ordered.

7. Promote adequate hydration. See *Forcing Fluids.*
8. Change and handle dressing with aseptic technique if incision and drainage has been done.
9. Teach parents home management.
   a. How to do warm soaks.
   b. How to administer medications. See *Administration of Medications, Parental.*
   c. Signs of spread of infection to report to the physician.

Cerebral palsy. Nonprogressive disorders created by damage to voluntary motor centers in the brain.

A. **General Considerations.**
   1. Damage may occur before, during, or after birth due to:
      a. Perinatal anoxia.
      b. Birth trauma.
      c. Postnatal infection.
      d. Kernicterus.
   2. The infant may exhibit:
      a. Asymmetry in motion or contour.
      b. Difficulty in sucking and swallowing.
      c. Listlessness or irritability.
      d. Seizures.
      e. Developmental delays.
      f. Persistence of primitive reflexes.
      g. Delay in appearance of later reflexes, e.g., Landau, parachute, labyrinth-righting, and body-righting.
   3. The majority of children have either spasticity (tension in certain muscle groups) or athetosis (involuntary or excess movements).
   4. The child's psychological and emotional problems may interfere with development more than motor difficulties.
   5. The intellectual development of the child with cerebral palsy may vary from below normal to above normal.
   6. Orthopedic appliances may be used to prevent or reduce deformity.
   7. Organic brain damage may cause abnormalities of behavior and personality.
   8. A multidisciplinary habilitation team should evaluate the child and recommend specific programs to:
      a. Establish locomotion, communication, and self-help skills.
      b. Correct defects in vision, hearing, and perception.
      c. Promote integration of motor functions.
      d. Identify educational resources appropriate to the child's potential.
   9. Orthotic appliances and/or orthopedic surgery may be necessary to prevent or correct deformities.
   10. Physical therapy is essential to accomplish muscle control, locomotion, skeletal alignment; to prevent contractures; and to alleviate motor dysfunction.

B. **Nursing Management.** See EXCEPTIONAL CHILD.
   1. Support the child and parents during hospitalization. See *Hospitalization, Support During.*
   2. Initiate discharge planning. *See Discharge Planning.*
   3. Find out how mother manages the child at home and record information on the Kardex.
      a. Feeding technique.
      b. Food preferences.
      c. Sleep patterns.
      d. Toileting needs.
      e. Daily routines.
      f. Self-care activities.
   4. Assess the child's and parent's understanding of diagnosis and treatment and provide information as needed.
   5. Initiate screening and evaluation methods to detect neuromuscular dysfunction early. See *Hearing Screening, Vision Screening, Appendix v,* and *Appendix vi.*
   6. Promote improved nutrition by establishing a feeding plan to be used by all caregivers (Rice, 1981).
      a. Obtain modified feeding utensils such as spoons with large handles, rimmed plates with suction cups, and covered cup with hole for inserting straw.
      b. Place child in sitting position, in chair if possible, with head stabilized and facing forward.
      c. Offer very small amounts of food from spoon tip.
      d. Encourage child to suck food from spoon as nurse closes his lips and withdraws spoon.
      e. Close jaw by raising mandible and stroking throat gently upward if child unable to close jaw voluntarily.
      f. Offer finger foods to develop independent eating skills.
      g. Provide consistent, positive reinforcement for cooperative behavior.
   7. Handle the young child with spasticity in a manner to counteract hyperreflexia and hyperextension (Davis and Hill, 1980).
      a. Place the child in a sitting position before lifting.
      b. Hold him under the armpits as the arms are lifted up.
      c. Place child's arms over nurse's shoulders while abducting the child's legs and flexing his knees.
      d. Place the child in a flexed sitting position,

support the upper extremities, and maintain the head and shoulders in a forward, semi-flexed position.
8. Handle the older child with spasticity or the child with athetosis in a manner to control movements and provide head support.
   a. Grasp the child under the arms from behind.
   b. Place the nurse's arms under his upper arms.
   c. Grasp the inner aspect of the child's thighs.
   d. Flex the child's knees and hips while lifting.
9. Prevent contractures.
   a. Reposition frequently.
   b. Use a high back chair with chest strap.
   c. Place a platform or stool for feet.
   d. Apply splints at night if ordered.
   e. Do passive stretching exercises if ordered.
10. Provide frequent rest periods in a quiet room.
11. Set consistent expectations and limits and record on Kardex.
12. Provide play and educational opportunities.
    a. Give toys that require eye–hand coordination, e.g., hammer, blocks, stacking rings.
    b. Balls.
    c. Mirrors.
    d. Stories.
    e. Word games (Barnard and Erickson, 1976).
13. Prepare the child and parents if surgical procedure is planned. See *Postoperative Care, Preoperative Care,* and *Preparation for Surgery.*
    a. Be sure that parents understand that surgery will improve function, but will not make the extremity normal.
    b. Teach cast care. See *Cast Care.*
14. Assist parents to identify community resources to help plan long-term program for habilitation.
15. Discuss with parents those aspects of a home management program that are essential for success (Barnard and Erickson, 1976).
    a. The program should use specific guidelines which break down developmental tasks into individual steps that are positively reinforced as they are accomplished.
    b. Parents should be included in observing and planning as well as implementing a consistent, systematic approach.

Cerumen. Ear wax.

A. **General Considerations.**
   1. Most children have some ear wax.
   2. The tympanic membrane is generally visible beyond wax.

3. Many parents fear ear wax will lead to loss of hearing.
4. Wax rarely accumulates enough to interfere with hearing.
5. Impacted ear wax may need to be removed by a physician or a nurse practitioner.

B. **Nursing Management.**
   1. Explain the function of ear wax to child and parent.
      a. Cleanses internal ear canal.
      b. Removes foreign objects and epithelial cells.
   2. Teach the child and parent not to insert swabs, bobby pins, or other objects into the ear.
   3. Teach child and parent safe ear cleaning.
      a. Wrap a finger in warm wet washcloth and wash ears.
      b. Do not clean ears with cotton-tipped applicators.
         1. Can scratch ear canal causing secondary infection.
         2. May push accumulated cerumen further in ear canal, causing plugging of wax.
   4. Observe consistency and quantity of wax in canal.
   5. Determine if wax interferes with hearing. See *Hearing Screening.*
   6. Remove ear wax.
      a. Discuss procedure with the child and parents. See *Preparation for Procedures.*
      b. Elicit cooperation.
      c. Restrain if necessary. See *Restraints.*
      d. Remove hardened large masses.
         1. Soften by instillation of mineral oil or detergent soap.
         2. Irrigate with warm water or other solution as instructed.
      e. Remove small masses with curet if ordered.
   7. Teach the child and parents that a constantly moist environment leads to external otitis.

Chalazion. Infection of meibomian glands within the tarsal cartilage of the eyelids.

A. **General Considerations.**
   1. Incidence is more common in adolescents because of hormonal influences.
   2. Pain is minimal.
   3. Causes include retention of gland secretions and/or chronic granulomatous inflammation.
   4. Symptoms include:
      a. Small, slow growing, hard, but painless nodule in the lid.
      b. Skin over nodule is freely moveable.
      c. No inflammation or edema.
   5. Hospitalization is not required.

B. Nursing Management.

1. Observe child's upper and lower lids for irregularity.
2. Discuss management with the child and parents.
   a. Goals of treatment are shrinking hard nodule and letting it absorb naturally.
   b. Discuss and demonstrate application of warm moist packs every 4 hours.
   c. Discuss and demonstrate administration of topical antibiotics if ordered, to keep nodule soft and to prevent secondary infection.
   d. Explain that treatment may last 4 to 6 weeks.
   e. Support referral for complete excision or incision and curettage if no response to medical treatment.
3. Elicit and discuss the child and parents' concerns.
4. Alleviate the child and parents' concern by providing factual information.
   a. Is not cancerous.
   b. Does not lead to blindness.
   c. Is correctable.
   d. Altered cosmetic appearance will improve with treatment.

Chemotherapy.
Use of immunosuppressive drugs for treatment of disease, most commonly malignancies.

A. General Considerations.

1. Most chemotherapeutic drugs destroy cells only when the cells are dividing.
2. Chemotherapy is frequently used in combination with surgery and/or irradiation.
3. More than one drug is usually used and they may be given in cyclic form, one drug following another, or in combined form.
4. Drugs given in combination:
   a. Act on the cell in different phases of division.
   b. Produce a greater reduction in the number of cells than the use of the drugs in cyclic form.
   c. Are selected to have different side effects or the same side effects at different times.
   d. Should not increase the incidence of toxic reactions.
5. All medications given must be considered in relation to chemotherapy, since other drugs may increase or decrease chemotherapeutic response.
6. Chemotherapy may be less effective in treatment of bone and/or brain tumors, since bone has poor blood perfusion and many drugs do not cross the blood-brain barrier.
7. There is a narrow margin between the therapeutic and toxic doses.

8. Most chemotherapeutic drugs are metabolized in the liver and excreted by the kidneys.
9. Zyloprim (allopurinol) may be given to block uric acid formation and therefore protect the kidneys from uric acid build-up due to cell destruction.
10. Nonmalignant cells are also destroyed by chemotherapy but regenerate more quickly.
11. The most rapidly dividing cells are the ones most affected, e.g., hair follicles, mucous membrane cells of gastrointestinal tract, bone marrow.
12. Certain chemotherapeutic drugs are used together in protocols for treatment of specific malignancies, e.g., mechlorethamine, Oncovin, procarbazine, prednisone (MOPP), for Hodgkin's disease.
13. Chemotherapy may be used in treatment of nonmalignant conditions, e.g., prednisone and/or cyclophosphamide for the nephrotic syndrome.
14. The physical effects of chemotherapy may have a profound impact on the child's/adolescent's body image (Griffiths, 1980). See *Body Image*.

B. Nursing Management.

1. Support the child and parents during chemotherapy.
   a. Find out what the child and/or parents have been told about the drugs and record on Kardex.
   b. Explain when and how the drug(s) will be administered.
   c. Discuss chemotherapeutic drugs.
      1. Explain expected side effects and teach when they may be expected to occur.
      2. Tell what will be done to eliminate or alleviate side effects, e.g., giving an antiemetic.
      3. Teach the child and/or parents what they can do to eliminate and/or alleviate side effects, e.g., drink lots of fluids.
   d. Answer all questions honestly.
   e. Permit the child some control if possible, e.g., let child decide what liquid he wants with a pill.
2. Assess and record baseline data about the following against which the child's response to chemotherapy can be measured:
   a. Nutritional state.
   b. Skin condition.
   c. Condition of mouth.
   d. Urinary pattern and output.
   e. Bowel elimination patterns.
   f. Level of hearing.

g. Lab values.

h. Energy/activity level.

i. Emotional state.

3. Observe, record, and report the child's response to chemotherapy and other medications.

4. Provide nursing care for the child who is experiencing side effects from the chemotherapy.

   a. Leukopenia.

     1. Use meticulous hand washing.

     2. Limit the number of visitors.

     3. Keep the child away from anyone with an infection.

     4. Double prep the skin with alcohol and Betadine before blood work, lumbar puncture, bone marrow aspiration, etc. is done.

     5. Observe, record, and report any sign of infection.

     6. Treat all infections immediately.

     7. Place the child on reverse isolation if ordered.

     8. Keep the child's fingernails short and clean.

     9. Monitor lab values and report abnormal values immediately.

   b. Thrombocytopenia.

     1. Observe, record, and report signs of bleeding in urine, stool, vomitus, skin, oral mucosa, and sclera.

     2. Avoid trauma, e.g., keep side rails up to prevent falls.

     3. Report joint pain that may represent bleeding in the joint capsule.

     4. Do not take rectal temperatures.

     5. Give injections only when absolutely necessary and apply pressure to the site for 5 minutes afterward.

     6. Use a toothbrush that has been softened in hot water or clean the mouth with cotton swabs and half strength mouthwash.

     7. Get any aspirin order changed to acetominophen to decrease bleeding tendencies.

     8. Have adolescent male, who shaves, use electric razor.

     9. Monitor lab values and report abnormal values immediately.

   c. Anorexia, nausea, and vomiting.

     1. Observe, record, and report presence of anorexia, nausea, and/or vomiting.

     2. Give antiemetic as ordered.

     3. Make child comfortable at meals.

     4. Provide frequent mouth care.

     5. Feed smaller, more frequent meals.

     6. Encourage the child to select foods he likes.

     7. Provide dry, bulky, and/or bland foods.

     8. Provide ice chips, jello, flat colas, water, etc.

     9. Let parents bring in foods from home.

    10. Remove upsetting sights, sounds, and/or odors from mealtime environment.

    11. Discuss giving drugs which cause nausea in evening so the child will sleep through period of side effects.

    12. Observe for dehydration in presence of vomiting.

    13. Monitor electrolyte values. See *Appendix ii.*

   d. Fluid retention.

     1. Observe, record, and report weight gain, signs of edema, and respiratory distress.

     2. Decrease or limit salt intake.

     3. Apply lotion to stretched skin.

     4. Change position frequently to prevent fluid from pooling.

     5. Observe, record, and report signs of potassium imbalance if the child is on diuretics.

   e. Diarrhea.

     1. Observe, record, and report all stools.

     2. Replace fluid loss.

     3. Decrease roughage in diet.

     4. Do not give fresh fruits and juices.

     5. Offer constipating foods.

     6. Give yogurt to restore normal bowel flora.

     7. Wash anal area and dry thoroughly after each stool.

     8. Sit the child in warm water to soothe anal area.

     9. Apply ointment to anal area to prevent skin breakdown.

   f. Neuropathy.

     1. Observe, record, and report decreased sensation, poor coordination, development of foot drop, and/or severe constipation.

     2. Provide safe environment.

     3. Increase fiber content in diet.

     4. Give stool softener as ordered.

   g. Stomatitis.

     1. Assess the condition of the child's mouth every day.

     2. Provide frequent mouth care.

     3. Rinse mouth after meals, and as needed, with saline mouthwash made from 2 teaspoons of salt in a quart of water.

     4. Avoid the use of milk of magnesia substrate and mouthwash with alcohol since these are drying, and hydro-

gen peroxide rinses since they predispose to the development of *Candida albicans* (Brown and Kiss, 1982).

5. Do not use glycerin and lemon swabs, since these alter pH, decrease saliva, and dry the mucous membranes.
6. Provide topical anesthetic prior to meals as ordered.
7. Offer bland foods at moderate temperatures.
8. Use soft toothbrush, toothette, or cotton swabs for cleaning teeth.

h. Personality changes.
   1. Observe, record, and report alterations in behavior, e.g., depression, euphoria.
   2. Be nonjudgmental of child's behavior.
   3. Use a kind, consistent approach to the child.
   4. Let the child and/or parents know that you know the child cannot control changes.

i. Alopecia.
   1. Observe, record, and report hair loss.
   2. Do not comment on child's lack of hair.
   3. Apply scalp tourniquet as ordered to decrease drug effect on hair follicles.
   4. Provide cap or bonnet to wear during sleep so hair does not get in mouth.
   5. Provide wigs, hats, scarves, etc. to cover head when child is up.
   6. Wash scalp to prevent development of cradle cap.
   7. Explain hair regrows in about 2 months after therapy stops but may be changed in color and/or texture.
   8. Reassure child and/or parents by showing a child whose hair has regrown.

j. Fatigue.
   1. Observe, record, and report observations related to child's activity level.
   2. Plan care in blocks.
   3. Schedule rest periods.
   4. Provide quiet activities.
   5. Remember the fatigued child may react with hyperactive behavior.

k. Rectal ulcers.
   1. Clean the anal area carefully after each stool.
   2. Provide warm sitz baths.
   3. Expose ulcerated area to dry heat.
   4. Apply ointment to rectum prior to bowel movements to decrease discomfort.
   5. Avoid ointments/creams which promote moisture retention which supports bacterial growth.
   6. Monitor number of stools since the

child may hold back on defecating to avoid pain.
   7. Take an oral or axillary temperature.

l. Anemia
   1. Monitor hemoglobin and hematocrit values.
   2. Explain that fatigue is normal.
   3. Encourage increased rest periods.
   4. Observe for dyspnea and tachycardia.
   5. Promote intake of iron rich foods, if tolerated.

m. Irritation of vein used for injection may be reduced by application of warm, moist heat.

5. Meet the child's nutritional needs. See *Nutrition.*
   a. Encourage a high caloric intake, e.g., milk shakes with added egg, custards, etc.
   b. Provide food preferences.
      1. Talk with the dietician.
      2. Have parents bring favorite foods.
   c. Get order for commercial dietary supplement if needed.
   d. Freeze diet supplements and use in milk shakes.
   e. Provide mouth care before meals.
   f. Make meal time as pleasant as possible.
      1. Serve food in an attractive manner.
      2. Eliminate offensive sounds and odors.
      3. Provide companionship at meals.
      4. Position child as comfortably as possible.

6. Encourage a high fluid intake and administer allopurinol as ordered to prevent uric acid buildup.
7. Force fluids and have the child void frequently to protect the bladder mucosa from Cytoxan which can produce hemorrhagic cystitis.
8. Teach parents home management of the child receiving chemotherapy.
   a. Use comfort measures for side effects.
   b. Call the physician if:
      1. Medications to decrease nausea and vomiting are ineffective.
      2. Signs of infection develop or the child is exposed to a contagious disease.
      3. Mouth and/or anal sores develop.
      4. The child runs a fever.
      5. Fluid intake does not keep urine a light amber color.
      6. Diarrhea occurs.
      7. Signs of bleeding develop.
   c. Teach parents safety measures to use to decrease chances of bleeding episodes.

Chicken pox. A highly communicable disease caused by the varicella-zoster virus.

A. **General Considerations.**
   1. Low grade fever and malaise progress to high fever, irritability, and lymphadenopathy.
   2. The disease is characterized by the presence of four stages of lesions (macule, papule, vesicle, crust) all at the same time.
   3. The rash is extremely pruritic.
   4. Chicken pox can be severe or even fatal to a child receiving high doses of steroids or immunosuppressive drugs.
   5. The child should not resume peer contact for 5 to 7 days after onset of rash.
   6. Complications of pneumonia, secondary infection, Reye's syndrome or encephalitis are rare.
   7. The hospitalized child must be nursed in strict isolation to prevent exposure of the immunosuppressed patient.

B. **Nursing Management.** See HOME MANAGEMENT OF MINOR ILLNESSES.
   1. Promote comfort.
      a. Administer antihistamines, if ordered, or analgesics such as acetominophen. See *Administration of Medications, Parental.*
      b. Bathe in lukewarm water with one cup of cornstarch, baking soda, or oatmeal per half-tub of water.
      c. Pat dry.
      d. Dress the child in lightweight, soft clothing.
      e. Do not overheat with clothing or excess blankets, etc.
      f. Apply calamine lotion or paste of baking soda and water with patting rather than rubbing motion.
      g. Use rinses or gargles to relieve discomfort of mouth lesions.
      h. Apply saline soaks to ease discomfort of perineal lesions.
   2. Reduce fever. See *Fever Reduction.*
   3. Prevent infection.
      a. Encourage frequent handwashing.
      b. Keep the child's fingernails short and clean.
      c. Use mitts or gloves if needed to prevent scratching.
   4. Encourage fluid intake. See *Forcing Fluids.*
   5. Provide diversional activities which occupy the hands.
      a. Puzzles.
      b. Modular toys.
      c. Sewing.
      d. Coloring.
   6. Prevent scarring by explaining to the older child the outcome of continued scratching.
   7. Inform the parents of symptoms which should be reported to the physician.
      a. Purulent drainage from lesions.
      b. Elevated temperature.
      c. Persistent vomiting.
      d. Headache.
      e. Seizures.
      f. Behavior changes.
   8. Observe for symptoms of encephalitis after the first week.
      a. Headache.
      b. Elevated temperature.
      c. Behavior changes.
      d. Hyperactivity.
      e. Seizures.
      f. Speech disorder.
      g. Muscle weakness.

Child abuse See *Abused Child.*

Child care. See *Day Care Center.*

Chordee. See *Hypospadias.*

Chorea. See *Rheumatic Fever.*

Christmas disease See *Hemophilia.*

Chronic illness. A long-term disorder that can be progressive and fatal or that can be associated with a normal life span despite physical or mental handicaps (Mattsson, 1972).

A. **General Considerations.** See EXCEPTIONAL CHILD and HANDICAPPED CHILD.
   1. Parents who have limited socioeconomic resources, limited health knowledge, and unfavorable attitudes toward health care are less likely to maintain long-term health supervision for their chronically ill child.
   2. When the child develops a chronic illness, his role in the family will be altered causing stress on family relationships.
   3. Family equilibrium is affected when the child develops a long-term illness or when the chronically ill child improves (Steele, 1983).
   4. Parents of chronically ill children may decrease their participation in community activities and social events.
   5. In some families, chronic illness may strengthen family ties and/or make support systems more visible.
   6. Siblings of chronically ill children may develop emotional problems in response to family stress.
   7. The attitude of the family toward the child's illness/disability is more significant to the child's coping than the severity of the diagnosis.

8. Symptoms of depression are not uncommon in the school-aged child or adolescent who has a chronic illness or handicap (Rodgers et al., 1981).
   a. Sad, unhappy, pessimistic attitude.
   b. Social withdrawal.
   c. Negative self-concept.
   d. Sleep disturbance or complaints of fatigue.
   e. Unusual alteration in appetite or weight.
   f. Disruption in school performance.
   g. Emotional lability or aggressive behavior.
   h. Somatic complaints.
9. Support groups for parents of chronically ill children help the parents gain more understanding of the disease as well as improve their coping skills (Johnson, 1982).
10. Specific efforts should be made to support the father as well as the mother in coping with the illness and its implications (McKeever, 1981).
11. Programs which involve the child and family as self-care agents may decrease episodes of illness and resultant hospitalization (Pierce and Giovinco, 1983).
12. Many chronically ill children do not receive ongoing health care. See *Dental Care, Health Promotion and Maintenance,* and *Immunizations.*
13. Making the older child responsible for taking medications, carrying out procedures, etc. decreases the likelihood that these areas will become a focus of adolescent rebellion.
14. The adolescent may need guidance to make an appropriate career choice.

B. Nursing Management. See *Body Image.*
1. Find out how the mother manages the child at home and record information on the Kardex.
   a. Feeding techniques.
   b. Food preferences.
   c. Sleep patterns.
   d. Toileting needs.
   e. Daily routines.
   f. Self-care activities.
2. Set consistent limits and expectations and record plan on Kardex. See *Discipline.*
   a. Encourage the withdrawn or nonresponsive child by gradually increasing his exposure to new people and activities.
   b. Channel the child's natural aggression into appropriate outlets.
   c. Discuss the limits with the child so he knows what is expected of him so attempts to manipulate the staff are minimized.
3. Maintain treatment routines, since the child may become very anxious when changes are made.
4. Meet the child's need for privacy and for a secure place for possessions.

5. Recognize that dependency and regression are normal, but encourage independence.
   a. Assign simple chores.
   b. Allow choices whenever possible.
   c. Encourage the child's participation in planning care.
   d. Allow the older child to help formulate rules.
6. Provide undisturbed, quiet period for schoolwork for the older child.
7. Create altered and/or increased stimuli by arranging for walks, field trips, weekend passes for visits home, etc.
8. Observe, record, and report signs that the child has progressed too rapidly in physical activities.
   a. Increased pulse.
   b. Rise in evening temperature.
   c. Fatigue.
   d. Disturbed sleep.
9. Establish short-term goals with the child and family, for example, stages of ambulation, increased socialization, responsibility for activities of daily living.
10. Establish long-term goals that include discharge planning, e.g., independent ambulation, maintaining the child as part of his family, self-care.
11. Assist the child and parents to establish a realistic view of the child's illness or disability.
    a. Educate the family about the illness or disability.
    b. Provide information on normal growth and development. See *Appendix v.*
    c. Evaluate the parent's understanding of recommendations of all health team members.
    d. Explore the family's plans for education, vocation, residential placement as appropriate.
12. Assist the older child/adolescent to decide what information to give peers about his illness.
13. Identify specific parent teaching needs.
    a. Write down instructions since anxiety decreases comprehension.
    b. Have parents return demonstration of procedures.
    c. Help family incorporate child's care into home routine.
    d. Help the parents discuss the child's needs with siblings. See *Siblings.*
    e. Assist the parents to identify resources to cope with their own feelings.
       1. Physical activities for frustration outlet.
       2. Respite care.
       3. Group support from parents whose children have similar problems.

14. Provide for follow-up.
    a. Identify where, when, and by whom child will receive routine health supervision.
    b. Act as a liaison to coordinate the child's health care.

Cleft lip.
Failure of the maxillary processes to unite during fetal life.

A. General Considerations.
1. Cleft lip can be unilateral or bilateral and may occur separately or in association with a cleft palate.
2. The parents may have a severe emotional response to the baby's appearance at birth. See *Exceptional Child.*
3. Surgical repair may be done in the first few days of life or when the infant is 1 to 3 months of age.
4. Revision of the lip scar may be necessary in early school years for cosmetic reasons.
5. A thin metal wire called a Logan bow may be taped to each side of the suture line to decrease tension.
6. Habilitation of the child requires an interdisciplinary approach, particularly if the child has an associated cleft palate.

B. Nursing Management.
See EXCEPTIONAL CHILD.
1. Support the child and parents during hospitalization. See *Hospitalization, Support During.*
2. Initiate discharge planning. See *Discharge Planning.*
3. Meet the needs of the child preoperatively. See *Preoperative Care* and *Preparation for Surgery.*
    a. Feed the baby with the method to be used postoperatively.
        1. Feed in an upright position.
        2. Use a feeding or medicine dropper or bulb syringe with rubber tubing attached.
        3. Place the dropper or tubing on top of the tongue.
        4. Direct the flow of formula to the side and back of the mouth.
        5. Feed a small amount at a time and feed slowly.
        6. Burp frequently with the infant in an upright position.
        7. Feed more slowly if choking occurs.
    b. Cleanse the lip frequently with water or half strength peroxide to prevent infection.
    c. Apply baby or mineral oil to the lip area if it is very dry.
    d. Observe for symptoms of otitis media if the child has an associated cleft palate which may interfere with action of the eustachian tube.
        1. Fever.
        2. Pain.
        3. Pulling on ear.
        4. Discharge from ear.
        5. Vomiting and diarrhea.
    e. Prepare parents for what to expect in postoperative period.
4. Meet the needs of the child postoperatively. See *Postoperative Care.*
    a. Observe for respiratory distress, since baby must adjust to breathing through a smaller airway.
    b. Have laryngoscope and endotracheal tube available on nursing unit.
    c. Observe for hemorrhage at operative site.
    d. Reposition infant every 2 hours on side, back, or upright in infant seat.
    e. Explain purpose of mist tent to parents if needed. See *Mist Tent.*
    f. Suction carefully with bulb syringe if necessary.
    g. Remove arm or elbow restraints one at a time every 4 hours. See *Restraints.*
    h. Feed on demand rather than on a schedule.
    i. Place the dropper or rubber tubing at the corner of the mouth; do not touch the suture line.
    j. Follow feeding with sterile water to rinse mouth.
    k. Place on right side after feeding to reduce possibility of aspiration.
    l. Prevent scarring by cleansing suture line immediately after feeding and PRN with ordered solution.
    m. Dab suture line with solution, do not rub.
    n. Apply antibiotic ointment or mesh gauze strip to suture line if ordered.
    o. Anticipate infant's needs to minimize crying which increases suture line tension.
5. Teach the parents home management.
    a. Help parents feel comfortable in caring for infant.
        1. Have parents return feeding demonstration.
        2. Demonstrate cleansing of suture line.
        3. Discuss need for and use of restraints.
        4. Discuss prevention of infection, especially otitis media.
    b. Tell parents that bottle feeding can be resumed when sutures are removed in 12 to 14 days.
    c. Explain that the operative site may be red for as long as a year.
    d. Refer parents for genetic counseling if appropriate. See *Genetic Counseling.*
    e. Help parents anticipate needs if child has an associated cleft palate. See *Cleft Palate.*
        1. Begin solids at same time as parent would a noncleft child.

2. Dilute strained foods with formula and feed with a spoon.

3. Avoid acid and spicy foods and those which stick to the palate such as peanut butter, creamed dishes, cooked cheese dishes (Berkowitz, 1971).

4. Feed small amounts slowly and frequently.

5. Wean the child from the bottle before palate surgery.

6. Encourage parents to stimulate normal speech development by playing vocal games such as "pat-a-cake."

7. Encourage words with vowel or vowel-like sounds such as new, you, low, one (Snyder et al).

Cleft palate. Failure of the soft or hard palate or both to unite during fetal life.

A. General Considerations.

1. Cleft palate may be unilateral or bilateral and may occur separately or in association with a cleft lip.

2. The parents may have a severe emotional response to the baby's defect. See *Exceptional Child.*

3. Surgical repair is usually begun around 12 to 18 months and may be performed in stages.

4. Family guidance can be provided best by a team approach to habilitation.

5. Extensive orthodontics and prosthodontics may be required to correct malposition of teeth and maxillary arches.

6. Special dental plates or obturators may be used to close the severe cleft mechanically to facilitate feeding and speech production until surgery can be performed.

7. The child should be referred to a cleft palate center for interdisciplinary team approach to habilitation if at all possible.

B. Nursing Management. See EXCEPTIONAL CHILD.

1. Support the child and parents during hospitalization. See *Hospitalization, Support During.*

2. Initiate discharge planning. See *Discharge Planning.*

3. Meet the needs of the child preoperatively. See *Preoperative Care* and *Preparation for Surgery.*

a. Observe, record, and report signs of infection.

b. Report abnormal clotting and bleeding times to the surgeon.

c. Feed the child from a cup since this method will be used postoperatively.

d. Ascertain fluid preferences so these can be provided postoperatively.

e. Introduce the child to the elbow restraints since these will be used postoperatively.

f. Prepare the parents for what to expect in the postoperative period.

4. Meet the needs of the child postoperatively. See *Postoperative Care.*

a. Observe, record, and report symptoms of respiratory distress or hemorrhage.

b. Suction nasopharynx carefully if absolutely necessary.

c. Position on abdomen with foot of bed slightly elevated and the child's head to one side.

d. Keep the child dry in mist tent, if used. See *Mist Tent.*

e. Remove elbow restraints one at a time every 4 hours. See *Restraints.*

f. Offer preferred fluids frequently. See *Forcing Fluids.*

g. Feed from a cup or side of a spoon or allow self-feeding if the child can cooperate.

h. Rinse mouth with sterile water after each feeding.

i. Prevent trauma to the suture line.

1. Do not give straws or ice chips.

2. Choose large toys such as rubber balls which cannot be placed in the mouth.

3. Choose toys that do not require sucking or blowing.

4. Administer sedative PRN to prevent irritability and crying.

j. Provide quiet diversion such as stories, coloring, etc. See *Stimulation.*

5. Teach the child and parents home management.

a. Help parents feel comfortable in caring for the child.

1. Continue feeding with cup or side of spoon.

2. Give a soft diet offering no food harder than mashed potatoes.

3. Rinse mouth after every feeding, including between meals.

4. Continue to use restraints.

5. Assure adequate sleep and nutrition.

b. Encourage parents to observe for hearing loss, since frequent ear infections may result when the cleft palate interferes with eustachian tube function.

c. Tell parents to schedule hearing tests on a routine basis.

d. Teach the parents proper dental hygiene so they may teach the child. See *Dental Care.*

e. Encourage parents to continue stimulation of speech development after sutures are removed.

1. Refer to speech pathologist for evaluation.

2. Encourage dramatic play such as puppets or acting out stories.
3. Have the child blow feathers or ping-pong balls.
4. Encourage words beginning with the letters P, B, F, and T.
5. Exercise muscles by giving foods which require chewing and frequent swallowing.
  f. Help parents to treat the child as normally as possible.

Clothing. Protective garments.

A. General Considerations.
1. Keep clothing comfortable and simple.
2. No shoes are needed until the child walks.
3. Study labels of all clothes to determine care needed and flammability.

B. Nursing Management.
1. Teach parents to consider safety.
   a. Avoid purchasing a slippery nylon snowsuit for a baby, because the child could slip out of the parents' arms.
   b. Buy bright colors for outerwear and bathing suits for easy identification.
   c. Buy nonflammable clothes.
   d. Put strip of adhesive tape across bottom of baby's leather soled shoes to prevent a slip.
   e. Guide infant's arms and legs through openings of shirt and pants.
   f. Put long legged pants on the creeping infant to protect the knees.
2. Teach parents to save money by buying clothes that can be easily coordinated and easily laundered.
3. Teach parents to protect a child from the elements.
   a. Buy a jacket with hood attached to avoid cold drafts.
   b. Carry a sweater to protect the child from overcooled supermarkets in summer.
   c. Put on a shirt and hat at beach to protect tender skin.
   d. Buy water repellent garments for dryness.
   e. Dress boys and girls in long pants in cold weather.
   f. Dress in several layers of clothing in winter.
   g. Teach children to remove outerwear when indoors.
   h. Dress children in pajamas with feet.
4. Teach parents to prevent clothing loss.
   a. Pin mittens to cuffs of snowsuit or run a length of yarn through the sleeves and pin mittens on each end.
   b. Label with indelible ink pen or buy three-line

labels with name, address, and phone number to sew on clothing.
5. Teach parents that newborn's clothes:
   a. Should be comfortably warm.
   b. Should allow infant freedom to move and exercise.
6. Teach parents that an infant's clothes:
   a. Should be simply constructed to avoid struggle during dressing.
   b. Should allow infant to kick and to develop gross body movements.
   c. Need to include only socks or soft-soled shoes to keep feet warm if infant is not walking.
   d. Should include shoes firm enough to protect against rough surfaces if walking.
7. Teach and discuss with parents that adolescents:
   a. Are acutely aware of what others are wearing.
   b. Demand clothing that is often unreasonable in terms of family's financial situation.
   c. Feel special clothing is important.
   d. Spend a considerable amount of time selecting clothing.
8. Teach the parents how to purchase shoes.
   a. Purchase shoes with pliable soles that allow a wide range of foot motion when the infant begins to walk.
   b. Do not hand down shoes, since each child's foot is different.
   c. Purchase new shoes when the big toe is less than a thumb's width from the end of the shoe when the child is standing.
   d. Purchase shoes from a store where a trained salesperson can fit the child correctly.

Clubfoot (talipes equinovarus). Foot deformity consisting of inversion of the foot, adduction of the forefoot, and plantar flexion.

A. General Considerations.
1. Treatment should begin in the newborn period.
2. The inversion and adduction of the foot are corrected first.
3. Correction of the plantar flexion follows.
4. Gentle manipulation of the feet is followed by immobilization.
5. If conservative treatment is ineffective after 3 to 5 months, surgery will probably be necessary.
6. Surgery may also be necessary for the older child whose defect recurs or is resistant to correction.

B. Nursing Management.
1. Support the child and parents during hospitalization. See *Hospitalization, Support During.*

2. Initiate discharge planning. See *Discharge Planning*.

3. Help the parents cope with the diagnosis. See *Exceptional Child*.

4. Have the mother demonstrate manipulation of feet if she is to perform this at home.
   a. Do not release grasp of foot during this procedure.
   b. Do not allow foot to resume deformed position.
   c. Carry out the manipulation in one smooth flowing motion.

5. Assist with immobilization procedure selected by orthopedic surgeon.
   a. Adhesive strapping.
      1. Have the mother return demonstration of strapping procedure.
      2. Tell the mother to manipulate and renew strapping every 2 to 3 days.
   b. Plaster casts. See *Cast Care*.
      1. Tell parents the cast extends to midthigh to keep the child from kicking off the cast.
      2. Prepare parents for the necessity of cast changes weekly or biweekly due to the infant's rapid growth.
      3. Use disposable diapers or plastic pants to protect the cast from urine.
      4. Teach parents how to check the adequacy of circulation.
   c. Denis-Browne Splints.
      1. Reinforce the physician's directions for how and when splints should be applied.
      2. Protect infant's feet with socks.
      3. Teach the parents to observe the feet for swelling, irritation, or discoloration.
      4. Instruct the parents not to reposition the shoes on the bar.
      5. Show parents how to tighten shoes against the bar with a splint key.
      6. Encourage parents to hold the child and to change position frequently.
   d. Kite or wedge cast.
      1. Tell parents the long leg cast will be wedged frequently to correct the deformity.
      2. Teach parents how to check the adequacy of circulation.
      3. Tell parents the final cast will be in place for 4 to 8 weeks.

6. Reinforce the explanation to parents that the feet must be maintained in an overcorrected position with casts or splints for 5 to 6 months after correction is obtained.

7. Explain that special shoes may be worn during the day and a Denis-Browne Splint worn at night to prevent recurrence after the final cast is removed.

8. Discuss with parents the need for periodic orthopedic reevaluation.

9. Prepare the child and parents for the operative procedure if this becomes necessary. See *Preparation for Surgery* and *Preoperative Care*.

Coarctation of the aorta. See *Congenital Heart Disease*.

Cognitive development. See *Appendix v*.

Colds, common (acute nasopharyngitis).
Viral infections of the upper respiratory tract which affect the nose and pharynx.

A. **General Considerations.**
   1. Signs and symptoms include:
      a. Malaise.
      b. Irritability.
      c. Head congestion.
      d. Sore throat.
      e. Cough.
      f. Clear, watery nasal discharge.
      g. Moist, boggy mucous membranes.
      h. Low grade fever; infant may have subnormal or markedly elevated temperature.
   2. Reinfections occur throughout life.
   3. Infant may aspirate secretions from nasopharynx.
   4. Overuse of salicylates can result in salicylate poisoning. See *Poisoning*.
   5. The activity of the virus in the upper respiratory tract impairs defenses and predisposes the child to secondary bacterial infections, e.g., otitis media, sinusitis (DeAngelis, 1979).
   6. A productive cough should not be suppressed except when it is interfering with the child's sleep.
   7. Antibiotics are only used to treat secondary bacterial infections.
   8. Saline nose drops are effective in relieving nasal congestion in all age groups, drops containing phenylephrine should be used only with older children because they cause tachycardia in infants.
   9. Saline nose drops can be made by dissolving 1 teaspoon of table salt in 8 ounces of tepid tap water.
   10. The use of single agent, rather than fixed combination over-the-counter cold products, is recommended so that the appropriate dose of a drug can be given for a specific symptom (Clark, Queener, Karb, 1982).

B. Nursing Management. See PHARYNGITIS, VIRAL.
1. Discuss control of contributing factors.
    a. Provide adequate nutrition. See *Nutrition*.
    b. Prevent chilling. See *Clothing*.
    c. Assure adequate rest and sleep. See *Sleep*.
    d. Help the child cope with stressful situations. See *Coping*.
    e. Protect infants from contact with infected persons.
2. Teach the child and parents symptomatic treatment.
    a. Offer small frequent feedings of the child's preferred foods.
    b. Increase clear fluid intake in order to thin secretions. See *Forcing Fluids*.
    c. Keep the child at rest during febrile stage.
    d. Relieve nasal congestion.
        1. Place a warm washcloth over nares to promote drainage.
        2. Use nasal syringe to aspirate.
        3. Use a cool mist vaporizer to increase humidity.
        4. Use nose drops: administer 15 to 20 minutes before feedings; use for a maximum of 3 days to prevent "rebound" effect of increased edema and congestion.
    e. Administer antipyretics. See *Administration of Medications, Parental*.
        1. Use for 24 to 48 hours only unless otherwise ordered.
        2. Overuse of salicylates results in salicylate poisoning.
    f. Teach other methods of reducing fever. See *Fever Reduction*.
    g. Do not use antibiotics for routine treatment.
    h. Explain that nasal decongestants, antihistamines, and expectorants are not particularly helpful.
    i. Avoid use of over-the-counter cough medicines to suppress a productive cough.
    j. Plan rest periods.
    k. Apply vaseline to lips.
    l. Reposition the child frequently to prevent pooling of secretions.
    m. Prevent secondary bacterial infections.
        1. Use good handwashing.
        2. Keep the child away from family members who are infectious.
3. Teach parents, who use over-the-counter medicines, to purchase single agent rather than fixed combination cold products.

Colic. Paroxysmal abdominal pain felt to be due to excessive accumulation of gas in the intestines or in the stomach.

A. General Considerations.
1. Symptoms usually occur at the same time each day and include:
    a. Long periods of intense crying.
    b. Abdominal distention.
    c. Legs drawn up on abdomen.
    d. Flushed face.
2. There is no specific etiology, but factors that may predispose to colic include:
    a. Emotional tension.
    b. Immaturity of the digestive system.
    c. Excessive air swallowing.
    d. Too rapid feeding.
    e. Overfeeding.
    f. Excessive carbohydrate intake that promotes gas formation.
    g. Food allergies.
3. Different formulas may be tried.
4. The infant is not ill and actually appears to be thriving.
5. Treatment is aimed at prevention and/or symptomatic relief; antispasmodics or sedatives may be used.
6. Colic disappears at about 3 to 4 months of age with or without specific treatment.

B. Nursing Management.
1. Prevent build-up of gas.
    a. Provide a quiet, relaxed setting for feeding.
    b. Feed infant slowly.
    c. Burp after every ounce of formula.
    d. Do not overfeed.
    e. Position infant in upright position for half hour after feeding.
    f. Offer pacifier to calm tense infant.
2. Promote relief of abdominal distention.
    a. Change infant's position, e.g., place on abdomen.
    b. Apply low temperature, covered hot water bottle or heating pad on low setting on abdomen.
    c. Insert bulb of rectal thermometer just past anal sphincter to mechanically facilitate expulsion of gas.
    d. Observe, record, and report the child's response to antispasmodic and/or sedative drugs.
3. Assist parents in dealing with stress produced by colicky infant.
    a. Emphasize the successes parents are having in infant care.
    b. Encourage a break from infant care.
    c. Assist couple in supporting each other in coping with infant.
4. Teach parents.
    a. Management techniques as stated above.
    b. How to administer medications if ordered. See *Administration of Medications, Parental*.

Colostomy. See *Anorectal Malformation* and *Hirschsprung's Disease.*

Concussion. See *Home Management of Minor Emergencies.*

Congenital heart disease. Anatomic malformation of the heart.

A. **General Considerations.**
  1. Congenital heart defects are commonly divided into two categories on the basis of the alterations in circulation.
    a. Acyanotic defects which:
      1. Result from the shunting of oxygenated blood from the left side to the right side of the heart (from a higher to a lower pressure gradient).
      2. The pulmonary circulation is increased.
      3. There is no mixing of unoxygenated blood in the systemic circulation.
    b. Cyanotic defects in which:
      1. A shunting of unoxygenated blood from the right to the left side of the heart through an abnormal opening and/or an abnormal vessel configuration occurs.
      2. There is mixing of unoxygenated blood in the systemic circulation.
  2. Eisenmenger's complex (syndrome) occurs when progressive pulmonary vascular resistance causes a severe acyanotic left-to-right shunt to become a cyanotic right-to-left shunt.
  3. The two major manifestations of congenital heart disease in children are cyanosis and congestive heart failure.
  4. Cyanosis becomes apparent when there is a venous arterial shunting of blood or an obstruction of blood flow to the lungs.
  5. Congestive heart failure occurs when cardiac output is unequal to body requirements; blood dams up in the heart and the pulmonary vasculature becomes engorged. See *Congestive Heart Failure.*
  6. Ventricular septal defect (VSD): Abnormal opening in the ventricular septum with an acyanotic right-to-left shunt.
    a. Characteristics:
      1. May improve or close spontaneously in first year of life.
      2. With a large defect the child may develop: pulmonary vascular disease and pulmonary artery hypertension leading to the development of cyanosis, congestive heart failure, and/or bacterial endocarditis.
    b. Signs and symptoms may include:
      1. Loud, harsh, pansystolic murmur not necessarily related to the size of the defect.
      2. Right ventricular hypertrophy and possible right atrial hypertrophy, with more severe defects.
      3. Slow growth, shortness of breath, easy fatigability with exercise.
    c. Treatment includes:
      1. Observation of children with small defects since 50 percent close in first 3 years of life.
      2. Open heart surgery with repair of defect by suturing or use of a patch for large defects.
      3. Pulmonary banding to decrease pulmonary blood flow and the development of increased pulmonary resistance in infants unable to tolerate corrective surgery.
  7. Atrial septal defect (ASD): Abnormal opening between the left and right atria with acyanotic left-to-right shunt.
    a. Characteristics include:
      1. Possible spontaneous closure during first year of life.
      2. Possible interference with normal heart rhythm or conduction system.
      3. Complications which may occur include: pulmonary thrombosis or embolus; pulmonary infections; rupture of pulmonary artery.
    b. Signs and symptoms include:
      1. Crescendo–decrescendo systolic ejection murmur.
      2. Wide, fixed splitting of second heart sound.
      3. Dyspnea on exertion.
      4. Growth retardation.
    c. Treatment includes the use of a surgical procedure similar to that used for a VSD and is done when the defect is moderate to large.
  8. Patent ductus arteriosus (PDA): Acyanotic defect in which there is a patent duct between the descending aorta and pulmonary artery bifurcation resulting in an increased left heart work load.
    a. Characteristics include:
      1. May remain asymptomatic.
      2. Complications which may develop include pulmonary artery hypertension with right-to-left shunt, congestive heart failure, right atrial and ventricular hypertrophy.
    b. Signs and symptoms include:
      1. Machinery-like murmur.
      2. Widened pulse pressure.
      3. Hypertrophy of the left atrium and ventricle.

4. Easy fatigability.
5. Dyspnea on exertion.
6. Respiratory infections.
7. Growth retardation.
c. Treatment includes:
  1. Surgical division or ligation of the patent vessel usually between one and two years of age.
  2. Attempts at pharmacological closure by the use if indomethacin (Indocin) in seriously ill neonates.

9. Coarctation of the aorta (COA): Narrowing of the aorta which may occur anywhere on the aortic arch.
a. Characteristics include:
  1. Development of collateral circulation which minimizes pressure changes.
  2. Development of complications such as congestive heart failure, endocarditis, cerebral vascular accidents.
b. Signs and symptoms include:
  1. High blood pressure and bounding pulses in areas proximal to the defect, headache, dizziness, nosebleeds.
  2. Decreased blood pressure and cooler skin distal to the defect, weak or absent femoral pulses.
  3. Soft, high frequency murmur.
c. Treatment includes:
  1. Surgical resection of the defect usually about 4 years of age when adequate vessel growth is more likely to occur.
  2. Use of prostaglandins to maintain patency of the ductus arteriosus to provide adequate circulation in infants with serious defects until corrective surgery can be done.

10. Pulmonic stenosis: Narrowing at the entrance of the pulmonary artery.
a. Characteristics include:
  1. Low or normal pulmonary artery pressure.
  2. Possible complications include: right ventricular hypertrophy, congestive heart failure, cyanosis.
b. Signs and symptoms include:
  1. Systolic ejection murmur with associated thrill.
  2. Dyspnea and fatigue on exertion.
  3. Right ventricular hypertrophy.
c. Treatment includes:
  1. Continued observation in asymptomatic child whose right ventricular function is overcoming the obstruction.
  2. Surgery to remove stenosis (pulmonary valvotomy) in children who demonstrate an increased pressure gradient.

11. Aortic stenosis: Narrowing of the aortic valve or left ventricular outflow obstruction.

a. Characteristics include:
  1. Remains acyanotic unless defect is severe.
  2. Often is asymptomatic in infants and young children.
  3. Possible development of left ventricular hypertrophy.
  4. Intractable congestive heart failure may develop in infants.
  5. Sudden death may occur due to ischemia after severe exertion.
b. Signs and symptoms include:
  1. Systolic ejection murmur with an associated thrill.
  2. Left ventricular failure in severe cases.
  3. Fainting.
  4. Epigastric pain.
  5. Angina.
  6. Exercise intolerance.
  7. Dizziness associated with prolonged standing.
c. Treatment includes:
  1. Surgical opening of the valve (commissurotomy).
  2. Treatment rarely results in a complete repair of the valve and strenuous activity may be contraindicated (Moss, 1979).

12. Tetralogy of Fallot: Cyanotic defect comprised of the following: ventricular septal defect, pulmonic stenosis, overriding aorta, and right ventricular hypertrophy.
a. Characteristics include:
  1. Increased right ventricular pressure from obstructed pulmonary outflow.
  2. Complications such as polycythemia, iron deficiency anemia, cerebral infarctions, and cerebral abscesses.
b. Signs and symptoms include:
  1. Cyanosis.
  2. Hypoxic ("blue spells").
  3. Squatting or assumption of knee–chest position.
  4. Clubbing of fingers and toes after 1 year of age.
  5. Marked growth retardation.
  6. Pansystolic murmur.
  7. Respiratory distress and fatigue on feeding.
c. Treatment includes:
  1. Medical management of paroxysmal dyspnea and cyanotic spells.
  2. Palliative procedures to increase the flow of unsaturated blood through the lungs for relief of severe cyanosis and/or hypoxia in infants. (Blalock-Taussig, Potts anastomosis, Waterston anastomosis) (Moss, 1979).
  3. Corrective surgery done when the child is older.

13. Truncus arteriosus: Cyanotic defect in which there is fusion of the aorta and pulmonary artery into a single vessel which overrides both ventricles and transports blood from the pulmonary and systemic circulation.
   a. Characteristics include:
      1. Death within first 6 months of life from congestive heart failure, if not treated.
      2. Single component to second heart sound due to presence of single valve in a common trunk.
   b. Signs and symptoms include:
      1. Cyanosis.
      2. Fatigue.
      3. Dyspnea.
      4. Growth retardation.
      5. Tachypnea.
      6. Rales.
      7. Congestive heart failure.
      8. Recurrent respiratory infections.
      9. Decrescendo murmur.
   c. Treatment includes:
      1. Surgical intervention in the first 6 months of life.
      2. Repeated surgical procedures to replace blood conduits as the child grows.
14. Transposition of the great vessels: Cyanotic defect in which the aorta leaves the right ventricle and the pulmonary artery leaves the left ventricle.
   a. Characteristics include:
      1. A ventricular septal defect, atrial septal defect, or patent ductus arteriosus is required to connect the two independent circulations to prevent death.
      2. May cause premature cardiac contraction and escape beats.
   b. Signs and symptoms include:
      1. Cyanosis.
      2. Congestive heart failure within the first day of life.
      3. Poor feeding.
      4. Hepatomegaly.
      5. Metabolic acidosis from hypoxia.
   c. Treatment includes:
      1. Palliative surgery to relieve cyanosis (Waterston-Cooley shunt).
      2. Corrective surgery (Mustard or Rastelli procedure).
15. Cyanosis and congestive heart failure are the two most common signs of congenital heart disease. See *Congestive Heart Failure.*
16. The diagnosis of congenital heart disease is a crisis.
17. Children with congenital heart disease are prone to developing bacterial endocarditis because bacteria may lodge on damaged or abnormal valves.
18. A team approach to care is necessary.

B. **Nursing Management.** See LIFE-THREATENING ILLNESS.
   1. Support the child and parents during hospitalization. See *Crisis Intervention* and *Hospitalization, Support During.*
   2. Initiate discharge planning. See *Discharge Planning.*
   3. Allow a grief period for parents/family when the diagnosis is made. See *Crisis Intervention, Exceptional Child.*
   4. Observe, record, and report the following about all children with congenital heart disease.
      a. Color of skin and mucous membranes at rest and during activity.
      b. Respiratory rate, depth, and symmetry.
      c. Blood pressure.
      d. Apical and peripheral pulses; noting any discrepancies.
      e. Daily weight.
      f. Response to activities of daily living.
      g. Interaction with family visitors, and peers when appropriate.
   5. Assess for cyanosis, making sure:
      a. You use a good, natural light source.
      b. The child's temperature is not subnormal.
      c. Check mucous membranes, blanching of fingernails and toenails, conjunctiva and lips of dark-skinned children.
   6. Observe, record, and report signs and symptoms of congestive heart failure. See *Congestive Heart Failure.*
   7. Provide care to decrease demands on the heart.
      a. Feed.
         1. Feed the infant on demand with a soft nipple.
         2. Allow the infant to set his own feeding pace.
         3. Burp after every ounce or oftener.
         4. Feed the older child smaller, more frequent meals.
      b. Promote rest.
         1. Schedule care in blocks to allow rest in between, e.g., weight, bathe if condition warrants, feed, then put down for rest.
         2. Position the child for comfort, e.g., knee chest if cyanotic, elevated 30 to 60 degrees in infant chair if dyspneic, or lying on side.
         3. Provide quiet activities for the older child.
      c. Bathe.
         1. Bathe only as necessary, i.e., infant may only need face, hands, and perineal area washed.
         2. Avoid chilling during bath since this increases oxygen needs.
      d. Promote comfort.

1. Control environmental temperature so child is neither over heated nor chilled.
2. Do not allow infant to cry for long periods.
3. Position appropriately, i.e., knee chest, semi-Fowler's.
4. Meet the child's needs on a consistent basis, e.g., hold, rock to relieve tension.
   e. Avoid constipation. See *Constipation*.
   f. Administer humidified oxygen as ordered.
   g. Give oxygen during painful procedures to meet increased oxygen needs.
8. Administer medications as ordered and observe for side effects.
9. Provide oral fluids within set limits.
10. Prevent infection.
    a. Prevent contact with other children, staff, and visitors who have infections.
    b. Wash hands before all contact with the child.
    c. Teach the child hygienic practices.
11. Prevent bacterial endocarditis.
    a. Promote/maintain optimal dental health. See *Dental Care*.
    b. Encourage the use of antibiotic prophylaxis with dental procedures or surgery.
    c. Use correct techniques in caring for all intravenous infusion lines to prevent bacterial entry.
12. Prepare the child and parents for all procedures. See *Preparation for Procedures*.
13. Support normal growth and development.
    a. Provide diversional activities appropriate to age and exercise tolerance level.
    b. Do not limit exercise, child will set own limits (Roberts, 1972).
    c. Be consistent.
    d. Set behavioral limits. See *Discipline*.
    e. Assess body image concept due to psychological ramifications of heart defects. See *Body Image*.
14. Support parents.
    a. Include parents in the assessment process.
    b. Point out "normal" features of the child.
    c. Facilitate verbalization of concerns.
    d. Answer all questions truthfully.
    e. Do not give false reassurance.
15. Record plan of care on Kardex to promote consistent physical and psychological care.
16. Teach parents home management.
    a. Assess the child for change in cardiac status and notify physician.
    b. Teach about digitalis. See *Administration of Medications, Parental*.
       1. Give only as ordered.
       2. Check with physician before giving if pulse is altered.
       3. Report observable toxic signs of anorexia, vomiting, and irregular pulse.

    c. Make the child a part, rather than the center, of the family.
    d. Do not restrict activity unless ordered.
    e. Use consistent approach to the child and set limits to provide security.
    f. Prepare the child and parents for palliative or corrective surgery. See *Preoperative Care* and *Preparation for Surgery*.

Congenital hip dysplasia. Congenital abnormality of one or both hips.

A. **General Considerations.**
   1. The classification of the anomaly will determine treatment.
      a. Unstable or dysplastic hip will be treated by using double or triple diapers, Frejka pillow, or abductor splint.
      b. Subluxation (partial dislocation) will be treated as above or with traction followed by closed reduction and hip spica cast.
      c. Luxation (complete dislocation) will be treated by traction followed by closed or open reduction and hip spica cast.
   2. The unstable or subluxated hip may deteriorate if the untreated child begins weight bearing.
   3. The diagnosis of hip dysplasia may be overlooked if the newborn has congenital anomalies or life-threatening illness that delays routine newborn assessment.
   4. An arthrogram may be necessary to confirm the diagnosis since x-rays may be unreliable because the femoral head has not ossified completely.
   5. With proper instruction, parents may be able to maintain traction at home and decrease prolonged hospitalization (Joseph, MacEwen, and Boos, 1982).
   6. The prognosis is poor and surgical correction is usually necessary if the diagnosis is delayed until school age.

B. **Nursing Management.**
   1. Support the child and parents during hospitalization. See *Hospitalization, Support During*.
   2. Initiate discharge planning. See *Discharge Planning*.
   3. Observe, record, and report symptoms in the infant:
      a. Limitation in abducting hip.
      b. Shortening of the affected leg when the infant is supine with hips and knees flexed at 90 degrees (Galeazzi's sign).
      c. Positive Barlow's modification of Ortolani's sign.

4. Observe, record, and report symptoms in the toddler:
   a. Limp characterized by lurching or swaying toward the affected side.
   b. Downward tilt of the pelvis toward the unaffected side when the child stands on the affected leg and raises the normal leg (Trendelenburg sign).
5. Record what parents have been told about anomaly and planned treatment on Kardex or clinic record.
6. Teach parents how to care for the infant in a Frejka pillow or splint.
   a. Apply the splint over the diaper and shirt.
   b. Use disposable diapers or plastic pants to protect the splint.
   c. Provide meticulous skin care.
   d. Encourage the parents to hold and cuddle the infant frequently.
   e. Discuss the baby's need for normal developmental stimulation. See *Stimulation.*
7. Provide care for the child in traction. See *Traction, Care of Child.*
8. Meet the needs of the child who requires surgery. See *Postoperative Care, Preoperative Care,* and *Preparation for Surgery.*
9. Teach the parents cast care. See *Cast Care.*
10. Initiate referral to state crippled children's services or other community agency if appropriate.
11. Help parents understand the need for long-term follow-up.

Congestive heart failure. Syndrome in which the heart cannot supply enough blood flow to the body tissues or can sustain a normal output only by the use of compensatory mechanisms which cause further problems.

A. **General Considerations.**
   1. Congestive heart failure occurs when there is a failure of the compensatory mechanisms of the sympathetic nervous system and the renal system to maintain metabolic requirements.
   2. Signs and symptoms which develop when decompensation occurs include those related to:
      a. Decreased myocardial function:
         1. Restlessness.
         2. Tachycardia.
         3. Fatigue, e.g., infant tires easily when feeding.
         4. Anorexia.
         5. Poor peripheral circulation with pale, cool extremities and weak pulses.
         6. Cardiomegaly.
      b. Pulmonary congestion.
         1. Dyspnea.
         2. Orthopnea.
         3. Tachypnea.
         4. Retractions.
         5. Wheezing.
         6. Rales.
         7. Coughing.
         8. Grunting respiration.
         9. Cyanosis.
      c. Systemic congestion.
         1. Hepatomegaly (usually first sign).
         2. Periorbital edema (seen more often than neck vein engorgement).
         3. Diaphoresis.
         4. Sudden weight gain of 200 Gm or more in 24-hour period (Modrcin, Schott, 1979).
         5. Ascites and dependent edema (rare).
   3. Diagnosis is made on the basis of clinical signs and symptoms.
   4. Treatment is directed toward:
      a. The improvement of cardiac function.
      b. Decreasing sodium and water retention.
      c. Decreasing the cardiac workload.
      d. Improvement of tissue oxygenation.
      e. Promotion of adequate nutrition.
      f. Promotion of normal growth and development.
   5. Treatment includes:
      a. Drugs.
         1. Digitalis preparation to improve cardiac function (most commonly Digoxin).
         2. Diuretics to remove accumulated water and sodium.
      b. Measures to decrease cardiac workload.
         1. Maintenance of a neutral thermal zone.
         2. Rest.
         3. Prevention or immediate treatment of any infection.
         4. Placement in semi-Fowler's position.
         5. Mild sedation for the highly active child.
      c. Measures to increase tissue oxygenation.
         1. Administration of cool, humidified oxygen.
         2. Placement in semi-Fowler's position.
         3. Suctioning of oral secretions.

B. **Nursing Management.**
   1. Support the child and parents during hospitalization. See *Hospitalization, Support During.*
   2. Initiate discharge planning. See *Discharge Planning.*
   3. Administer digitalis preparation as ordered.
      a. Do not give digitalis preparations without a specific order for the heart rate at which drug is to be omitted.
      b. Take apical pulse for 1 full minute before giving.
      c. Observe, record, and report signs of digitalis toxicity.

1. Cardiac arrhythmias, especially bradycardia.
2. Gastrointestinal symptoms such as anorexia, nausea, and vomiting.
3. Neurological symptoms such as headache and blurred vision which are difficult to evaluate objectively.

d. Observe, record, and report signs of therapeutic response to digitalis preparation.
   1. Weight loss from diuresis.
   2. Improved circulation due to increased cardiac output.
   3. Decreased pulse rate.
   4. Decreased fluid in lungs.
   5. Greater tolerance to activity.

4. Administer diuretics as ordered.
   a. Observe, record, and report child's response.
      1. Note exact time of administration.
      2. Record exact times of voiding.
      3. Measure urinary output accurately.
      4. Note changes in edema.
      5. Notify physician if child's urinary output following dose of diuretic differs from prior response to same dose.
   b. Schedule administration of diuretic, if possible, so the maximum response time does not disturb child's sleep.

5. Monitor electrolyte levels, especially potassium, since hypokalemia increases the occurrence of digitalis toxicity. See *Fluid and Electrolyte Imbalance*.

6. Measure intake and output accurately.
   a. All sources of intake must be totalled, e.g., oral intake from water and food source, I.V. fluids, and fluids used to administer I.V. medications (often a significant source which is not considered).
   b. Measure output: 1 to 2 cc per Kg. per hour is normal in presence of normal intake.
      1. Weigh the child as ordered.
         a. At the same time.
         b. On the same scale.
         c. Nude, or in the same amount of clothing.
      2. Include estimations of nonmeasurable fluid loss, e.g., diaphoresis.
      3. Weigh diapers of child who is not toilet trained: weigh dry diaper and mark weight, weigh same diaper when wet: 1 Gm change in weight equals 1 cc of urine.

7. Support additional fluid loss by:
   a. Restricting fluids if ordered.
      1. Explain rationale for fluid restriction.
      2. Remove fluids from bedside table.
      3. Allocate fluid amounts to cover a 24-hour period.
      4. Serve favorite fluids in small cups.
      5. Let older child record fluid amounts taken to permit some control of situation.
   b. Restricting salt intake as ordered.
      1. Identify sources of salt in diet which can be eliminated, e.g., bacon, luncheon meats, potato chips.
      2. Remove salt shaker from tray.
      3. Teach parents about low-sodium cooking; involve nutritionist.

8. Provide care to decrease demands on the heart. See *Congenital Heart Disease*.

9. Promote adequate nutrition.
   a. Determine child's caloric needs. See *Appendix vii*.
   b. Avoid the use of pacifiers since this reduces infant's sucking at feeding time.
   c. Place child in 20 to 30-degree elevated position after feeding to decrease chance of vomiting.
   d. Monitor daily caloric intake to determine whether other measures may be needed, e.g., feeding via nasogastric tube, parenteral nutrition.

10. Promote normal growth and development. See *Stimulation, Appendix v*.

11. Remain alert to signs and symptoms of increasing heart failure.
   a. Continued tachycardia.
   b. Increased liver size; mark edge of liver margin each day to determine change.
   c. Continued or progressive tachypnea.
   d. Increased peripheral vasoconstriction.

12. Teach parents home management.
   a. Assessment of child for signs and symptoms of congestive heart failure.
   b. Promotion of comfort.
   c. Administration of medications. See *Administration of Medications, Parental*.

Conjunctivitis. Inflammation of the conjunctival sac of the eye.

A. **General Considerations.**
   1. Common causative agents include bacteria and viruses, but it may be due to chemicals, physical irritation, or allergens.
   2. Signs and symptoms include:
      a. Redness.
      b. Mucoid or purulent discharge depending on the causative agent.
      c. Eyelids stuck together on awakening.
      d. Sensation of something in the eye.
      e. Itching.
      f. Photophobia.
      g. Burning sensation in eye(s).
   3. The child is able to see.

4. A culture may be done to determine the causative agent.
5. Bacterial conjunctivitis, commonly called "pink eye" is:
   a. Easily spread from one eye to another.
   b. Transmitted by hands, towels, wash cloths, etc.
   c. Commonly found in epidemic form in schools.
6. Treatment of the causative agent includes:
   a. Local and/or systemic antibiotics for bacterial infection.
   b. Topical antibiotics to prevent secondary bacterial infection.
   c. Ophthalmic vasoconstrictors.
   d. Steroid ophthalmic ointments for chronic allergic problems.
7. Complications include:
   a. Corneal invasion.
   b. Cellulitis of the eyelids.
8. Viral conjunctivitis is self-limiting and treatment is the removal of the accumulated secretions and avoidance of pharmaceutical preparations.
9. Compresses should not be kept on the eye since the occlusive covering promotes bacterial growth.

B. Nursing Management.
1. Obtain culture of the exudate prior to start of ophthalmic ointments. See *Preparation for Procedures*.
2. Teach parents to:
   a. Clean the eye before instilling medication.
   b. Apply ophthalmic ointments as instructed. See *Administration of Medications, Parental.*
   c. Clean the affected eye(s) by:
      1. Using a separate damp cotton ball for each eye.
      2. Wiping from the medial to the lateral canthus of the eye.
   d. Separate the child's towel and washcloth from the others.
   e. Use meticulous handwashing when caring for the child's eyes.
   f. Keep the child home from school during the acute stage.
   g. Call the physician if the child develops:
      1. Pain.
      2. Fever.
      3. Edema and redness of the eyelid.
3. Teach the child to:
   a. Avoid touching the eyes.
   b. Wash hands if eyes are touched.
   c. Use only his own towel and washcloth.
4. Manage the hospitalized child who has conjunctivitis by:
   a. Use of isolation technique as ordered.

b. Observing, recording, and reporting the response to medications.
c. Using meticulous handwashing when caring for the child.

Constipation. Consistent passage of firm or hard stools.

A. General Considerations.
1. Factors that cause constipation include:
   a. Emotional problems.
   b. Inappropriate toilet training techniques.
   c. Inadequate diet.
      1. Excessive milk intake.
      2. Lack of bulk.
      3. Inadequate fluid intake.
   d. Overuse of laxatives and enemas.
2. Normal developmental patterns may be misinterpreted as constipation.
   a. Newborn "pushing movements," red face, and grunting noises are normal.
   b. The toddler may be unwilling to stop play in order to eliminate.
   c. Older children may refuse to eliminate bowels at school or in social situations.
3. Constipation is common in children who have locomotion problems.

B. Nursing Management.
1. Obtain an accurate history to help determine the etiology.
   a. Find out what the term constipation means to the mother.
   b. Obtain information on number, consistency, and frequency of bowel movements.
   c. What management has the mother tried and what have results been?
   d. Find out how the child was toilet trained.
   e. Complete a nutritional assessment.
   f. Evaluate the child's activity level.
   g. Assess the child's interpersonal relationships.
2. Administer enemas if ordered. See *Preparation for Procedures.*
   a. Remember that this is an intrusive procedure.
   b. Explain how the child will feel during the enema.
   c. Reassure him that the procedure is not a punishment.
   d. Explain to the mother that tap water enemas should not be used since they cause electrolyte imbalance.
3. Administer stool softeners as ordered.
   a. Give a double-dose of water-soluble vitamins if mineral oil is ordered.
   b. Mineral oil is more palatable in orange juice.
4. Adjust the diet if appropriate.

a. Add corn syrup or increase the fluid in infant's formula.
b. Reduce the milk or protein intake if either is excessive.
c. Increase bulk in diet.
   1. Whole grain cereals.
   2. Fruit juices and fresh fruits except apples and bananas.
   3. Raw vegetables.
5. Help the child establish a normal bowel pattern. See *Toilet Training*.
   a. Establish what is normal for this child.
   b. Take the child to the toilet at regular times every day.
   c. Provide privacy during elimination.
   d. Praise the child for his cooperation in attempting elimination, not just for successful bowel movements.

Convulsions. See *Seizures*.

Coping. Process by which the child tries to deal with new and/or stressful experiences.

A. **General Considerations.**
1. Coping patterns developed in infancy remain characteristic of the individual throughout life.
2. Three major coping strategies are:
   a. Withdrawal from new people or new experiences.
   b. Interpretation of new experiences as a challenge.
   c. Toleration of new experiences without becoming involved with them.
3. Many factors influence the child's coping pattern:
   a. Level of development.
   b. Adaptability to change.
   c. Environmental support.
   d. His past experiences.
   e. His perception of events.
   f. His innate resources.
4. Successful coping is essential to the development of self-esteem.
5. The child's range of coping behaviors will be influenced by sex-role stereotyped expectations, e.g., girls may cry, boys should not.
6. The child must have experiences which give him an opportunity to practice coping behavior.
7. The child may use defense mechanisms such as regression, denial, or projection in the coping process.
8. The child's response to stressful situations depends on his perception of what is happening, not what is actually happening.

9. Hospitalization can assist the child to develop more mature coping behaviors if positive support is available to him.

B. **Nursing Management.**
1. Allow the child to become comfortable in the new environment/situation. See *Admission to Hospital, Elective*.
2. Ask the parents how the child usually deals with new situations and record information on the Kardex.
3. Follow home routines as much as possible.
4. Encourage family participation in care to increase the child's feeling of security.
5. Prepare the child and parents for all procedures. See *Preparation for Procedures*.
6. Meet the child's physical needs so that his energy can be used for coping.
7. Assess the child's behavior during:
   a. Play.
   b. Self-care activities.
   c. Social interactions.
   d. Painful procedures.
8. Identify and support the child's coping strategies.
   a. Motility, i.e., fight or flight response.
   b. Control of others.
   c. Resisting control of others.
   d. Cooperating or complying.
   e. Aggression.
   f. Regression.
   g. Delaying tactics.
   h. Sleep.
   i. Humor.
   j. Identification with others, particularly peers.
9. Involve the child as an active participant in his care.
   a. Allow dependency, but encourage independency.
      1. Cuddle and hold the child to convey love and affection.
      2. Feed the child if he wants you to, but also give him finger foods.
      3. Bathe the child, but have him put soap on the washcloth.
   b. Offer appropriate choices.
   c. Consider his developmental level when establishing goals.
10. Encourage the child to express feelings.
    a. Provide therapeutic play for the young child. See *Play, Therapeutic*.
    b. Ask the older child what he thinks has happened or will happen.
11. Provide an outlet for direct release of aggression.
    a. Water play.
    b. Bean bag toss.
    c. Sponge balls, airplanes, etc.

d. Ring toss game.
e. Pounding board.
f. Tearing paper.
g. Balloon throwing.
12. Support the child during painful procedures.
a. Tell the child to squeeze your hand hard.
b. Tell him he can cry as loud as he wants.

Coxa vara. See *Slipped Femoral Epiphysis.*

Cradle cap. See *Dermatitis, Seborrheic.*

Crib death. See *Sudden Infant Death Syndrome.*

Crisis intervention. Use of therapeutic techniques to assist the child and parents in coping with a crisis situation.

A. **General Considerations.**
1. A crisis situation develops when a stressful event produces disequilibrium, and the child and/or parent is unable to restore equilibrium using previously learned problem solving techniques.
2. Balancing factors that affect the ability to solve the problem and restore balance include (Ageulera and Messick, 1978):
a. Perception of the event.
b. Available support systems.
c. Coping mechanisms.
3. The individual or family in crisis has (Ageulera and Messick, 1978):
a. Distorted perception of the stressful event.
b. Inadequate situational support.
c. Absent or inadequate coping mechanisms (most common).
4. Behaviors exhibited by individuals experiencing a crisis include:
a. Anxiety.
b. Tension.
c. Depression.
d. Disorganization.
e. Anger.
5. Crisis situations may be (Burgess and Baldwin, 1981):
a. Dispositional: distress results from a situation which is viewed as a problem, e.g., child hospitalized for diagnostic tests.
b. Crisis of anticipated life situations: crises which reflect anticipated life transitions over which the individual has no control, e.g., adolescence.
c. Crises resulting from sudden traumatic stress: crisis is precipitated by unexpected situations which overwhelm the individual, e.g., diagnosis of a life-threatening illness.
d. Maturational/developmental crises: crises resulting from the individual's attempt to deal with interpersonal situations in a manner that reflects an earlier, unresolved developmental issue, e.g., the adolescent's assertion of independence.
e. Crises resulting from psychopathology: psychopathology has been a precipitating factor.
f. Psychiatric emergencies: severely impaired general functioning precipitates a crisis situation.
6. The simultaneous occurrence of a dispositional and a developmental crisis situation may be overwhelming to a child.
7. Crisis situations:
a. Are self-limiting to between 4 and 6 weeks.
b. Will be resolved in a manner that is:
1. Adaptive: individual learns new and more effective coping behaviors which make him less vulnerable to future stressors.
2. Maladaptive: individual continues to use old ineffective coping behaviors or learns new coping behaviors which are self-defeating or neurotic and leave him increasingly vulnerable to stress.
c. Decreases psychic defense mechanisms and bring about increased cognitive and affective awareness.
d. Make the individual more receptive to learning in both the cognitive and affective areas.
8. A crisis is time limited and the child and parents are most receptive to help at the time the crisis occurs.
9. Use of the nursing process is an effective approach in crisis intervention.

B. **Nursing Management.** See COPING.
1. Use the nursing process.
a. Assess the child and parents and the problem.
1. What type of crisis situation appears to be present?
2. How is the stressful event being perceived? (e.g., realistically or distorted).
3. What support systems are available and how adequate are they?
4. What coping methods are usually used to deal with a problem?
5. How effective are the coping methods being used?
6. What behaviors are being exhibited?
b. Plan nursing interventions based on assess-

ment of type of crisis situation (Burgess and Baldwin, 1981):

1. Dispositional: assist in problem identification and provide service needed, e.g., referral, patient education.
2. Crises of anticipated life situations: explain expected changes, provide support and anticipatory guidance so child/parents can plan adaptive coping behaviors.
3. Crises resulting from sudden traumatic stress: provide or mobilize support for the child/parents when they cannot mobilize own coping mechanisms, provide anticipatory guidance to help child/parents develop new coping mechanisms.
4. Maturational/developmental crises: child/parents need support and guidance in dealing with current problem and the earlier unresolved maturational/developmental issue which precipitated or contributed to the current crisis.
5. Crises resulting from psychopathology and psychiatric emergencies: provide a safe, supportive environment for child/parents and obtain assistance from health care professional trained to handle these crises.

c. Intervene on basis of the above using the following behaviors as appropriate:
1. Encourage the expression of feelings.
2. Talk about the event with the child and parents in a realistic manner.
3. Provide facts.
4. Present information in manageable amounts.
5. Use short, direct, concise statements.
6. Discourage blaming of self or others.
7. Encourage the child and parents to accept support available.
8. Assist the child and parents in identifying additional support systems.
9. Reinforce appropriate coping behaviors.
10. Assist the child and parents to develop additional appropriate coping behaviors.

d. Evaluate the effectiveness of the intervention in terms of the ability of the child and parents to cope successfully with the crisis and alter plans accordingly.

2. Assign staff members who have the best rapport with the child and parents to care for the child during the crisis situation.
3. Record crisis intervention plan on Kardex to promote consistency in care.
4. Review with the child and parents how effective or ineffective the coping behaviors were when the crisis has passed.

Crossed eyes. See *Strabismus*.

Croup, acute spasmodic. Acute inspiratory obstruction occurring at the level of the vocal cords.

A. **General Considerations.**
1. Must be differentiated from acute epiglottitis and acute laryngotracheobronchitis which also present with inspiratory stridor and altogether comprise the croup syndromes (Lipow, 1977).
2. Signs and symptoms include a barking, metallic sounding cough, hoarseness, and marked inspiratory stridor.
3. There is no elevation of temperature with acute spasmodic croup.
4. Severe supraclavicular and substernal retractions are rare but can occur.
5. The onset of symptoms is sudden, usually occurs late at night, and tends to recur for several nights.
6. The causative organism is unknown but allergy and mild viral infection are suspected.
7. Treatment measures include:
   a. Exposure to increased humidity, e.g., steam from hot running shower at home, cool mist tent in the hospital.
   b. Aerosol racemic epinephrine via intermittent positive pressure (usually terminates an attack).
8. Home management is usually possible but hospitalization is required for severe symptoms.

B. **Nursing Management.**
1. Support the child and parents during hospitalization. See *Hospitalization, Support During*.
2. Initiate discharge planning. See *Discharge Planning*.
3. Increase environmental humidity.
   a. Cool steam vaporizer at bedtime.
   b. Mist tent. See *Mist Tent*.
4. Promote hydration to liquefy secretions. See *Forcing Fluids*.
   a. Encourage oral fluids.
   b. Avoid cold fluids that may cause spasm.
5. Provide someone to stay with the child to decrease anxiety since stress may increase symptoms.
6. Observe, record, and report signs that may indicate the presence of one of the more serious croup syndrome diseases.
   a. High fever.
   b. Sore throat.
   c. Difficulty swallowing.
   d. Increasing restlessness due to air hunger.
   e. Severe supraclavicular or substernal retractions.
7. Teach parents home management.
   a. Increase humidity in environment.

1. Run hot shower in bathroom with door closed.
2. Use cool mist vaporizer at bedside.
3. Ride the child in car with windows down.
   b. Advise parents of signs that indicate the child should be seen by a physician.
   c. Do not induce vomiting since aspiration may occur.

Cryptorchidism. Failure of one or both testes to descend into the scrotum.

A. **General Considerations.**
1. Cryptorchidism can be subdivided into three types (Toguri, 1982):
   a. Undescended—lie on the posterior abdominal wall.
   b. Ectopic—found in the interstitial portion of the superficial inguinal pouch.
   c. Retractile—observed in the scrotum, but become hidden because of an active cremasteric reflex precipitated by fear or cold.
2. The young child is concerned about how he is different from his peers even though the fears are not expressed to parents.
3. Secondary sex characteristics will develop normally.
4. Hormonal injections to stimulate descent may be tried if there is no coexisting hernia.
5. Injection of human gonadotropin may be administered to stimulate testes descent in the retractile type, but cannot be used if there is a coexisting hernia/hydrocele.
6. Surgical intervention may be done in infancy or preschool years or at puberty.
7. Although rare, testicular cancer is more common in undescended testes.
8. Orchiopexy, surgical descent of the testes, does not prevent testicular cancer, but the incidence of malignancy is less if the repair is done before the age of 5 years.

B. **Nursing Management.**
1. Support the child and parents during hospitalization. See *Hospitalization, Support During.*
2. Initiate discharge planning. See *Discharge Planning.*
3. Prepare the child and parents for the results of surgery. See *Preoperative Care* and *Preparation for Surgery.*
   a. Use pictures to show the child the operative site.
   b. Assume the preschool child is worried about having his penis cut off and tell him directly that this will not happen.
   c. Clarify with the surgeon whether the child will have a rubber band traction suture or other device postoperatively and tell the child and parents.

4. Meet the needs of the child postoperatively. See *Postoperative Care.*
   a. Clean fecal material from the perineum carefully to prevent contamination of the suture line.
   b. Apply a small ice pack to decrease swelling if ordered.
   c. Administer antibiotics as ordered.
5. Teach the child and parents home management.
   a. Maintain the child on limited activity for 2 to 7 days as ordered.
   b. Provide age-appropriate play to help the child deal with immobilization and with emotionally traumatic surgery. See *Play, Therapeutic.*
   c. Encourage parents to discuss emotional aspects with surgeon or nurse.
      1. Possible fear of homosexuality.
      2. Possible fear of sterility.
   d. Teach the adolescent to perform testicular self-exam. See *Appendix viii.*

Cultural aspects of health care. Cultural beliefs and practices that should be considered in the development of health care.

A. **General Considerations.**
1. Nurses should study the predominant cultural groups in their practice area.
2. There is variation in health care beliefs and practices among different cultures, and not all people within the culture hold the same beliefs and practices.
3. Conflict arises when the demands of the dominant culture are at variance with the subculture and there is no flexibility.
4. Delivery of safe, effective nursing care to members of a different cultural group requires knowledge of their:
   a. Beliefs and customs.
   b. Health care practices.
   c. Language.
   d. Dietary preferences.
   e. Physical differences, e.g., appearance of cyanosis is different in blacks.
5. Family ties within many subcultures are extremely strong and should be seen as a sign of strength.
6. A family group, rather than the parents may make decisions relating to health care sought and/or accepted for a child, e.g., the Latino/Chicano mother may consult with the family before giving the child a medication which has been prescribed.
7. An individual other than the parent may be the person who is accepted as the decision

maker in matters relating to the child, e.g., in some Indian tribes the grandmother assumes authority (Primeaux, 1977).

8. The concept of who constitutes "family" varies among cultures and often extends to persons not related by bloodline, e.g., an Indian child may have several women referred to as "mother" (Primeaux, 1977).

9. Use of folk healers and folk medicines is common among different cultural groups, e.g., Chinese herb pharmacist, Indian medicine man, Latino/Chicano curandero.

10. The concept of illness as a result of an imbalance in opposing forces within the body is held by several cultural groups, e.g., Chinese balance of Yin, cold, and Yang, hot; and Latino/Chicano balance of "good" and "evil" (Branch and Paxton, 1976).

11. Foods, some of which may be indigenous to a particular culture, are often used to restore the perceived bodily imbalance causing illness, e.g., Chinese child with an earache which is considered a hot disease would not be given scrambled eggs, a hot food (Campbell and Chang, 1973).

12. Religious beliefs and health care practices are frequently intertwined in cultures, e.g., religious healing services practiced by blacks (Branch and Paxton, 1976).

13. Health maintenance activities may be valued but not used due to a "present" rather than "future" orientation produced by the stresses of poverty, poor housing, and inadequate public services.

14. A family may use medicine prescribed by a physician along with folk remedies.

15. Beliefs about causes of illness may be inconsistent with known scientific facts.

16. Some cultures may view and/or value male and female children differently.

B. **Nursing Management.** See ADVOCATE.

1. Talk to individuals and families from the predominant cultural groups in your practice area to learn about their health values, beliefs, and practices.

2. Examine your own beliefs, attitudes, behaviors toward, and willingness to interact with an ethnic group before becoming involved in delivering health care services to a child or family who is a member of that group.

3. Include the following in a nursing assessment (Branch and Paxton, 1976):
   a. Cultural practices and beliefs.
   b. Cultural preferences in terms of food, recreation, grooming products, dress, etc.
   c. Behaviors that are valued by the culture.
   d. Cultural taboos and sanctions.

e. Adherence of the child and/or parent to the cultural system.
   f. Differences in skin color that affect nursing assessment.
   g. Use of folk medicines along with prescribed medications.

4. Focus on identified strengths of the child and/or parents in developing care.
   a. Meaningful family relationships.
   b. Membership in ethnic organizations or clubs.
   c. Life experiences within an ethnic community.

5. Serve as a patient advocate in developing care that is consistent with the culture of the child and parent.
   a. Arrange visiting patterns congruent with cultural beliefs about family.
   b. Plan care for the child with the family member(s) recognized as the decision maker(s).
   c. Encourage the use of cultural practices related to health care that are not detrimental to the child.
   d. Permit the bringing of foods from home or arrange with dietician to provide appropriate ethnic foods.
   e. Arrange for a caregiver who speaks the same language, if possible, or work with family to locate a translator.
   f. Be willing to meet with indigenous health care workers to discuss care.
   g. Establish goals that are mutually agreed upon as being realistic.

6. View all behavior in relationship to the culture and avoid judgmental labels.

7. Record the plan of care on the Kardex in order to promote continuity of care.

Cyanotic heart disease. See Congenital Heart disease.

Cystic fibrosis. An autosomal, recessive disorder characterized by dysfunction of the mucus secreting glands.

A. **General Considerations.**

1. Absent or decreased secretion of pancreatic enzymes causes malabsorption, possible meconium ileus in infancy, and failure to thrive.

2. An overproduction of secretions in the respiratory system causes expiratory obstruction.

3. Thick secretions block the pancreatic ducts interfering with the flow of enzymes to the duodenum.

4. Fat and protein digestion and absorption is markedly decreased as a result.

C

5. The elevated sodium and chloride content of the saliva and sweat in children with cystic fibrosis serves as the basis of the sweat chloride test which is used for diagnosis.
   a. 40 mEq or below is normal.
   b. 40–60 mEq is questionable.
   c. Over 60 mEq is diagnostic.
6. Other diagnostic criteria are:
   a. Positive family history.
   b. Absence of pancreatic enzymes.
   c. Chronic pulmonary involvement.
7. Initial symptoms frequently include bulky, foul smelling stools; poor weight gain; and frequent respiratory infections.
8. Treatment is symptomatic.
9. Most hospitalizations are due to respiratory infections.
10. The prognosis is generally dependent on the damage to the tracheobronchial tree at the time of diagnosis.
11. As diagnosis and treatment improve, more patients are surviving through adolescence and young adulthood.
    a. Females have thick cervical mucus and may have difficulty conceiving.
    b. Males are almost always sterile due to aspermia and absence of the vas deferens.

B. **Nursing Management.** See *Chronic Illness, Genetic Counseling,* and *Life-Threatening Illness.*
   1. Support the child and parents during hospitalization. See *Hospitalization, Support During.*
   2. Initiate discharge planning. See *Discharge Planning.*
   3. Prepare the child and parents for the sweat test. See *Preparation for Procedures.*
      a. A plastic sweat-generating electrode is placed on the skin.
      b. The electrical current involved is not hazardous to the child.
      c. The concentration of sodium and chloride is not related to severity of the disease.
      d. The procedure is not painful and is completed in about 30 minutes.
   4. Help the child and parents adjust to the diagnosis.
      a. Encourage parents to verbalize their concerns about handling care at home.
      b. Recognize that the child and parents may have anticipatory anxiety if a sibling has died from the disease.
      c. Refer to the social worker, state Crippled Children's Commission, or community agencies for financial assistance.
   5. Meet nutritional needs.
      a. Administer replacement pancreatic enzyme.

      1. Mix with applesauce or pudding for infant or young child.
      2. Do not add to warm or hot food since this deactivates the enzyme.
      3. Do not add until the child is ready to eat.
      4. Give during middle of meal.
      b. Provide a higher than normal salt intake to counter salt depletion due to sweating.
      1. Have the breast-feeding mother discuss sodium needs with the physician since breast milk is lower in sodium (Laughlin, Brady, and Eigen, 1981).
      2. Discusss the use of regular canned foods rather than natural packed without sodium.
      3. Allow the older child to salt food generously, particularly in hot weather.
      c. Give skim or low-fat milk if a decrease in fat content is desired.
      d. Include a large amount of protein.
      1. Lean meat.
      2. Cottage cheese.
      3. Add skim milk powder to infant formula or use Probana.
      4. Diet supplements such as Instant Breakfast, Ensure, or Sustacal.
      e. Help the child match the amount of replacement enzymes to fat intake if no dietary restriction is ordered.
      f. Administer water-miscible vitamins and iron supplement.
   6. Observe, record, and report the following:
      a. Character of feces.
      b. Respiratory status.
      1. Rate and rhythm.
      2. Color of skin.
      3. Dyspnea.
      4. Cough.
      c. Signs of cardiac failure.
      1. Increased pulse.
      2. Decreased urinary output.
      3. Diaphoresis.
      4. Fatigue.
      5. Anorexia.
      6. Abdominal pain.
      7. Dilated neck veins.
      d. Response to aerosol therapy and postural drainage.
   7. Keep the child comfortable in mist tent. See *Mist Tent.*
   8. Meet comfort needs.
      a. Reposition frequently to prevent skin breakdown and to aerate lungs.
      b. Give frequent mouth care.
      c. Provide a room deodorizer.
      d. Treat rectal prolapse that occurs because of weak rectal muscles.

1. Place the child in Trendenlenberg position.
2. Replace prolapse with lubricated, gloved hand.
3. Tape buttocks to maintain pressure.
   e. Schedule postural drainage before meals.
   f. Maintain a comfortable room temperature.
   g. Provide rest periods before meals.
9. Administer antibiotics as ordered.
   a. Monitor blood serum levels of antibiotics and notify physician of toxic levels.
   b. Observe for side effects since high doses are usually ordered.
10. Observe for iodide sensitivity if expectorants are being used.
11. Prevent infection.
   a. Protect from staff and visitors who have respiratory infections.
   b. Use good handwashing technique.
12. Teach the child and parents home management.
   a. Help parents integrate the child's care into family life-style.
   b. Encourage the child to assume as much responsibility for his own care as possible to increase his independence.
     1. Food selection.
     2. Use of pancreatic enzymes.
     3. Use of equipment.
     4. Breathing exercises.
   c. Have parents return demonstration of postural drainage.
   d. Discuss measures to prevent infection.
     1. Appropriate clothing.
     2. Immunizations. See *Immunizations*.

   e. Explain care of mist tent or aerosol equipment if used at home.
   f. Help the child and parents with breathing exercises.
     1. Blowing feathers, pinwheels, ping-pong balls for young children.
     2. Calisthenics for older child.
     3. Encourage swimming.
   g. Review dosage, time, actions, and side effects of medications to be given at home. See *Administration of Medications, Parental.*
     1. The child should not be given antihistamines or cough suppressants.
     2. Prophylactic antibiotics may be ordered.
   h. Encourage regular school attendance and peer contacts.
     1. Initiate contact with school nurse.
     2. Explain the child's individual needs to teacher.
   i. Explore community agencies which could offer family support.
     1. Community health nurse for general supervision.
     2. Babysitters so parents have time alone.
     3. Day care centers for young siblings. See *Day Care Center.*
     4. Agencies to assist with equipment purchase/rental.
     5. Family support groups.
13. The older adolescent needs an opportunity to discuss feelings about reproductive difficulty or inability.

Dandruff. See *Dermatitis, Seborrheic.*

Day care center. A facility that provides child care, usually for a set fee.

  A. General Considerations.
    1. The terms *day care* and *nursery school* are frequently used interchangeably.
    2. A day care center denotes a facility whose main purpose is child care for employed parents.
    3. A nursery school denotes a preschool facility dedicated to:
      a. Stimulating the child's sense of creativity and initiative.

      b. Introducing the child to new experiences and social contacts he would not have in the home.
    4. A low child–caretaker ratio increases the likelihood of individual attention for the child.
    5. Licensing of day care centers and nursery schools varies from state to state.

  B. Nursing Management.
    1. Discuss with parents the difference between day care and nursery school.
    2. Teach parents they cannot depend on the name of the facility to define its purpose.
    3. Urge parents of children under 1 year of age to

D

find a facility that keeps the caregiver–child ratio as low as possible.

    a. The establishment of basic trust depends on a consistent one-to-one relationship.

    b. Stranger anxiety occurs during the latter half of the first year.

4. Teach parents that during the preschool period peer exposure appears to have positive effects.

    a. The child approaches school comfortably and ready to learn if he has already learned to be at ease in a group.

    b. The child will interact positively with others if he has had early peer experiences.

5. Discuss with parents how to assess if their child needs a nursery school experience.

    a. Evaluate the age groups in the neighborhood with which the child has daily contact.

    b. Determine if some parent in the neighborhood can supervise organized play so the child has peer contact.

6. Suggest that parents review the licensing criteria for child care facilities.

    a. Call the agency responsible for licensing facilities and get names of licensed centers or schools.

    b. Request criteria for licensing.

7. Encourage the parent to visit the prospective day care center or nursery school without an appointment.

    a. Observe the child–caretaker ratio.

    b. Observe if the personnel attend to the needs and developmental tasks of specific age groups.

    c. Observe the reaction of children to caretakers and vice versa.

        1. Do the caretakers respond warmly to the children?

        2. Do the caretakers seem interested in the children?

        3. Are the physical needs of the children being met?

        4. Is there a nonpressure atmosphere?

        5. Do the children appear happy?

    d. Observe if indoor and outdoor play areas are available.

    e. Observe if toys are available to inspire creativity, e.g., fingerpaints, free form blocks, play stove, and refrigerator.

    f. Look at the menu for meals and snacks for evidence of a nutritious diet.

    g. Look for a safe and clean environment.

    h. Observe for a fire exit plan, fire extinguishers, smoke alarms, and posted emergency numbers.

    i. Request to see health certificates of employees if required for licensure.

    j. Inquire about the policy regarding a sick child.

    k. Determine if any employee is qualified to administer first aid.

    l. Request written information about hours, cost, etc.

    m. Discuss the criteria for and methods of discipline.

    n. Determine if the facility meets the child's needs.

        1. Talk to parents familiar with the facility.

        2. Visit several facilities and compare.

        3. Visit the facility again with an appointment to talk with the director and caretakers about any unresolved questions.

8. Help the parents to prepare the child for the experience.

    a. Visit the facility for a short period with the child so he can become familiar with the surroundings.

    b. Discuss the positive aspects of the experience with the child.

        1. New friends.

        2. New activities.

    c. Discuss the child's experiences with him at the end of each day.

    d. Elicit the caretaker's feelings about the child's adjustment.

Deafness. Inability to hear.

A. **General Considerations.**

1. Deaf children have the same basic needs as children who can hear.

2. Hearing plays a vital part in:

    a. Speech acquisition.

    b. Providing continuity to events, e.g., a cake becomes associated with a birthday party by the conversation accompanying the two events.

    c. Detecting safety hazards in the environment.

    d. The development of human relationships.

3. There are two types of hearing loss: conductive and sensorineural.

4. Normal hearing is present when the child hears in the 0–20 decibel range.

5. Hearing deficits are defined as:

    a. Mild: hears only in the 20–40 decibel range.

    b. Moderate: hears only in the 40–65 decibel range.

    c. Severe: hears only in the 65–85 decibel range.

    d. Profound: hears only over 85 decibels.

6. Hearing aids:

    a. Can help children with conductive hearing losses.

b. Cannot help children with sensorineural hearing losses.

c. Do not restore normal hearing but amplify the sounds the child hears.

d. Can be fitted on an infant as young as 1 month of age (Schmitt, 1976).

7. Signing and lip reading can be taught to young children.

8. Deaf children may appear retarded, since they lack the speech necessary to communicate their thoughts.

9. Voice volume control is difficult for the deaf child who learns to speak since he cannot hear himself.

10. Public Law 94-142 effective September, 1977 mandates free and appropriate education for all handicapped children.

B. **Nursing Management.** See EXCEPTIONAL CHILD.

1. Focus nursing care on the child not his deafness.

2. Meet the special needs of the deaf child in the hospital or clinic setting. See *Hospitalization, Support During.*

   a. Record on the Kardex.
      1. How the child communicates, e.g., reads lips, signs.
      2. Special gestures for common activities.
      3. Whether or not the child wears a hearing aid.

   b. Use pictures of equipment and procedures to help prepare the child. See *Preparation for Procedures.*

   c. Demonstrate procedures before you perform them and repeat as needed.

   d. Take the child on tour of hospital areas he will go to and demonstrate what equipment will be used, e.g., x-ray, physical therapy, recovery room.

   e. Assign a minimal number of persons to care for the child to reduce the new people with whom he must communicate.

   f. Do not restrain both hands unless absolutely required.

   g. Keep a nightlight in the room, since the deaf child relies on sight to tell him about his environment.

   h. Permit as much activity as possible, since the child relates to his environment in this manner.

   i. Place the child in an area of the unit where activity can be observed.

   j. Awaken the child gently.

   k. Provide additional play time for the child to work through feelings he cannot express. See *Play, Therapeutic.*

   l. Do not use the intercom, since it distorts sound and even the child with some hearing will not understand you.

3. Support the development of speech.
   a. Face the child when you speak and get down so you are face to face.
   b. Say a word and then demonstrate it.
   c. Repeat words and phrases while the child watches your face.
   d. Build on the child's interests and experiences to teach words.

4. Discuss with parents.
   a. Safety factors related to care of the deaf child.
   b. The need to provide age-appropriate activities.
   c. Ways to promote speech development.
   d. The importance of allowing the child age-appropriate independence.
   e. The importance of having a specialist fit the child with a hearing aid that meets the specific needs of the child.
   f. The need for periodic evaluation of the child's hearing and hearing aid.

5. Support the parents in accepting their child's handicap.

Death, concept development of. The child's progression in understanding death.

A. **General Considerations.**

1. Life experiences and cultural background influence the child's understanding of death.

2. Maturation of the concept of death occurs as part of normal development.

   a. Birth to 3 years.
      1. Movement between sleep and wakefulness gives the child a sense of being and nonbeing.
      2. Differentiation of self from the environment is confirmed by the game peek-a-boo in which the baby observes the object appear and disappear.
      3. The young child also experiments with separation by making things "all gone."

   b. 3 to 5 years.
      1. Death is denied.
      2. Death is equated with sleep and separation.
      3. Death is reversible.
      4. Life and consciousness are attributed to the dead, e.g., the dead can feel, cry, eat, drink, etc.
      5. The immobility is due to the coffin.

   c. 5 to 6 years.
      1. Death is gradual or temporary.
      2. There are degrees of death, e.g., "not very badly killed."

D

3. Life and death are interchangeable, e.g., "when he's tired of being dead, someone else goes in the coffin."
  d. 7 to 9 years.
    1. Death is personified, e.g., "boogie man," skeleton.
    2. Death can be avoided by "being good."
  e. 9 years and older.
    1. Death is cessation of corporal life.
    2. Death is universal and inevitable.
    3. The school-age child confirms his aliveness by dare-devilry and jokes about death.
  f. Adolescent.
    1. Concept approaches adult perception.
    2. Searches for meaning and values related to death.

B. Nursing Management.
1. Help parents evaluate their own feelings about death.
2. Encourage parents to maintain open communication with the child.
3. Explain that avoiding the subject of death denies the child the opportunity to master a painful experience.
4. Refer parents to books which can be read to the child as an introduction to the subject. See *Appendix viii.*
5. Help parents recognize the value of teaching factual information in small amounts over time.
6. Discuss with parents how the child can be helped to deal with actual death.
  a. Explain the child will perceive the parents' grief even if they do not discuss it with him.
  b. The preschooler who experiences the death of the opposite sex parent or a sibling should be reassured that his magical thoughts are not responsible for the death. See *Preschooler.*
  c. Pets may serve as an object of affection when there is death of a loved one.
  d. Include the young child in family rituals at the time of death.
  e. Avoid explanations that associate death with sleep, since the child may then fear going to bed.
  f. Explain that the child may become angry with God if he is told that the death is God's will.
  g. Encourage the child to talk about the event before and after if he attends the funeral.
  h. Answer the child's questions honestly.
  i. Encourage the parents to verbalize to the child that their sadness is due to the loss of the relationship with the loved one.
  j. Explain that the young child's response is not an accurate reflection of his true feelings.

1. The level of psychosocial development will affect his response.
2. The child's usual coping behaviors will be part of his response to this stress.
3. The child cannot stop the process of development in order to mourn.
4. The child has a short tolerance for sadness and pain.
5. The child may develop somatic symptoms such as regression, aggression, etc.
  k. The schoolage child will ask many questions about the deceased and what happens to the body, etc., as he tries to understand about death.
  l. The child needs physical gestures of affection from parents to know he is still loved.
  m. The child needs opportunities to express his feelings as much as he needs explanations.

Dental care. Measures to ensure healthy teeth.

A. General Considerations.
1. Deciduous ("baby") teeth act as pathfinders for permanent teeth.
2. Children from lower socioeconomic families have more caries and missing teeth due to lack of good nutrition and lack of proper instruction in care of teeth.
3. The initial dental examination should be when the child is around 18 to 36 months of age at the latest.
4. Caries in deciduous teeth should be repaired even though the child will lose these teeth.
5. Failure to repair caries can result in:
  a. Poor chewing, resulting in poor digestion.
  b. Abscess.
  c. Pain.
  d. Osteomyelitis.
6. Comprehensive oral health programs include:
  a. Regular dental examinations.
  b. Removal of plaque.
  c. Use of fluoride.
  d. Low cariogenic diet.
7. Dental caries can be caused by frequent use of sugar containing medication (Babington and Spadaro, 1982).
8. The chronically ill child or multiple handicapped child is at high risk for caries because of poor nutrition, long-term medication therapy, and lack of ability to be responsible for his own dental health. See *Chronic Illness* and *Handicapped Child.*
9. The infant or very young child's teeth should be brushed with an extremely small amount of fluoride toothpaste or a nonfluoride toothpaste.
10. The frequency of the child's sugar intake has more effect on causing caries than does the total amount of sugar eaten.

B. Nursing Management.

1. Observe and record the number and condition of teeth and condition of gums.
2. Teach the child and parents the importance of daily dental care at all ages.
   a. Tell parents dental care should begin when the first tooth erupts.
   b. Demonstrate to parents how to clean the child's tooth/teeth with gauze wrapped around the parent's finger until the child is about 18 months of age.
      1. Gingival teeth are too tender to brush.
      2. The use of toothpaste is not necessary.
      3. Clear water should be offered after each feeding to rid the mouth of carbohydrate.
      4. Position the child supine on the parent's lap or on the floor in front of the parent with his back to the parent and his body between the parent's legs (Kilmon and Helpin, 1981).
   c. Demonstrate to the child and parents how to floss and brush the child's teeth after 18 months of age.
      1. Tell the child not to swallow the toothpaste.
      2. Use a small, soft medium toothbrush.
      3. Use unwaxed dental floss.
      4. Stress the importance of the mechanical action to remove food.
3. Teach the parents to make dental care an enjoyable experience so that oral hygiene can be viewed positively.
   a. Allow plenty of time for tooth brushing.
   b. Provide a stool for the child for easier access to the sink.
   c. Encourage the parents to brush the child's teeth and then let the child brush.
   d. Allow the child to watch the parents brush their teeth.
   e. Allow the child to choose the toothbrush and toothpaste.
   f. Use disclosing tablets to assess effectiveness of brushing.
   g. Praise the child for his efforts.
4. Inform the parents that until the child is 5 years of age he usually lacks the fine motor coordination required for adequate brushing.
5. Teach the child and parents that optimum general health reduces the probability of caries.
   a. Proper nutrition. See *Nutrition.*
   b. Adequate rest. See *Sleep.*
   c. Protection from mouth injuries.
6. Urge the parents to call their family dentist or a pedodonist regarding the age of the child at the first visit.
7. Teach the parents to prepare the child for the initial dental visit.
   a. Discuss the purpose of the visit in terms that the child can understand.
   b. Approach the subject matter-of-factly and positively.
   c. Discuss what will happen.
   d. Encourage the child to ask questions and answer them truthfully.
   e. Visit the dentist's office prior to the appointment for exploration of the office and equipment, if possible.
   f. Visit the library and select a book about a dental visit.
   g. Allow the child to take his security blanket or animal.
8. Teach parents to observe and report abnormal conditions of the teeth and gums.
   a. Drifting of permanent teeth caused by loss of deciduous teeth.
   b. Darkening spots, pits, or fissures indicating decay.
   c. Bleeding gums.
9. Teach expectant parents and parents of infants the perils of the "Nursing Bottle Syndrome." See *Nursing Bottle Syndrome.*
10. Teach the child and parents that foods such as raw carrots and apples promote cleaning effect of the teeth when chewing.
11. Instruct the parents that the child's teeth should be brushed after each meal, snack, and administration of medication.
12. Encourage parents to teach the older child to rinse the mouth well with water if brushing is impossible, e.g., at school.
13. Encourage parents to discuss with the dentist or physician methods of providing fluoride if the water supply is not fluoridated.
14. Teach the child and parents to limit refined sugar intake as well as intake of natural foods such as honey, molasses, corn syrup, and dried fruits such as raisins which are high in sugar.
15. Discuss the special needs for dental care with the parents of the chronically ill or handicapped child.
16. Teach the child and parents about resources for dental education and service.
    a. School dental health program.
    b. Media advertisements.
    c. Dental insurance plans.
    d. Health department.

Dermatitis, atopic (eczema). Chronic superficial skin inflammation of unknown etiology.

A. General Considerations.

1. Infantile eczema usually begins at 2 to 3 months of age and resolves around 3 years of age.
   a. The cheeks and scalp are affected first.

D

  b. Extensor aspects of the extremities are involved next.
 2. About one-third of the children will progress to childhood eczema which may last from 2 years to adolescence.
  a. Antecubital and popliteal fossae are involved.
  b. Neck, wrists, hands, and feet may be affected.
  c. Enlargement of lymph nodes is common adjacent to affected sites.
 3. Pathogenic factors may include:
  a. Environment: heat, humidty, and external irritants.
  b. Immunological factors: food allergies.
  c. Emotional factors: response to stress.
  d. Heredity: family history of allergies.
  e. Genetically abnormal (dry) skin.
 4. Infants are most commonly allergic to foods such as cow's milk, egg albumin, or wheat.
 5. Environmental inhalants and pollen become stronger allergens as the child grows older.
 6. The disease is characterized by exacerbations and remissions.
 7. Secondary bacterial infection is common.
 8. Treatment is primarily supportive with the first goal the removal of the offending allergens.
 9. Breast feeding and hypoallergenic diets may be beneficial to infants with a family history of allergy.
 10. Treatment failure is usually due to noncompliance.

B. Nursing Management.
 1. Support the child and parents during hospitalization. See *Hospitalization, Support During.*
 2. Initiate discharge planning. See *Discharge Planning.*
 3. Obtain a thorough nursing history which includes a nutritional assessment.
 4. Help parents adjust to the diagnosis.
  a. Encourage them to verbalize their feelings.
  b. Identify positive aspects of the child's growth and development.
  c. Answer questions honestly.
  d. Record what parents have been told on the Kardex or clinic record.
 5. Apply steroid or coal tar ointment as ordered.
  a. Apply a thin film.
  b. Apply with an ungloved hand.
   1. Thickness of medication can be gauged more accurately.
   2. Skin changes can be assessed.
   3. Using gloves may suggest to the child that he is "untouchable."
  c. Do not apply steroid creams around the eyes.

  d. Wash hands thoroughly after the procedure.
 6. Apply wet dressings as ordered.
  a. Use clean, not sterile technique.
  b. Moisten the dressing and squeeze out excess.
  c. Cover dressings immediately with dry flannel to retain warmth.
  d. Pin dressings snugly to prevent chilling.
  e. Do not allow pins to touch patient.
  f. Use stockinette or cotton socks to cover arm or leg dressings.
 7. Observe, record, and report the child's response to medications, e.g., antipyretics, sedatives, and antibiotics. See *Administration of Medications, Parental.*
 8. Bathe in tepid water without soap.
 9. Add emollient lotion or oil half-way through the bath after skin has been hydrated.
 10. Pat skin dry, do not rub.
 11. Promote rest.
  a. Avoid scheduling potentially traumatic treatments at nap or bedtimes.
  b. Administer sedation prior to bedtime if ordered PRN.
  c. Give soothing bath before sleep.
 12. Meet emotional needs.
  a. Provide frequent physical contact.
  b. Provide consistent nursing care.
  c. Provide release from tension and frustration.
   1. Pacifier for infant.
   2. Pounding board.
   3. Bean bags to throw.
   4. Ring toss game.
  d. Provide age-appropriate stimulation. See *Stimulation.*
 13. Prevent secondary bacterial infection.
  a. Use good handwashing technique.
  b. Keep the child's nails clipped and clean.
  c. Apply elbow or mitt restraints if absolutely necessary when the child cannot be supervised. See *Restraints.*
  d. Provide diversionary activities which require use of the hands.
   1. Puzzles.
   2. Coloring.
   3. Blocks.
 14. Observe, record, and report changes in the appearance and location of skin lesions.
 15. Protect the child from sunlight since coal tar ointments increase photosensitivity.
 16. Check dietary tray before serving patient if food allergens have been identified.
 17. Help the older child deal with altered body image. See *Body Image.*
 18. Teach the child and parents home management.

a. Review nursing care meaures described above.

b. Help the mother plan ways to incorporate treatment regimen into family routine.

c. Encourage the mother to dress the child appropriately.
   1. Avoid wool and rough synthetic clothing.
   2. Wash new clothes before the child wears them.
   3. Rinse clothing well after laundering.
   4. Do not overdress since heat will cause itching.

d. Discuss the purchase of a humidifier for the bedroom if the skin is dry.

e. Discuss dietary restrictions if appropriate.

f. Assist the mother to treat the child as normally as possible.
   1. Reinforce the positive ways she interacts with her child.
   2. Help her set age-appropriate limits on behavior.
   3. Help parents understand that the child's irritability is caused by his discomfort and that he is not an "irritable" child.
   4. Encourage the parent to provide body contact and cuddling.

g. Teach the mother to remove coal tar ointment from sheets by rubbing both sides with lard or cooking oil.

h. Suggest that the mother bathe child in starch or oatmeal baths to relieve itching.

19. Discuss with the parents that negative feelings toward the child's disease and treatment required are normal, but must be dealt with to assure a positive parent–child relationship.

20. Initiate a referral to the public health nurse if parents have trouble coping or if the child has required repeated hospitalizations.

Dermatitis, contact.
Delayed hypersensitivity response of the skin to contact with an allergen.

A. **General Considerations.**
   1. Distribution of the lesions on the body aids in diagnosis, e.g., face lesions due to cosmetics, arm lesions due to poison ivy.
   2. Intense itching is characteristic.
   3. Patch testing may be done to identify allergens if elimination of suspected agents is unsuccessful.
   4. Skin reaction may progress from erythema to papules, vesicles, and frank weeping.
   5. The goal of treatment is to prevent further skin exposure to the offending substance.
   6. The skin will usually heal without further treat-

ment unless the child is exposed again or a secondary infection develops.

7. One of the most common examples of contact dermatitis is poison ivy which is treated with steroids to reduce inflammation, cool compresses, an antihistaminic/sedative or analgesic.

B. **Nursing Management.**
   1. Obtain a thorough history of exposure.
   2. Teach the child and parents to avoid offending substances.
      a. Teach the child how to recognize poison ivy.
      b. Encourage thorough washing after suspected contact.
      c. Dress the child appropriately for outdoor activity.
      d. Read fabric labels.
      e. Wash new clothing prior to first wearing.
      f. Use hypoallergenic skin cleansers and makeup if the rash is on the face.
      g. Rinse all laundry thoroughly.
      h. Use a minimum number of household cleaning products.
   3. Teach the mother how to apply wet soaks if ordered.
      a. Use clean, not sterile technique.
      b. Moisten the dressing and squeeze out excess.
      c. Cover dressings immediately with dry flannel to retain warmth.
      d. Pin dressings snugly to prevent chilling.
      e. Do not allow pins to touch the child.
      f. Use cotton socks to cover arm or leg dressings.
   4. Teach the mother to apply lotion or pastes by patting, not rubbing.
   5. Avoid all secondary irritation such as detergents, wool, etc.
   6. Review dose, time, action, and side effects if antibiotics, antihistamines, or steroids are ordered. See *Administration of Medications, Parental.*
   7. Prevent infection.
      a. Wash hands frequently.
      b. Keep the child's fingernails short and clean.
      c. Keep skin clean and dry.
      d. Allow vesicles to rupture spontaneously.
   8. Provide comfort measures.
      a. Bathe in lukewarm water with starch, baking soda, or oatmeal, and pat dry.
      b. Dress in lightweight, soft clothing.

Dermatitis, diaper.
Inflammation of the skin in the diaper area due to contact with urine and/or feces.

A. **General Considerations.**
   1. Signs and symptoms include an initial redness

of the skin followed by the development of red bumps and a thickened appearance of the skin.

2. It must be differentiated from a fungal infection caused by *Candida albicans*. See *Candida albicans*.
3. Predisposing factors include:
   a. Poor hygienic practices.
   b. Irritating laundry substances retained in the diaper fabric.
   c. Increased urine ammonia levels.
4. Treatment involves symptomatic relief and elimination of the causative factor(s).
5. Disposable diapers may act as irritants to some infants' skin.

B. Nursing Management.
   1. Prevent skin irritation and breakdown.
      a. Change diapers frequently.
      b. Wash the diaper area with clear water with each diaper change.
      c. Dry the area thoroughly, especially in folds.
      d. Avoid the use of rubber pants.
      e. Apply protective skin ointments or lotions, e.g., Vaseline, Desitin, A and D ointment.
   2. Promote healing.
      a. Wash with clear water, thoroughly dry, and expose the diaper area to:
         1. The air for 20 minutes two to three times a day.
         2. A 20-watt bulb in a gooseneck lamp placed at least 12 inches from the diaper area for 20 minutes two to three times a day.
      b. Apply ointment or lotion as needed to form a moisture barrier.
      c. Use talcum powder if powder is used, since it takes up moisture.
      d. Do not use cornstarch, since it promotes the growth of *Candida albicans* (Weston, Philpott, and Philpott, 1976).
      e. Do not use powder when either lotions or ointments are used since this blocks pores.
   3. Make sure that the light bulb in the lamp is covered by a small mesh screen so that if breakage occurs the child will not be injured.
   4. Prevent inhalation of talcum powder by shaking powder into your hand and then rubbing on infant.
   5. Observe, record, and report signs of secondary infection by *Candida albicans* which include a deep red, raised area surrounded by small, pustular satellite lesions.
   6. Teach the parents:
      a. How to prevent skin irritation and breakdown.
      b. Methods to promote healing.
      c. Laundering techniques to use for diapers.
         1. Soak diapers in a gallon of water with half cup of Borax before washing (Brown and Murphy, 1975).
         2. Use a mild soap.
         3. Double rinse diapers.
         4. Do not use fabric softeners, since these decrease absorbency and may be irritating.
         5. Hang diapers in the sun to dry if possible.
      d. To try cloth diapers if disposables cause irritation.
      e. Signs of *Candida Albicans* infection to report to the physician or nurse practitioner.

Dermatitis, seborrheic. Erythematous, nonpruritic, scaly condition of the face, scalp, or perineum.

A. General Considerations.
   1. Accumulations of high levels of sweat, sebum, and dirt are thought to be partially responsible.
   2. The problem is commonly seen in infants whose mothers are afraid to wash their heads.
   3. Variations in the disease include:
      a. Cradle cap in the infant.
      b. Dermatitis of the diaper area in the infant.
      c. Blepharitis marginalis.
      d. Otitis externa.
      e. Dandruff.
      f. Dermatitis of the midsternum, upper midback, or head of the older child.
   4. The lesions are characteristic in appearance.
      a. Salmon colored erythema.
      b. Greasy scales.
      c. Yellow crusty patches.
   5. The lesions may start at the scalp and spread to the entire body if untreated.
   6. Treatment includes:
      a. Selenium sulfide shampoo.
      b. Sulfur and salicyclic acid ointments.
      c. Coal tar bath solutions.
      d. Steroid creams.
      e. Antibiotics for secondary infections.

B. Nursing Management.
   1. Observe the scalps of infants, children, and adolescents as part of the nursing assessment.
   2. Teach the child and parents to administer and to observe for response to medications.
   3. Teach the child and parents management of the lesions.
      a. Apply petroleum jelly or mineral oil to loosen the scales in severe cases.
      b. Brush the hair or use a fine toothed comb to remove the scales.
      c. Shampoo the hair and rinse well.
      d. Keep the nails clipped and clean.
      e. Apply topical medications to other parts of the body as instructed.

f. Dress the child in soft, loose, absorbent clothing.
4. Teach the child and parents to recognize and report signs of secondary infection.
   a. Inflamed sores.
   b. Accumulation of pus.
   c. Constant itching.
5. Teach the child and parents preventive measures.
   a. Demonstrate proper headwashing to the child and/or parents.
   b. Encourage daily cleansing with a mild soap or shampoo and thorough rinsing and drying.
   c. Review principles of general hygiene.

Diabetes mellitus. Metabolic disease of unknown etiology resulting from a deficiency of insulin and irregularity in glucagon release.

A. **General Considerations.**
1. The onset of symptoms of overt diabetes is usually acute.
   a. Fatigue.
   b. Enuresis resulting from polyuria.
   c. Polyuria.
   d. Polyphagia.
   e. Polydypsia.
   f. Weight loss.
2. An oral glucose tolerance test with insulin assay is used to confirm the diagnosis.
3. The goals of management are to promote normal growth and development, to prevent or delay possible complications, and to allow the child as normal a life style as possible.
4. Most children have insulin dependent diabetes and oral hypoglycemic agents are not effective treatment.
5. The amount of insulin required by the child will vary in some circumstances.
   a. Exercise decreases the body's insulin requirements.
   b. Trauma, stress, and infection increase the body's requirements.
6. Early and adequate insulin therapy may stimulate insulin production and decrease the insulin requirements for a temporary period called the "honeymoon" phase.
7. Some children require two injections a day to achieve metabolic control.
8. Most children receive a combination of rapid- and intermediate-acting insulin.
9. The child and parents must learn to manage a continuum of acute episodes due to the disease and its treatment.
   a. Diabetic ketoacidosis (DKA): the most acute state of glucose intolerance which includes dehydration and resultant fluid and electrolyte imbalance.
      1. Hyperlipidemia, hyperkalemia, or hypokalemia and CNS depression may occur.
      2. Kussmaul (deep and rapid) respirations and acetone smell of the breath are classic symptoms.
   b. Diabetic ketosis: glucose and ketones are present in the blood and urine, but the child is not acidotic.
   c. Hyperglycemia: glucose is present in the blood and urine, but ketones are not.
10. Insulin is not well absorbed from hypertrophied or atrophied injection sites so the child's response to the same dosage will vary with the condition of the site.
11. The short-term complications in juvenile diabetes mellitus are:
    a. Diabetic ketoacidosis. Because glucose is unavailable for cells, the body breaks down protein and fat resulting in ketone bodies in the bloodstream and urine.
    b. Hypoglycemia (insulin shock). Low blood sugar level.
12. Diabetic ketoacidosis is usually secondary to infection which causes dehydration, not dietary indiscretion.
13. Hypoglycemia is due to overdosage or improper distribution of insulin or to imbalance of food and exercise.
14. When differentiation between hyperglycemia and hypoglycemia is in doubt, the child should be treated for hypoglycemia to prevent brain damage from lack of glucose.
15. If it is difficult to maintain metabolic control, special equipment may be necessary such as the blood glucose testing meter and the insulin pump.
16. Rapid swings from marked glycosuria to hyperglycemia may be due to the Somogyi reflex.
    a. Counterregulatory hormones are triggered by a decrease blood glucose level.
    b. The blood sugar level then rises above normal for a period of time.
    c. The treatment is to decrease the insulin, or preferably, to increase the food.
17. The adolescent who has not been allowed the responsibility of administering insulin, checking urine, and controlling his diet may rebel against parental control by refusing to follow treatment regimen resulting in ketoacidosis.
18. The child who is in poor control is more vulnerable to infection, since white blood cells phagocytize bacteria less well in a high glucose environment.
19. Long-term or chronic complications include:
    a. Retinopathy.

b. Nephropathy.

c. Neuropathy.

B. Nursing Management. See CHRONIC ILLNESS and LIFE-THREATENING ILLNESS.

1. Support the child and parents during hospitalization. See *Hospitalization, Support During.*
2. Initiate discharge planning. See *Discharge Planning.*
3. Meet the physical needs of the child in ketoacidosis.
   a. Administer insulin as ordered.
      1. One-half of dose I.V. by constant infusion pump.
      2. One-half of dose SQ or I.V. bolus.
      3. Rotate injection sites.
   b. Monitor I.V. rate accurately.
   c. Monitor vital signs as ordered.
      1. Decreased respirations indicate profound acidosis.
      2. Increased pulse occurs as epinephrine is released in response to hypoglycemia.
   d. Do not add potassium to the I.V. fluid until the child has voided since potassium is excreted by the kidneys.
   e. Check sugar and acetone levels in urine every hour.
   f. Maintain strict I and O records.
   g. Observe, record, and report the following symptoms of hypokalemia:
      1. Cardiac arrhythmia.
      2. Gastric atony.
      3. Ileus.
      4. Leg cramps.
      5. Weakness.
      6. Muscle paralysis.
   h. Observe, record, and report infection symptoms.
   i. Begin oral feedings as ordered.
      1. Offer clear fluids frequently. See *Forcing Fluids.*
      2. Progress to four equal feedings or three feedings plus a midnight snack.
4. Meet the physical needs of the child in ketosis.
   a. Administer regular insulin every 4 to 6 hours as ordered.
   b. Rotate injection sites.
   c. Check urine sugar and acetone levels as ordered.
      1. Clarify with the physician whether first or second voided specimens should be checked.
      2. Check first specimen even if double voiding is desired, since the child may be unable to void again.

d. Begin regular diet as ordered.
   1. Give feeding 20 to 30 minutes after the injection of regular insulin.
   2. Institute usual three meal-three snack pattern when hyperglycemia is controlled.
5. Meet the physical needs of the child with hyperglycemia.
   a. Administer small doses of regular insulin as ordered.
   b. Rotate injection sites.
   c. Check urine sugar and acetone levels as ordered.
   d. Institute oral feedings as ordered.
6. Meet the physical needs of the child when initial stabilization is achieved.
   a. Encourage the child to eat all food sent on the diet tray.
   b. Have the child empty his bladder, then collect fractional urines, single-voided or double-voided specimens as ordered.
   c. Record the results of the sugar and acetone tests of urine.
   d. Rotate injection sites.
7. Meet the psychological needs of the child and family.
   a. Support the child's and parents' need to adjust to the diagnosis, since the demands of coping may not leave energy for learning new tasks.
   b. Record what the child and parents have been told about the diagnosis on the Kardex.
   c. Answer all questions honestly.
   d. Explain there may be a "honeymoon" period in which the insulin dosage is reduced, but this is a temporary phase.
8. Teach the child and parents about hyperglycemia.
   a. Review symptoms.
      1. Flushed face.
      2. Fatigue.
      3. Double or blurred vision.
      4. Irritability.
      5. Fruity smelling breath.
      6. Nausea and vomiting.
      7. Thirst.
      8. Hunger.
      9. Frequent urination.
      10. Headache.
      11. Coma.
   b. Explain how to manage hyperglycemic episodes.
      1. Increase insulin dosage as instructed by physican when the child has an infection.
      2. Decrease food intake during an infection.

c. Explore the child's and parent's understanding of when the physican should be notified.

9. Teach the child and parents about hypoglycemia.
   a. Review symptoms.
      1. Pallor.
      2. Staggering gait.
      3. Seizures.
      4. Yawning.
      5. Dilated pupils.
      6. Behavior changes.
      7. Trembling.
      8. Cold, clammy sweat.
      9. Difficulty in talking.
      10. Headache.
      11. Coma.
   b. Explain how to manage hypoglycemic episodes.
      1. Administer pure glucose tablets since the amount of glucose given can be controlled.
      2. Give milk, food, or juice if glucose pills are unavailable.
      3. Give I.M. glucogon if the reaction is severe and/or the child cannot swallow.
      4. Provide the school-age child with glucose pills or hard candy so he does not have to leave the classroom.

10. Initiate teaching about insulin therapy. See *Preparation for Procedures.*
    a. Discuss with parents that insulin is a life-giving medication.
    b. Assess the child's developmental level and fine-motor coordination before deciding if he should give his own insulin.
    c. Assist the child and parents in developing a rotation pattern.
       1. A site should be used only once every 60 to 90 days.
       2. Atrophy or fibrosis of the site may occur if the sites are not rotated.
       3. Absorption from fibrotic areas is slow and incomplete.
    d. Explain that parents should give the injection in sites the child cannot reach so they can keep in practice.
    e. Insert the needle into a subcutaneous pocket and aspirate before injecting.
    f. Tell parents that at some time a painful injection will occur and support will be needed to allay the child's fears.
    g. Teach the child and parent to withdraw insulin from the same bottle first each time to prevent contamination of both bottles.
    h. Store the bottle of insulin in daily use away from heat and at room temperature.
    i. Review guidelines for adjustment of insulin dosage if ordered by physician.
    j. Teach the child and parents about the use of the insulin pump and/or blood glucose testing meter according to instructions and hospital policy.

11. Teach the child and parents the dietary management.
    a. Review dietary plan ordered by the physician.
    b. Help the family incorporate the child's management into their normal life style.
    c. Anticipate that the schoolchild and adolescent will have some problem with dietary restrictions.
       1. Encourage fruit rather than candy if the child is hungry.
       2. Suggest the child exercise, preferably with a friend, to balance the intake.
       3. Encourage the child to give the body time to absorb the snack before eating additional food.
       4. Encourage the child to talk with the physican about a diet change if constant hunger is a problem.
    d. Encourage the child and parents to use "free" foods creatively, e.g., unsweetened gelatin blocks, raw group A vegetables.
    e. Teach the child and parents that food intake must be balanced with exercise.
       1. Addition or deletion of food in relation to more or less exercise can only be determined by trial and error.
       2. Results of urine testing and absence of hypoglycemic symptoms are important in determining this balance.

12. Teach the child and parents about urine testing.
    a. Be aware that double voiding is seldom practical for home management.
    b. Teach the two- or five-drop Clinitest method depending on which will be used at home.
    c. Explain that touching the Clinitest tablet may give a false result and may cause a caustic burn.
    d. Instruct the child and parents to keep their eyes on the test tube to detect a "pass through" color change.
    e. Explain that tape or stick methods are more convenient, but may be less accurate.
    f. Prevent faking of the results by praising the child for testing the urine accurately rather than obtaining negative sugar and acetone.
    g. Recognize that urine testing will become a chore even if the child is enthusiastic initially.

13. Teach the child and parents about the importance of good hygiene and routine health promotion.
  a. Encourage frequent bathing to decrease skin bacteria.
  b. Explain that foot care is important, since circulation to the lower extremities may be impaired.
    1. Apply lotion to keep the skin soft.
    2. Trim nails straight across.
    3. Purchase proper size shoes of materials other than plastic or vinyl to permit ventilation.
    4. Purchase cotton and/or white socks to decrease problems with lack of absorption and dyes.
    5. Avoid calluses and blisters.
  c. Maintain good dental hygiene to prevent abscesses. See *Dental Care.*
  d. Keep immunization status current.
  e. Have eyes examined regularly, since retinopathy is a long-term complication.
14. Teach parents to keep daily records so problems can be prevented by altering management.
  a. Daily urine checks.
  b. Insulin dosage.
  c. Variations from usual food and activity.
  d. Hypoglycemia.
15. Help parents to relinquish control and to let the child assume more responsibility for his own care as he matures.
16. Reassess the child's and parent's knowledge of the disease and its treatment and observe their technical skills periodically to assure there are no knowledge/skill gaps.
17. Plan separate teaching and/or review sessions with the adolescent regardless of how long he has been diagnosed, since he may be facing new problems in management. See *Adolescent.*
18. Encourage parents to explain to the child's teacher what is necessary in relation to lunch time, physical education, snacks, symptoms of hypoglycemia, and hyperglycemia.
19. Assist the parents to explore the possibility of outpatient management of ketoacidosis in the pediatric outpatient clinic or in the emergency room to prevent the trauma and expense of hospitalization (Lille and Mosteller, 1982).
20. Talk with the schoolager or adolescent about what he will tell his peers about his health problem.
  a. What the disease is.
  b. It is not contagious.
  c. How they can help by having sugar-free soda and sugar-free foods on hand.
21. Encourage the parents to provide the child

with a Medic-Alert identification, preferably a bracelet which is less likely to be missed in an emergency situation.
22. Refer the child and family to community agencies and the American Diabetes Association for assistance.
23. Assess the home environment if the adolescent experiences more than one hospitalization per year.
  a. Determine the general adolescent–parent relationship.
  b. Identify family stresses, e.g., parental separation, divorce, serious illness, death, etc.
  c. Evaluate the kind of support given by parents and other family members.
24. Refer the adolescent and family for various types of counseling, as appropriate.
  a. "Forgetting" to take insulin and extreme dietary indiscretions may be suicide attempts.
  b. The older adolescent may need vocational counseling to plan for a career.

Diaper dermatitis. See *Dermatitis, Diaper.*

Diarrhea. Accelerated excretion of the intestinal contents resulting from malabsorption of water and electrolytes.

A. General Considerations.
  1. Diarrhea may be acute or chronic in nature.
  2. Acute diarrhea may be caused by a number of conditions including:
    a. Viral gastroenteritis (most common cause).
    b. Bacterial gastroenteritis.
    c. Contaminated food stuffs.
    d. Dietary indiscretions or inappropriate feeding.
    e. Milk protein allergy.
    f. Other illnesses such as respiratory or urinary tract infections.
    g. Use of antibiotics.
  3. Chronic diarrhea may be seen with such conditions as:
    a. Carbohydrate intolerance.
    b. Milk protein allergy.
    c. Parasites.
    d. Cystic fibrosis.
    e. Maternal deprivation.
  4. There is a wide range of normal stool patterns in infants and children, and the following criteria are used to identify diarrhea:
    a. Increased frequency of stools.
    b. Watery consistency.
    c. Color of stool becomes green.
  5. The child with diarrhea may also have:
    a. Fever.
    b. Anorexia.

c. Irritability.

d. Dry mucous membranes.

e. Decreased skin turgor.

f. Blood and/or mucus in the stool.

g. Failure to gain weight or weight loss.

h. Vomiting.

i. Decreased urine volume and an increased specific gravity.

6. Complications of acute diarrhea include:

a. Dehydration.

b. Metabolic acidosis.

c. The development of chronic diarrhea.

7. Complications of chronic diarrhea include:

a. Dehydration.

b. Metabolic acidosis.

c. Poor nutritional status due to malabsorption of nutrients.

d. Delayed growth and development.

8. Complications are more common if the child:

a. Is less than a year of age.

b. Has a poor nutritional status.

c. Has had severe diarrhea.

d. Has had diarrhea for a long period of time.

9. Lab studies which may be done to determine the etiology of the diarrhea include:

a. Stool cultures.

b. Tests for fecal blood, pH, and/or reducing and nonreducing sugars, fat, and leucocytes.

c. X-ray studies of the upper and lower gastrointestinal tract.

d. Sweat chloride test for cystic fibrosis.

10. Treatment includes:

a. Placing the bowel at rest.

b. Replacement of fluid and electrolyte losses.

c. Elimination or management of the underlying cause.

11. No potassium should be given to replace losses until the child has voided, since potassium is excreted by the kidneys.

12. Home management is usually possible except for the child who is dehydrated or acutely ill.

13. Antidiarrheal drugs are not usually given since they slow intestinal motility and may prolong the course of some infectious diarrheas (Fitzgerald, 1978).

14. Lactose intolerance due to a disturbance of normal enzyme activity may persist for a period of time following cessation of the diarrhea and a lactose-free formula may be required.

15. Feedings should be infrequent and relatively large to decrease bowel stimulation.

B. **Nursing Management.** See *Gastroenteritis* and *Vomiting.*

1. Support the child and parents during hospitalization. See *Hospitalization, Support During.*

2. Initiate discharge planning. See *Discharge Planning.*

3. Isolate the child to prevent cross-contamination in cases of infectious diarrhea. See *Isolated Child.*

a. Use enteric isolation.

b. Wash hands thoroughly between contact with children.

4. Keep the child NPO as ordered to rest the gastrointestinal tract.

5. Meet the needs of the child who is NPO.

a. Give frequent mouth care.

b. Provide a pacifier for the infant to meet sucking needs.

6. Tell parents the rationale for keeping the child NPO.

7. Provide basis for calculating fluid needs.

a. Record intake and output accurately.

b. Weigh the child daily.

c. Weigh diapers as ordered.

8. Weigh child.

a. At the same time each day.

b. Before feeding.

c. Nude.

d. On the same scale.

9. Promote fluid and electrolyte balance.

a. Maintain I.V. or give P.O. fluids in amount ordered.

b. Maintain a stable environmental temperature to decrease insensible water loss.

10. Advance the diet as ordered adding milk and milk products last.

11. Observe, record, and report the following:

a. Characteristics of stools.

1. Number.

2. Color.

3. Consistency.

4. Odor.

5. Presence of blood and/or mucus.

b. Signs and symptoms of fluid and electrolyte imbalance. See *Fluid and Electrolyte Imbalance.*

12. Prevent irritation and breakdown of anal mucosa and perineum.

a. Take axillary temperatures.

b. Change diapers as soon as possible after they are wet or soiled.

c. Wash and thoroughly dry the perineum after each stool.

d. Expose the perineal area to the air.

13. Test stools as ordered for the presence of blood and/or glucose using a fresh specimen.

14. Collect stool specimens as ordered.

15. Teach parents enteric isolation technique.

16. Teach parents home management of diarrhea as follows, unless otherwise instructed.

a. Progress diet as follows.

1. Stop all milk and milk products.

2. Give sips of clear liquids every ½ to 1

D

hour and increase as tolerated for the first 24 hours, e.g., give flat, diluted coke, gingerale, diluted sweetened tea, Gatorade, or a commercial electrolyte solution.

3. Add plain solids after 24 hours if diarrhea is improving, e.g., bananas, rice cereal, applesauce, etc.
4. Increase plain solids on third day, e.g., dry toast, saltines, plain baked potato, etc.
5. Add milk and milk products last, starting with half-strength formula and progressing to full strength if tolerated.
6. Offer yogurt when milk products are added. This helps to restore normal bowel flora.

b. Stop all solids and milk if diarrhea recurs and start again with sips of liquids.

c. Explain the rationale for milk-free formula if this is ordered.

d. Call the doctor if the child does not respond to dietary management within 12 hours if under age 3 months, 24 hours if the child is under 1 year, 48 hours if the child is over 1 year, or if the child:

1. Refuses liquids.
2. Shows signs of dehydration. See *Fluid and Electrolyte Imbalance.*
3. Develops a fever over 102°F rectally.
4. Has a distended abdomen.
5. Develops vomiting.
6. Urinates less than twice between 8:00 A.M. and 8:00 P.M.
7. Has blood and/or mucus in the stool.

Diet. See *Nutrition.*

Discharge from the hospital. Procedures related to sending the child home.

A. General Considerations.

1. The child who has been hospitalized for a period of time and/or has an altered body image may be reluctant to leave the hospital, since it has become a "safe place."
2. Children may have concerns about being accepted by their siblings, peer group, classmates.
3. Parents may have many concerns about their ability to care for the child at home.
4. Children and parents may be happy to go but may have difficulty saying goodbye to staff members with whom they have developed relationships.
5. Once home, children may exhibit a variety of behaviors in response to the hospitalization, for example, withdrawal, sleep disturbances, regression, clinging, aggression, etc. See *Sleep* and *Regression.*

6. The child between 6 months and 4 years of age is most vulnerable to the effects of separation and may exhibit the most pronounced behavior changes.
7. Adolescents may have mixed emotions about being discharged; pleasure at the thought of increased independence may be mixed with concern about return to peer group and school.

B. Nursing Management.

1. Inform the child and parents of the discharge date as soon as known if the physician has not already done so.
2. Check the Kardex for any teaching and referral needs that have not been met and plan for their completion. See *Discharge Planning.*
3. Accept any negative response to the planned discharge in a nonjudgmental manner.
4. Support the parents if they express concern about being able to cope at home.
   a. Do not give false reassurance.
   b. Review what they have learned to do while in the hospital.
   c. Assess the parents for additional teaching and/or referral needs.
   d. Make sure they have the name and phone number of someone they can call for assistance.
5. Explain your agency's discharge procedure to the parents so they know what to do, e.g., where the cashier's office is, how they can handle their bill, what time they should get the child, where they can park, etc.
6. Support the child if he expresses concern about being accepted at home.
   a. Do not give false reassurance.
   b. Remind him of signs that he has not been forgotten, e.g., cards, phone calls, visits, etc.
   c. Help the child identify activities he might plan that would include a friend or classmate.
   d. Assist the child in deciding how and what he will tell his peers about his illness and hospitalization.
7. Support the adolescent.
   a. Encourage verbalization of feelings.
   b. Take a positive approach but do not offer false reassurance.
   c. Assist in the identification of things adolescent might do to facilitate adjustment to home, school, and peers, e.g., invite a few close friends over to talk before returning to school, arrange to talk with teachers privately about making up any missed work.
   d. Tell adolescent that he/she is welcome to call the unit after discharge to discuss concerns.

8. Reassure the child and parents that you will not forget them as soon as they are gone.
9. Teach the parents how to cope with the behaviors exhibited following discharge (Wilkinson, 1978).
   a. Discuss developmental principles and the effects of illness and hospitalization on the child's development. See *Hospitalization, Response to.*
   b. Stress that some behavioral change is normal.
   c. Tell them that some leniency during the adjustment phase is a good idea but that the child needs consistent limit setting to feel secure.
   d. Tell them that the child should not be punished for his behavior nor should it be reinforced.
   e. Encourage parents to start out leaving the child for short periods and slowly increase the time until the child can tolerate the separation.
   f. Encourage them to provide the child with play materials that he can use to work through his feelings about hospitalization, e.g., doctor/nurse play kits, paper and crayons, clay, play hospital, etc. See *Play, Therapeutic.*

Discharge planning. A systematic approach to assisting the child and parents in their readjustment to the home environment.

A. **General Considerations.**
   1. Planning for discharge is an ongoing process that should be initiated at the time of admission.
   2. The objectives of discharge planning include:
      a. Providing for continuity of care so that there is a smooth transition from the hospital to the home setting.
      b. Giving the child and parents the information and instruction they need in order to promote optimal home care, since they may have many concerns about their ability to manage.
      c. Initiating referrals to agencies or persons in the community who can assist the child and/or parents in meeting their ongoing health care needs.
   3. Achievement of discharge planning objectives is most likely to occur if the nurse and family have worked together to develop mutual goals.

B. **Nursing Management.** See *Discharge from the Hospital.*
   1. Develop an optimal discharge plan.
      a. Have one nurse coordinate the plan.
      b. Involve the child and parents in the development of the plan.
         1. Ask about specific concerns and needs and include them in the plan.
         2. Identify mutual short- and long-term goals.
         3. Consider the family's life style, culture, religious beliefs and practices, support system, and financial resources.
      c. Include the child's ongoing health care needs in the plan as well as needs related to the current diagnosis, e.g., need for immunizations, vision screening, etc.
      d. Identify individuals and/or agencies to whom referrals will need to be made.
      e. Record the plan on the Kardex as it is developed and implemented.
   2. Carry out the plan.
      a. Use teaching principles to give information and/or help the child and parents learn treatments and procedures.
         1. Identify what it is the child and parents want to learn and need to learn.
         2. Record teaching areas on the Kardex as they are identified.
         3. Start with the topic about which the child and/or parents are most motivated to learn and then include essential content.
         4. Provide factual information and explain the implications of what you teach so the child and parents can see the relationship to their situation.
         5. Assess the capabilities of the child and parents and help them to learn to do what they can for themselves.
         6. Use language that is understood by the child and parents.
         7. Write out information or provide printed materials if the material presented is difficult to remember.
         8. If you cannot provide the information or answer, say so and then find someone to help you.
      b. Use developmental guidelines in teaching children (Pidgeon, 1977).
         1. Do not rely on verbal communication with the preschool child but also use visual, tactile, auditory, and motor learning experiences, e.g., use puppets to demonstrate bandage changes, or a tape recording of the sounds associated with cast removal.
         2. Explain the causation of and treatment rationale for the school-age child's illness, since he can often understand causation.
         3. Move from teaching the concrete and tangible (e.g., how to do a procedure) to

D

the abstract and intangible (e.g., why the procedure is done) when teaching the school-age child, since he remains absorbed with concrete reality.

4. Explain the rationale for and significance of a procedure and then proceed to the details of performance when teaching an adolescent, since he is capable of abstract thinking and very interested in theories.

c. Teach the child and parents the following, if applicable:

1. Facts about the illness and injury and the implications for the child and family.
2. Administration of medications.
3. Dietary requirements and/or restrictions.
4. Activities in which the child may or may not engage.
5. When the child may return to school.
6. How to carry out treatments, procedures, and/or exercises at home.
7. How to modify activities of daily living and/or the environment to meet the child's needs.
8. Signs and symptoms related to the disease and/or medications which should be reported to the physician.
9. How to contact the physician and/or nurse for assistance.
10. When they are to bring the child back to the hospital, clinic, or office for follow-up care or evaluation.
11. Age-appropriate play activities to promote development.
12. How to contact any referral agency or when they have an appointment if one has been made.

d. Initiate referrals as the need is identified with the child and parents.

1. Follow the referral system of your agency.
2. Obtain a referral directory for your unit if one is not available, e.g., Medicare and Medicaid Directory.
3. Give the child and family specific written information about any referral which is completed, e.g., agency, date, time, person to see at agency.
4. Assist the parents if they are to make contact with the agency by providing the name, location, and phone number of agency and person with whom to make contact.

e. Summarize the discharge plan in writing and give a copy to the parents and any referral agency and keep one with the child's records.

f. Initial each part of the plan on the Kardex as it is carried out so that the staff knows what has been taught and can reinforce learning.

3. Evaluate the plan.

a. Review the summary with the child and parents, validate their understanding of each area, and date and initial each item.
b. Ask for feedback from the child, parents, and any referral agencies in order to improve discharge planning.

Discipline. Guidance to help the child learn to control his own behavior and to get along with others and action taken by adults when the child has not complied with behavioral limits.

A. General Considerations.

1. Discipline is a part of a socialization process begun by parents.
   a. The child must learn to reach his goals by methods that are not destructive to himself or to others.
   b. The child needs to understand social standards of behavior.
2. As a rule, the clearer the limits set for the child, the less discipline is needed.
3. Parents are most likely to use disciplinary measures used by their own parents.
4. Parents may need assistance in identifying alternative disciplinary measures.
5. The child will feel more secure in the long run if parents set realistic limits.
   a. The young child does not have the knowledge or experience to make safe judgments.
   b. Limit-setting by parents helps the child learn right from wrong.
   c. The child will demonstrate anger initially when denied something he wants.
   d. Limits on behavior must be appropriate to the child's level of development.
6. Both parents must agree on the expectations for the child and on actions to be taken if the child misbehaves.
7. Punishment is a positive aspect of discipline if it resolves the conflict between the child's behavior and parental expectations.
   a. Punishment must be associated immediately with the child's action, since the young child quickly forgets his misbehavior.
   b. Delaying punishment until the father is home can jeopardize a good father–child relationship.
   c. The selection of a punishment must be one that is consistent with the severity of the

child's action, e.g., verbal scolding for breaking an object carelessly; withdrawal of a privilege for actively breaking a family rule.

d. The child should be helped to understand that the punishment is a logical consequence of his error in decision making.

e. Parents should avoid using the same punishment for every offense, e.g., limiting television viewing regardless of whether that is related to the child's misbehavior.

f. Time out (placing the child in an isolated or unstimulating place) is effective because it involves no physical punishment, no reasoning or scolding, and is easy to apply consistently.

8. The child who has done something wrong for which he was not punished may misbehave in order to be punished for the first offense.

9. Children who are not given attention for positive behavior may misbehave just to get attention.

10. Limit-setting should be reserved for those situations in which the child's welfare is affected, rather than every aspect of his behavior.

11. The love, trust, and discipline provided in early childhood is the foundation for the adolescent's socially acceptable behavior.

B. **Nursing Management.** See BEHAVIOR PROBLEMS.

1. Teach the parents the principles of discipline with the infant.

a. Begin to use the word "no" when the infant reaches 8 to 9 months of age.

b. Remove the infant from an unsafe environment and/or remove unsafe objects from the infant's environment rather than relying on the frequent use of the word "no."

c. Set limits that are few in number and are consistent.

d. Maintain the limits even if the older infant displays negativism or temper tantrums. See *Temper Tantrums.*

2. Teach parents the principles of discipline with the toddler.

a. Anticipate that the child will not comply immediately with the parent's request.

b. Restrict the use of "no" to important actions.

c. Remember that positive reinforcement for cooperation is more effective than negative reinforcement for misbehavior.

d. Be consistent with limits and punishment for misbehavior to avoid confusing the child.

e. Make it clear to the child that the parent does not like the child's behavior, but still loves the child.

f. Remove breakable or tempting objects from the child's reach, because this is easier on the parent and child than saying "no" constantly.

g. Remember that learning self-control is difficult for the toddler and takes time.

h. Give the child something positive to do, since this is more effective than telling him "don't," e.g., "please put the wagon where no one will fall over it," rather than "don't leave your wagon on the sidewalk."

3. Teach parents the principles of discipline with the preschooler.

a. Educate the child by telling him why he should or should not do something.

b. Help the child identify alternatives to his misbehavior.

c. Be clear about what is expected of him so that he can feel good about meeting parents' wishes.

d. Admit any incorrect or inappropriate reactions to the child's behavior and apologize to the child.

e. Be consistent in setting and enforcing limits.

4. Teach parents the principles of discipline with the schoolchild.

a. Involve the child in setting reasonable rules of behavior and in deciding punishment for infractions of agreed-upon rules.

b. Trust the child to behave in a socially acceptable manner when away from parents.

c. Talk with the child about the relationship of his decisions to the outcomes.

d. Recognize that when the child learns that the parents are capable of making errors he may challenge them on their decisions.

5. Teach parents the principles of discipline with the adolescent.

a. Involve the teenager in setting rules of behavior and in deciding punishment for infractions of the rules.

b. Talk with other parents of adolescents to determine if family rules are in line with peer group limits.

1. This approach is helpful for the parent who is told by the teenager "Everybody else can do it."

2. This gives parents an opportunity to learn that differences between teenager and parent are not unique to their family.

c. Expect the teenager will not accept parental values without question and open discussion may or may not be helpful in decreasing conflict.

Dislocated hip. See *Congenital Hip Dysplasia.*

Diverticulum, Meckel's. See *Meckel's Diverticulum.*

Divorce. See *Single Parent Families.*

Down's syndrome. See *Mentally Retarded Child.*

D

Drug abuse (drug dependence). Use of drugs for nontherapeutic purposes to the extent that physical and/or psychological harm affects the user.

A. **General Considerations.**
1. Many preadolescents and adolescents experiment with drugs but never suffer effects which require health care.
2. Use moves to abuse because of the stresses of adolescence, lack of alternatives for problem solving, as well as the sensations caused by drugs.
3. The first drug abused by most teenagers is alcohol. See *Alcoholism.*
4. Adolescents should be considered at high risk if they (Tennant and LaCour, 1980):
   a. Smoke cigarettes before age 12 years.
   b. Have a family history of substance abuse.
   c. Exhibit behavior problems at school; e.g., poor grades, hyperactivity, vandalism, truancy, aggressiveness, etc.
5. Peer, family, and personality appear to act independently as causes of drug abuse.
   a. Family members' use of drugs may be related to adolescent drug abuse despite "normal" peer and personality factors.
   b. Peer pressure may lead to drug abuse even when the family and personality traits do not place the teenager at risk.
   c. Personality traits may be associated with drug abuse when the family and peer factors are benign.
6. The adolescent may have an underlying depressive disorder but the symptoms are rarely recognized and the teenager is brought to treatment because of his school behavior (Rice and Kibber, 1983).
7. The adolescent may not wait passively to be offered drugs but may actively seek them.
8. Classes of psychotropic drugs frequently abused and their effects include:
   a. Stimulants: agitation, euphoria, increased pulse, fever, hallucinations.
   b. Depressants: emotional lability, ataxia, red eyes, decreased pulse, decreased appetite.
   c. Antidepressants and tranquilizers: decreased blood pressure, lethargy, decreased respirations.
   d. Hallucinogens and psychoactive drugs: nausea and vomiting, dry mouth, disorientation, delusions, aggressive behavior.
9. Inhalants, e.g., airplane glue, which cause slurred speech, dizziness, drowsiness, and decreased coordination are more commonly used by schoolchildren.
10. It is often impossible to determine which drug the child has taken.
11. Adverse reactions that precipitate seeking medical attention include:
   a. Panic states ("bad trips").
   b. Drug psychoses.
   c. Homicidal or suicidal thoughts.
   d. Respiratory depression.
12. A goal of total drug abstinence may not be reasonable from the adolescent's point of view.
13. Drug education programs are effective when they focus on helping the adolescent cope with the drug environment.
14. Actions to prevent drug abuse include:
   a. Legislation to limit drug advertising.
   b. Counseling programs for teenagers.
   c. Teenage employment programs.
15. Treatment for the adolescent drug abuser may necessitate family as well as individual therapy.

B. **Nursing Management.** See ADOLESCENT and COPING.
1. Observe, record, and report signs and symptoms of possible drug abuse.
   a. Signs and symptoms of psychotropic drugs.
   b. Erratic behavior.
   c. School absenteeism.
   d. Drop in school performance.
   e. Somatic complaints.
   f. Mood swings.
   g. Needle tracks on extremities.
   h. Wearing long sleeved shirts at all times.
   i. Lack of interest in appearance.
   j. Change in peer group.
2. Discuss with the adolescent the family, peer, and community support that is available to help him cope with stresses of adolescence.
   a. Hotlines.
   b. Group therapy.
   c. Outpatient drug action centers.
   d. Residential therapeutic communities.
3. Focus on the teenager's present problems, feelings, and relations, rather than past difficulties.
4. Help the teenager identify his own strengths as a way of improving his self-image.
5. Meet the needs of the adolescent admitted with an adverse drug reaction.
   a. Support the adolescent and parents during hospitalization. See *Hospitalization, Support During.*

b. Initiate discharge planning. See *Discharge Planning.*

c. Obtain as accurate a history as possible regarding the drug(s) taken. See *History Taking.*

  1. Interview the adolescent separately from his parents.

  2. Talk to the teenager's friends to get additional history data.

d. Decrease the auditory and visual stimuli.

e. Stay with the adolescent or have a peer remain in the room.

f. Try to focus the communication on positive, reality-oriented topics but change the subject if the adolescent becomes more upset.

g. Avoid physical restraint since this increases the panic response.

h. Observe, record, and report the adolescent's response to diazepam (Valium) if administered for sedation.

6. Meet the needs of the adolescent admitted with a drug overdose.

a. Support the adolescent and parents during hospitalization. See *Hospitalization, Support During.*

b. Initiate discharge planning. See *Discharge Planning.*

c. Assist with administration of oxygen and initiation of I.V. fluid if appropriate.

d. Assist with gastric lavage and send the contents for laboratory analysis if ordered.

e. Observe, record, and report:

  1. Respiratory rate.

  2. Other vital signs.

  3. Urinary output.

  4. Level of consciousness.

f. Reposition the adolescent every 2 hours.

g. Initiate actions to prevent infection, since the drug-dependent adolescent's poor physical condition makes him vulnerable to infection.

h. Reduce fever if necessary. See *Fever Reduction.*

i. Initiate seizure precautions. See *Seizures.*

j. Observe, record, and report signs and symptoms of opiate withdrawal.

  1. Anxiety.

  2. Yawning.

  3. Rhinorrhea.

  4. Sweating.

  5. Trembling.

  6. Vomiting and diarrhea.

  7. Abdominal cramps.

  8. Restlessness.

  9. Insomnia.

k. Observe, record, and report signs and symptoms of barbiturate withdrawal.

  1. Anxiety.

  2. Twitching.

  3. Intention tremor.

  4. Weakness.

  5. Dizziness.

  6. Distorted vision.

  7. Nausea and vomiting.

  8. Insomnia.

  9. Orthostatic hypotension.

  10. Convulsions.

l. Observe, record, and report the teenager's response to methadone if administered as part of the withdrawal regimen.

m. Promote the adolescent's self-esteem.

  1. Provide toothbrush, comb, etc., and encourage parents to bring the teenager's own clothing so he can feel more positive about appearance.

  2. Allow him to make as many decisions about his care as possible.

  3. Recognize need for privacy.

  4. Respect need for confidentiality.

  5. Involve him in setting limits on behavior which respect the rights of others.

  6. Use a positive approach that conveys your expectation that he can and will cooperate with nursing measures.

n. Provide a high calorie bland diet.

o. Be alert for signs that the adolescent is receiving drugs from visitors.

p. Support the adolescent and his family when referral alternatives are presented.

7. Initiate discussions with the adolescent about those situations which induce him to use drugs.

a. Changing the peer group may eliminate the problem.

b. Learning how to say "No" without excuses or lengthy explanations can help.

c. Identifying other ways to increase self-esteem can decrease the need for drugs.

d. Becoming involved in activities, clubs, exercise, etc. can reduce boredom.

8. Refer the adolescents to Ala-Teen for assistance with drug abuse as well as alcoholism.

Dying child, care of the. Physical care and emotional support of the child which allows the child to die with dignity within the context of his family.

  A. General Considerations.

  1. Consistent, competent physical and emotional care are supportive to both the dying child and his family.

  2. Complete physical dependency develops as death approaches, and care must be adjusted accordingly.

3. The use of complex monitoring machines should never replace nursing care of the child.

4. Parents may be unsure of how to provide care even though they may wish to participate.

5. The child fears regression, and meeting his increasing physical needs as they arise assists him in coping. See *Coping*.

6. The child needs to be permitted to talk about his concerns about dying.

7. The wishes of the parents concerning what the child is told about dying must be respected, but they should be encouraged to be open and honest in responding to their child's questions, since this is supportive to the child.

8. Research shows that a child may understand that he is going to die before he is able to say so (Spinetta, Rigler and Karon, 1973)

9. A major nursing role is the support of parents so that they are able to support their child and other family members.

10. Religious and/or cultural practices of the family relating to death should be incorporated into the child's care. See *Cultural Aspects of Health Care* and *Religious Aspects of Health Care*.

11. Parents should be involved in decisions about what procedures will continue to be performed and what, if any, life support systems will be used.

12. The sense of touch becomes a major form of communication as death approaches.

13. The sense of hearing may remain until death occurs even though the child is unable to respond.

14. The dying child may fear sleeping and/or being immobilized since mobility represents life.

15. Caring for a dying child is emotionally draining, and the family and staff need opportunities to discuss their feelings.

16. The amount of pain the child will experience is the prime concern of most children and parents (Gyulay, 1978).

17. Parents should be supported in a decision to take their child home to die.

18. It is appropriate for staff to grieve over the approaching death of a child, and it helps families to know that others share their grief.

B. **Nursing Management.** See CRISIS INTERVENTION.
1. Meet the physical needs of the dying child.
   a. Find out how needs were met at home and record on the Kardex to promote consistency and continuity of care.
   b. Relieve pain.
      1. Observe nonverbal cues that the child needs pain medication, since the child may fear receiving medication, and become restless, irritable, and withdrawn.
      2. Give pain medication as ordered.
      3. Tell the child the route of administration.
      4. Provide analgesia before performing painful procedures.
      5. Do not hold back on giving analgesics, since prompt relief of pain reduces anxiety, and the child may require less medication.
      6. Use nonmedical measures of reducing discomfort, e.g., repositioning, providing companionship, suctioning, backrubs.
      7. Move the child slowly and gently.
      8. Observe, record, and report signs and symptoms which indicate a need for alteration in analgesia, e.g., child unable to sleep, pain not relieved, etc.
   c. Promote rest and sleep.
      1. Position child for comfort.
      2. Provide pain relief.
      3. Have someone stay with child.
      4. Give the child favorite toy, blanket, or other security object.
      5. Place call bell within reach and reassure the child that you will come when he calls.
      6. Make sure bedding is clean and free of wrinkles.
      7. Dim the lights.
      8. Decrease environmental noise.
      9. Explain unfamiliar sounds to decrease anxiety.
      10. Plan care so that child can have periods of uninterrupted sleep.
   d. Maintain an open airway.
      1. Suction the child as needed.
      2. Give tracheotomy or endotracheal tube care as needed if these are present.
      3. Position the child with his head slightly extended, e.g., parent's lap, on side with a towel rather than a pillow under the head.
      4. Observe, record, and report signs and symptoms that indicate an airway may be needed, e.g., stridor, irregular respiratory rate, increasing secretions, etc.
      5. Position the child so aspirations will not occur if the child is vomiting.
   e. Provide for nutritional needs but do not force the child to eat.
      1. Offer small amounts.
      2. Provide favorite foods.
      3. Let parents bring favorite foods from home.

4. Give mouth care prior to meals.
5. Use topical anesthetic for sore throat or mouth discomfort prior to meals as ordered.
6. Schedule treatments and medications away from mealtime when possible.

f. Maintain skin integrity.
1. Use clear warm water to bathe the child.
2. Dry skin thoroughly, giving careful attention to skin folds.
3. Apply lanolin rich lotion, especially over pressure areas.
4. Remove all drainage from skin surfaces as it occurs.
5. Change the child's position on a regular basis to prevent stasis.
6. Place a pillow between the child's legs when lying on side.
7. Promote hydration.
8. Avoid injections when possible.
9. Do not give an injection at an edematous site.
10. Move the child gently using the palms of your hands.

g. Meet elimination needs.
1. Offer to take the child to the bathroom or offer the bedpan and/or urinal since the child may not ask.
2. Support the child's level of development, e.g., let the child use the bathroom for as long as able, help the child accept the use of bedpan and/or urinal or diapers if this becomes necessary.
3. Provide privacy.
4. Avoid verbal and nonverbal communication that indicates a negative reaction to the child's elimination.
5. Observe, record, and report:
   a. Signs and symptoms of urinary retention and/or constipation.
   b. Incontinence of urine or stool.
   c. Number of stools and times voided.
6. Plan food and fluid intake to promote bowel and bladder function, e.g., increased fluids and fruits if constipation is a problem, decreased roughage if diarrhea is present.
7. Administer stool softener as ordered.

h. Promote temperature control as ordered. See *Fever Reduction*.
1. Administer antipyretics.
2. Sponge the child.
3. Use a cooling mattress and change the child's position so no one body part becomes too cool.
4. Promote hydration. See *Forcing Fluids*.

i. Administer medications.
1. Allow the child some choice when possible, e.g., "Do you want water or juice with the pill?"
2. Follow home routine for taking medications if possible.
3. Let the parents give the medications if they wish.

j. Control seizure activity.
1. Administer anticonvulsants as ordered.
2. Monitor temperature accurately to assess when antipyretic may be needed.
3. Avoid loud environment noises and rough handling when caring for the child.

k. Prevent contractures.
1. Include active range of motion in your care as long as the child is able to move.
2. Provide passive range of motion.
3. Use a footboard to prevent food drop.

l. Observe, record, and report signs and symptoms that indicate that death is approaching.
1. Cheyne-Stokes breathing.
2. Increasing cyanosis and/or mottling of the skin.
3. Weak irregular pulse.
4. Decreasing body temperature.
5. Fighting sleep and asking to be taken from the room and moved about.

2. Meet the emotional needs of the dying child. See *Death, Concept Development of.*
a. Find out what the child has been told and what the family wishes him to be told.
b. Answer the child's questions as openly and honestly as possible.
c. Explain everything you do right up until the time of death.
d. Attend to physical needs in a consistent, caring manner as they arise.
e. Be nonjudgmental of the child's behavior.
f. Set consistent limits for the child in order to provide security.
g. Spend time with the child when you are not directly involved in giving care, e.g., sit with or read to him.
h. Promote parental participation in the care of their child.
i. Reassure the child that he is loved and that he has not been the cause of what is happening to him.
j. Include the child in the ongoing activities of the unit for as long as possible.
k. Avoid a "death room" look in the child's environment, e.g., keep the room light, talk in a normal tone.
l. Limit the number of procedures to those which are essential.

D

m. Continue to talk to the child even when he does not respond.
3. Include the physical needs of the parents in your plan of care.
   a. Encourage parents to take time to eat, sleep, and get some exercise.
   b. Provide a cot and pillow for sleeping in the child's room.
   c. Provide bathroom facilities, including showers.
4. Meet the emotional needs of the parents and other family members.
   a. Explain all aspects of your care.
   b. Explain all changes in the physical condition of the child.
   c. Involve parents and other family members in decisions to be made concerning the child's care.
   d. Teach parents how to give care they wish to give.
   e. Do not force parents to become more involved in the child's care than they indicate they can handle.
   f. Accept the behavior of parents and other family members in a nonjudgmental manner.
   g. Support the family in carrying out religious and/or cultural practices as they request, e.g., calling clergyman, preparing the child's body, etc.
   h. Provide privacy for the family and arrange for periods of time when you can talk with them.

i. Let the parents know that those who care for the child share their grief.
j. Support the parents in giving explanations to other family members, especially siblings.
k. Encourage talking to the child.
l. Support a decision to take the child home to die and assist the family in developing a plan of care (Martinson, 1976).
   1. Teach parents the physical care the child requires and provide opportunities for them to demonstrate care.
   2. Provide names and phone numbers of professionals so family can reach someone at anytime.
   3. Maintain contact with the family on a prearranged basis, e.g., daily phone call from a staff member.
   4. Initiate a referral for a community health nurse to visit if necessary.
   5. Tell the family that they can return to the hospital with the child.
   6. Give parents written instructions of what to do and who to call when the child dies.

Dysmenorrhea. See *Menstruation*.

Dysplasia, hip. See *Congenital Hip Dysplasia*.

Ear wax. See *Cerumen*.

Earache. See *Otitis Media*.

Eczema. See *Dermatitis, Atopic*.

Education, sex. See *Sex Education*.

Electrolytes. See *Fluid and Electrolyte Imbalance*.

Emergency admission. See *Admission to Hospital, Emergency*.

Emotionally disturbed child. The child who is unable to establish inner controls and/or relate to others at a developmentally appropriate level.

A. **General Considerations.**
   1. The child may be seen in a health care agency with symptoms or illnesses of an emotional origin.
      a. Language delay.
      b. Stuttering.
      c. Abdominal pain.
      d. Headaches.
      e. Peptic ulcer.
      f. Obesity.
      g. Anorexia nervosa.
   2. The child with an emotional disturbance may be admitted for treatment of the physical man-

ifestations of his emotional illness or for a totally unrelated illness.

3. The child with an emotional illness often functions at a developmental level below his chronological age.

4. Professional counseling for the child and family members is usually necessary.

5. The child and the parents need support in adjusting to the diagnosis and in accepting the need for long-term therapy.
   a. Referral is necessary for many other kinds of problems, e.g., a dermatological problem.
   b. Confidentiality will be maintained by the therapist.

B. **Nursing Management.** See *Behavior Problems.*
   1. Find out the child's home or institutional routines and record on the Kardex.
   2. Establish consistent limits and approaches for the child and his parents. See *Discipline.*
      a. Involve the child and family in setting the limits if possible.
      b. Share the information with all health team members in a team conference.
      c. Identify and support the child's coping behaviors. See *Coping.*
      d. Expect the child to cooperate with requests.
      e. Reinforce positive behavior and ignore negative behavior unless it is dangerous to the child or to others.
      f. Praise the child for attempting new skills rather than criticizing imperfect performance.
   3. Observe, record, and report behavior that may aid in diagnosis.
      a. Interactions with other people.
      b. Response to limit setting.
      c. Response to procedures and treatments.
      d. Feeding, sleeping, and elimination habits.
      e. Play activities.
   4. Observe, record, and report the child's behavior after therapy sessions.
   5. Clarify with the child's therapist whether or not problem areas should be explored or avoided in discussions with the child.
   6. Provide explanations about procedures and support based on the developmental level at which the child is functioning.
   7. Provide activities in which the child can be successful in order to build his self-esteem.

Encephalitis. Inflammatory process of the brain caused by protozoa, bacteria, fungi, or viruses.

A. **General Considerations.**
   1. Encephalitis in children is usually caused by a virus.
      a. Primary viral encephalitis: direct viral invasion of the central nervous system causing inflammation and neuronal injury.
      b. Postinfectious encephalitis: an indirect mechanism such as an antigen–antibody response occurs and the virus cannot be recovered from the nervous system.
   2. Signs and symptoms of primary encephalitis include:
      a. Fever.
      b. Headache.
      c. Meningeal signs: stiff neck, Kernig and Brudzinski signs.
      d. Ataxia.
      e. Drowsiness and lethargy, followed by stupor and coma.
      f. Excitation, irritability, and disorientation.
      g. Convulsions.
      h. Respiratory difficulty.
      i. Hyperthermia.
      j. Paralysis.
   3. Viruses that may cause primary encephalitis include:
      a. Enteroviruses.
      b. Herpes.
      c. Mumps.
      d. Arborviruses, arthropod-borne.
      e. Infectious mononucleosis.
   4. Signs and symptoms of postinfectious encephalitis usually occur during the convalescent period.
      a. Fever.
      b. Headache.
      c. Vomiting.
      d. Stiff neck.
      e. Convulsions.
      f. Drowsiness.
      g. Stupor or coma.
      h. Respiratory difficulty.
      i. Swallowing difficulty.
   5. Postinfectious encephalitis can occur after:
      a. Measles.
      b. Varicella.
      c. Rubella.
      d. Vaccinations.
         1. Rabies.
         2. Pertussis.
   6. If the child becomes comatose, this stage can last from 12 hours to a month or more.
   7. The child should be isolated if hospitalized during the acute stage of an infectious disease.
   8. Treatment for either type is symptomatic.
      a. Sedatives.
      b. Tracheotomy or ventilator if respiratory paralysis occurs.
      c. Tube feedings if swallowing difficulty occurs.
      d. Hypothermia.
      e. Anticonvulsants if seizures occur.

9. Residual effects of the disease can include:
   a. Seizure disorders.
   b. Behavior disorders.
   c. Learning disorders.
   d. Partial or generalized paralysis.
   e. Mental retardation.
   f. Hydrocephalus in infants.
10. The mortality varies with the causative organism, e.g., extremely low in mumps; high in herpes simplex.

B. Nursing Management.

1. Assign the child to a room near the nurses' station to ensure close observation and have the following equipment ready:
   a. Tracheotomy set.
   b. Ambu bag.
   c. Emergency cart.
   d. Oxygen.
2. Support the child and parents during hospitalization. See *Hospitalization, Support During.*
3. Prepare the child and parents for the diagnostic procedures which include (See *Preparation for Procedures*):
   a. Lumbar puncture (spinal tap).
   b. Blood culture.
   c. EEG.
   d. Skull and chest x-rays.
   e. Oropharyngeal or nasopharyngeal cultures.
   f. Stool cultures.
4. Initiate fever reduction measures. See *Fever Reduction.*
5. Find out what the child and parents have been told about the diagnosis and prognosis and record on the Kardex.
6. Provide opportunities for the parents to discuss their feelings about the possibility for slow recovery and long-term sequelae.
7. Observe, record, and report signs and symptoms of increasing involvement.
   a. Seizure activity. See *Seizures.*
   b. Signs and symptoms of increased intracranial pressure. See *Increased Intracranial Pressure.*
   c. Decreased urinary output.
   d. Altered level of consciousness.
   e. Swallowing difficulty.
   f. Inability to handle secretions.
   g. Febrile episodes.
8. Restrain the child only if necessary since resisting restraint may increase intracranial pressure. See *Restraints.*
9. Reposition the child every 2 hours.
10. Monitor the I.V. accurately to prevent cerebral edema.
11. Orient the child to time, place, and person if needed.
12. Observe, record, and report the child's response to medications.
13. Involve the parents and child in planning approaches to meet the child's nutritional needs.
14. Provide play activities appropriate to the child's age and physical progress.
    a. Activities that stimulate gross motor function, e.g., throwing a ball, climbing stairs.
    b. Activities that stimulate fine motor activity, e.g., play dough, puzzles.
15. Meet the needs of the child who is comatose.
    a. Talk to the child the same as to the conscious child, e.g., explain all procedures.
    b. Promote adequate respirations.
       1. Administer oxygen as ordered.
       2. Suction as needed.
       3. Perform chest physiotherapy or observe, record, and report the child's response if performed by the respiratory therapist.
       4. Encourage coughing and deep breathing as the child's level of consciousness improves.
    c. Provide good skin care.
       1. Obtain an alternating pressure mattress, sheepskin, etc., to prevent skin breakdown.
       2. Change the child's position every 1 to 2 hours.
       3. Massage bony prominences twice a day.
    d. Promote comfort.
       1. Provide eye irrigations, drops, or dressings as ordered.
       2. Provide mouth care every 4 hours.
       3. Put lubricant on the child's lips.
    e. Promote adequate nutrition.
       1. Administer tube feedings as ordered after checking placement.
       2. Remove the tube and insert a new one in the opposite nostril every 5 days or according to hospital policy.
       3. Tape the tube so it does not cause pressure on the nares.
       4. Elevate the child's head during feeding.
       5. Follow the feeding with water.
    f. Prevent contractures.
       1. Provide passive range of motion to extremities every 2 hours.
       2. Maintain good body alignment.
       3. Ask the parents to bring in hard soled shoes and put them on for 2 hours, then remove for 2 hours, since foot boards are usually ineffective in preventing foot drop in the child.
    g. Prevent infection.
       1. Wash hands before all care.
       2. Provide catheter care twice a day.
       3. Use sterile technique when changing the urinary drainage bag.

4. Use sterile technique when suctioning the tracheotomy.

5. Prevent exposure to staff or visitors who are infectious.

6. Treat all areas of skin breakdown immediately.

h. Promote bladder tone by clamping the catheter if ordered and draining every 3 to 4 hours.

i. Provide sensory stimulation through stories, books, radio, records, or television. See *Stimulation.*

j. Coordinate weekly patient-centered conferences with nursing staff, physician(s), social worker, teacher, all therapists, and nutritionist so that all team members have compatible goals for the child and family.

16. Initiate discharge planning when it is clear what the child's home care will require. See *Discharge Planning.*

a. Develop a home program which includes specific instructions from each discipline that has participated in the child's care.

b. Discuss how the child's care can be incorporated into the family's life style.

c. Initiate referrals to community agencies for physical therapy, homebound teacher, equipment rental, etc.

d. Have the parents demonstrate how to perform nursing measures if necessary.

e. Encourage the parents to maintain follow-up of developmental progress.

Encopresis.
Repeated voluntary or involuntary passage of feces of normal or near-normal consistency into places inappropriate for that purpose in the child's cultural setting and not a result of organic disease (American Psychiatric Association, 1980).

A. **General Considerations.**

1. The condition is classified as:
   a. Primary encopresis if the child has never been continent of stool.
   b. Secondary encopresis if the child has been continent of stool prior to the development of the condition.

2. A child may develop encopresis when:
   a. A disturbed parent–child relationship exists (most common cause).
   b. Toilet training has been particularly rigid.
   c. Situational stress occurs, e.g., birth of a sibling, hospital admission.
   d. There is fear of using the bathroom, e.g., toilet is too large for the child, schoolchild is intimidated by older child.
   e. Chronic constipation is present and painful

anal fissures develop causing the child to seek to avoid pain by holding the stool until it is passed involuntarily.

3. Encopresis may be associated with enuresis.

4. Treatment measures are directed toward establishing normal bowel patterns and improved family and interpersonal relationships through counseling.

5. Establishing normal bowel elimination patterns requires time and may include:
   a. Enemas to clear the bowel; should be used only at the start of treatment and only if absolutely necessary.
   b. Mineral oil and stool softeners.
   c. Alterations in diet to increase natural laxatives and food roughage.
   d. Behavior modification techniques which reward the child for not soiling.

6. If enemas are necessary they should be administered by a health care provider and not a parent because:
   a. The child may view the administration of an enema as punishment because of the intrusive nature of the procedure.
   b. It prevents further conflict over bowel control between parent(s) and child.

7. Rectal leakage of mineral oil may occur, and this can be as upsetting to the child and/or parents as the encopresis.

8. Hospitalization may be required for initial evaluation and treatment, but the child can usually be managed at home.

9. Further evaluation will be needed if poor physiological sphincter control is present.

B. **Nursing Management.** See BEHAVIOR PROBLEMS.

1. Support the child and parents during hospitalization. See *Hospitalization, Support During.*

2. Initiate discharge planning. See *Discharge Planning.*

3. Obtain a nursing history to help determine the etiology.
   a. Assess parent–child relationships.
   b. Identify the presence of stress factors in the child's environment.
   c. Find out the:
      1. Current status of toilet training.
      2. Word(s) used for defecation.
      3. Assistance the child needs in using the bathroom.
      4. Time of day the child has or attempts to have a bowel movement.
   d. Complete a nutritional assessment, since poor nutritional habits can cause constipation. See *Appendix vii.*

4. Involve the child and parents in the development of a flexible bowel training program.

5. Teach parents to:

a. Refrain from threatening, demeaning, or punishing the child.
b. Prevent siblings from teasing the child.
c. Administer stool softener as ordered. See *Administration of Medications, Parental.*
d. Administer mineral oil as ordered:
1. Give between meals to decrease loss of fat-soluble vitamins A, D, E, and K.
2. Support the child if leaking occurs.
3. Notify health care provider if leakage is a problem.
4. Administer supplemental vitamins if ordered.
e. Reward the child for cooperating with a bowel training program.
f. Include foods with increased roughage and natural stool softeners/laxatives in the child's diet.
g. Use developmental norms as a basis for interpreting the child's behavior. See *Appendix v.*
6. Care for the hospitalized encopretic child. See *Hospitalization, Support During.*
a. Prepare the child for administration of enemas, if ordered. See *Preparation for Procedures.*
b. Observe, record, and report the child's response to medications.
c. Find out what routines are followed at home and record on the Kardex.
d. Use the same techniques as those which would be taught to parents of the encopretic child.
7. Promote the development of a bowel elimination schedule but do not force the child. See *Toilet Training.*
a. Take or have the child go to the bathroom at set times.
b. Provide privacy.
c. Schedule bathroom times so the child is not rushed.
8. Encourage the intake of fluid, fruits, and high fiber foods to stimulate peristalsis if constipation is a problem. See *Constipation.*
9. Observe, record, and report the parent–child relationship in order to assess if intervention is needed. See *Parenting.*
a. Support the parent–child relationship in a positive manner.
b. Support the child and parents in accepting professional help if indicated.
10. Teach the parents as indicated.
a. How to administer an enema.
b. To observe and report leakage of mineral oil if this is used.
c. Dietary management of constipation.
d. Developmental norms for their child to provide a better basis for understanding behavior. See *Appendix v.*

Enucleation. See *Neuroblastoma* and *Retinoblastoma.*

Enuresis. Absence of bladder control at an age when control would be expected.

A. **General Considerations.**
1. The child must be able to retain 300 to 350 ml of urine before he can sleep through the night without voiding.
2. The condition is classified as:
a. Primary enuresis if the child has never achieved control.
b. Secondary enuresis if the child achieved control but reverted to wetting.
3. Enuresis may be seen in a child with:
a. A small functional bladder capacity.
b. Stressful life experiences, e.g., arrival of a new sibling, hospitalization.
c. Diabetes, sickle cell anemia, urinary tract obstruction or infection, or myelomeningocele.
d. An emotional disorder.
e. Food allergies.
f. Consumption of foods or medications with diuretic action.
4. Enuretic children tend to come from homes which are socially handicapped.
5. Enuresis may predispose a child to urinary tract infection due to the warm, moist environment it creates (Kolvin, McKeith, Meadow, 1973).
6. Diagnostic studies:
a. A urinalysis and culture should be done on all children with enuresis to rule out organic disorders.
b. An intravenous pyelogram (IVP) and voiding cystourethrogram (VCUG) are indicated when the history or physical exam indicate urologic pathology (Chen, 1980).
7. Treatment of enuresis due to an organic problem involves management of the underlying condition.
8. Treatment of functional (nonorganic) enuresis may include the use of:
a. Imipramine (Tofranil) given at bedtime to decrease bladder contractions.
b. Bladder stretching exercises which involve:
1. Keeping a record of intake and output to establish a baseline.
2. Having the child drink increasing amounts of fluids and holding the urine for as long as he can.
c. Attempts to reduce identified stress factors in the child's environment.
d. Counseling to improve parent–child relationships.

e. Behavior modification which rewards the child for each dry night.

9. Bladder stretching exercises require several months to be effective, and the child may have many "accidents" during this time.

10. Children respond best to a treatment program that actively involves them and gives them some responsibility for management.

11. Use of mail order "Wet Alarms," limiting the child's fluid intake, and getting the child up to void during the night are of questionable value and may intensify parent-child conflict over the problem.

12. Many enuretic children come from families with a history of enuresis, and this may influence the child and parents' response to the condition and treatment.

B. **Nursing Management.** See BEHAVIOR PROBLEMS.
1. Use a nursing history to assess:
    a. Parent-child relationships.
    b. Presence of stress factors in child's life.
    c. Factors related to the enuresis including:
        1. How long the condition has been present.
        2. What has/have the child/parents been doing about the condition.
        3. How do the child and parents feel about the enuresis.
2. Teach the parents to:
    a. Recognize that the occurence of illness, fatigue, stressful situations, and the introduction of new foods may cause regression during treatment.
    b. Refrain from teasing or punishing the child.
    c. Prevent the child's siblings from embarrassing the child.
    d. Bathe the child in the morning to remove urine that may cause odor and skin breakdown.
    e. Use plastic sheeting on the bed covered by several layers of absorbent material.
    f. Use a room deodorizer.
    g. Light the route from the child's room to the bathroom so the child will not avoid using the bathroom due to fear of the dark.
    h. Keep the child warm at night, since cold increases the urge to urinate.
    i. Administer drugs as ordered and observe for side effects. See *Administration of Medications, Parental.*
    j. Keep imipramine (if used) out of reach of small children since fatal poisoning can occur.
    k. Carry out bladder stretching exercises if prescribed.
    l. Avoid waking the child in the night and/

or restricting fluids, since they have not been proven to be effective.
    m. Permit the child to handle his own linens and wash if old enough, since this decreases embarrassment.
    n. Involve the child in any treatment program undertaken and ignore "accidents" and reward progress in staying dry.
3. Support the child and parents.
    a. Prepare the child and parents for intravenous pyelogram and voiding cystourethrogram which may be done to detect any underlying urinary tract abnormality. See *Preparation for Procedures.*
    b. Reassure the child that enuresis does not mean he is a "bad" child.
    c. Tell them that the problem is common and is usually outgrown (Tsai, 1976).
    d. Accept feelings of guilt, anger, frustration, and embarrassment in a nonjudgmental manner.
    e. Initiate referral for counseling if further assistance seems necessary.
4. Care for the hospitalized enuretic child. See *Hospitalization, Support During.*
    a. Find out what routines are followed at home and record on the Kardex.
    b. Orient to bathroom facilities on the unit.
    c. Keep extra linens and gowns in the room for the child to use.
    d. Use the same techniques as those which would be taught to parents when caring for the child with enuresis.

Epiglottitis. A medical emergency in which there is inflammation and swelling of the epiglottis usually due to a bacterial infection which causes laryngeal obstruction.

A. **General Considerations.**
1. Signs and symptoms develop rapidly over a period of 4 to 12 hours and include:
    a. Rapidly increasing inspiratory stridor with retractions.
    b. Fever.
    c. Sore throat.
    d. Drooling due to dysphagia.
    e. Assumption of a classic posture in which the child sits up with his head and neck extended forward to open the airway ("sniff position").
    f. Coughing.
    g. Muffling of voice sounds.
    h. Restlessness due to air hunger.
2. Complete airway obstruction may occur suddenly from either examination of the throat or from making the child lie down.
3. Treatment includes:

E

a. Hospitalization; in an intensive care area if symptoms are severe.
b. Intravenous antibiotic therapy.
c. Cold mist and oxygen.
d. Measurement of arterial blood pH, PO_2, and $pCO2$.
e. Continuous cardiac and respiratory monitoring.
f. Endotracheal intubation or tracheotomy if there is severe obstruction.

4. Nasopharyngeal and blood cultures may be done to determine the causative organism, usually *Haemophilus influenzae* type B.

5. The decision to treat the child conservatively or to perform a tracheostomy or intubation will be based upon the:
a. Severity of the symptoms.
b. Age of the child. (Younger children have smaller airways.)
c. Availability of an anesthesiologist and/or surgeon.

6. The child and parents are often extremely frightened and require constant, consistent support.

7. Epiglottitis must be differentiated from acute spasmodic croup and laryngotracheobronchitis which also present with inspiratory stridor.

8. Most children have only mild to moderate symptoms.

B. **Nursing Management.**

1. Support the child and parents during hospitalization. See *Hospitalization, Support During.*

2. Initiate discharge planning as child's condition indicates. See *Discharge Planning.*

3. Meet the needs of the child receiving conservative therapy.
a. Do not attempt to examine the child's throat.
b. Do not make the child lie down.
c. Have someone stay with the child at all times to:
1. Observe any changes since they may occur suddenly.
2. Decrease anxiety.
d. Support the parents in being able to stay with their child.
e. Explain all procedures to decrease anxiety. See *Preparation for Procedures.*
f. Use mist tent to increase environmental humidity and to decrease swelling and liquify secretions. See *Mist Tent.*
g. Administer oxygen through mist tent as ordered for hypoxia.
h. Initiate fever reduction measures. See *Fever Reduction.*
i. Observe, record, and immediately report signs and symptoms of increasing airway obstruction which include:

1. Increasing retractions.
2. Flaring nares.
3. Increasing stridor.
4. Restlessness due to air hunger.
5. Fatigue.
6. Increasing pulse rate.
7. Circumoral pallor.
8. Cyanosis.
j. Monitor I.V. accurately.
k. Observe, record, and report the child's response to medications.
l. Keep an endotracheal tube and/or tracheotomy tray at the bedside.
m. Schedule care in blocks of time to promote rest.

4. Meet the needs of the child who is to be treated by surgical intervention.
a. Prepare the child and parents for surgery. See *Postoperative Care, Preoperative Care,* and *Preparation for Surgery.*
b. Explain everything you do.

5. Meet the needs of the child with a tracheotomy or endotracheal tube.
a. Support the child and parents.
1. Explain all procedures.
2. Keep the child under direct observation at all times to assess when care and/or help is needed.
3. Provide a means of communication for the child, since he cannot talk or cry, e.g., bell.
4. Meet the child's security needs, since he may be very frightened.
b. Prevent obstruction of the airway.
1. Suction the child as needed.
2. Restrain the child as needed to prevent removal of the tube.
3. Keep the child well hydrated to help liquify secretions.
4. Provide humidified air or oxygen as ordered.
5. Tie tracheotomy ties at the side of the neck to avoid accidental untying when the child's gown is changed.
6. Keep small objects which might be aspirated away from the child.
c. Prevent pooling of respiratory secretions.
1. Change the child's position every 2 hours.
2. Carry out coughing and postural drainage techniques as ordered.
d. Prevent aspiration during feeding by positioning the child in a semi-Fowler's position.
e. Prepare the child and parents for removal of the tube, usually 3 to 5 days.

6. Teach the child and parents home care of the child who is:
a. Managed conservatively.

1. Provide increased humidification.
2. Promote hydration. See *Forcing Fluids.*
3. Administer medications as ordered. See *Administration of Medications, Parental.*
4. Call the physician if symptoms increase.
  b. Managed with surgical intervention.
   1. Keep the incision clean and dry.
   2. Promote hydration.
   3. Provide humidification.
   4. Report any signs of infection to the physician.

Epilepsy. See *Seizures.*

Epistaxis. See *Home Management of Minor Emergencies.*

Equinovarus, talipes. See *Clubfoot.*

Erythema infectiosum. See *Fifth Disease.*

Esophageal fistula. See *Tracheoesophageal Fistula.*

Ethnic groups. See *Cultural Aspects of Health Care.*

Ewing's sarcoma Malignant tumor of the shafts of long bones, the metatarsals, and/or the ileum.

A. General Considerations.
  1. Signs and symptoms include:
    a. Pain.
    b. Tenderness.
    c. Fever.
    d. Leukocytosis.
  2. Pathological features may occur at the tumor site due to invasion of the bone by malignant cells.
  3. Metastasis occurs early to the lungs, other bones, and lymph nodes.
  4. Treatment is with high-dose radiotherapy combined with chemotherapy. See *Radiation Therapy* and *Chemotherapy.*
  5. Lesions in expendable bone (rib, fibula, clavicle) may be surgicaly resected (Pritchard, 1980).
  6. Amputation of an extremity may be necessary if radiation is not expected to produce the desired results.
  7. Approximately one-half of the patients survive 2 years if the disease is localized at diagnosis (Gaddy, 1982).

8. The adolescent who faces the diagnosis of this potentially fatal disease must cope with specific problem areas (Nilson, 1982). See *Adolescence.*
    a. Desire for independence.
    b. Heterosexual peer adjustment.
    c. Body image.
    d. Change in vocational/educational goals.

B. Nursing Management. See LIFE-THREATENING ILLNESS and CRISIS INTERVENTION.
  1. Support the child and parents during hospitalization. See *Hospitalization, Support During.*
  2. Initiate discharge planning. See *Discharge Planning.*
  3. Support the child and parents when the diagnosis is made.
    a. Find out what the child and parents have been told about the diagnosis and treatment and record on the Kardex.
    b. Answer all questions honestly.
    c. Use terminology that the child understands.
    d. Arrange for uninterrupted periods of contact with the child and parents so supportive discussions can be held.
    e. Maintain continuity in assignment of nursing personnel.
  4. Observe, record, and report side effects of chemotherapy and/or radiation therapy. See *Chemotherapy* and *Radiation Therapy.*
  5. Observe, record, and report the following symptoms of lung metastasis:
    a. Chest pain.
    b. Coughing.
    c. Expectoration of blood.
  6. Move the patient carefully to prevent pain and pathological fractures.
  7. Provide comfort measures for patient receiving chemotherapy.
  8. Supervise the child when ambulating.
    a. Protect from falls.
    b. Report symptoms of a fracture if the child does fall.
  9. Meet the needs of a child who requires an amputation.
    a. Provide preoperative care. See *Preoperative Care* and *Preparation for Surgery.*
     1. Check the stump for bleeding every 15 minutes for 4 hours, then hourly for the first 24 hours.
     2. Elevate the stump, but avoid causing contractures.
     3. Turn the patient frequently without causing indentations on the cast or disturbing the compression bandage depending on which is used.
     4. Administer pain medication as ordered,

since the child's phantom pain is a normal phenomenon.

5. Treat the stump matter-of-factly to help the child accept it.

6. Encourage the child to examine the stump for irritation and breakdown and to bathe it with soap and water daily.

7. Support the child in exercises for muscle strengthening.

8. Discuss with the child and his parents how the child will modify clothing, manuever at school, etc., after discharge.

9. Teach the child how to use crutches.

10. Meet the child's nutritional needs, since chemotherapy may adversely affect the child's intake.

11. Obtain an order for a stool softener if needed.

12. Help the child and parents deal with body image changes. See *Body Image*.

13. Teach the child and parents home management.

   a. Encourage the parents to help the child and the family to make home life as normal as possible.

   1. Have the child resume normal activities such as play groups or school.

   2. Encourage normal peer relationships.

   3. Maintain normal discipline.

   4. Encourage adequate rest and nutrition for all family members.

   b. Help the child continue to work through feelings about intrusive procedures, since chemotherapy may continue on an outpatient basis.

14. Assist the child and family to cope with failure to respond to therapy when this happens. See *Dying Child, Care of the*.

Exanthem. See *Rash*.

Exanthem subitum. See *Roseola*.

Exceptional child. The child who is significantly different from normal.

A. **General Considerations.**
1. Parents expect to reproduce themselves by giving birth to a perfect child.
2. The parents may interpret the child's birth as punishment for their sins, particularly if the pregnancy were unplanned.
3. Reactions to the birth of a baby with one or more defects includes:
   a. Disappointment.
   b. Frustration.
   c. Grief.
   d. Anxiety.
   e. Anger.
   f. Guilt.
   g. Denial.
4. The parents must go through mourning the loss of the perfect child they expected (Young, 1977).
   a. Feelings of loss.
   b. Longing for the desired child.
   c. Resentment.
   d. Guilt.
5. Factors which affect the family's adjustment to the child's diagnosis include:
   a. Available support systems.
   b. Perception of the child's illness/handicap.
   c. Coping patterns as individuals and as a family.
6. Grieving by parents of a defective child cannot be finally resolved unless the child dies.
7. Fathers have fewer opportunities to help the child directly and are offered less assistance by parent organizations and service agencies.
8. The response of parents may vary from one extreme of overprotection to the other extreme of intolerance or abandonment.

B. **Nursing Management.** See CRISIS INTERVENTION and GENETIC COUNSELING.
1. Acknowledge that your feelings may be similar to those experienced by the parents.
   a. Recognize that there are normal responses.
   b. Discuss your responses with peers or instructor/supervisor.
2. Find out what the parents have been told about the diagnosis and prognosis and record on the Kardex or clinic record.
3. Support the parents in adjusting to the diagnosis.
   a. Identify which coping mechanisms are being used by each parent.
   1. Respect the parent's need for withdrawal initially.
   2. Gently and consistently stress reality if the parent is using denial.
   3. Avoid taking the parent's anger as a personal attack.
   4. Expect that parents will ask the same questions repetitively until they can deal with the answers.
   b. Convey warmth and caring by sitting quietly in the room or by touching the parent(s).
   c. Provide the parents with opportunities to discuss their feelings.
   d. Ask them to tell you more about their thinking rather than saying that you understand their feelings when you cannot.
   e. Recognize that your facial expressions and

any sign of revulsion or withdrawal will influence the parents' feeling about their child.

    f. Avoid false reassurances and attempts to make parents feel it could have been worse, since this is not possible from their perspective.

    g. Be alert for signs that the parent is ready to learn to care for the child.
      1. Demonstrate and discuss the child's care.
      2. Encourage parent participation in care.
      3. Support the parent assuming responsibility for providing care.
      4. Praise the parent's success in physical care.
      5. Reinforce the parent's positive interactions with the infant.

4. Discuss with the parents how they will share the information with siblings, other family members, and friends.

5. Help the mother plan how to incorporate the child's care into the family lifestyle.
    a. Plan time for the mother to be relieved from child care.
    b. Plan time for interaction with the father and siblings.

6. Provide anticipatory guidance in relation to the child's expected developmental progress in the next 6 to 12 months.

7. Encourage parents to use limit-setting along with positive reinforcement for behavior control of the older infant and child. See *Discipline.*

8. Be alert to the parents' readiness for help from others:
    a. Introduce them to parents of a child with a similar defect.
    b. Tell them about community organizations for parents with special problems.

9. Encourage the parents to continue with routine health supervision for the child.

Exercise.
Activity directed toward the promotion of health.

A. General Considerations.
  1. Exercise helps to:
    a. Increase muscle development.
    b. Promote adequate circulation.
    c. Improve digestion.
    d. Improve respiratory function.
    e. Use up calories to prevent or control obesity.
    f. Release tension.
    g. Provide a sense of accomplishment.
  2. Exercise teaches body:
    a. Control.
    b. Coordination.
    c. Balance.

3. Exercise should be incorporated into the child's daily routine from the time of birth.
4. Formal exercises are not recommended for the child under 5 years of age.
5. All exercise should be geared to the developmental level of the child.
6. The child who sees his parents enjoying regular exercise is more likely to follow an exercise routine, since children copy what they see their parents do.
7. Postural problems are not outgrown.
8. Boys and girls should have the same and equal exercises in the prepubertal period.
9. Hospitalized children should have exercise included in the plan of care.

B. Nursing Management. See IMMOBILIZED CHILD.
  1. Discuss with parents the part exercise plays in their child's development.
  2. Explain to parents how they can provide areas for exercise for their child.
    a. Indoors.
      1. Clear furniture from an area to provide space.
      2. Use a rug or several thicknesses of blankets on the floor for padding.
      3. Use the bathtub, under supervision with a young child, to provide for exercise free of the pull of gravity.
    b. Outdoors.
      1. Set up a gym set or improvise equipment, e.g., a board, suspended between two blocks becomes a balance beam.
      2. Take the child to a local park.
  3. Teach parents to dress their child appropriately for exercise.
    a. Use loose, absorbent clothing.
    b. Cover knees and elbows in situations where the skin may be scraped, e.g., infant crawling on rough surface, or an older child climbing trees.
    c. Provide old clothes so the child feels free to be active.
    d. Dress the child in the same weight clothing the parent would wear for the activity and environmental temperature.
  4. Encourage parents to ease the child into the exercise program and present exercises as "games" to the younger child.
  5. Tell the following to the parents:
    a. Do not force the child to do an exercise that is beyond his ability.
    b. Stop exercises before the child becomes fatigued.
    c. Do not allow the child to stand on his head, since the neck is never capable of safely supporting the body.
    d. Avoid exercises that require the child to place undue strain on muscles such as:

E

1. Those exercises that require using muscles on only one side of the body.
2. Lifting weights.
3. Pulling heavy objects.
4. "Duck walking" in a squatting position.
5. Bending over backward.
6. Lifting both legs straight off the ground at the same time.

6. Teach parents what they can do to promote exercise for the infant.
   a. Keep the infant out of confining spaces as much as possible, e.g., playpen, crib, infant seat.
   b. Change the infant's position to encourage the use of different muscle groups.
   c. Let the infant crawl instead of carrying him around the house.
   d. Provide bright objects that will encourage the child to explore his environment.
   e. Hang a "bouncer seat" from the doorway.
   f. Let the infant splash in the bathtub, under strict supervision.
   g. Move the infant's arm and legs in a rhythmic maner, e.g., play "pat-a-cake."

7. Teach parents what they can do to promote exercise for the toddler and preschooler.
   a. Allow time outside each day, if possible, for the increased activity needs of this age child.
   b. Provide push toys to stimulate walking.
   c. Let the child walk when the parent goes out even though it may slow progress a little bit.
   d. Provide climbing activities.
   e. Let the child play in the bathtub or a wading pool under supervision.
   f. Play active games with the child, e.g., ball, tag, "ring-around-the-rosy."
   g. Provide active toys such as tricycles, scooters, and slides.

8. Teach parents what they can do to promote exercise for the schoolchild.
   a. Involve the child in a planned period of exercise each day.
   b. Participate in an exercise program with the child.
   c. Let the child walk as long as he can do so safely instead of driving him everywhere.
   d. Encourage peer group participation in such activities as bicycle riding and basketball.
   e. Provide for independent active play such as jumping rope or playing hopscotch.
   f. Praise the child for exercise activities.
   g. Let the child go to the playground.

9. Teach parents what they can do to promote exercise for the adolescent.
   a. Let the child walk instead of driving him everywhere.
   b. Encourage participation in structured athletic activities.
   c. Support the child's desire to be involved in safe competitive sports, e.g., track.
   d. Give the adolescent a series of lessons in an active sport as a gift, e.g., tennis.
   e. Let the adolescent buy the clothes needed for the sport if possible, e.g., running shorts, sneakers.

10. Encourage parents to participate in activities with their children and to exercise daily.

11. Provide exercise for the hospitalized child as his condition permits.
    a. Include active and/or passive range of motion exercises in the daily care of each child.
    b. Obtain permission to take the child outside if his condition and the situation permits.
    c. Provide for large muscle activities in the playroom, e.g., throwing a sponge through a hoop.
    d. Ask the physical therapist to conduct exercise periods for children whose conditions permit.

Exopthalmos. See *Hyperthyroidism*, *Neuroblastoma*, and *Retinoblastoma*.

Eye, foreign bodies. See *Eye Injury*, and *Home Management of Minor Emergencies*.

Eye injury. Trauma to the eye by a blunt or pointed object.

A. **General Considerations.**
1. Trauma to the eye with a blunt object may result in harm ranging from pain to intraocular destruction.
2. Hemorrhage into the anterior chamber of the eye as a result of blunt trauma is called hyphema.
   a. Repeated or delayed hemorrhage may occur several days after the accident.
   b. Secondary glaucoma may develop.
3. Treatment for hyphema includes:
   a. Hospitalization.
   b. Sedation.
   c. Binocular bandages.
   d. Bed rest.
4. Serious complications of hyphema may occur immediately or at a later time.
   a. Impaired vision.
   b. Cataract formation as a result of poor lens nutrition from damage to the ciliary body.
   c. Permanently dilated pupil as a result of a tear of the iris sphincter.
5. Pointed objects may penetrate the eyeball and

cause serious injury that may necessitate enucleation.

6. Symptoms of penetrating injuries include:
   a. Red and soft eye.
   b. Prolapsed iris due to loss of aqueous fluid.
   c. Hemorrhage into the entire eye.
7. Ophthalmological examination of the eye may be very difficult so that accurate assessment of damage to the lens, retina, and choroid may be impossible.
8. Treatment for penetrating injuries may require 2 to 3 weeks.
   a. Hospitalization.
   b. Binocular bandages.
   c. Bed rest.
   d. Sedatives.
   e. Local or systemic antibiotics.
9. A sensitivity reaction (sympathetic uveitis) can develop in the uveal tract of the uninjured eye and cause blindness.
10. If the injured eye does not respond to treatment, enucleation should be performed before uveitis occurs and bilateral blindness results.

B. **Nursing Management.** See ADMISSION TO HOSPITAL, EMERGENCY.
   1. Support the child and parents during hospitalization. See *Hospitalization, Support During.*
   2. Initiate discharge planning, when appropriate, see *Discharge Planning.*
   3. Find out what the ophthamologist has told the child and parents about the bandages and the treatment and record on the Kardex.
   4. Be sure that the child and parents understand the restrictions on activity.
   5. Elevate the head of the bed 30 degrees or as ordered.
   6. Encourage a family member to stay with the child if possible.
      a. The child will be very frightened with both eyes bandaged.
      b. The use of restraints can be minimized.
   7. Provide continuity of nursing personnel, particularly if a family member is unable to stay.
   8. Provide nursing care measures that will prevent an increase in intraocular pressure.
      a. Introduce fluids gradually to prevent vomiting.
      b. Provide a diet high in bulk, fruits, and fruit juices to prevent straining with bowel movement.
      c. Tell the child not to blow his nose forcefully.
      d. Apply restraints gently to decrease resistance and use only if absolutely necessary.
   9. Assist the child in adapting to loss of vision.
      a. Explain new sounds, e.g., "The bell you hear tells the nurse to come."

   b. Let the child handle all materials and equipment that will be used in his care.
   10. Encouarge adequate nutrition.
      a. Allow the child adequate time to eat.
      b. Select foods with distinct smells to stimulate the child's appetite.
      c. Name the foods on the child's plate so he can identify specific tastes with the food.
      d. Tell the child which foods are hot and which are cold.
      e. Tell the child what food is in each spoonful if you are feeding the child.
      f. Place the younger child's food in small bowls and have the child use a spoon if approved by the physician.
      g. Offer finger foods for the young child who is allowed to feed himself.
      h. Tell the older child who is allowed to feed himself where things are located on the plate according to the time on a clock face, e.g., eggs are at 6 o'clock.
   11. Provide verbal cues where visual ones would normally be used by the child.
      a. Identify yourself when you enter the room and tell the child when you are leaving.
      b. Speak to the child before you touch him.
      c. Tell the child what you are doing in the room as you work.
   12. Describe the room and equipment to the child, e.g., "there are two beds, one for you and one for a roommate, a chair for your mother, etc."
   13. Observe, record, and report the child's response to medications.
   14. Darken the room and prepare the child in advance before eye drops are instilled. See *Preparation for Procedures.*
   15. Organize nursing care so that the effects of the sedative are not counteracted by disturbing the child unnecessarily.
   16. Provide the child and parents with opportunities to verbalize the guilt, anger, hostility, or other emotions that they may be experiencing.
   17. Provide diversion that does not overstimulate the child.
      a. Story telling.
      b. Radio.
      c. Record player.
      d. Reading to the child.
      e. Modeling clay.
      f. Play dough.
   18. Teach the child and parents home management.
      a. Review activity restrictions.
      b. Review administration of medications. See *Administration of Medications, Parental.*
      c. Discuss measures used in the hospital for feeding, orientation to the environment, diversion, etc.

19. Meet the needs of the child and parents if the child requires enucleation of the eye. See *Preparation for Surgery.*
    a. Provide opportunities for the child and parents to verbalize their concerns about disfigurement and loss of some vision.
        1. Prepare the child and parents through explanations and interviews.
        2. Anticipate that the child may handle his fears of disfigurement by becoming angry and irritable.
    b. Provide information about the prosthesis.
        1. The prosthesis will be fitted when the edema subsides.
        2. The child will not be able to see with the new eye.
        3. The artificial eye can be attached to the eye muscles so that it moves in coordination with the real eye.
    c. Meet the needs of the child preoperatively. See *Preoperative Care.*
    d. Meet the needs of the child postoperatively. See *Postoperative Care.*
        1. Observe, record, and report hemorrhage, edema, or signs of infection of the orbit.
        2. Reinforce the dressing if necessary, but do not change unless ordered.
        3. Help the child cope with body image changes. See *Body Image.*
    e. Teach care of the artificial eye.
        1. Review the physician's guidelines about whether the prosthesis should be removed for sleep or other specific instructions.
        2. Wash hands before beginning the procedure.
        3. Irrigate the socket with normal saline.
        4. Clean the socket and eye when excessive tearing or crusting occur.
        5. Wipe away the normal watery discharge with sterile, disposable tissues.
        6. Clean the prosthesis with soap and warm water only.
        7. Store a plastic prosthesis in a container with plain tap water.
        8. Store a glass prosthesis in its own case after drying.
    f. Teach measures for eye safety.
        1. Wear safety glasses or goggles if prescribed as a method of protecting the normal eye.
        2. Do not carry sharp objects while walking or running.
        3. Avoid rubbing the eyes when a foreign body is present.
        4. Seek medical assistance promptly for any injuries or infections.

Eyeglasses. See *Strabismus.*

Eyelid, infection of. See *Dermatitis, Seborrheic.*

Failure to thrive, nonorganic. Condition in which the child's weight is below the third percentile on a growth chart and there is no chronic, organic, or metabolic disease present.

A. **General Considerations.**
    1. Physical causes must be ruled out before a diagnosis of nonorganic failure to thrive can be made.
    2. Characteristic of parents who are at risk for having a child who fails to thrive include:
        a. Inadequate parenting as a child.
        b. Inadequate support systems.
        c. Acute or chronic stress which may be emotional, social, financial, or physical.
        d. Inability to perceive the child's needs accurately.
    3. Characteristics of the child who fails to thrive include:
        a. Body posturing which is stiff and rigid or floppy.
        b. Difficult to feed.
        c. Lack of eye contact with caregiver.
        d. Irregularity in activities of daily living.
        e. Delayed structural growth.
        f. Developmental delays in language, motor, and social and adaptive areas.
        g. Diminished response to stimulation.
    4. A "mismatching" of the mother and child is another factor in failure to thrive, e.g., quiet, passive mother and an active, assertive infant.
    5. Severe failure to thrive in early life can result in permanent neurological damage.

6. Parents of these children tend to feel inadequate and they are threatened by authority figures.
7. Treatment is directed at:
   a. Promotion of age-appropriate growth and development.
   b. Development of parenting capabilities consistent with the child's needs.
   c. Support of the parents while they develop parenting skills.
8. Hospitalization is usually necessary to rule out organic disease and initiate weight gain in the infant.
9. The prognosis depends on the severity and duration of the condition and on the response of the child and parents to intervention.
10. If there is no intervention, or if intervention is unsuccessful, the child suffering from nonorganic failure to thrive may later be abused.

B. Nursing Management.
1. Support the child and parents during hospitalization. See *Hospitalization, Support During.*
2. Initiate discharge planning. See *Discharge Planning.*
3. Observe, record, and report factors in the home and family that are known to contribute to failure to thrive.
4. Promote consistency in the care of the child.
   a. Develop a plan of care and record it on the Kardex.
   b. Assign the same caregiver to the child.
   c. Have team conferences to discuss the child's care.
5. Support the development of mothering skills. See *Parenting.*
   a. Assign someone to work with the mother who can:
      1. Listen to what the mother has to say.
      2. Relate to the mother in a warm positive manner.
      3. Avoid being an authority on child care or giving directions on what the mother should do for her child.
      4. Assess and respond to the mother's needs as well as the child's.
      5. Collaborate with the mother in developing plans which meet the child's needs.
      6. Encourage others to support the mother.
      7. Make home visits to maintain continuity of care.
   b. Help the mother learn to respond to her child in order to promote maternal–child bonding.
      1. Point out skills that the child has developed, e.g., "he sucks very well, he must enjoy the bottle you're feeding him."
      2. Praise the mother for signs of appropriate parenting.
      3. Involve the mother in planning care, e.g., ask her "what do you think will work best?"
      4. Demonstrate appropriate interaction with the child, e.g., playing games, talking to the child during a feeding.
      5. Provide information about growth and development norms so the mother knows what is normal. See *Appendix v.*
      6. Provide anticipatory guidance about growth and development.
   c. Validate with the mother aspects of the child's behavior that may make him difficult to manage, e.g., "you're right, he certainly does take a long time to drink a bottle."
   d. Talk with the mother about ways she might cope with the child's behavior, e.g., have someone else feed the child occasionally.
6. Promote weight gain. See *Nutrition.*
   a. Offer food when the child indicates hunger.
   b. Let the child set the pace.
   c. Do not force the child to eat more than desired.
   d. Help the child to associate eating with pleasant experiences.
   e. Have mother feed whenever possible.
      1. Hold, cuddle, rock, and/or sing to the infant during feeding.
      2. Feed the older child in pleasant, age-appropriate surroundings, e.g., in the playroom at a table, with peers.
      3. Interact in a positive way with the child at mealtimes.
      4. Do not schedule procedures and/or medications to coincide with mealtime.
      5. Involve the older child in selecting and/or preparing some of his food.
      6. Find out daily caloric needs of the child and work with the dietician to plan an adequate caloric intake.
7. Weigh the child each day:
   a. At the same time.
   b. On the same scale.
   c. Nude.
8. Promote adequate sleep since human growth hormone is released during sleep. See *Sleep.*
   a. Schedule care to permit naps.
   b. Make sure the infant is dry and fed before you put him down for sleep.
   c. Allow the toddler to carry out presleep rituals, e.g., getting a drink of water, reading a favorite story.
   d. Check that the child is neither too hot nor too cold.

e. Decrease environmental stimulation as much as possible, e.g., dim lights, close door.
9. Promote development.
   a. Assess child's developmental level. See *Appendix v.*
   b. Provide developmentally appropriate stimulation. See *Stimulation.*
   c. Interact actively with the child, e.g., roll ball back and forth with the toddler, do not just give him a ball.
   d. Place the child in an activity area or place where he can observe activity involved in his care.
   e. Provide the parents with specific suggestions to promote development at home.

Fallot, tetrology of. See *Congenital Heart Disease.*

Falls. See *Accident Prevention* and *Head Injury.*

Family. See *Adoption; Aggression, Parental; Anxiety, Parental; Parenting; Siblings;* and *Single-Parent Families.*

Fatal illness. See *Dying Child.*

Father. See *Parenting* and *Single-Parent Families.*

Fears. An emotional response to an anticipated danger or pain.

A. General Considerations.
1. Many fears are unique to children.
2. Specific fears are characteristic of the child's developmental level.
   a. Infant.
      1. Separation from mother.
      2. Strangers.
   b. Toddler and Preschooler.
      1. Separation or abandonment.
      2. Dark.
      3. Intrusive procedures.
      4. Mutilation of body parts.
      5. Monsters and ghosts.
      6. Unknown.
   c. Schoolchildren and adolescents.
      1. Disability.
      2. Loss of a body part.
      3. Loss of control.
      4. Loss of friends.
      5. Loss of status with peers.
      6. Loss of life.
3. Children need more support and active intervention from others to cope with their fears.
4. Children need more preparation for procedures because of their fears. See *Preparation for Procedures.*
5. Parental fear and anxiety is readily perceived by children.

B. Nursing Management.
1. Orient the child as thoroughly as possible to the pediatric unit, clinic, or physician's office.
2. Ask the child's parents about specific fears and record on the Kardex or patient record.
3. Encourage parental participation in the child's care.
4. Encourage the child to express his fears.
   a. Use therapeutic play for the younger child. See *Play, Therapeutic.*
   b. Discuss the older child's fears with him.
      1. Ask him how he thinks he can learn to cope with his fears.
      2. Let him know that other children have the same fears if that is true.
5. Identify and support the child's coping behavior. See *Coping.*
6. Teach parents how to help the child cope with age-appropriate or illness-related fears.
   a. Do not ignore the fear or force the child to confront a feared object.
   b. Give the child an opportunity to be near a feared object and then inspect it, e.g., stethoscope.
   c. Encourage the parents to help him participate in the feared activity or use the feared object.
7. Provide physical comfort for the child during and after a painful procedure.
8. Obtain oral or axillary rather than rectal temperatures, since this is a particularly intrusive procedure for most children.
9. Provide the toddler or preschooler with a band-aid after an injection or blood withdrawal, since this will help preserve his feeling of body wholeness.
10. Anticipate that suture removal will be frightening to the young child, since he fears that his "insides will come out."
11. Explain to the child that his body part is present under his bandage or cast.
12. Discuss the older child's disease and its treatment with him using pictures, diagrams, body outlines, etc.
13. Allow the child to maintain control by offering choices whenever possible.
14. Encourage the older child to continue peer relationships.
   a. Encourage phone calls or letters.

b. Arrange for children of the same age to share a room.

c. Encourage shared mealtimes, games, and activities.

15. Help the child maintain his status by helping with schoolwork and teaching him about his body and his illness.

16. Provide some means of mobility to counteract the older child's fear of disability.

Feeding. See *Feeding Problems* and *Nutrition*.

Feeding problems. Difficulties related to the feeding situation.

A. **General Considerations.**

1. The development of mutually satisfying feeding experiences in infancy serves as a basis for a trusting relationship between the parent and child.

2. Parents may perceive normal developmental changes in feeding behaviors as if they were feeding problems.

3. Feeding problems develop when the infant/child:

    a. Does not take in enough food to meet age-appropriate nutritional requirements.

    b. Does not receive satisfaction from the feeding situation.

    c. Does not exhibit age-appropriate feeding behaviors.

    d. Refuses an entire food category or all new foods for an extended period of time.

    e. Uses the feeding situation to control parental behavior.

4. Feeding problems develop when the parent:

    a. Does not take into consideration the developmental level of the child in relationship to intake and eating behaviors.

    b. Expects the child to eat more or less than the child can or desires to eat.

    c. Insists on feeding the child when he can feed himself.

    d. Insists on table manners to the point where the child loses interest in eating.

    e. Does not understand that illness often decreases a child's appetite.

5. The presence of feeding problems may indicate the presence of other problems within the family.

6. Treatment consists of:

    a. Providing information on norms of growth and development.

    b. Providing information on nutrition.

    c. Helping the child and parents identify and eliminate the underlying cause.

d. Helping parents set consistent, appropriate limits.

B. **Nursing Management.** See BEHAVIOR PROBLEMS; FAILURE TO THRIVE, NON-ORGANIC and NUTRITION.

1. Assess if a feeding problem actually exists.

    a. Do a nutrition history to see what the child is actually eating.

    b. Ask the parents to describe:

        1. How the child reacts to the feeding situation.

        2. How they feel about the feeding situation.

        3. Eating behaviors exhibited by the child.

        4. What feeding behaviors they expect from the child.

        5. Whether any foods or food groups are totally refused.

        6. Rewards or punishments associated with the feeding situation.

    c. Assess the child's developmental level.

    d. Observe the child and parent during a feeding, if possible.

2. Support the parents in developing a mutually satisfying feeding experience with the infant.

    a. Provide information on development as needed.

        1. Pushes food from mouth until 3 to 4 months due to tongue extrusion reflex.

        2. Starts sips from cup between 6 to 8 months.

        3. Begins to feed self crackers between 6 to 7 months.

        4. Holds own bottle between 6 to 8 months.

        5. Feeds self finger foods using pincer grasp (thumb and index finger) between 9 to 11 months.

        6. Chews firm foods well between 2½ and 3 years of age.

    b. Praise parenting behaviors that encourage the child to feed well.

    c. Observe a feeding and point out developmental behaviors as they occur.

    d. Role model a feeding for the parents if needed.

    e. Point out cues of hunger and satiation exhibited by the infant.

    f. Give parents a sample menu for the child and indicate age-appropriate amounts of foods.

    g. Discuss adaptations necessary to improve feeding behaviors.

        1. Decrease the noise level in the room.

        2. Remove distractions, e.g., television, extra people.

        3. Use infant seat, feeding table, or high chair for the child's comfort.

    h. Support the parent in seeking assistance

with feeding the infant in order to obtain an occasional break from the routine.

3. Support the toddler and parents in coping with feeding problems.

   a. Provide information on development related to feeding skills and behaviors.

      1. Begins to use spoon, but turns it over before reaching mouth around 15 months.
      2. Controls spoon better, but still spills around 18 months.
      3. Uses spoon correctly and holds own glass around 2 years.
      4. Feed self completely if food is prepared for him around 3 years.

   b. Provide information on development related to feeding behaviors.

      1. Eats decreased amounts of food because growth rate has decreased.
      2. Runs everywhere and is always active which leads to the child being "too busy to eat."
      3. Asserts self in the feeding situation and may develop food jags as a result of a growing sense of autonomy.
      4. Demands certain foods and the serving of meals in a certain way due to the ritualistic behavior of the toddler.

   c. Praise parents for behaviors that reinforce positive eating behaviors.

   d. Observe a feeding and point out developmental behaviors as they occur.

   e. Discuss with the parents adaptations in the feeding situations that encourage appropriate eating behaviors.

      1. Let the child feed himself.
      2. Offer small portions of food and let the child ask for seconds.
      3. Cut up fruits, vegetables, and meats into pieces or strips and offer to the child as a snack midway between meals.
      4. Let the toddler help get ready for a meal, e.g., put napkins on table and put foods out.
      5. Give the toddler his own place and utensils at the table.
      6. Schedule mealtimes early enough for the child not to be overtired.
      7. Continue to offer a wide variety of foods, but do not force the child to eat.
      8. Include the child in family conversations.
      9. Praise the child for completing a meal, but say nothing if he does not finish everything.
      10. Offer food choices but make them equally nutritious.

   f. Assist parents in coping with food jags (Henneman and Koziol, 1980).

      1. Tell them that jags are usually short lived unless an issue is made of it.
      2. Explain that jags are not harmful if other foods groups are still eaten.
      3. Tell them to try meeting the child halfway, e.g., provide half the preferred food and half other food.

   g. Explain that bribes, threats, and punishment should be avoided, since this reinforces negative rather than positive behavior.

   h. Give parents a sample menu and indicate age-appropriate amounts of each food group. See *Appendix vii.*

   i. Explain decreased need for milk during the toddler period.

4. Support the preschool child and parents in dealing with problems related to eating.

   a. Provide information on development of the preschooler related to eating behaviors.

      1. Eats less due to increased motor activities and interest in the environment.
      2. Gains weight on an erratic basis and therefore has a variable appetite.
      3. Desires more independence in the selection, preparation, and consumption of food due to an increasing sense of initiative.

   b. Discuss adaptations that encourage appropriate eating behaviors.

      1. Keep a supply of nutritious snacks on hand, e.g., cheese cubes, peanut butter crackers, fresh fruits.
      2. Let the child assist in preparation of snacks and meals and serve himself.
      3. Offer snacks between, not just before, meals so they do not dull the appetite.
      4. Have the child set the table.
      5. Introduce new foods in an attractive manner.

   c. Give parents a sample menu and indicate age-appropriate amounts of each food group. See *Appendix vii.*

5. Support the schoolchild and his parents in dealing with problems related to eating.

   a. Provide information on development related to eating behaviors.

      1. Gains weight slowly which leads to a decreased appetite.
      2. Being in school decreases parental control of foods eaten.
      3. Identifies with the peer group which causes some foods to be accepted and others to be rejected.
      4. Develops a sense of industry which causes the child to want to play a larger role in the management of his nutrition.

   b. Discuss adaptations in the eating situation

that encourage appropriate eating behaviors.
1. Let the child serve himself the amount of food he desires.
2. Let the child select and prepare a dish for a meal.
3. Teach the child the basic food groups and praise his ability to select a well-balanced meal.
4. Make realistic allowances for likes and dislikes.
6. Support the adolescent and his parents in dealing with problems related to eating.
  a. Provide information on development related to eating behaviors.
    1. Growth spurts lead to an increased appetite.
    2. Worries about body size and skin conditions lead to some foods being accepted or rejected.
    3. Identifies with the peer group and demands certain "in" foods.
    4. Develops a sense of role identity which may lead to the rejection of traditional family foods and eating patterns.
  b. Assist the adolescent in assuming responsibility for his nutrition.
    1. Provide factual information.
    2. Permit choice of foods.
    3. Explain relationship of food to skin problems. See *Acne.*
    4. Explain the relationship of necessary nutrients to the promotion and maintenance of health.

Fever of unknown origin (FUO). The presence of a temperature of 100.4 F. (38 C.) or higher for 2 weeks or more not explained by history, physical exam, or laboratory findings.

  A. **General Considerations**
    1. Fever is a symptom and the degree of fever does not necessarily indicate the severity of the illness.
    2. Causes of a fever of undetermined origin include:
      a. Infection.
      b. Neoplasm.
      c. Autoimmune or collagen disease.
      d. Miscellaneous conditions, e.g., granulomatous diseases, drug ingestion, abnormal circadian temperature cycle.
    3. Causes of fever of unknown origin vary for different age groups:
      a. Children under six years of age; most common causes include:
        1. Viruses.
        2. Urinary tract infections.
        3. Pneumonia.
      b. Children over six years of age; most common causes include:
        1. Infections.
        2. Autoimmune diseases (juvenile rheumatoid arthritis is most common).
    4. Diagnostic tests include:
      a. Repeated physical examinations.
      b. Followup of any abnormal findings.
      c. Laboratory tests:
        1. CBC and differential.
        2. Cultures: blood, urine, cerebrospinal fluid, nasopharyngeal, stool, wound, etc.
        3. Erythrocyte sedimentation rate (ESR).
        4. Computerized tomographic scanning (CT).
    5. Treatment consists of the use of antipyretics which:
      a. Will not be started until the cultures are obtained.
      b. Are usually given when the rectal temperature is greater than 102 F.
      c. Should be acetaminophen rather than aspirin so that the diagnosis of juvenile rheumatoid arthritis is not missed.
    6. The infant under a year with FUO is usually hospitalized for further evaluation whereas an older child may be observed for a longer period at home.
    7. In approximately 10 percent of cases of FUO, the cause of the fever remains undiagnosed despite exhaustive clinical evaluations.
    8. Parents may report a fever in an infant/child when none is present as a means of gaining attention from a health care professional.

  B. **Nursing Management.**
    1. Support the child and parents during hospitalization. See *Hospitalization, Support During.*
    2. Initiate discharge planning as appropriate when diagnosis and specific needs are determined. See *Discharge Planning.*
    3. Explain to the child and parents (See *Preparation for Procedures*):
      a. Antipyretics may be withheld until tests are done.
      b. Why tests will be performed.
    4. Observe, record, and report other signs and symptoms which may lead to a diagnosis, e.g., rash, vomiting, diarrhea, bleeding, etc.
    5. Promote hydration. See *Forcing Fluids.*
    6. Monitor intake and output accurately.
    7. Use comfort measures related to fever such as:
      a. Tepid bath water.
      b. Light weight absorbent clothing.
      c. Adequate room ventilation.

F

8. Meet the child's nutritional needs. See *Nutrition.*
   a. Offer small, frequent feedings.
   b. Do not force the child to eat solids but encourage fluids.
9. Initiate fever reduction measures as ordered and observe, record, and report the child's response. See *Fever Reduction.*
10. Assist with lab tests as ordered.
11. Observe, record, and report signs and symptoms of dehydration and/or seizure activity. See *Fluid and Electrolyte Imbalance* and *Seizures.*

F

Fever reduction. Measures taken to reduce a fever.

A. **General Considerations.**
   1. The temperature regulating mechanism is not mature until the child is approximately 8 years old.
   2. Young children may run high fevers with relatively benign diseases.
   3. A child is considered to be febrile with a rectal temperature of 100°F but intervention is frequently delayed until the temperature is 102°F.
   4. Fever reduction is done to:
      a. Promote comfort.
      b. Reduce the occurrence of dehydration.
      c. Prevent, or reduce the number of, febrile seizures.
      d. Prevent central nervous system sequelae.
   5. There is no evidence that brain damage occurs with rectal temperatures less than 105°F (Frothingham, 1977).
   6. Cool sponges should not be used for longer than 20 to 30 minutes at a time, since vasoconstriction may develop preventing further heat loss.
   7. Parents need to know how to use a thermometer.
   8. Parents need to be taught how to reduce the child's fever.
   9. Aspirin and acetaminophen may be alternated every 2 hours or used in combination to provide for longer periods between antipyretics, e.g., 6 to 7 hours rather than 4 hours between doses (Frothingham, 1977).
   10. Aspirin and acetaminophen preparations can both produce toxicity.
   11. Isopropyl alcohol is not added to the water, since it may be inhaled and cause coma.

B. **Nursing Management.**
   1. Support the child and parents.
   2. Monitor the child's temperature accurately.
   3. Use a cool sponge bath as ordered.
      a. Keep the water temperature between 85 and 90°F.
      b. Do not add ice or alcohol to the water.
      c. Place a cool cloth on the child's forehead.
      d. Use one of the following methods.
         1. Place the child in a tub and squeeze the water over his chest and back.
         2. Sponge portions of the body in sequence, drying each portion before proceeding to the next.
         3. Wrap the child in cool, moist towels, changing them as they become warm.
      e. Sponge for 20 to 30 minutes.
      f. Take the temperature ½ hour later, since it continues to decrease after the sponge bath.
      g. Repeat the sponge bath as ordered if the temperature is still elevated.
      h. Give waterproof toys to the child in the tub to distract him during the sponging.
   4. Administer antipyretics as ordered.
   5. Dress the child in light weight, absorbent pajamas, or diaper and shirt.
   6. Keep the room temperature between 68 and 72°F, if possible.
   7. Force fluids or monitor I.V. accurately to prevent dehydration.
   8. Cover the child with a sheet or leave uncovered, since bed clothes hold heat in the body.
   9. Use a hypothermia mattress as ordered making sure to change the child's position so no one part becomes too cold.
   10. Teach parents home management of fevers.
      a. Instruct parents to take the child's temperature when he feels warm or complains of a headache.
      b. Encourage parents to ask their physician about what fever reduction methods should be used.
      c. Teach parents methods of fever reduction.
         1. Sponge bath techniques.
         2. Forcing fluids.
         3. Administration of antipyretics. See *Administration of Medications, Parental.*
      d. Advise parents not to give antipyretic:
         1. More often than ordered.
         2. In greater amounts than ordered.
      e. Tell parents to keep a record of:
         1. Each temperature taken.
         2. The time of day each temperature was taken.
         3. Any associated signs and symptoms.
         4. When, how much, and what types of medication the child received.
      f. Remind parents that children can run high fevers without being seriously ill.
      g. Call the physician if the child develops signs and symptoms of dehydration or seizures. See *Fluid and Electrolyte Imbalance* and *Seizures.*

Fever, scarlet. See *Scarlet Fever.*

Fifth disease (Erythema Infectiosum). A viral disease of childhood transmitted by personal contact.

A. **General Considerations.**
1. The disease begins with an intensely erythematous, slightly raised rash on the face which has a "slapped face" appearance.
2. One day later, the rash appears on the extensor surfaces of the extremities, followed the next day by involvement of the flexor surfaces and trunk.
3. The fading of the lesions from the center out gives the lesions a lace-like pattern.
4. The rash may reappear intermittently for several weeks if precipitated by such factors as trauma, heat, cold, or sunlight, which irritate the skin.
5. There are no complications or sequelae, and medical treatment is unnecessary.

B. **Nursing Management.**
1. Tell the child and parent the stages of the rash.
2. Teach comfort measures for the rash. See *Rash.*

Fibrosis, cystic. See *Cystic Fibrosis.*

Fistula, tracheoesophageal. See *Tracheoesophageal Fistula.*

Fluid and electrolyte imbalance. Disturbance of the body's normal fluid and electrolyte balance.

A. **General Considerations.**
1. Electrolyte balance is dependent on fluid balance and the regulatory action of cardiovascular, renal, pulmonary, adrenal, and parathyroid mechanisms.
2. Fluid and electrolyte balance in children differs from that in adults in the following ways.
   a. Total body water is greater in the child.
   b. A greater proportion of the child's body water is in the extracellular space leaving a smaller intracellular fluid reserve.
   c. The child's metabolic rate is two to three times that of the adult, creating a tendency toward metabolic acidosis.
   d. A greater volume of urine is required to excrete waste products produced by the higher metabolic rate.
   e. The child's kidneys do not concentrate urine, excrete excess fluid, or conserve water effectively.
   f. Greater fluid losses may occur because the child has a greater body surface area in proportion to his mass.
   g. Buffer systems are less mature in children.
3. The younger the child the more significant the differences from the adult and the more rapidly problems develop.
4. Acid-base balance is dependent upon chemical buffers, the action of the renal and respiratory systems, dilution of strong acids and bases in the blood, and maintenance of a 20:1 ratio of base bicarbonate to carbonic acid.
5. Acid-base imbalances of the extracellular fluid include:
   a. Metabolic acidosis from a base bicarbonate deficit, e.g., decreased food intake, ketogenic diet, diabetic acidosis, etc.
   b. Metabolic alkalosis from a base bicarbonate excess, e.g., vomiting, gastrointestinal suction, potassium-free intravenous solution, etc.
   c. Respiratory acidosis from a carbonic acid excess, e.g., asthma, pneumonia, etc.
   d. Respiratory alkalosis from a carbonic acid deficit, e.g., fever, encephalitis, intentional overbreathing, etc.
6. The use of a nursing history will assist in determining the possible cause(s) of fluid and electrolyte and/or acid-base imbalance. See *Apendix iv.*
7. The use of a nursing assessment of the following in conjunction with a review of laboratory findings will assist in determining the type of fluid and electrolyte and/or acid-base imbalance.
   a. Behavioral changes.
      1. Irritable and lethargic: fluid volume deficit.
      2. Restlessness: hyperkalemia.
      3. Convulsions: fluid volume overload.
      4. Coma: severe acidosis/alkalosis; fluid volume overload.
   b. Temperature.
      1. Elevated: sodium excess.
      2. Subnormal or elevated: dehydration.
   c. Pulse.
      1. Increased: severe potassium excess or deficit.
      2. Decreased: sodium excess; magnesium excess or deficit.
      3. Bounding: fluid volume excess.
      4. Rapid, weak, thready: circulatory collapse.
   d. Respiration.
      1. Slow, shallow: compensatory mechanism in respiratory alkalosis (watch for decreased ventilation leading to the development of metabolic acidosis).
      2. Rapid, deep: compensatory mechanism

in metabolic acidosis (watch for hyperventilation and the development of respiratory alkalosis).
3. Dyspnea: generalized edema; pulmonary fluid volume excess.
4. Rales: fluid excess.
5. Shallow: potassium excess or deficit.
6. Stridor: severe calcium deficit.

e. Blood pressure (not a good indicator of fluid volume because the elastic nature of the child's blood vessels may permit them to constrict and keep blood pressure up until shock occurs).
1. Increased: fluid volume excess.
2. Decreased: sodium deficit; decreased plasma volume.

f. Weight.
1. Loss: 2 to 4 percent loss = mild dehydration; 5 to 9 percent loss = moderate dehydration; 10 percent or greater = severe dehydration.
2. Gain: ascites; edema.

g. Urine.
1. Increased: interstitial-fluid-to-plasma shift; increased renal solute load; diabetes.
2. Decreased: mild fluid deficit.
3. Oliguria: moderate to severe fluid deficit; plasma-to-interstitial fluid shift; deficit or severe excess of sodium; potassium excess.
4. Specific gravity: low in the presence of fluid excess, severe potassium deficit or renal disease; high in the presence of fluid deficit, sodium excess, glycosuria, and proteinuria.
5. pH: acid in the presence of acidosis (metabolic or respiratory) or diarrhea; alkaline in the presence of alkalosis (metabolic or respiratory).
6. Glucose: increased in the presence of diabetes mellitus or glucose infusions.
7. Ketones: positive in the presence of ketoacidosis or starvation.
8. Osmolality: increased in the presence of dehydration, syndrome of inappropriate antidiuretic hormone (SIADH), or hyperglycemia with glycosuria; decreased in the presence of excessive water intake or use of I.V. 5 percent dextrose/water solutions.

h. Skin.
1. Pale: protein loss; fluid compartment shift.
2. Flushed: sodium excess.
3. Dry: fluid deficit; sodium excess.
4. Thickened: sodium excess.
5. Poor turgor: dehydration.

6. Cold, clammy: sodium deficit; plasma-to-interstitial fluid shift.
7. Dry mucous membranes: fluid volume deficit; sodium excess.
8. Gray color: dehydration.

i. Fontanels: depressed in moderate fluid volume deficit; bulging in fluid volume excess.

j. Tears and salivation: absent in fluid volume deficit.

k. Eyeballs: sunken in fluid volume deficit.

l. Neurological signs.
1. Weakness: metabolic acidosis.
2. Twitching: hypocalcemia; magnesium deficit; alkalosis.
3. Decreased muscle tone: hypocalcemia.
4. Increased muscle tone: tremors, tetany = alkalosis with decreased calcium ionization; positive Chvostek's sign = hypocalcemia.
5. Combination of headache, blurred vision, vomiting, cramps, muscle twitching: overhydration.

m. Sensory alterations.
1. Thirst: fluid deficit; sodium or calcium excess.
2. Nausea: potassium deficit; calcium or potassium excess.
3. Muscle cramps: calcium or potassium deficit.
4. Abdominal cramps: sodium deficit; potassium excess.
5. Tingling in fingers and/or toes: calcium deficit; alkalosis.
6. Lightheaded sensation: respiratory alkalosis.

n. Alterations in blood chemistries.
1. Serum osmolality: increased in dehydration; decreased in overhydration.
2. Serum sodium: increased when water loss exceeds sodium loss or dietary intake increases without an increase in water intake; decreased when sodium loss exceeds water loss.
3. Serum potassium: increased with acidosis, renal failure, overtreatment with potassium supplement, and intestinal obstruction; decreased with direct loss of potassium or poor dietary intake.
4. Serum chloride: increased in dehydration and metabolic acidosis; decreased in vomiting, gastric suction, sodium losing conditions, excessive perspiration, and excessive use of diuretics, alkalosis.
5. Serum calcium: increased with increased vitamin D intake, fractures, long-term immobilization, use of thia-

zide diuretics; decreased with poor nutrition, inadequate vitamin D intake, and acidosis.

6. Blood urea nitrogen (BUN): increased with dehydration and poor renal blood flow or urine production.

7. Hematocrit: decreased with loss of red blood cells or water excess; increased with dehydration.

o. Alterations in arterial blood gas values: occur in different combinations according to the type of acidosis or alkalosis present and are best understood when viewed in relation to one another. See *Appendix ii.*

8. Dehydration is the most common fluid and electrolyte imbalance in children and:

a. Results from loss of fluid and electrolytes from the extracellular fluid due to:
1. Vomiting.
2. Diarrhea.
3. Burns.
4. Diaphoresis.
5. Excessive urinary output.
6. Wound drainage.
7. Malnutrition (food and fluid).

b. Is classified according to the serum concentration of sodium and each classification is associated with different degrees of intracellular fluid (ICF) and extracellular fluid (ECF) shift in order to maintain serum osmolality.
1. Isonatremic (isotonic): serum sodium between 130 and 150 mEq/L.
2. Hypernatremic (hypertonic): serum sodium above 150 mEq/L.
3. Hyponatremic (hypotonic): serum sodium below 130 mEq/L.

c. Isonatremic dehydration:
1. Occurs when losses of water and sodium are proportionately equal and there is no shift from ICF to ECF; hypovolemic shock may occur from the decreased circulating blood volume.
2. Is most commonly caused by diarrhea, vomiting, and malnutrition.
3. Is characterized by weight loss, lethargy, pale or gray color skin, dry mucous membranes, poor skin turgor, absence of tearing and salivation, and decreased urine output.
4. Treatment involves the use of iso-osmolar solutions to correct hypovolemic shock and replace losses over a 24-hour period.

d. Hypernatremic dehydration:
1. Occurs when water loss is greater than sodium loss; increased ECF osmolality

causes shift from ICF to ECF and results in severe cellular dehydration.
2. Is most commonly caused by severe diarrhea and a high solute intake without adequate water intake; other causes include fever and poor renal function.
3. Is characterized by weight loss, avid thirst, confusion, convulsions, tremors, thick and firm skin turgor, sunken eyeballs and fontanels, absence of tearing, increased pulse and respiration; the blood pressure and urine output may be normal or decreased.
4. Intracranial hemorrhage is a late sign and occurs in the presence of severe hypernatremic dehydration.
5. Treatment involves gradual reduction in sodium, replacement of fluid, and calcium gluconate to prevent convulsions.

e. Hyponatremic dehydration.
1. Occurs when sodium loss is greater than water loss; the osmolality of the ECF is lower than that of the ICF and there is fluid shift from the ECF to the ICF.
2. Is most commonly caused by severe diarrhea, excessive water intake, infusion of electrolyte free fluids, sodium losing renal disease, and use of diuretics.
3. Is characterized by thirst, weight loss, lethargy, clammy skin with poor turgor, soft sunken eyeballs, symptoms of shock, and decreased urine output.
4. Treatment is with Ringer's lactate or use of a 5 percent dextrose solution with varying amounts of sodium depending upon the serum sodium level.

9. Treatment measures for other forms of fluid and electrolyte imbalances and acid-base imbalances will be directed at eliminating their underlying cause.

10. The major extracellular electrolytes are sodium and chloride.

11. Potassium is excreted via the kidneys and should not be:
a. Added to an I.V. until it has been determined that the child is voiding.
b. Continued in an I.V. in the presence of oliguria or anuria.

12. A cardiac monitor may be used if the child is receiving potassium.

13. Overhydration occurs if the child receives too much intravenous fluid or tap water enemas are used.

14. Fluid and electrolyte replacement therapy is aimed at:

a. Meeting daily fluid requirements from sensible and insensible losses.
b. Correcting fluid deficits.
c. Replacing continued losses.

15. A 5 percent glucose solution is required to:
a. Keep the child from being hungry.
b. Spare protein.
c. Prevent ketosis.

16. With fluid restriction or long-term therapy, additional calories will be needed to spare protein.

17. The nurse must be especially observant of fluid and electrolyte imbalance, because children do not describe thier symptoms.

18. Blood products may be administered as part of a therapeutic regimen and agency policy for their use should be followed strictly.

B. Nursing Management.

1. Obtain a nursing history. See *Appendix iv.*
2. Review normal blood chemistry, blood gas, and urine values. See *Appendix ii.*
3. Carry out a nursing assessment, as above, in conjunction with a review of the child's laboratory values and observe, record, and report deviations from normal values.
4. Observe, record, and report signs and symptoms of overhydration such as:
a. Headache.
b. Nausea.
c. Vomiting.
d. Blurred vision.
e. Cramps.
f. Muscle twitching.
g. Convulsions.
h. Rales.
5. Weigh the child each day:
a. At the same time.
b. On the same scale (note on the Kardex which scale is used).
c. Nude.
6. Record output accurately as this serves as a basis for replacement.
a. Amount voided.
b. Number and character of stools.
c. Amount and character of vomitus.
d. Fluid lost through fistulas, tubes, and suction.
7. Observe, record, and report the following signs and symptoms of blood transfusion reactions:
a. Chills.
b. Fever.
c. Headache.
d. Nausea and vomiting.
e. Pruritis.
f. Urticaria.
g. Flushing.
h. Asthmatic wheezing.
i. Confusion.
j. Hypotensive shock.
k. Flank pain.
l. Shock and/or renal failure.
8. Stop the transfusion immediately if signs or symptoms of transfusion reaction are noted.
9. Monitor I.V. accurately.
a. Use only the solution ordered.
b. Run at rate ordered.
c. Do not increase rate to catch up, since this may cause overhydration.
d. Keep an hourly record of fluid absorbed.
e. Observe frequently for infiltration, disconnection due to the child's activity, or kinks in the tubing.
f. Use a pediatric fluid administration set.
g. Do not irrigate a blocked I.V. since it may dislodge a clot.
10. Do not add potassium to an I.V. until the child has voided twice (one voiding is not sufficient evidence of urinary function; a child may have had a full bladder on admission).
11. Add heparin as ordered to the I.V. fluid to prevent clotting.
12. Use a fluid infusion pump as ordered.
a. Check that tubing is in correct place in pump.
b. Observe insertion site frequently for infiltration, since the pump will continue to push fluid into the tissue.
13. Support the child with an I.V. See *Preparation for Procedures.*
a. Restrain only those body parts that must be restrained for the child's safety. See *Restraints.*
b. Release restraints periodically to promote range of motion.
c. Provide mouth care for the child who is NPO.
d. Provide extra time for sucking, cuddling, etc., for the restrained infant.
e. Make sure the I.V. tubing is long enough so the child can have some movement.
f. Request I.V. not be placed in arm older child uses to write with if possible.
g. Explain to the child that I.V. is not punishment.
14. Support the parents.
a. Find out what they have been told about why their child has an I.V. and clarify as necessary.
b. Explain how the equipment works.
c. Encourage them to participate in the child's care.

Folk practices. See *Cultural Aspects of Health Care.*

Forcing fluids. Therapeutic increase of oral fluid intake.

A. **General Considerations.**
  1. Increased fluid intake is an important therapeutic intervention in a number of disease processes.
  2. The goal for fluid intake should be realistic in terms of the child's age and condition.
     a. Daily water intake varies from 50 ml/kg for adolescents to 150 ml/kg for infants.
     b. Fluid losses as a result of fever, diarrhea, etc., must be considered.
  3. Fluid requirements increase approximately 10 percent for each degree of temperature elevation.
  4. Fluid requirements may be met partly through other sources.
     a. Baby foods are high in moisture content and may meet fluid requirements.
     b. Jello, popsicles, and soup are recorded as fluid intake in some hospitals.

B. **Nursing Management.**
  1. Discuss with the child and parents what the fluid goal is and why.
  2. Find out the child's preferences for kind and temperature of fluids and record on Kardex.
  3. Consider the child's developmental level.
     a. Make a game of increasing the intake of the young child, e.g., pretend the child is a car that needs frequent stops at a gas station for "gas."
     b. Give the older child some responsibility for recording intake, e.g., marking a colored "X" on a chart to indicate that a glass of fluid was partially or completely drunk or recording the number of ml drunk.
  4. Offer fluids in a small cup so the child can feel successful in emptying it.
  5. Praise the child's effort for drinking, not just meeting the goal.
  6. Encourage the young child to drink with a straw so he can hear the "slurp" when the cup is empty.
  7. Offer saltine crackers to increase thirst if allowed on the child's diet.
  8. Keep fluid in the child's room and encourage frequent sips.
  9. Enlist the parents' cooperation in recording intake.

Foreign bodies in eye. See *Home Management of Minor Emergencies* and *Eye Injury*.

Formula feeding. See *Nutrition*.

Fracture. A break in a bone.

A. **General Considerations.**
  1. Fractures in childhood are more difficult to diagnose.
     a. The x-ray appearance of the growth plate may resemble a fracture.
     b. Children commonly have greenstick fractures in which one side of the bone is broken and the other only bent.
     c. Greenstick fractures may present with minimal pain, swelling, or deformity.
     d. The child may continue to use the involved extremity, since childhood fractures are usually stable.
  2. Minor twists and falls may cause a greenstick fracture, since the child's bone is more porous.
  3. Fractures can usually be reduced and immobilized by traction or by manipulation and casting so open reduction is rarely necessary except for fractures which cannot be maintained by conservative methods or which have caused injury to tissue, nerves or arteries.
  4. A long leg cast-brace with knee hinges is often used to treat fractures of the distal femoral shaft in older child or adolescent (Meggitt, Juett, and Smith, 1981).
  5. Desired alignment of bone fragments is often side-to-side rather than end-to-end in many childhood fractures.
  6. Blood loss secondary to fractured femur may necessitate transfusion.
  7. Once the fracture is immobilized, irritability, crying, and complaints of pain by the child are indicative of complications.
  8. Healing is rapid and nonunion of bone is rare.
  9. Early mobilization and active range of motion are used to prevent joint stiffness although prolonged stiffness is rare in children.
  10. Kidney stones are a rare complication due to prolonged nonweightbearing.
  11. Pulmonary emboli can occur in a child with multiple fractures.
  12. Permanent damage to the growth plate can result in progressive deformity although this is uncommon.

B. **Nursing Management.** See CAST CARE and TRACTION, CARE OF CHILD.
  1. Support the child and parents during hospitalization. See *Hospitalization, Support During*.
  2. Initiate discharge planning. See *Discharge Planning*.
  3. Administer antitetanus vaccine if ordered.
  4. Prepare the child for surgery if appropriate. See *Preparation for Surgery, Preoperative Care*, and *Postoperative Care*.
  5. Observe, record, and report the following (Webb, 1974):
     a. Pain.
        1. Be alert for behavioral symptoms of pain in the infant or young child. See *Pain*.

2. Determine exact area of pain.
3. Assess any increase in pain or lack of relief from analgesics.
   b. Pulse.
   1. Check brachial, radial, ulnar, and digital pulses if upper extremity is involved.
   2. Check femoral, popliteal, posterior tibial, and dorsalis pedis pulses if lower extremity is involved.
   c. Paresthesia.
   1. Check for diminished sensation, numbness, and lack of sensation.
   2. Check nerve functioning of the hand by pricking the web space between the thumb and index finger, the distal fat pad of the small finger, and the distal surface of the index finger.
   3. Check nerve functioning of the foot by pricking the web space between the first and second toe.
   d. Paralysis.
   1. Assess hand function by asking the child to hyperextend his thumb or wrist, to oppose his thumb and little finger, and to abduct all his fingers.
   2. Assess motor function of the foot by asking the child to dorsiflex and plantarflex his ankles and to flex and extend his toes.
   e. Pallor.
   1. Note color of the extremity distal to the fracture site.
   2. Assess capillary return of the nail beds following blanching.

3. Assess temperature of affected extremity in comparison to the unaffected extremity.
6. Observe, record, and report symptoms of Volkmann's contracture of the forearm if the child has an upper extremity fracture.
   a. Increased pain and hyperextension of the wrist.
   b. Increased pain with passive extension of the fingers.
   c. Absent radial pulse.
7. Observe, record, and report symptoms of anterior compartment syndrome if the child has a fractured proximal tibia.
   a. Increased pain and tenderness.
   b. Induration at the fracture site.
   c. Inability to extend the great toe.
   d. Decreased sensation in the web space between the first and second toes.
8. Initiate immediate action for symptoms of Volkmann's contracture or anterior compartment syndrome if present.
9. Meet comfort needs.
   a. Assess the child's need for pain medication, since the child may fear injections more than pain. See *Pain*.
   b. Discuss the child's perception of what has and will happen.
10. Teach the child and parent home management. See *Cast Care*.

Fungal infections. See *Candida Albicans* and *Tinea*.

Gait, disturbances in. See *Congenital Hip Dysplasia, Legg-Perthes Disease,* and *Slipped Femoral Epiphysis.*

Gastric acid, reflux of. See *Gastroesophageal reflux.*

Gastric malformation. See *Pyloric stenosis.*

Gastritis, acute. See *Gastroenteritis, infectious.*

Gastroenteritis, infectious. Infections of the gastrointestinal track caused by either bacteria or viruses.

A. General Considerations.
   1. Staphlococcal gastroenteritis (food poisoning).
      a. Follows the ingestion of an enterotoxin found in contaminated foods which have not been properly refrigerated.

b. Signs and symptoms appear suddenly about 2 to 6 hours after eating and include:
   1. Diarrhea (variable) lasting approximately 24 hours.
   2. Nausea.
   3. Vomiting.
   4. Pronounced abdominal cramping.
   5. Fatigue.
c. Treatment is symptomatic and directed at maintaining fluid and electrolyte balance.

2. Salmonella gastroenteritis.
   a. Sources of infection include:
      1. Contaminated water or food.
      2. Contact with a carrier or mildly infected person.
      3. Contact with a contaminated object.
   b. Signs and symptoms appear after an incubation period that varies from 1 to 4 days or more:
      1. Fever.
      2. Vomiting.
      3. Rhinorrhea.
      4. Diarrhea: stools are loose, green, slimy, and smell like spoiled eggs.
   c. Diagnosis is made on the basis of identification of one of the species of the organism in a stool culture.
   d. Treatment is symptomatic and directed at preventing fluid and electrolyte imbalance.
   e. Most cases are self-limiting and resolve within a few days.
   f. Patients convalescent from salmonella may excrete the organisms in their stools for up to a year.
   g. Salmonella infection may spread to distant locations and cause osteomyelitis, pyelonephritis, meningitis, and arthritis (most common) (Nete, Faden, 1979).

3. Shigella gastroenteritis (bacillary dysentery).
   a. Follows the ingestion of contaminated food or water.
   b. Signs and symptoms appear after an incubation period of 8 to 40 hours and include:
      1. Fever.
      2. Vomiting.
      3. Watery diarrhea progressing in severe cases to bloody, mucoid diarrhea.
   c. Stool examination shows marked leukocytosis.
   d. Diagnosis is based on identification of one of the four different shigella organisms in the stool.
   e. Treatment includes the use of antibiotics and symptoms usually subside in 4 to 10 days.

4. Enteropathogenic *Escherichia coli* gastroenteritis.
   a. The causative organism is spread via contaminated hands, linen, and equipment.

b. Signs and symptoms develop after an incubation period of a few hours and include:
   1. Diarrhea.
   2. Anorexia.
   3. Vomiting.
   4. Fever: may be absent in mild cases.
c. Diagnosis is made by stool culture.
d. Treatment measures include:
   1. Fluid and electrolytes to avoid imbalance.
   2. Antibiotics (debated).

5. Viral gastroenteritis (rotavirus diarrhea).
   a. Most common cause of diarrhea in infants and children.
   b. Signs and symptoms develop after a 1- to 3-day incubation period and include:
      1. Vomiting: may be severe.
      2. Diarrhea.
   c. Diagnosis is made by detecting virus particles in the stool.
   d. Treatment is symptomatic and directed at prevention of fluid and electrolyte imbalance.

6. Compazine is not given to children because it may produce adverse behavioral symptoms.

7. Mild cases of gastroenteritis can usually be managed at home, but infants and children with severe cases may need to be hospitalized.

8. Enteric isolation precautions should be followed to prevent the spread of infection.

9. Inflammatory lesions of the stomach (acute gastritis) may occur in the presence of severe gastroenteritis.

B. **Nursing Management.**
   1. Support the child and parents during hospitalization. See *Hospitalization, Support During.*
   2. Initiate discharge planning. See *Discharge Planning.*
   3. Explain the isolation procedure and its rationale.
   4. Explain the rationale for placing the child NPO for a period of time, e.g., it prevents loss of more fluid and electrolytes.
   5. Observe, record, and report the child's response to antiemetic medication if given.
   6. Observe, record, and report the following:
      a. Number and character of stools.
      b. Amount and character of stools.
      c. Frequency and amount of urination.
      d. Temperature: take axillary if anal area excoriated or diarrhea present.
      e. Daily weight.
      f. Signs and symptoms of fluid and electrolyte imbalance. See *Fluid and Electrolyte Imbalance.*
      g. Skin condition in perineal area.

h. Abdominal pain.

7. Monitor I.V. accurately if this route is used to maintain hydration until oral intake is adequate.

8. Initiate fever reduction measures if the temperature is elevated. See *Fever Reduction*.

9. Progress the child's diet as ordered.

10. Withhold fluid and food and notify physician if vomiting and/or diarrhea recur. See *Diarrhea* and *Vomiting*.

11. Provide for sucking needs of the infant who is NPO.

12. Give frequent mouth care.

13. Prevent skin breakdown.

14. Teach the child and parents home management.

    a. Explain the rationale for keeping the child NPO for a period of time if ordered.

    b. Withhold food and fluids for the time period ordered.

    c. Progress diet as ordered. See *Vomiting*.

    d. Stop feeding if vomiting and/or diarrhea recur and start diet progression over again after a period of being NPO.

    e. Do not boil skim milk, since this produces a hypertonic solution.

    f. Do not use over-the-counter medications for vomiting or diarrhea unless so instructed by the physician.

    g. Explain the administration of antiemetic suppositories if ordered. See *Administration of Medications, Parental*.

       1. Lubricate or wet the suppository as needed.

       2. Insert the suppository just past the internal anal sphincter.

       3. Hold buttocks together until the urge to defecate passes.

    h. Call the physician if symptoms continue or signs and symptoms of dehydration develop.

Gastroesophageal reflux.

Condition resulting from a relaxed or incompetent cardiac sphincter which allows regurgitation of stomach contents into the esophagus or pharynx; frequently associated with hiatal hernia.

A. **General Considerations.**

1. Reflux is common in newborns because of immature neuromuscular control, but becomes a concern if it continues for several months.

2. Laryngospasm, induced by gastroesophageal reflux (GER), is characterized by choking and apnea and may be related to sudden infant death syndrome (Seashore, 1982).

3. Severe reflux may cause:

    a. Failure to thrive.

    b. Recurrent pneumonitis.

    c. Esophagitis.

    d. Gastrointestinal blood loss.

    e. Pain.

    f. Esophageal stricture.

4. Older children frequently have a history of chronic cough, wheezing, and recurrent pneumonia.

5. Diagnostic work-up may include:

    a. History of postprandial regurgitation becoming more severe between 4 and 8 weeks of age as the volume per feeding increases.

    b. Observation of feeding habits.

    c. Barium esophagram.

    d. Manometric tests of esophageal motility.

    e. Acid reflux tests to measure intraesophageal pH.

    f. Isotope scanning.

    g. Gastric emptying studies.

    h. Endoscopy.

6. Treatment goals are to decrease the episodes of reflux and to coat the esophagus with a neutral material.

    a. Positioning prone at an elevation of 30 to 45 degrees 24 hours a day.

    b. Small, frequent feedings of thickened formula.

    c. Antacids may be given 15 to 30 minutes after feeding if the above have been ineffective.

7. Conservative therapy of 6 to 8 weeks is successful in the majority of infants.

8. Some infants and most older children will require surgical correction.

9. Nissan fundoiplication entails wrapping the fundus of the stomach around the distal esophagus.

10. Complications of the fundoplication include:

    a. Esophageal perforation.

    b. Gastric bloat syndrome.

    c. Herniation of the plication.

11. A child who has aspirated feedings preoperatively may have slow clearing of the pneumonitis and require feeding gastrostomy for several months.

12. The child who is severely brain damaged has a higher incidence of reflux and usually requires surgical intervention (Wesley et al., 1981).

13. Dilatations may be required postoperatively in a few patients.

B. **Nursing Management.**

1. Support the child and parents during hospitalization. See *Hospitalization, Support During*.

2. Initiate discharge planning. See *Discharge Planning*.

3. Prepare the older child and parents for the di-

agnostic procedures. See *Preparation for Procedures.*

4. Observe the feeding technique of the parent(s) to assist in the diagnosis.
5. Teach the parents home management if conservative treatment is recommended.
   a. Keep the infant in an upright position or over the shoulder in a "burp" position whenever holding or carrying.
   b. Bathe the baby in a sitting position in the tub.
   c. Add rice cereal to thicken feedings; feed smaller volumes more frequently and in an upright position and burp frequently.
   d. Make a wedge of folded beach towels to prop the infant in an upright position for diaper changing (Boyd, 1982).
   e. Encourage the parents to stimulate the baby by use of mobiles, pictures, and toys tied to the rim of a play pen. See *Stimulation.*
   f. Provide the parents with instructions on making a bed or antireflux saddle, etc. at all times.
6. Inform the parents that discontinuing the postural therapy after 6 asymptomatic weeks will involve slow change in position from upright to flat.
7. Prepare the older child and parents if surgery is necessary. See *Preparation for Surgery.*
8. Provide appropriate preoperative and postoperative care. See *Preoperative Care* and *Postoperative Care.*
9. Teach the child and parents home management.
   a. Inform parents to notify the surgeon of fever, persistent cough, recurrence of reflux, or symptoms of wound infection.
   b. Have the parents demonstrate gastrostomy feeding techniques if appropriate.
   c. Reinforce the need for follow-up care.
   d. Explain the procedure for dilatations if these are necessary postoperatively.
10. Initiate referral to the community health nurse or other agencies as needed.

Gastrostomy. See *Burns, Chemical,* and *Tracheoesophageal Fistula.*

Genetic counseling. Use of knowledge of human genetics in providing information about inheritable abnormalities.

A. General Considerations.
1. Most individuals or couples seek counseling after having had a child with a defect.
2. The disorders for which counseling may be sought result from four different mechanisms (Wood, 1974):
   a. Single pair mutations: autosomal dominant and autosomal recessive, and sex linked which are Mendelian patterns of inheritance, e.g., cystic fibrosis.
   b. Chromosomal abnormalities: usually not inheritable except in cases of translocations, e.g., Down's syndrome.
   c. Multifactorial: complex interaction of multiple genetic and environmental factors, e.g., pyloric stenosis.
   d. Environmental factors: agents in the environment produce nonheritable disorders which mimic genetic diseases.
3. The probability that a specific disorder will occur can be stated most accurately for those which follow Mendelian patterns, less accurately for chromosomal abnormalities, and least accurately for the remainder.
4. The chances of having a defective child are expressed as probabilities, not as absolutes and are the same for each pregnancy.
5. A highly detailed history of both maternal and paternal sides of the family is the basis for detecting specific patterns of disorders.
6. Amniotic fluid obtained by amniocentesis can be subjected to chromosomal and biochemical analysis to detect many, but not all, defects.
7. Many genetic disorders are treatable, e.g., phenylketonuria.
8. Genetic counseling represents a situational crisis because the individual or couple has to:
   a. Cope with feelings related to the actual or potential birth of a defective child.
   b. Divulge information about themselves and their family which they may not have shared with their mate or others.
   c. Decide whether to, depending on the situation:
      1. Attempt to have a child or another child.
      2. Undergo lab tests which may detect a defect.
      3. Continue with pregnancy or have an abortion if amniocentesis verifies a defect.
9. The actual decision about future actions must be left up to the individual or couple.

B. Nursing Management. See CRISIS INTERVENTION and EXCEPTIONAL CHILD.
1. Find out what the individual or couple has been told already about the defect and what they wish to know.
2. Validate your information about the specific defect before doing any counseling.
3. Offer appropriate counseling (Sahin, 1976).
   a. See both parents together if possible so they both hear the same information.

b. Provide for privacy and adequate time.

c. Do not have an affected child present, if possible, when you talk with the parents.

d. Provide information requested but do not push information on parents.

e. Explain that no one is to blame for the defect.

f. Facilitate verbalization of parental feelings.

g. Explain treatment modalities available in appropriate situation, e.g., diet treatment in phenylketonuria.

h. Summarize the counseling session in written form, since anxiety reduces retention of information.

4. Make sure parents understand the concept of statistical probability related to their situation, e.g., use checkerboard square diagram to show Mendelian inheritance.

5. Prepare parents for diagnostic procedures which may be ordered for them or their child, e.g., amniocentesis or chromosomal studies. See *Preparation for Procedures.*

6. Initiate referrals for further assessment and/or support as indicated. See *Discharge Planning.*

German measles. See *Rubella.*

Glasses, eye. See *Strabismus.*

Glomerulonephritis, acute. Inflammation of the kidneys following infection of the pharynx or skin by certain strains of the group A beta hemolytic streptococcus.

A. **General Considerations.**

1. The disease results from an altered immune response in which antigen–antibody complexes produce glomerular changes.

2. Signs and symptoms include:

a. Headache.

b. Malaise.

c. Red- or "coke"-colored urine.

d. Anorexia.

e. Nausea.

f. Vomiting.

g. Diarrhea.

h. Hypertension.

i. Periorbital edema.

j. Decreased urinary output.

3. Severe signs and symptoms include:

a. Convulsions secondary to cerebral ischemia and/or hypertension.

b. Pulmonary congestion.

c. Acute renal failure.

4. Complications may occur during the acute phase.

a. Hypertensive encephalopathy.

b. Acute cardiac decompression.

c. Acute renal failure.

5. Laboratory studies include:

a. Urinalysis that will show:

1. Protein.

2. Red blood cells.

3. White blood cells.

4. Casts.

b. Blood studies that will show:

1. Decreased serum complement level.

2. Mild anemia.

3. Elevated BUN.

4. Elevated serum creatinine level.

5. Elevated antistreptolysin O titer.

6. Elevated erythrocyte sedimentation rate.

7. Decreased hemolytic complement activity and C_3 levels.

6. Treatment is symptomatic and home management is often possible.

7. Bed rest is recommended during acute phase.

8. Antibiotics will be used to treat any remaining streptococcal infection.

9. A "no added salt" diet is usual since severe sodium restriction is rarely necessary, and children will not eat a severely restricted diet.

10. The prognosis for complete recovery is generally favorable.

B. **Nursing Management.**

1. Support the child and parents during hospitalization. See *Hospitalization, Support During.*

2. Initiate discharge planning. See *Discharge Planning.*

3. Assess fluid retention.

a. Compare the child's admission weight with preillness weight.

b. Weigh daily and record.

1. Use the same scale.

2. Weigh at the same time each day.

3. Weigh the child nude or in underpants.

c. Observe for edema, especially periorbital.

4. Assess renal function.

a. Measure intake and output accurately.

b. Collect a urine sample each morning for visual comparison with previous day's specimen.

c. Test urine for protein.

d. Check reports of lab values for renal function.

5. Monitor vital signs and blood pressure accurately.

a. Report any alterations from norms.

b. Check blood pressure every 1 to 2 hours if the diastolic pressure is greater than 90 mm Hg.

6. Observe, record, and report the child's level of consciousness.

7. Observe, record, and report signs and symptoms of hypertensive encephalopathy.
   a. Headache.
   b. Drowsiness.
   c. Restlessness.
   d. Double vision.
   e. Seizures.
   f. Coma.
8. Institute seizure precautions as needed. See *Seizures.*
9. Observe, record, and report signs and symptoms indicative of heart failure.
   a. Tachycardia.
   b. Tachypnea.
   c. Dyspnea.
   d. Restlessness.
   e. Poor feeding.
   f. Easy fatigability.
   g. Distended abdomen.
   h. Dependent edema.
   i. Pulmonary edema.
10. Observe, record, and report signs and symptoms of renal failure.
    a. Headache.
    b. Fatigue.
    c. Anorexia.
    d. Pallor.
    e. Hypertension.
    f. Decreased urinary output.
11. Observe, record, and report the child's response to antihypertensive and/or diuretic drugs if these are given.
12. Observe, record, and report the child's response to antibiotics if these are given.
13. Prevent infection.
    a. Avoid chilling.
    b. Prevent contact with individuals with infections, especially upper respiratory infections.
14. Restrict sodium intake as ordered.
15. Promote adequate nutrition. See *Nutrition.*
    a. Record on Kardex and provide foods the child likes.
    b. Feed smaller, more frequent meals.
    c. Provide companionship at meal times.
16. Maintain bedrest if ordered.
17. Provide age-appropriate diversional activities. See *Play.*
18. Encourage school age child to keep up with schoolwork as condition permits.
19. Teach the child and parents home management.
    a. Administration of medications. See *Administration of Medications, Parental.*
    b. Dietary restrictions if required.
    c. Signs and symptoms to report to the physician:
       1. Blood in urine.
       2. Decreased urinary output.
       3. Increased weight.
       4. Signs and symptoms of infection, especially upper respiratory, e.g., fever, sore throat, cough.
    d. Activity restrictions, if any.
20. Explain the importance of returning for follow-up visits so renal function can be assessed.

Gonorrhea. See *Sexually Transmitted Diseases.*

Grafts, skin. See *Burns.*

Graves' disease. See *Hyperthyroidism.*

Grief. See *Dying Child, Exceptional Child,* and *Life-Threatening Illness.*

Growing pains. Chronic, intermittent limb pain.

A. **General Considerations.**
   1. The site of the pain may be the front of the thighs, calves, behind the knees, or in the groin.
   2. Pain is characteristically described as outside the joint area.
   3. Pain usually occurs in the late afternoon or evening, although it may awaken the child from sleep.
   4. Pain may be accentuated by running, but specific trauma or infection is denied.
   5. The peak incidence is in the preschooler, but the pain may begin as early as infancy (Peterson, 1977).

B. **Nursing Management.**
   1. Obtain an accurate history from the parents and child if old enough.
      a. Location of pain.
      b. Child's activity level.
      c. Time of day pain occurs.
   2. Teach parents home management.
      a. Administer aspirin or aspirin substitute.
      b. Initiate massage of the affected muscles.
      c. Apply heat to the affected muscles being sure that safety measures are followed.
         1. Wrap the leg(s) in a hot, wet towel.
         2. Cover the towel with waterproof plastic wrap.
         3. Cover the wrapping with a dry towel.
      d. Refer to a physician if:
         1. Pain persists.
         2. Medication is required more than occasionally.
         3. Symptoms such as swollen, red, or warm joints occur.

Growth and development. See *Appendix v.*

Halo femoral traction. See *Scoliosis.*

Hand-foot syndrome. See *Anemia, Sickle Cell.*

Handicapped child. The child who is disadvantaged because of a congenital or acquired physical condition.

A. **General Considerations.**
1. The family must deal with the loss of the anticipated normal child and the reality of parenting a handicapped child. See *Exceptional Child.*
2. Factors which affect the family's adjustment to the child's diagnosis include:
   a. Available support systems.
   b. Perception of the illness/handicap.
   c. Coping patterns as individuals and as a family.
3. The child's ability to cope with his handicap is primarily determined by the parents' ability to cope.
4. The child who acquires a serious disability proceeds through three stages (Whaley and Wong, 1983).
   a. Withdrawal—the child is depressed and unresponsive.
   b. Preoccupation with self—the child focuses on his disability and loss of previous abilities.
   c. Gradual return to reality.
5. The child who has an obvious handicap such as congenital absence of a limb will more likely accept his condition than the child with an invisible handicap such as diabetes or hemophilia.
6. The problems facing the family of the handicapped child are numerous and significant (Pless, 1980).
   a. Day-to-day stresses of the child's need for attention, reactions of others, social relations, effect on siblings and marital relations.
   b. Life maintenance stresses of finances, housing, transportation, clothing, and appliances.
   c. Concerns about the future such as additional children, education and vocational training, and residential care.
7. Parents must also cope with the repeated and numerous hospitalizations and surgeries.

8. The overwhelming difficulties of managing the handicapped child and the feelings of failure on the part of parents often leads to family disharmony and subsequent divorce.
9. Fathers have fewer opportunities to help the child directly and are offered fewer services by parent organizations and service agencies.
10. Siblings of the handicapped child may be tremendously affected in a negative way.
    a. Anger and resentment over added responsibilities and loss of parental attention.
    b. Fear for their own health.
    c. Feelings of isolation.
11. Siblings can be helped to view the family's coping with the handicap as a positive experience if they are praised and given attention for their contributions.
12. A collaborative, multidisciplinary team effort is essential to providing optimal care for the handicapped child.
13. The nurse should consider the following information when planning intervention:
    a. The parents may have recurrence of grieving reactions as the child encounters difficulty as he reaches different developmental levels, e.g., entering school, reaching puberty, etc.
    b. Parents have difficulty in establishing discipline which is not too lenient or too restrictive and consistent with that of the nonhandicapped sibling(s).
    c. Conflict with educators about the child's abilities and the educational prescription can be avoided by good communication between parents and teachers.
    d. Parents need relief from the stress of the handicapped child to avoid emotional and physical exhaustion.

B. **Nursing Management.**
1. Support the child and parents during hospitalization. See *Hospitalization, Support During.*
2. Initiate discharge planning. See *Discharge Planning.*
3. Individualize nursing care to the needs of the child. See *Chronic Illness.*
   a. Assess the child's developmental level. See *Appendix v.*
   b. Evaluate the child's understanding of his handicap and add to his knowledge as his comprehension increases.
   c. Provide meticulous personal hygiene and

help the older child and parents to understand how important this is to social acceptance.

d. Involve as many disciplines as necessary to help the child learn to be independent in cleanliness and grooming.

e. Follow the child's preferences for how procedures and routines are performed as much as possible.

f. Arrange for the child to learn relaxation techniques to decrease stress (Steele, 1983).

g. Encourage exercise to increase the child's body awareness (Bernard et al., 1981).

h. Involve the child in food selection to improve his knowledge of nutrition. See *Nutrition.*

i. Help the older child to identify peer group activities such as Amputee Camp, Hemophilia Camp, camp for asthmatics, Special Olympics, wheelchair basketball, etc.

j. Encourage play and diversionary activities which have some potential for the child to be successful.

4. Assess the family's understanding of the handicap and specific treatment goals in order to supply information they lack and to clarify any misconceptions.

5. Review the child's general health history and make sure the child is receiving appropriate well-child care, e.g., immunizations, health screening, dental care. See *Appendix vi, Dental Care, Health Promotion and Maintenance.*

6. Evaluate the parents' ability to prioritize their own needs and if appropriate, refer to community mental health agencies for counseling or to the family physician for health care.

7. Assist the family to identify community resources for financial help, e.g., state Crippled Children's Services, Supplementary Social Security benefits, etc.

8. Identify ways in which families can increase peer acceptance of the child and family through summer camp activities, parent or sibling groups, mainstreaming in the educational setting.

9. Explore resources which can help the family cope if constant, total care is unrealistic.
   a. Day care centers.
   b. Home health aides.
   c. Respite care.
   d. Institutionalization.

10. Encourage parents to facilitate management of the child (Zamerowki, 1982).
    a. Keep their own records regarding physician visits, evaluation, etc.
    b. Ask questions of health professionals when they do not understand.
    c. Use parent groups to gain support and to learn more about the handicap.

d. Evaluate recommended treatment programs in perspective for their own child; not every program works for every child.

Head injury. Trauma to any area of the scalp, skull, and/or brain.

A. General Considerations.

1. Children's response to head injuries differs from those of adults.
   a. Symptoms may be exaggerated, since the child's general physiological response is more labile.
   b. Neurological signs secondary to increased intracranial pressure may be delayed or absent, since the skull is more expandable.
   c. The incidence of associated seizure activity is more frequent.

2. Categorization of head injuries is based on significant clinical and pathological findings.
   a. Mild.
      1. Characterized by transient loss of consciousness, amnesia for the event, and no demonstrable neurological signs.
      2. The young child may resume playing with minimal complaints of pain after brief loss of consciousness.
      3. Sequelae may be nonexistent or mild.
      4. Concussion, mild contusions, and limited subarachnoid bleeding are associated with mild head injuries.
      5. Most children with mild injury can be managed at home.
   b. Moderate.
      1. Characterized by disturbance of or loss of consciousness from several minutes up to an hour.
      2. Abnormal neurological signs are frequent, although transient.
      3. Sequelae are moderate and of 12- to 36-hour duration.
      4. Cerebral edema, contusions, and lacerations are associated with moderate head injuries.
   c. Severe.
      1. Unconsciousness may be immediate or may occur after an initial lucid period.
      2. Abnormal neurological signs may persist from hours to days or may be permanent.
      3. Sequelae may be significant.
      4. Extensive cerebral edema, contusions, and lacerations of the brain, intracranial bleeding, and brainstem damage are associated with severe head injuries.
      5. Hospitalization will be necessary to initiate treatment and to diagnose other injuries.

3. Diagnostic procedures may include one or more of the following.
   a. Skull x-rays.
   b. Cervical and spine films.
   c. Cerebral angiography.
   d. CAT scan.
   e. Brain scan.
   f. Echoencephalography.
   g. Subdural taps.
   h. Exploratory burr holes (trephines).
   i. EEG for defining seizure activity in the recuperative stage.
4. Complications and sequelae include:
   a. Posttraumatic seizures.
      1. More common in younger children.
      2. Usually transient and require no treatment if they occur in the first 48 hours (Singer and Freeman, 1968).
      3. Use of prophylactic anticonvulsants is controversial.
   b. Epidural or subdural hematomas.
   c. Subarachnoid hemorrhage.
   d. CSF rhinorrhea and otorrhea.
   e. Hydrocephalus.
   f. Mental retardation.
   g. Postconcussion syndrome.
      1. Behavior disturbances, e.g., aggressiveness, regression, withdrawal.
      2. Sleep disturbances.
      3. Irritability.
      4. Emotional lability.
      5. School difficulties.
      6. Phobias.
5. Evoked potential monitoring may be used to determine the extent of a severe head injury.
6. The majority of children with mild head injury and simple linear skull fractures have no sequelae.
7. Most sequelae are the behavioral and emotional difficulties which disappear within a few months or a year.

B. **Nursing Management.** See *Home Management of Minor Emergencies* for care of the child with a mild head injury.
   1. Support the child and parents during hospitalization. See *Hospitalization, Support During.*
   2. Initiate discharge planning. See *Discharge Planning.*
   3. Maintain an adequate airway.
   4. Monitor the child's physiological function as ordered.
      a. Vital signs.
      b. CVP.
      c. Intracranial pressure monitoring.
      d. Specific gravity of urine.
      e. Hourly intake and output.
5. Observe, record, and report signs and symptoms of increased intracranial pressure. See *Increased Intracranial Pressure.*
6. Administer medications as ordered.
   a. Anticonvulsants.
   b. Sedatives for restlessness.
   c. Aspirin or aspirin substitute for headache.
   d. Tetanus prophylaxis for scalp wound.
   e. Antibiotics for "dirty" wound or CSF rhinorrhea or otorrhea.
   f. Steroids or hypertonic solutions for cerebral edema.
7. Initiate fever reduction measures as ordered. See *Fever Reduction.*
8. Monitor I.V. accurately to prevent increased intracranial pressure.
9. Report clear, colorless fluid drainage from the ear(s) or nose.
   a. Check drainage for glucose with Dextrostix to determine if CSF.
   b. Place in high Fowler's position if glucose test is positive.
   c. Do not suction nasally since the catheter might enter the brain through the fracture site.
10. Turn the child frequently to protect pressure points and to minimize the risk of orthostatic pneumonia.
11. Apply antiembolic stockings as ordered.
12. Promote comfort.
    a. Provide irrigations, eye drops, or eye dressings as ordered.
    b. Use cool compresses to reduce edema if ordered.
    c. Provide mouth care.
    d. Provide meticulous skin care.
13. Perform passive range of motion exercises.
14. Provide quiet stimulation, e.g., radio, records, holding and rocking, etc.
15. Promote adequate nutrition.
    a. Offer food in an attractive manner.
    b. Feed via nasogastric or gastrostomy tube as ordered.
16. Assure adequate elimination.
    a. Provide appropriate fluid intake as ordered. See *Forcing Fluids.*
    b. Administer stool softener.
    c. Administer suppositories or enemas as ordered.
17. Check the child for bladder distention if restlessness is noted.
18. Restrain the child only if absolutely necessary.
    a. Restraints may increase the child's frustration and result in increased intracranial pressure.

b. Use elbow restraints or mitts if restraints are required.

19. Meet the special needs of the child who requires surgery.
    a. Position the child with the bed flat or slighly elevated as ordered.
        1. Move the head and neck as a single unit if surgery was performed in the low occipital area.
        2. Position on unoperative side unless ordered otherwise.
        3. Do not lower the head of the bed or elevate the foot of the bed.
        4. Change position hourly with slow, careful movements.
    b. Observe, record, and report the following:
        1. Rapid increase in drainage or bright red blood on head dressing.
        2. Increase in facial or neck edema.
        3. Urinary incontinence or retention.
    c. Reinforce the head dressing with sterile towel or pads if needed.
        1. Use a ballpoint pen to outline drainage, since fluid from a felt tip pen may penetrate the dressing.
        2. Clarify with the surgeon how much drainage should be expected.

20. Encourage the child's return to normal functioning when his condition improves.
    a. Explain that edema and/or surgical trauma make return to normal functioning a slow process.
    b. Support the parents in order that they do not overprotect the child.
    c. Help the child adjust to changes in body image. See *Body Image.*
        1. Obtain a cap, scarf, or ruffled sleeping bonnet.
        2. Have the child wear a wig until hair grows.
    d. Refer the family to the community health nurse if appropriate.
    e. Initiate contact with the child's teacher and school nurse.
        1. Classmates need to expect change in the child's behavior and/or appearance.
        2. Activity restrictions must be explained.
        3. Rest periods should be planned initially.

21. Support the parents whose child's recovery is prolonged or indefinite.
    a. Explain the role of the allied health therapies.
    b. Assist them in evaluating placement alternatives.
    c. Support their decision if residential placement outside the home is necessary.
    d. Arrange community follow-up if the child is taken home.

e. Teach procedures and equipment management.

f. Identify resources for supplies.

g. Encourage the parents to maintain contact with the hospital staff if there are management problems at home in the first few weeks.

Headache. Discomfort stemming from pain-sensitive structures of the head.

A. **General Considerations.**
1. Headaches in the older child are common and usually benign.
2. Headaches in the young child are rare and more often indicative of pathology.
3. Early morning headaches accompanied by vomiting and no nausea is characteristic of brain tumors.
4. Young children may report "headache" in imitation of adults.
5. The infant or toddler with a headache may be irritable and/or restless and rub his head.
6. Headaches can be categorized as follows (McCarthy, 1982):
    a. Migraine (also called vascular).
    b. Tension (also called psychogenic or muscle contraction).
    c. Traction/inflammatory (caused by brain lesions or inflammatory processes).
7. Diagnostic studies may include:
    a. EEG, if seizures are a possibility.
    b. CAT scan.
    c. Skull films.
8. A thorough history of the child's headache pattern and family headache history is valuable to establishing a diagnosis. See *Nursing History.*
9. Migraine headaches are characterized by:
    a. Family history of migraines.
    b. Nausea and vomiting.
    c. Presence of a visual aura such as diplopia or zigzag patterns across the field of vision.
10. Tension is usually the cause of headaches assumed to be due to refractive error, so glasses are seldom helpful.
11. Treatment is directed toward the primary disorder if a specific intracranial disorder or systemic disease is diagnosed.
    a. Hypertension.
    b. Allergies.
    c. Epilepsy.
    d. Emotional distubance.
    e. Dental problems.
9. Treatment of primary headache varies.
    a. Tension headaches may be relieved by salicylates or antianxiety drugs, but primary

attention is given to reducing emotional strain.

b. Migraine headaches are treated with salicylates, Cafergot P-B, phenytoin, or methysergide maleate.

B. **Nursing Management.** See SCHOOL PHOBIA, SEIZURES, and SINUSITIS.

1. Support the child and parents if diagnostic procedures are necessary. See *Preparation for Procedures.*
   a. Explain the procedure and the rationale for performing it.
   b. Discuss the implications of the results.
2. Reinforce the physician's explanation of the cause and treatment once the diagnosis has been established.
3. Meet the needs of the child and family when tension headaches are diagnosed.
   a. Provide opportunities for the child and parents to express their feelings about the diagnosis.
   b. Explore with the child and parents how the child's environment can be less stressful.
      1. Discuss the need for expectations based on the child's individual and developmental abilities.
      2. Discuss community resources that may relieve family stress.
      3. Discuss proper posture for studying to reduce contracture of neck muscles.
   c. Support the need for professional counseling if appropriate.
4. Meet the needs of the child and parents when migraine headaches are diagnosed.
   a. Reassure the child and parents that even severe migraines are benign and are not symptomatic of brain tumor.
   b. Encourage the child to avoid foods which may trigger the headache; e.g., aged cheese, chocolate, vinegar, cured meats, alcohol for the adolescent (McCarthy and Mehegan, 1982).
   c. Discuss measures that may relieve the intense pain.
      1. Prescription medications. See *Administration of Medications, Parental.*
      2. A quiet, dark room.
      3. Rest or sleep.
      4. Biofeedback or relaxation techniques.
   d. Explore ways to decrease environmental stress. See above.
   e. Discuss with the parents that how the adults in the family cope with their migraines will influence how the child copes, e.g., the mother who remains in bed for 3 days with a migraine will find it difficult to convince the child to attend school when he has a migraine.

Health promotion and maintenance. Activities of the family and/or health care professional that are directed at the attainment or continuation of optimal health.

A. **General Considerations.**
   1. A nursing history serves as the basis for identifying health promotion and maintenance needs.
   2. The following needs must be provided for in the promotion and/or maintenance of health (Murray and Zentner, 1975).
      a. Regular health assessment.
      b. Primary, secondary, and tertiary preventive measures aimed at avoidance, early treatment, or prevention of progression of a disease.
      c. The avoidance of extremes in behaviors or emotions.
      d. Care of the body and its functions.
      e. Adequate nutrition.
      f. Talking care of illness or injury as it occurs.
      g. Health education and anticipatory guidance.
      h. Continuity of care for the individual, family, or social group.
   3. In order to promote and maintain health effectively the nurse must:
      a. Value the prevention of injury and illness as much as its treatment and cure.
      b. Be willing to be an advocate for the patient/client and his family.
   4. Health promotion and maintenance is a joint responsibility of the individual, the individual's family, and other support groups, and health care professionals.
   5. The way in which a patient/client and his family use, or accept the use of, health promotion and maintenance practices will be influenced by their:
      a. Culture.
      b. Religion.
      c. Life style.
      d. Educational level.
      e. Financial status.
      f. Existing unmet needs.
   6. Health promotion and maintenance needs should be included in every plan of care for the patient/client and his family.

B. **Nursing Management.** See CULTURAL ASPECTS OF HEALTH CARE, RELIGIOUS ASPECTS OF HEALTH CARE, and WELL-CHILD CARE.
   1. Obtain a nursing history to identify health promotion and maintenance needs of the child and his family and record the needs on the chart or Kardex. See *History Taking.*
   2. Assist the child and parents in understanding and valuing health promotion and maintenance.

a. Discuss the importance of regular health care visits even when the child feels well.

b. Teach the child and parents behaviors they can use to promote and maintain health, e.g., receive immunizations, see a dentist on a regular basis, eat well-balanced meals, etc.

c. Explain that the purpose of health education and anticipatory guidance is to help the child and parents help themselves.

3. Involve the child and parents in the development of any plan.

4. Consider the following when developing a plan with the family:
   a. Cultural patterns.
   b. Religious practices.
   c. Life style.
   d. Educational level.
   e. Financial status.
   f. The presence of immediate unmet needs.

5. Be realistic in your plan and set priorities based initially on what must be done and then on what would be nice to do in terms of health promotion and maintenance.

6. Accept the fact that not all children and their parents will be able to accept and/or use health promotion and maintenance behaviors because their immediate needs are so great that they are unable to be future oriented.

7. Encourage the child to assume increasing responsibility for his own health promotion and maintenance needs as he matures.

Hearing screening. Use of one or more techniques to determine whether or not the child is able to hear.

A. General Considerations.

1. Hearing screening tests can detect the presence of, but not the severity of, a hearing deficit.

2. Hearing is essential to the child's development of language and socialization, and, therefore, hearing screening should be a part of every well-child evaluation.

3. Screening tests employed will vary according to the age of the child and the qualifications of the person doing the screening.

4. Brainstem evoked audiometry (BSER) permits detection of hearing loss in children too young (under age 3) or unable to participate in the use of pure-tone audiometry (Adams and Roser, 1979).

5. Infants and/or children should be suspected of having a hearing deficit if one or more of the following is present:
   a. Parents feel that their child does not hear.
   b. The infant never awakens to sound.
   c. Speech development is delayed.

d. The child does poorly in school.

6. Any infant whose history reveals a high-risk factor for hearing loss should have a complete hearing evaluation.
   a. Prematurity or low birth weight.
   b. Bilirubin level greater than 20 mg per dl in the first week of life.
   c. Rubella or other nonbacterial intrauterine infections, e.g., herpes simplex, cytomegalovirus.
   d. Congenital defects of the ear, nose, and throat.
   e. Familial history of deafness.

7. The sense of hearing is fully developed at birth.

8. A child who fails a hearing screening should be referred for complete audiometric evaluation.

9. Hearing losses may be either conductive, those which involve the middle ear structures; or sensorineural, those which involve the organ of Corti or the eighth nerve system.

10. How loud a child plays the radio, television, or phonograph is not reliable, since many children tend to turn up the volume.

B. Nursing Management. See WELL-CHILD CARE.

1. Screen the newborn by use of the Crib-o-gram.

2. Assess the presence or absence of risk factors in older children by asking for a history of:
   a. Viral infections, e.g., measles, mumps.
   b. Meningitis.
   c. Encephalitis.
   d. Use of ototoxic drugs, e.g., sulfa drugs, Kanamycin.
   e. Chronic respiratory infection and/or allergy.
   f. Impacted ear wax.

3. Assess behavioral cues that the child may not hear well such as:
   a. Failure to react to a sudden, loud noise.
   b. Not attempting to localize the source of the sound.
   c. Continuing to babble when speech sounds should be developng.
   d. Cessation of babbling.
   e. Inability to cope with situations which demand attentive listening.
   f. Inappropriate response to a situation because verbal cues are given but visual cues are lacking.
   g. Withdrawn or aggressive behavior.
   h. Poor school performance.

4. Prepare the child and/or parents for the hearing screening procedure.

5. Screen the infant (Caufield, 1978).
   a. Use several noisemakers since not all will attract his attention, e.g., bell, rattle, spoons.

b. Schedule tests between meals when he is neither too sleepy nor too hungry.

6. Screen the infant under 4 months.
   a. Make a loud noise and observe for a blink response.
   b. Be sure that a positive response is not due to the infant picking up vibrations or visual cues.

7. Screen the infant between 4 months and 18 months (Downs and Silver, 1972).
   a. Test hearing in a quiet room.
   b. Let the infant/child remain in the mother's lap.
   c. Get the child's attention visually.
   d. Make a sound with a bell or squeeze a toy out of the child's vision.
   e. Observe response.
      1. Infant of 4 months should show widening of eyes, some turning toward the sound, and/or listening behavior.
      2. Infant of 6 months should turn head to the sound but need not recognize if it is above or below him.
      3. Infant of 8 months or more should turn head 45 degrees or more in the direction of the sound and usually determines if sound is above or below him.

8. Screen the older child (Chinn and Leitch, 1979).
   a. Rub fingers together in front of the child's ears to test for higher frequencies.
   b. Have the child listen to a ticking watch.
   c. Perform the Weber test using a tuning fork.
      1. Strike tuning fork.
      2. Place the handle on the center of the forehead.
      3. Ask the child where he hears the sound; the sound should be equal in each ear.
   d. Perform the Rinne test on both ears using a tuning fork.
      1. Strike tuning fork.
      2. Place handle on the mastoid process.
      3. Ask the child to indicate when sound stops.
      4. Move handle in front of ear.
      5. Ask the child to indicate when sound stops. The child should hear the sound in each position, but air conduction is longer than bone conduction.

9. Refer any child with a sign of impaired hearing for full evaluation.

10. Prepare the child for an audiometric screening test.
    a. Explain that he will go to a quiet room with the tester.
    b. Tell him that he will wear earphones and listen for special sounds that will come from the machine on the table in the room.
    c. Tell him that he can raise his hand or say "now" or "I hear" when he hears the sound.
    d. Make a game of it for the young child, e.g., pretend to be an astronaut or a telephone operator.

11. Prepare the child and/or parents for the use of brainstem evoked response audiometry. See *Preparation for Procedures.*
    a. Electrodes are placed over each mastoid bone and at the vertex of the skull.
    b. Wires are connected to an oscilloscope and waves are recorded.
    c. A sound stimulus of 20 clicks per second at 60 decibels is delivered to each ear.
    d. Waves from the brainstem are analyzed by computer and the presence or absence of normal hearing can be determined.

Heart failure. See *Congestive Heart Failure.*

Heat rash. See *Prickly Heat.*

Hemophilia. A bleeding disorder characterized by a deficiency of a factor necessary for clotting.

A. **General Considerations.**
   1. The majority of children with hemophilia have a deficiency of antihemophilic factor (AHF).
      a. This bleeding disorder is also called Hemophilia A, AHF or AHG deficiency, or Factor VIII deficiency.
      b. Treatment is by infusion of fresh whole blood, cryoprecipitate, or Factor VIII concentrate.
      c. Children can develop serum inhibitors to AHF that necessitate treatment with prothrombin complex concentrates.
   2. The second most common deficiency is that of plasma thromboplastin component (PTC).
      a. This bleeding disorder is also called Hemophilia B, Christmas disease, or Factor IX deficiency.
      b. Treatment is by infusions of plasma, Factor IX concentrate or lypholized whole plasma.
   3. Laboratory tests to identify an abnormal clotting or hemostasis mechanism include:
      a. Prothrombin consumption.
      b. Thromboplastin generation.
      c. Partial thromboplastin time.
      d. Prothrombin time.
      e. Fibrinogen levels.
      f. Specialized assays to determine factor deficiencies.

4. The risk of hepatitis is greater with factor concentrates because of the larger donor pool.
5. Home administration of plasma concentrate prophylactically and as treatment for bleeding episodes is preferable since it results in earlier treatment, decreased emotional trauma, and decreased financial cost.
6. Lacerations, epistaxis, or bleeding from tooth extraction may be treated with local hemostatic agents.
7. Corticosteroid therapy may be used in the treatment of recurrent joint bleeding or renal bleeding.
8. Hemophilia A and Hemophilia B are usually transmitted to males as a sex-linked recessive trait although mutations may occur. See *Genetic Counseling*.
9. The severity of the disease may vary from severe with many spontaneous bleeding episodes to mild with bleeding only at times of severe trauma or surgery.
10. Signs and symptoms include:
    a. Bleeding in the newborn after circumcision.
    b. Excessive bruising after minor falls.
    c. Bleeding into joints (hemarthrosis).
       1. Knees.
       2. Elbows.
       3. Ankles.
    d. Bleeding from minor lacerations.
11. The disease is often not discovered until the child becomes active and experiences falls and bruises.
12. Repeated hemarthroses can result in degenerative changes, osteoporosis, and fixed, unusable joints.
13. Reconstructive surgery may be indicated for severe joint involvement.
14. The adolescent may rebel by engaging in high risk activities such as motorcycle riding, drag racing, etc.

B. **Nursing Management.**
   1. Meet the needs of the child with a bleeding episode.
      a. Support the child and parents during hospitalization. See *Hospitalization, Support During*.
      b. Initiate discharge planning. See *Discharge Planning*.
      c. Immobilize the affected part.
      d. Apply ice and pressure to the affected area.
      e. Elevate the joint and support in a slightly flexed position.
      f. Provide a bed cradle to keep bedclothes off the affected part.
      g. Allow the child to decide what is the least painful method of repositioning.
      i. Protect the child from further injury.
         1. Pad the infant's crib or playpen.
         2. Remove hazardous toys.
         3. Supervise ambulation.
      j. Administer analgesics or narcotics orally, if possible.
      k. Use precautions with I.M. injections.
         1. Rotate injection sites.
         2. Inject medication slowly.
         3. Apply pressure on injection site for at least 5 minutes.
      l. Observe, record, and report the following.
         1. Signs of shock.
         2. Increased warmth or joint swelling.
         3. Increased pain.
         4. Discoloration of skin.
         5. Severe limitation of motion.
      m. Meet the need for sensory stimulation of immobilized child. See *Immobilized Child* and *Stimulation*.

      n. Initiate range of motion when the bleeding is controlled around 48 hours after therapy is started.
      o. Provide ways for the older child to keep up with schoolwork.
         1. Arrange for peers or parents to obtain homework assignments.
         2. Provide time for completion of homework.
         3. Arrange for a tutor or homebound teacher.
   2. Explore the emotional aspects of the disease with the child and his parents.
      a. Encourage an attitude of appropriate supervision without overprotection.
      b. Help parents deal with the child's need for limits. See *Discipline*.
      c. Discuss ways that the child can accomplish developmental tasks of initiative, independence, identification, etc.
      d. Identify age-appropriate, nonhazardous activities such as swimming, sports team manager, or scorekeeper.
      e. Encourage the parents to talk with school personnel if there are difficulties in enrolling the child in a school with normal, rather than handicapped children.
      f. Explore alternatives for handling financial difficulties related to treatment costs and initiate referrals as needed.
      g. Allow the older child/adolescent to express frustration with the restrictions necessitated by his "invisible" disease. See *Handicapped Child*.
         1. Help identify an adult with whom the adolescent can discuss problems; e.g., school counselor, athletic coach, scout leader, clergy, etc.
         2. Help the teenager to see that assuming

responsibility for own safety will lead to more freedom from parental restrictions.

3. Discuss home management with the child and parents.
   a. Explore ways to make the home safe. See *Accident Prevention.*
      1. Pad the infant's crib or playpen.
      2. Pad the knees and elbows of the toddler's clothing.
      3. Keep the floors free of toys, scatter rugs, etc.
   b. Teach management of minor trauma.
      1. Cleanse the wound thoroughly.
      2. Immobilize the affected part.
      3. Apply pressure to the area.
      4. Apply a hemostatic agent to the wound.
      5. Administer plasma concentrate as instructed.
   c. Discuss long-term physical needs of the child.
      1. Review the need for and the elements of good dental hygiene. See *Dental Care.*
      2. Discuss the importance of a diet high in iron to prevent anemia and adequate in calories to promote growth, but prevent obesity.
      3. Encourage normal health supervision. See *Well-child Care.*
   d. Support the child and parents who enter a home-treatment program.
      1. Assess the child's and parent's readiness to assume the responsibility.
      2. Evaluate their knowledge about the disease and its treatment.
      3. Teach venipuncture technique, reconstitution, syringe preparation, and infusion technique (Sergis-Deavenport and Varni, 1982).
      4. Discuss guidelines for when and how much plasma concentrate to administer.
      5. Review complications such as intracranial bleeding or psoas hematoma.
      6. Encourage the child and parents to maintain telephone contact frequently.
   e. Refer the family to a hemophilia care center for a comprehensive program and to the National Hemophilia Foundation for support.

Hepatitis, viral. Infection with hepatitis A or B virus.

A. **General Considerations.**
   1. Characteristics of type-A infection include:
      a. Transmission by a fecal to oral route among persons in close contact or through contaminated water or shellfish.
      b. An incubation period of 2 to 6 weeks.
      c. A mild clinical course seldom requiring hospitalization.
   2. Characteristics of type-B infection include:
      a. Transmission by transfusion of blood or blood products, by parenteral drug abuse, or by contact with the body fluids of an infected person.
      b. An incubation period of 6 weeks to 6 months.
      c. A severe clinical course, which may necessitate prolonged hospitalization and convalescence.
   3. Symptoms are similar for both types although they are more rapid in type-A and jaundice may not occur in type-A.
   4. Signs and symptoms of the prodromal period include:
      a. Fever.
      b. Fatigue.
      c. Anorexia.
      d. Nausea and vomiting.
      e. Loss of taste for cigarettes.
      f. Dull epigastric or right upper quadrant pain.
      g. Headache.
      h. Tenderness of the liver and/or **hepatomegaly.**
      i. Generalized lymphadenopathy.
      j. Splenomegaly.
   5. Signs and symptoms of the icteric phase include:
      a. Dark urine.
      b. Light-colored stools.
      c. Icterus of the skin and sclera (jaundice).
   6. Diagnostic evaluation includes:
      a. History which confirms exposure to hepatitis virus.
      b. Dectection of hepatitis A antigen, hepatitis B surface antigen, or the antibody to this antigen.
      c. Liver function studies: serum bilirubin, cephalin flocculation, BSP excretion, prothrombin time, serum protein, blood ammonia, alkaline phosphatase, SGOT, SGPT, and LDH levels.
      d. Urine bilirubin and urobiligen levels.
      e. Stool sample.
      f. Liver biopsy, if diagnosis in doubt.
   7. Treatment is symptomatic.
      a. Bed rest.
      b. High-caloric diet.
   8. Hospitalization is not always necessary, but isolation techniques must be maintained if the child is treated at home.

9. Prednisone may be used in type-B if blood chemical values are abnormal.

10. Neomycin or kanamycin may be ordered to decrease flora in the gastrointestinal tract if hepatic coma is likely.

11. Complications can occur in both types, but are more common in type-B.
   a. Hepatic encephalopathy.
   b. Gastrointestinal bleeding.
   c. Ascites.
   d. Chronic hepatitis.
   e. Fulminant hepatitis.

12. Prophylactic I.M. gamma globulin may be effective in preventing the infection if given to contacts early.

13. Alcohol intake may not be permitted for the adolescent for up to 6 months or until the liver has fully recovered.

14. Adolescents are at higher risk for hepatitis B due to drug abuse and/or sexual contact with carriers.

B. Nursing Management. See DRUG ABUSE.

1. Support the child and parents during hospitalization. See *Hospitalization, Support During.*

2. Initiate discharge planning. See *Discharge Planning.*

3. Maintain limited activity level as ordered.
   a. Meet the needs of the immobilized child if bed rest is ordered. See *Immobilized Child.*
   b. Plan specific rest periods if the child is allowed out of bed.
      1. Plan care in blocks of time.
      2. Make the environment conducive to rest by darkening the room or turning off the television and radio.

4. Meet the child's nutritional needs for increased protein and carbohydrate and decreased fat.
   a. Inform the dietician of the child's preferences and also record them on the Kardex.
   b. Offer frequent small feedings.
   c. Avoid scheduling traumatic procedures at mealtime.
   d. Make the food tray as attractive as possible.
   e. Stay with the child during mealtime.
   f. Have the parents bring in food from home.

5. Use precautions when handling I.V. equipment or syringes.

6. Follow hospital procedure for enteric isolation.
   a. Provide extra stimulation for the child since he lacks peer contact. See *Isolated Child.*
   b. Explain to the older child and adolescent why isolation is necessary.

7. Prepare the child for a liver biopsy if ordered. See *Preparation for Procedures.*

8. Observe, record, and report symptoms of hepatic encephalopathy.
   a. Unusual somnolence.
   b. Mental confusion.
   c. Extreme anorexia.

9. Measure the abdominal girth as ordered since ascites can occur.

10. Provide good skin care, since decreased protein synthesis by the liver lowers colloid osmotic pressure resulting in fluid leaking into interstitial tissues.

11. Observe, record, and report signs and symptoms of gastrointestinal bleeding.
   a. Nosebleed.
   b. Blood in the stool.
   c. Chills.
   d. Diaphoresis.
   e. Cold, clammy skin.

12. Observe, record, and report the child's response to medication.

13. Teach the child and parents home management.
   a. Do not allow the child to kiss anyone.
   b. Have the child use a separate toilet or disinfect the toilet after each use.
   c. Encourage the family members to wash their hands frequently.
   d. Launder the child's clothing and linen in an automatic washer with hot water to destroy the virus.
   e. Wash the child's dishes and eating utensils in a dishwasher or use disposable dishes.
   f. Discuss how to meet the child's dietary needs.
      1. Consider when the child tends to be hungry.
      2. Consider food preferences.
      3. Consider family lifestyle.
   g. Avoid involving the child in food preparation.
   h. Involve the child in planning adequate rest periods.
   i. Discuss the physician's recommendations about alcohol intake with the child.
   j. Discuss with the child and parents that nonprescription drugs should be avoided, since the liver may be unable to detoxify them, e.g., Tylenol.

14. Identify resources in the community for the older child or adolescent who has a suspected history of illicit drug use. See *Drug Abuse.*

15. Inform the adolescent nondrug user that he may contract the virus through oral contamination with semen, saliva, and vaginal secretions, including menstrual blood of carriers of hepatitis B (Whaley and Wong, 1983).

Hernia, inguinal. Protrusion of a portion of the bowel through the inguinal ring into a patent processus vaginalis.

A. General Considerations.

1. A hernia usually presents as painless inguinal bulge that increases with coughing, crying, straining, or standing.
2. Constipation, anorexia, and irritability due to pain may occur when the bowel slips into the hernial sac and partial obstruction develops.
3. Diagnosis may be made on the basis of the parent's report of seeing a bulge and the physician detecting a "silk glove" sign when an empty hernial sac is rolled between the fingers.
4. A diagnostic herniogram may be done by injecting radiopaque dye into the peritoneal cavity 2 cm below the umbilicus in order to visualize the hernial sac(s).
5. Surgery to remove the hernial sac is done as soon as possible after diagnosis to prevent a loop of bowel from becoming incarcerated in the hernial sac.
6. Bowel resection may be required if the blood supply to the incarcerated bowel has been decreased to the point where tissue damage occurs.
7. In the male there may be an associated hydrocele.

B. Nursing Management.

1. Support the child and parents during hospitalization. See *Hospitalization, Support During*.
2. Initiate discharge planning. See *Discharge Planning*.
3. Meet the needs of the child preoperatively. See *Preoperative Care* and *Preparation for Surgery*.
   a. Prevent crying as much as possible to decrease the chance of bowel being pushed into the hernial sac, e.g., hold, rock, feed when hungry.
   b. Provide a diet that promotes neither constipation or diarrhea to avoid straining.
   c. Find out what parents know about the surgical procedure and postoperative care and provide information as needed.
   d. Observe, record, and report signs of partial obstruction.
   e. Observe, record, and report signs and symptoms of incarceration.
      1. Firm irreducible mass below the external inguinal ring.
      2. Irritability and crying.
      3. Vomiting.
      4. Absence of bowel movements.
      5. Fever.
4. Meet the needs of the child postoperatively. See *Postoperative Care*.
   a. Keep surgical incision site clean and dry.
      1. Leave waterproof collodion dressing in place until it peels off naturally.
      2. Fold diaper down below incision site or leave open.
      3. Sponge bathe infant until incision is healed.
   b. Hold the infant for feedings; decrease strain on the incision and promote comfort when he is fretful.
5. Teach the parents home management.
   a. Keep the incision area clean and dry.
   b. Call the physician if signs of infection develop.

Hernia, umbilical. Protrusion of a portion of the intestines or omentum through the umbilical ring.

A. General Considerations.

1. Coughing, straining, and crying increase intra-abdominal pressure causing increased protrusion of the hernia.
2. Incarceration is rare.
3. Walking strengthens the abdominal muscles and usually promotes closure of the defect by school age if the fascial ring opening is less then 2 cm.
4. Surgical repair is indicated when:
   a. Incarceration occurs.
   b. The fascial ring is greater than 2 cm.
   c. Small hernias persist into school age and/or become larger.
5. Strapping, taping coins over the hernia, and other methods used to reduce the hernia are ineffective in promoting closure and may in fact cause incarceration.

B. Nursing Management.

1. Support the child and parents during hospitalization if surgery is required for closure. See *Hospitalization, Support During*.
2. Initiate discharge planning. See *Discharge Planning*.
3. Meet the needs of the child preoperatively. See *Preoperative Care* and *Preparation for Surgery*.
4. Meet the needs of the child postoperatively. See *Postoperative Care*.
   a. Keep the pressure dressing dry and intact.
   b. Allow normal activity.
5. Teach the parents to keep the surgical area clean and dry until healing occurs.
6. Teach the parents home management of the child who does not require surgery.
   a. Encourage age-appropriate exercise to promote closure. See *Exercise*.
   b. Avoid strapping since this does no good and may cause incarceration.
   c. Call the doctor if signs of incarceration develop.

1. Firm, irreducible mass through umbilical ring.
2. Vomiting.
3. Pain.
4. Irritability and crying.
   d. Have the child seen for well-child care to evaluate the status of the hernia.
   e. Explain when surgery would be indicated.

Herpes simplex gingivostomatitis.
Severe inflammation of buccal mucosa and lips caused by herpes simplex virus.

A. **General Considerations.**
1. This condition is:
   a. Usually caused by Type I herpes virus which produces lesions above the waist.
   b. May be caused by Type II herpes virus, which produces lesions below the waist, through orogenital sexual activity. See *Sexually Transmitted Diseases.*
   c. Spread by direct contact of the virus with the mucous membranes.
2. Antibodies develop after the primary infections but the child remains a carrier throughout life and recurrence of lesions is common.
3. Signs and symptoms associated with the primary infection include:
   a. Vesicles with yellowish membranes which rupture leaving small, shallow, painful ulcers.
   b. Submaxillary lymphadenopathy.
   c. High fever.
   d. Crusting of lips.
   e. Anorexia.
   f. Marked irritability.
4. Recurrent infections:
   a. Are usually milder.
   b. Are accompanied by painful vesicles on the lips (fever blisters).
   c. Do not produce systemic symptoms.
   d. Often follow physical or biochemical stress situations, e.g., illness, anxiety.
5. Treatment measures include:
   a. Application of 5 percent acyclovir (Zovirax) ointment.
   b. Topical anesthetics.
   c. Hydration; avoid acidic solutions.
   d. Analgesics.
   e. Antipyretics.
   f. Applying ice to painful lesions.
6. The infection can usually be treated at home but severe primary infections may require hospitalization.
7. The primary infection and recurrences run self-limiting courses in approximately 7 to 10 days.

B. **Nursing Management.**
1. Teach the child and/or parents to:
   a. Administer medication as instructed. See *Administration of Medications, Parental.*
   b. Employ comfort measures.
      1. Apply compresses of Burow's solution to weeping ulcers on lips.
      2. Apply ointment to crusted/cracking lesions to decrease bleeding.
      3. Use viscous Xylocaine as ordered.
      4. Have the child drink through a straw.
      5. Avoid acidic liquids.
   c. Maintain dental hygiene.
      1. Do not use a toothbrush since it is irritating.
      2. Have the child rinse mouth frequently with cool water or mild mouthwash.
      3. Use cotton swabs or gauze to remove food particles from teeth.
   d. Encourage fluids.
   e. Schedule rest periods, since the child may be irritable and not sleep well.
   f. Prevent secondary infection and avoid spreading infection to others.
      1. Apply medication with finger covered with finger cot or gloves.
      2. Practice good handwashing.
      3. Avoid touching the area.
      4. Do not kiss people.
   g. Promote nutrition but do not force feeding.
      1. Offer soft, nonacidic foods.
      2. Provide adequate time to eat.
      3. Administer analgesic prior to eating.
      4. Provide company for the child during mealtimes.
   h. Call the physician if the child:
      1. Appears dehydrated. See *Fluid and Electrolyte Imbalance.*
      2. Develops or continues to run a fever.
      3. Shows signs and symptoms of secondary infection.
2. Discuss with the child and parents the recurrent nature of the infection and ways of decreasing the stressors which precipitate a recurrence.
3. Provide for the hospitalized child:
   a. Support the child and parents during hospitalization. See *Hospitalization, Support During.*
   b. Initiate discharge planning. See *Discharge Planning.*
   c. Isolate the child as ordered. See *Isolated Child.*
   d. Observe, record, and report the child's response to medication.
      1. Apply topical anesthetic to lesions as ordered.
      2. Administer analgesics and antipyretics as ordered.

e. Prevent dehydration.
   1. Offer frequent, small sips of fluids.
   2. Assess what temperature fluid child takes best and record on Kardex.
   3. Provide nonacid fluids.
   4. Monitor I.V. accurately if this route becomes necessary.
f. Promote nutrition.
g. Maintain oral hygiene.

Herpes simplex. Infection caused by the herpes simplex virus.

A. **General Considerations.**
  1. A primary infection with the herpesvirus does not provide immunity to secondary herpes infections even though circulating antibodies can be identified and the individual harbors the latent virus for life.
  2. The herpesvirus may be either Type I, which causes lesions of the mouth, skin, or central nervous system, or Type II, which causes genital lesions and congenital or neonatal herpetic infection.
  3. Secondary herpes simplex infections are common and may be precipitated by:
    a. Fever.
    b. Menstruation.
    c. Severe infection.
    d. Stress.
    e. Trauma.
  4. Signs and symptoms of primary infections vary according to the type and location of the infection.
    a. Acute herpetic gingivostomatitis (Type I).
      1. High fever.
      2. Irritability and restlessness.
      3. Pain in mouth and throat.
      4. Shallow, yellow ulcers of the mouth, gums, and throat.
      5. Crusting of lips.
      6. Enlarged cervical lymph nodes.
    b. Acute herpetic vulvovaginitis (Type II).
      1. Erythema of the perineal area.
      2. Edema.
      3. Shallow ulcers.
      4. Fever.
      5. Painful urination.
      6. Enlarged inguinal lymph nodes.
    c. Eczema herpeticum (Type I).
      1. High fever.
      2. Prostration.
      3. Crops of vesicles in areas of eczematous lesions.
    d. Acute neonatal congenital or acquired generalized infection (Type II).
      1. High or low temperature.

      2. Crops of vesicles.
      3. Dyspnea.
      4. Purpura.
      5. Jaundice.
      6. Convulsions.
    e. Mild neonatal herpetic infection (Type I).
      1. Repeated crops of vesicles.
      2. Possible central nervous system impairment.
  6. Herpes infection may be spread by direct contact.
  7. The course of the infection is usually under 2 weeks except in the case of congenital or neonatal infection which is often fatal.
  8. Treatment measures include:
    a. Application of idoxuridine (IDU, Herplex, Dendrid) to the lesions.
    b. Maintenance of adequate hydration.
    c. Promotion of comfort.
  9. Cytosine arabinoside (Ara-C) has been used in treating congenital or neonatal herpes, but the best treatment is still prevention.
 10. Treatment of mild primary or secondary infection can be managed at home, but congenital, neonatal, or severe infections in young children require hospitalization.
 11. Encephalitis may occur as a complication.

B. **Nursing Management.**
  1. Support the child and parents during hospitalization. See *Hospitalization, Support During*.
  2. Initiate discharge planning. See *Discharge Planning*.
  3. Isolate the child as ordered. See *Isolated Child*.
  4. Observe, record, and report the child's response to medication.
    a. Apply topical anesthetic to lesions as ordered.
    b. Administer analgesics and antipyretics as ordered.
  5. Prevent dehydration.
    a. Offer frequent, small sips of fluids.
    b. Assess what temperature fluid child takes best and record on Kardex.
    c. Provide nonacid fluids.
    d. Monitor I.V. accurately if this route becomes necessary.
  6. Promote nutrition in the child with gingivostomatitis but do not force the child to eat.
    a. Offer soft, nonacidic foods.
    b. Provide adequate time to eat, since eating may be a slow, painful process.
    c. Administer analgesic prior to the mealtime.
    d. Provide company for the child when he eats.
  7. Maintain oral hygiene.

a. Do not use a toothbrush as this is too irritating.

b. Have the child rinse mouth frequently with cool water or mild mouthwash.

c. Use cotton swabs or gauze to remove food particles from teeth.

8. Promote perineal comfort in the child with vulvar infection.

a. Pour cool water over perineum when the child urinates so urine does not create burning.

b. Use sitz baths as ordered.

c. Pat, do not rub, the perineum dry.

d. Provide absorbent, all cotton pants.

9. Schedule rest periods, since the child may be irritable and not sleep well.

10. Reassure the child that the vesicles will heal and he will look the same as before.

11. Teach the child and/or parents to:

a. Administer medications as instructed. See *Administration of Medications, Parental.*

b. Employ comfort measures for mouth, skin, or perineal infection.

c. Maintain personal hygiene.

d. Encourage fluids. See *Forcing Fluids.*

e. Promote nutrition but do not force eating.

f. Do not touch the vesicles since secondary infection may occur.

g. Call the physician if the child:

1. Appears dehydrated. See *Fluid and Electrolyte Imbalance.*

2. Develops or continues to run a fever.

3. Shows signs and symptoms of secondary infection.

12. Discuss with the child and parents the recurrent nature of the infection and ways of decreasing the stressors which precipitate a recurrence.

Herpes zoster (shingles). A secondary infection caused by the varicella-zoster virus (viral infection of nervous system).

A. **General Considerations.**

1. Primary infection with the varicella-zoster virus causes chickenpox.

2. The secondary infection may be due to reactivation of a latent varicella-zoster virus or to a second, or later, invasion by the virus.

3. Signs and symptoms include:

a. Peripheral neuritis.

b. Crops of confluent vesicles on an erythematous base, which usually follow lumbar and thoracic nerve distribution and are unilateral.

c. Motor weakness and root pain in the affected area.

4. Treatment is symptomatic and can be managed at home.

B. **Nursing Management.**

1. Explain to the child and parents that this illness is caused by the same virus that gave the child chickenpox.

2. Tell the child and parents that the skin lesions will heal and leave no scars.

3. Teach the following to the child and parents.

a. Administer analgesic for pain as instructed. See *Administration of Medications, Parental.*

b. Wear loose, nonirritating clothes over the affected area.

c. Do not rub or scratch the area in order to prevent secondary infection.

Hip, dysplasia. See *Congenital Hip Dysplasia.*

Hirschsprung's disease. (congenital megacolon). Absence of ganglion cells in an intestinal segment resulting in lack of peristalsis.

A. **General Considerations.**

1. The normal intestine near the involved segment becomes dilated from the accumulated fecal mass.

2. Signs and symptoms result from lack of peristalsis.

a. Newborn.

1. Poor feeding.

2. Bile-stained vomitus.

3. Abdominal distention.

4. Respiratory difficulty.

b. Older infant and child.

1. Overflow diarrhea alternating with obstipation.

2. Malnutrition and anemia.

3. Failure to thrive.

4. Enlarged abdomen.

3. Anomalies of the gastrointestinal and genitourinary tract may accompany Hirschsprung's disease.

4. Diagnostic tests include a barium enema and balloon manometry followed by a rectal biopsy under anesthesia to confirm the diagnosis if manometry indicates abnormal internal anal sphincter (Rosenberg and Vela, 1983).

5. All of the barium must be removed by colonic irrigations unless the infant or young child is having an ostomy performed immediately.

6. The child who has not been repaired may die of hypovolemic shock secondary to enterocolitis thought to be caused by bacterial overgrowth in the stagnated feces.

7. The older infant or child may be placed on a regime to improve his condition before surgery.

a. Total parenteral nutrition. See *Total Parenteral Nutrition.*

b. Low-residue diet.
c. Stool softeners.
d. Vitamins.
e. Daily enemas or colonic lavage.
8. Surgical treatment will be required.
  a. Colostomy or ileostomy may be performed on the young infant or on the older child whose condition is poor.
  b. Dissection of the dilated bowel and segment of aganglionic bowel followed by anastamosis (pull-through procedure) is performed when the infant reaches 6 months of age or when the older child's condition improves.
  c. Colostomy closure may be done at the same time as the definitive repair or may be delayed for 2 months or so.
9. Postoperative complications include:
  a. Leakage at the anastomosis site.
  b. Pelvic abscess.
  c. Incontinence.
  d. Intestinal obstruction from adhesions.

B. Nursing Management.
1. Support the child and parents during hospitalization. See *Hospitalization, Support During* and *Handicapped Child.*
2. Initiate discharge planning. See *Discharge Planning.*
3. Meet the preoperative needs of the child who requires a colostomy. See *Preoperative Care* and *Preparation for Surgery.*
  a. Use diagrams or a doll to explain the colostomy to the older child and to the parents.
  b. Reinforce that the colostomy is only temporary if this is true.
  c. Explain that the stoma will be large, protruding, red, and raw looking.
4. Meet the postoperative needs of the infant/child who requires a colostomy or ileostomy. See *Postoperative Care.*
  a. Measure nasogastric drainage every 8 hours and replace it with I.V. fluids as ordered.
  b. Measure liquid ostomy drainage and replace with I.V. fluid if ordered.
  c. Observe, record, and report signs and symptoms related to fluid and electrolyte balance.
    1. Presence of water ring on the ostomy dressing, since this indicates liquid loss even if the stool has become solid (Jones, 1978).
    2. Significant increase or decrease in urinary output.
    3. Positive urine glucose which indicates osmotic diuresis.
    4. Increase in stool volume which may result in dehydration.
  d. Observe, record, and report prolapse, hemorrhage, pallor, or dusky color of the stoma.

e. Observe, record, and report signs and symptoms of sepsis.
  1. Subnormal temperature.
  2. Lethargy.
  3. Irregular respirations.
  4. Irritability.
f. Observe, record, and report signs and symptoms related to ostomy functioning.
  1. Passage of flatus.
  2. Abdominal distention.
  3. Characteristics of stools.
g. Begin glucose feedings and advance to formula or prescribed diet.
  1. Limit feeding to 20 minutes to avoid tiring the infant.
  2. Supplement oral feeding with gavage feedings if necessary.
  3. Offer an oral electrolyte solution between formula feedings if needed to restore water and electrolyte loss from the ileostomy.
h. Provide skin care around the colostomy site.
  1. Keep the area clean with soap and water.
  2. Apply zinc oxide or other ointment to protect the skin.
  3. Apply a collection bag or place gauze square over the stoma and secure by pinning a diaper folded lengthwise over the dressing.
  4. Change the bag or dressing as necessary to prevent skin breakdown.
i. Administer medications to decrease gastrointestinal motility as ordered.
j. Teach home management.
  1. Have the mother return a demonstration of ostomy care.
  2. Help the mother assess the volume of ostomy drainage.
  3. Explain that the stoma appliance will have to be remeasured after 4 to 6 weeks as the stoma shrinks.
  4. Tell the mother to report symptoms of dehydration, e.g., decreased output, poor skin turgor, sunken fontanel, or dry mucous membranes.
  5. Review administration of medications. See *Administration of Medications, Parental.*
4. Meet the needs of the older infant or child whose condition needs to be improved before surgery.
  a. Review the elements of low-residue diet with the child and parents.
  b. Teach the administration of vitamins and stool softeners. See *Administration of Medications, Parental.*
  c. Discuss methods of improving nutrition at home. See *Feeding Problems.*
    1. Make mealtime pleasant.

2. Offer frequent small feedings.
3. Involve the older child in food preparation.

d. Teach the parents the administration of colonic irrigations.
1. Use an isotonic electrolyte solution or skim milk as an irrigant to prevent water intoxication or cerebral edema.
2. Clarify with the surgeon what procedure should be taught to the mother or refer to hospital policy.
3. Have the mother return a demonstration of the procedure.
4. Teach the mother that irritability, distention, and poor feeding indicate that the lavage should be repeated.

5. Meet the preoperative needs of the child admitted for an abdominoperineal pull-through procedure. See *Preoperative Care* and *Preparation for Surgery*.
a. Obtain a thorough nursing history of the child's feeding and elimination pattern.
b. Observe, record, and report the following:
1. Description of stools.
2. Vomiting.
3. Abdominal distention.
4. Abdominal pain.
c. Provide a clear liquid or low-residue diet in frequent small feedings as ordered.
d. Support the infant or child in an upright position if abdominal distention is severe.
e. Provide adequate bowel preparation.
1. Add an antibiotic to the colonic irrigating fluid as ordered.
2. Administer an antibiotic solution through the ileostomy or colostomy segment(s) as ordered.
f. Administer oral antibiotics as ordered to decrease intestinal flora.

6. Meet the needs of the infant/child after the pull-through procedure. See *Postoperative Care*.
a. Administer I.V. antibiotics as ordered.
b. Record Foley catheter output.
c. Position the infant/child to alleviate tension on the abdominal muscles and to relieve pressure on the perineum.
1. Knee–chest.
2. Place a diaper roll under the thighs to keep the knees flexed if the child is supine.
d. Obtain axillary or oral temperatures according to the child's age.
e. Administer medication for pain relief as ordered. See *Pain*.
f. Provide skin care of the perineal area.
1. Cleanse frequently with soap and water.
2. Apply a protective ointment.
3. Avoid diapers or underpants which might irritate the suture line.

4. Place in a sitz bath as ordered.
g. Encourage improved eating habits.
h. Prepare the child and parents if a barium enema is performed before discharge to determine that the anastomosis is not leaking.
i. Teach the child and parents home management.
1. Discuss methods of improving nutrition at home, e.g., behavior modification techniques, maintaining stress-free meal times, creating foods appetizing in appearance.
2. Discuss the establishment of normal elimination patterns. See *Toilet Training*.
3. Refer to community health nurse or other agencies as needed.

History taking. The gathering of information about the child and his family.

A. **General Considerations.**
1. A nursing history should be done on all patients or clients and their families to:
a. Serve as the basis for planning individualized nursing care.
b. Improve the quality of care.
c. Help identify teaching and/or referral needs.
d. Document the nursing role in health care.
2. The focus and depth of the nursing history will vary depending on the setting and the particular situation. A hospital history, for example, may ask for different information than one done in a clinic; an initial well-child care history will be in much greater depth than one done for an acute illness.
3. The nursing interview can serve as a means of developing a sense of trust among the child, the parents, and the nurse.
4. Problems which can develop during history taking include communications difficulties and/or poor interaction between the nurse and the child/adolescent or parent(s).

B. **Nursing Management.**
1. Explain to the child and/or parents why you are taking a nursing history.
2. Obtain a nursing history which includes the following areas (See *Appendix iv*):
a. Chief complaint or concern.
b. Present illness or reason for visit.
c. Past health history.
d. Family history.
e. Eating patterns.
f. Sleeping patterns.
g. Elimination patterns.
h. Developmental status.
i. Play, day care, school.

j. Self-care activities.

k. Disciplinary methods employed.

l. Peer and family relationships.

m. Habits and mannerisms.

n. Review of systems.

3. Approach the interview session in a warm, relaxed, nonjudgmental manner.

4. Use appropriate interviewing techniques.

a. Take only that information you need and plan to use.

b. Tell the child and parents how the information will be used.

c. Provide as quiet and private a setting as possible.

d. Find out about the child's and/or parents' concerns or questions first.

e. Encourage the schoolchild to answer questions about himself.

f. Interview the adolescent separately from his parents.

g. Make brief notes as you go so you can fill in details later.

h. Listen to what you are told.

i. Use language the child and/or parents can understand.

j. Do not start with highly personal topics.

k. Do not rush the interview.

l. Call the child and parents by name.

m. Be nonjudgmental about what you are told.

n. Use the following type of questions:

1. Fact finding: appropriate for obtaining specific data, e.g., date of birth.

2. Open ended: allows for elaboration of a topic, e.g., "tell me what a typical day at home is like."

o. Do not use the following types of questions:

1. Compound questions which ask for information about two or more topics, e.g., "do you have headaches and blurred vision?"

2. Questions that are global, e.g., "tell me about your son."

3. Questions that imply an answer, e.g., "your child does not wet his bed, does he?"

p. Encourage the child and parents to talk during the interview.

5. Obtain the following additional material about the hospitalized child.

a. Coping patterns.

b. Preparation for hospitalization.

c. Knowledge about the illness or reason for admission.

d. Reaction to any previous hospitalizations.

6. Identify teaching and/or referral needs of the child and parents.

7. Include the history in the chart or have it available for review and additions.

8. Transfer information to the nursing Kardex to promote individualized care on a consistent basis.

9. Attempt to solve problems which may arise during history taking.

a. Obtain an interpreter if the family speaks a different language.

b. Work to clarify communication so that interviewer and interviewee understand one another.

c. Have another nurse work with the family if you cannot communicate effectively with them.

Hodgkin's disease. A form of cancer that affects the lymphatic system.

A. General Considerations.

1. Painless enlargement of one or more lymph nodes, usually in the cervical, axillary, or inguinal regions, is the most common sign.

2. Systemic symptoms, which disappear when treatment is begun, include:

a. Fever.

b. Night sweats.

c. Weight loss greater than 10 percent.

d. Fatigue.

e. Anorexia.

f. Itching.

g. Pain in the affected lymph node(s) when alcohol is ingested.

3. The finding of Sternberg-Reed cells in a biopsied node is diagnostic.

4. Surgical staging of the disease will be done to determine the extent of the disease using the Ann Arbor Staging Classification.

a. Stage I: involvement of a single lymph node region (I) or of a single extralympathic region or site (Ie).

b. Stage II: involvement of two or more lymph node regions on the same side of the diaphragm (II) or localized involvement of an extralymphatic organ or site and one or more lymph node regions on the same side of the diaphragm (IIe).

c. Stage III: involvement of lymph node regions on both sides of the diaphragm (III), which may also be accompanied by involvement of the spleen (IIIs) or by localized involvement of an extralymphatic organ or site (IIIe) or both (IIIse).

d. Stage IV: diffuse or disseminated involvement of one or more extralymphatic organs or tissue, with or without associated lymph node involvement.

5. The stages are subclassed as follows:

a. Substage A: absence of systemic signs and symptoms.

b. Substage B: presence of systemic signs and symptoms; fever, night sweats, weight loss of 10 percent or more within the past 6 months which cannot be accounted for on another basis.

6. The staging process may also include:
   a. Laboratory tests such as a CBC, SMA-12, and ESR.
   b. X-rays of the chest, metastatic bone surveys, and liver and spleen scans.
   c. Lymphangiography.
   d. Bone marrow biopsy.
   e. Intravenous pyelogram.
   f. Liver biopsy.
   g. Exploratory laparotomy with splenectomy.

7. Treatment includes:
   a. Megavoltage radiation therapy.
   b. Combined chemotherapy, e.g., with mechlorethamine, Oncovin, procarbazine, and prednisone (MOPP therapy or adriamycin, bleomycin, vincristine and daunomycin (ABVD therapy).

8. After initial staging and initiation of therapy, the child is managed on an outpatient basis.

9. Different pathological types which are of prognostic value include (Hoffman, 1983):
   a. Lymphocyte-predominant: good prognosis.
   b. Nodular sclerosing and mixed cellular: intermediate prognosis.
   c. Lymphocyte-depletion: poor prognosis.

10. The overall prognosis for Hodgkin's disease has improved markedly in the past few years.

11. The adolescent may find the side effects of treatment, e.g., baldness, aspermia, as difficult to deal with as the disease itself.

B. Nursing Management.
1. Support the child and parents during hospitalization. See *Hospitalization, Support During.*
2. Initiate discharge planning. See *Discharge Planning.*
3. Promote relief of systemic symptoms.
   a. Administer antipyretic as ordered for fever.
   b. Administer antihistamines as ordered for itching.
   c. Provide frequent skin care.
      1. Sponge bathe as needed for comfort.
      2. Do not use soap since it dries the skin.
      3. Use a lanolin rich, nonperfumed skin lotion.
   d. Leave extra gowns and bed linens in the room if the patient has fever and/or night sweats.
   e. Encourage optimal nutrition. See *Nutrition.*

1. Offer small, frequent feedings that are high in protein and calories.
2. Encourage the family to bring in the child's favorite foods.
3. Include the child in selecting a menu.
   f. Schedule care to provide rest periods.
   g. Position the child for comfort if enlarged nodes are causing pressure on internal organs.

4. Monitor vital signs accurately.
5. Meet the needs of the child preoperatively. See *Preoperative Care* and *Preparation for Surgery.*
6. Meet the needs of the child, postoperatively. See *Postoperative Care.*
7. Prepare the child and parents for radiation therapy and/or chemotherapy. See *Chemotherapy* and *Radiation Therapy.*
8. Meet the needs of the child receiving radiation and/or chemotherapy.

9. Support the child and parents in carrying out outpatient therapy.
   a. Involve the child, his parents, the physician, and others caring for the child in the development of an individualized plan of care.
   b. Make sure the child and parents understand:
      1. Necessity for continuing treatment for as long as required.
      2. Implications if treatment is not followed.
      3. Way to contact the hospital or clinic if they need assistance.
   c. Teach comfort measures related to the reduction of symptoms associated with radiation and/or chemotherapy.
   d. Teach signs and symptoms that should be reported to a physician.
      1. Recurrence of initial signs and symptoms.
      2. Infections.
      3. Bleeding.
      4. Lesions of the mucous membranes.
   e. Suggest ways of handling an altered body image due to hair loss or surgical scars, e.g., wig, high collar or turtlenecks. See *Body Image.*

10. Meet the special needs of the adolescent. See *Adolescent.*
    a. Encourage verbalization of feelings.
    b. Explain all procedures.
    c. Involve the adolescent in the planning of care.
    d. Explain the implications of radiation and/or chemotherapy in relation to sexual function.
       1. The menstrual cycle may be erratic or stop for periods of time during therapy.

2. Birth control measures should be used if the adolescent is sexually active.

3. Infants of mothers receiving chemotherapy may have congenital malformations.

4. Sterility may occur.

e. Discuss dietary needs and any restrictions and help the adolescent incorporate them into his life style.

Home management of minor emergencies.

Measures that parents can use to handle minor accidents or injuries.

A. **General Considerations.**

1. Parents can handle many childhood accidents and injuries at home if they are given proper instruction and support.

2. Many parents may want to pursue courses in first aid or emergency medical training and can be directed to community resources.

3. Emergency supplies for the home should include:

   a. A first-aid kit containing cotton, bandages, gauze, etc.

   b. Syrup of ipecac and activated charcoal or poison first-aid kit.

   c. Ammonia inhalant.

   d. Antihistamine lotion.

   e. Iodophor solution for cleansing wounds, etc.

   f. Rubber alcohol.

   g. Salt tablets for heat exhaustion.

   h. Thermometers, oral and rectal.

   i. Tweezers.

   j. Oil of cloves for toothache.

   k. Scissors.

4. Some injuries and accidents will require physician or nurse practitioner evaluation and treatment before parents assume responsibility for management, e.g., food poisoning in the infant, insect bites in the hypersensitive child.

5. Abrasions and cuts.

   a. Cause little bleeding.

   b. May become infected if dirt and bacteria are not removed properly.

6. Bites from humans, animals, and poisonous snakes require medical attention.

   a. Consult the physician for a human bite if the skin is broken, since the mouth contains many bacteria.

   b. Wild and domestic animals can transmit rabies, therefore, all animal bites require medical attention initially.

   c. Bites from poisonous snakes are characterized by:

      1. Rapid swelling at the site, skin discoloration, and marked pain.

2. Additional symptoms that occur in 1 to 2 hours, e.g., weakness, nausea and vomiting, shortness of breath, increased pulse, and shock.

7. Bites from insects may cause hypersensitive reactions that result in anaphylaxis or serum sickness.

8. Burns classified as first degree

   a. Are caused by sunburn, scalds from hot water or steam, or brief contact with hot objects.

   b. Are characterized by redness, mild edema, and pain.

9. Concussion is a head injury characterized by a transient loss of consciousness, amnesia for the event, and no demonstrable neurological signs.

10. Food poisoning results from eating food that contains bacterial toxin.

    a. Foods containing milk, eggs, or meat that have been inadequately refrigerated or unrefrigerated for too long.

    b. Foods that have been contaminated by a food handler who has a staphylococcal skin infection.

11. Foreign bodies of the eye may or may not require medical attention.

    a. Particles that lodge in the cornea must be removed by a physician.

    b. Particles of wood, plastic, metal, dirt, or paper that lodge in the conjunctival sac may be removed without causing damage.

12. Frostbite is more likely to occur if the child is exposed to cold, moist air, or to cold air while wearing wet clothes.

    a. Early signs and symptoms of frostbite include:

       1. Shivering.

       2. Numbness, but no pain.

       3. Low body temperature.

       4. Drowsiness.

       5. Muscle weakness.

       6. Loss of consciousness.

       7. Shock.

    b. Later, the skin of the nose, cheeks, ear, fingers, or toes become slightly flushed, then changes to white or grayish yellow.

13. Heat exhaustion symptoms are due to pooling of blood in the capillaries as the body attempts to lose heat.

    a. White, cool, and clammy skin.

    b. Fainting.

    c. Weakness.

    d. Nausea and vomiting.

    e. Abdominal cramps.

14. Nosebleeds usually result from injury such as falls, irritation during a cold, or nosepicking.

15. Sprains usually result from forcing joint

movement beyond the normal range of motion.

16. Strains usually result from overexertion of muscles.

B. **Nursing Management.** See ACCIDENT PREVENTION, FEVER REDUCTION, and FORCING FLUIDS.
   1. Teach management of abrasions and cuts.
      a. Wash own hands.
      b. Wash the abrasion or cut and the area around it, preferably with povidone iodine (Betadine, Isodine).
      c. Rinse the abrasion or cut thoroughly under running water if possible.
      d. Blot the wound dry with a sterile gauze or clean cloth.
      e. Apply a bandage or dressing and tape securely.
      f. Report signs and symptoms of an infection.
         1. Swelling and redness.
         2. Fever.
         3. Pus under the skin or draining from the site.
         4. Throbbing pain.
         5. Swollen lymph glands.
         6. Red streaks leading from the wound.
   2. Teach management of animal or human bites.
      a. Gather descriptions from any witnesses so that health professionals can be well-informed about the event.
      b. Seek medical attention if the skin is broken.
      c. Administer antibiotics as instructed.
      d. Prevent infection of the wound.
         1. Wash hands before caring for the wound.
         2. Apply a clean or sterile dressing as instructed.
      e. Observe for signs of infection. See above.
      f. Review safety measures with the child about animal contact.
         1. Do not touch strange cats or dogs.
         2. Do not touch or try to capture wild animals.
         3. Avoid animals which run blindly, stagger, or dribble saliva.
   3. Teach management of spider bites.
      a. Treat the black widow spider, brown recluse spider, or scorpion bites.
         1. Apply ice to slow the absorption, then seek medical attention.
         2. Provide pain relief through sodium bicarbonate or spirits of ammonia compresses, warm baths, and analgesics such as aspirin.
         3. Administer sedatives and steroids as instructed.
         4. Teach the child to avoid areas where

spiders and scorpions live, e.g., under rocks, boxes, logs, storage sheds, etc.
      b. Teach management of insect stings.
         1. Remove the stinger by rubbing briskly with a credit card or other stiff object.
         2. Apply ice to slow absorption.
         3. Relieve pain with sodium bicarbonate or spirits of ammonia compresses and analgesics.
         4. Teach the child to avoid insect bites by wearing light-colored clothing, avoiding insect-infested areas, and by using insect repellent.
         5. Encourage the hypersensitive child to wear a Medic-Alert tag, to inform the teacher and school nurse of the hypersensitivity, and to take a prophylactic antihistamine before a nature hike, etc.

   4. Teach management of snake bites.
      a. Do not allow the child to walk or to move the involved body part.
      b. Immobilize the extremity in a position below the level of the heart.
      c. Wash the wound and apply ice, but do not pack in ice.
      d. Seek medical assistance since death from snake bite rarely occurs immediately.
      e. Do not use a tourniquet unless a long trip is necessary for medical care.
      f. Encourage the child to talk about the experience so he can deal with the fear.
      g. Teach the child to avoid areas where snakes are likely to be found, e.g., under rocks, on ledges, in gardens.
   5. Teach management of first-degree burns.
      a. Apply cold water to the affected area or submerge the burned area in cold water.
      b. Do not apply butter, oil, etc., to the site.
      c. Pat dry with a sterile gauze or a clean cloth.
      d. Apply a dry dressing if needed.
      e. Discuss safety measures to prevent repetition of the burn.
   6. Teach management of a concussion.
      a. Rouse the child every 2 hours for at least 24 hours.
         1. Set the alarm clock to rouse during the night.
         2. Evaluate alertness by asking the child his name, about his favorite toy, or to identify a color.
      b. Administer sedatives as instructed.
      c. Give the child small amounts of clear fluids.
      d. Report complications to the physician.
         1. Leakage of spinal fluid from nose, ear, or mouth.
         2. Seizures.
         3. Difficulty in rousing.
         4. Muscle weakness.

5. Change in pupils.
e. Handle behavioral changes.
   1. Speak in a gentle, reassuring voice.
   2. Touch the child in a soothing manner.
   3. Do not restrain the child's hands.
   4. Reorient him to his surroundings.
   5. Do not reprimand him for immature or antisocial behavior.
   6. Stay with him.

7. Teach management of food poisoning caused by staphylococci.
  a. Withhold food and fluids for 3 to 4 hours.
  b. Institute feedings.
    1. Give 1 to 2 teaspoons of flat cola, ginger ale, or Gatorade every 20 to 30 minutes for 2 hours.
    2. Increase the amount of fluid gradually to several ounces every 30 to 45 minutes.
    3. Return to step (a) if vomiting or diarrhea recur.
    4. Add dry crackers, hot cereals, rice, broth, etc., to the diet if the child's vomiting and diarrhea do not recur.
    5. Seek medical assistance if the symptoms worsen within 12 hours or do not subside within 24 hours.

8. Teach management of foreign bodies in the eye.
  a. Take the child for medical attention if something is embedded in the eyeball.
  b. Keep the child from rubbing the eye.
  c. Wash own hands before touching the child's eye.
  d. Do not use any object such as a match or toothpick to remove the particle.
  e. Pull down the lower lid and remove any foreign matter with a damp, lint-free cloth.
  f. Evert the upper lid over an applicator or match stick and remove any foreign matter with a damp, lint-free cloth.
  g. Have the child look down to expose the eyeball.
  h. Flush the eye with water using a dropper or small bulb syringe.
  i. Cover the eye with a dry dressing and seek medical assistance if the above measures are not immediately successful.
  j. Distract the older child with activities that require use of the hands to prevent rubbing.
  k. Apply elbow restraints (magazines taped around the arms) or mitts to the infant or young child to prevent rubbing.
  l. Apply ophthalmic drops or ointment as instructed.

9. Teach parental management of first-degree frostbite.

  a. Do not rub the part with snow or ice or thaw in cold water.
  b. Dress the child in dry clothes or wraps.
  c. Give the child a warm drink.
  d. Immerse the body part in warm water.
  e. Handle the affected part gently and do not massage.
  f. Have the child exercise the part once it is thawed.
  g. Cleanse the area with soap and water and blot dry.
  h. Place dry, sterile gauze between fingers and toes, if involved.
  i. Do not sit the child near a radiator, stove, fire, etc.
  j. Use a cardboard box as a bed cradle to keep linen off the affected part.
  k. Do not allow the child to walk on an involved foot until adequate circulation returns.

10. Teach parental management of heat exhaustion.
  a. Move the child to a cooler place, if possible.
  b. Loosen clothing.
  c. Encourage sips of fluids, particularly salt water, colas, ginger ale, or Gatorade to a total of ¼ to ½ a glass per hour.
  d. Place a cool cloth on the child's forehead.
  e. Direct the air from a fan over the child's body or fan with a paper, magazine, etc.
  f. Elevate the child's legs.

11. Teach parental management of nosebleed.
  a. Have the child sit leaning forward or lay the child down with the head and shoulders raised.
  b. Apply pressure to the involved nares or pinch the nares together for about 15 minutes.
  c. Apply cold compresses to the bridge of the nose.
  d. Do not let the child blow his nose.
  e. Insert a small pad of gauze cloth (not a cotton ball) partially into the nares and apply pressure with the thumb and index finger for 10 minutes if bleeding persists.
  f. Seek medical assistance if the above measures are ineffective.

12. Teach parental management of a sprain.
  a. Do not let the child walk if the ankle or knee is sprained.
  b. Elevate the extremity.
  c. Apply cold wet packs or place a small bag of ice over a thin cloth to the area for 4 to 6 hours.
  d. Wrap the extremity in an elastic bandage for 10 to 14 days.
  e. Rewrap the elastic bandage twice a day.
  f. Seek medical assistance if pain or swelling do not subside within 12 to 24 hours.

13. Teach parental management of a strain.
    a. Rest the involved extremity.
    b. Apply ice or cold packs, since heat application will increase any internal bleeding.

Home management of minor illnesses. Caring for the sick child at home.

A. General Considerations.
   1. Parents can provide improved home care for their sick child if they are taught basic principles of home management of illnesses.
   2. Adequate home care of minor illness often keeps them from becoming major illnesses.
   3. Needed equipment can be improvised.
   4. Most minor illnesses are infectious and prevention of the spread of infection is important.
   5. Parents need to know when to call the physician.

B. Nursing Management.
   1. Teach parents to:
      a. Recognize signs that may indicate the onset of illness in the child.
         1. Changes in eating, sleeping, or elimination patterns, e.g., anorexia, wakefulness, diarrhea.
         2. Changes in behavior, e.g., irritability, lethargy.
         3. Elevated temperature or subnormal temperature especially in infants.
         4. Rash.
         5. Inflammation.
      b. Take the child's temperature, pulse, and respirations and keep a record of them.
      c. Keep a record of vomiting, bowel movements, food and fluids taken, and any unusual signs and symptoms.
      d. Keep a record of any medications, date medications given, number of doses, and child's reaction.
      e. Provide adequate fluids but do not force the child to eat solid food. See *Forcing Fluids.*
      f. Find out what the physician wants done in terms of fever reduction and follow instructions.
      g. Initiate fever reduction measures for rectal temperature greater than 102°F or as instructed. See *Fever Reduction.*
      h. Withhold solid food and fluids from the child with vomiting and/or diarrhea for a period of 3 to 4 hours, then slowly begin fluids to prevent dehydration. See *Vomiting.*
      i. Separate the child from family members until a diagnosis is made.
      j. Call the physician if the fever (Pantell, Fries, Vickery, 1977):
         1. Is present in a child under 4 months of age.
         2. Is accompanied by stiff neck, altered level of consciousness, or seizures.
         3. Has persisted for more than 24 hours in a child between 4 months and 1 year.
         4. Shows no improvement after 3 days or lasts more than 5 days.
      k. Call the physician if vomiting (Pantell, Fries, Vickery, 1977):
         1. Is accompanied by abdominal pain, lethargy, or irritability.
         2. Contains blood or is a coffee grounds color.
         3. Is accompanied by urinary tract symptoms, e.g., burning on urination.
         4. Is accompanied by signs of dehydration or the child does not retain fluid for 8 hours or more.
      l. Call the physician if diarrhea.
         1. Is accompanied by blood in the stool.
         2. Is accompanied by severe abdominal pain and/or vomiting.
         3. Produces signs and symptoms of dehydration.
         4. Persists without improvement after solid foods and/or milk are withheld.
      m. Call the physician for:
         1. Other symptoms which persist or increase, e.g., cough, sore throat, skin rash.
         2. Consultation about any concern in regard to handling the child's care.
   2. Teach parents to give medications as instructed. See *Administration of Medications, Parental.*
      a. Give only those medications prescribed for the child during this illness.
      b. Avoid the use of over-the-counter drugs unless ordered by the physician.
      c. Give medications accurately.
   3. Discuss how to provide comfort for the child on bedrest.
      a. Give a bedbath or back rub.
      b. Leave a pitcher of fluids at the bedside for the older child.
      c. Change the bed more frequently.
      d. Humidify the air by placing a cool mist vaporizer at the bedside of a child with an upper respiratory infection.
      e. Position for comfort if the child is not moving about in bed.
   4. Explain the need to keep the sick child quiet but do not insist on the child remaining in bed if he feels well enough to be up, since children usually limit their own activity.

5. Provide information about planning different types of diets.
   a. Clear liquid: can see through them and they contain no pulp, e.g., apple juice.
   b. Full liquid: cannot see through them, e.g., milk, cream soups, orange juice.
   c. Soft: foods requiring little or no chewing and are easily digested, e.g., custard, oatmeal, hamburger.
   d. Regular: foods normally eaten.
6. Help the parents meet the diversionary needs of the child. See *Stimulation* and *Toys.*
   a. Provide some new activity each day to prevent boredom.
   b. Spend some time in active play with the child when he feels well enough, e.g., checkers, cards.
   c. Place an overbed table in the bed for the older child to work on or place a card table at the side of the bed.
   d. Arrange for visitors, if the child is noninfectious, but limit them to a time period which will not tire the child.
7. Teach parents how to improvise equipment such as:
   a. Overbed table: cut the bottom and a portion of two sides off a box so it will fit over the child's legs.
   b. Back rest: use a:
      1. Table leaf, padded with towels tilted against the headboard.
      2. Cushion from a sofa or large chair.
   c. Urinal: cut off the spout from a well-rinsed laundry detergent or milk bottle with a handle and smooth any rough edges.
   d. Croup tent: place a blanket over the side and top two-thirds of the crib; anchor it in place by tying it to the frame, and place a cool steam vaporizer at the cribside.
   e. Bedside table: two straight back (kitchen) chairs with a shelf or board across the seats to provide storage for books, games, radio, etc.
8. Teach the child and parents how to prevent the spread of infection.
   a. Wash hands before and after caring for the child.
   b. Wash the child's hands, or have him wash, before meals and after using the bathroom.
   c. Provide tissues at the bedside.
   d. Place a paper bag at the bedside to serve as a receptacle for soiled tissues.
   e. Keep the child's eating utensils, towels, washclothes, and personal care items (comb, brush, etc.) separate.
   f. Limit the number of people in contact with the child.

9. Teach parents to meet the emotional needs of the sick child.
   a. Give an infant extra cuddling time.
   b. Accept regression which may occur with illness.
   c. Check on the child frequently so he knows he is not forgotten.
   d. Develop a schedule for the older child so he knows when to expect meals, visits, etc.
   e. Provide the child with a means of calling you, e.g., bell, spoon in a tin cup or pan, party noisemaker, whistle.
   f. Respond to the child's call as promptly as possible.
   g. Set realistic limits for the child and be consistent.
   h. Keep the child, who does not need to be isolated, in the living room on the couch so he feels he is part of the activities.
   i. Do household chores in the child's room if he must be in bed, e.g., mending, ironing, letter writing.
   j. Encourage peers/classmates of the older child to make cards or send notes.
10. Teach parents to meet the special needs of ill adolescents who will be cared for at home.
    a. Encourage them to assume responsibility in taking medications and adhering to other prescribed treatment.
    b. Teach them comfort measures as above.
    c. Place bed near phone so adolescent can keep up with friends.
    d. Encourage them to keep up with schoolwork, if possible.

Homosexuality. See *Sex Education.*

Hookworm. See *Worms.*

Hordeolum. See *Sty*

Hospitalization, response to. Behavioral reaction of the infant/child and parents to illness and hospitalization. See ADMISSION TO HOSPITAL, ELECTIVE and EMERGENCY.

A. General Considerations.
1. Beginning with toddlerhood, hospitalized children/adolescents are affected by fears of (See *Fears*):
   a. Separation.
   b. Loss of control.
   c. Bodily injury and pain.

2. Behavioral regression is most pronounced in the toddler period, although it may occur in any age group.

3. Interpreting illness and/or hospitalization as a punishment begins with the toddler and may be present through adolescence.

4. The infant from birth to 3 months tolerates hospitalization well if his needs are met consistently.

5. The older infant is adversely affected if his mother is not available to care for him.
   a. Stranger anxiety reaches a peak around 8 months of life.
   b. Hospitalization of more than 3 weeks may cause serious disturbance.

6. Separation from parents is the most traumatic aspect of hospitalization for the toddler.

7. The toddler's response to hospitalization includes three phases:
   a. Protest: crying, screaming, etc. may last from a few hours to several days.
   b. Despair: withdrawn, depressed behavior and refusal to relate to others may gradually replace protest.
   c. Denial: indiscriminate, superficial relationships with all adults and lack of response to parents may occur during prolonged hospitalization.

8. The despair phase may be misinterpreted by the nursing staff as "settling in."

9. The preschooler has new concerns about illness as well as a fear of abandonment by his parents.
   a. The preschooler has trouble understanding how and why he became ill.
   b. The child may experience physical symptoms such as nausea, pain, etc. for the first time.

10. The young schoolchild may have much difficulty with separation from parents during hospitalization.

11. The schoolchild has little knowledge of his body and its functions or how illness is caused.

12. The most stressful part of hospitalization for the schoolager is immobilization. See *Immobilized Child.*

13. The schoolaged child believes in "illness as punishment" and the "germ theory" as the causes of illness, but his comprehension of the mechanism of infection is often inaccurate (Wood, 1983).

14. The adolescent who is struggling for independence finds the enforced dependency of illness and hospitalization very difficult.
   a. Parents may be overprotective and allow the teenager no decision making or withdraw and give no support.
   b. The adolescent needs much support from the nurse during procedures which result in exposure of the body.

15. Parents may be as anxious or more anxious than the child. See *Anxiety, Parental.*

B. Nursing Management. See HOSPITALIZATION, SUPPORT DURING.

1. Meet the needs of the infant. See *Infant.*
   a. Sit beside the parent during the first contact so the infant sees both of you at the same time. This helps the infant feel that you are a safe person.
   b. Adapt your usual feeding technique to that technique used by the parents unless their technique is unsafe or inappropriate.

2. Meet the needs of the toddler. See *Toddler.*
   a. Help the toddler during the protest phase.
      1. Allow the toddler to cry, but stay with him when possible.
      2. Recognize that the toddler's inability to be consoled is a response to separation, not a rejection of your nursing care.
   b. Help the toddler during the despair phase.
      1. Sit quietly by the crib until the child is able to accept interaction and comfort.
      2. Talk with him about his home and family.
      3. Follow his home routine and rituals.
      4. Set consistent limits on behavior.
      5. Provide age-appropriate stimulation.
      6. Provide outlets for aggressive feelings.
      7. Ask the mother to tell the child honestly when she is leaving.
      8. Explain to the mother that the toddler may turn away from her when she visits because the child feels he has been abandoned.
      9. Interpret to ancillary personnel that the child's lack of crying is evidence of grieving for his parents, not adjustment to the hospital.
   c. Help the child during the denial phase.
      1. Initiate specific nursing action if the child does not react positively when the parents arrive or negatively when the parents leave.
      2. Give high priority to consistency in assignment of one nurse per shift with a designated relief person.
      3. Facilitate more frequent visits by the parents by referrals for assistance with transportation, care of siblings, etc.

3. Meet the needs of the preschool child. See *Preschooler.*
   a. Ask the parents how the child usually copes with new situations.
   b. Tell the child he or she did not cause the illness.

c. Help the child learn terminology for the symptoms and let the child know what can be done to relieve them.

4. Meet the needs of the schoolchild. See *Schoolchild*.
    a. Discuss with parents the child's need for their physical presence and support.
    b. Use diagrams, pictures, etc. to explain the child's illness and treatment.
    c. Help the child cope with immobilization.

5. Meet the needs of the adolescent. See *Adolescent*.
    a. Admit to an adolescent unit or assign to a room with another teenager if possible.
    b. Ask the adolescent how he or she usually handles new situations.
    c. Support the adolescent's independence by permitting as many decisions as possible about nursing care to be made by the adolescent.
    d. Encourage physicians to discuss the treatment plans with the adolescent as well as with the parents.
    e. Involve the adolescent in setting limits on privileges, bedtime, snacks, etc.
    f. Encourage peer contact via visits, phone calls, letters, etc.

6. Meet the needs of the parents.
    a. Discuss the response to hospitalization characteristic of the child's age group.
    b. Explore with the parents what they believe will ease the trauma of hospitalization for the child and family.
    c. Encourage parent participation in care and 24-hour visiting.
    d. Support the parent who is not able to stay with the child.
       1. Ask the parents to tell the child and the nurse when the parents will leave and return.
       2. Stay with the child when the parents leave.
       3. Record the information on the parent's visiting plans on the Kardex so all staff can answer the child's questions honestly.
       4. Draw a clock for the young child which depicts when the parents will return or explain their return in relation to familiar routines such as meals, bath, or nap time.

Hospitalization, support during. Meeting the needs of the child and the parents.

A. General Considerations.
1. Illness and hospitalization are traumatic for the child.

    a. The child's normal growth and development are interrupted.
    b. The child is separated from daily routine and from supportive people in environment.
    c. The child will have to meet many strangers and experience intrusive and painful procedures.

2. The admission procedure sets the tone for the entire hospitalization. See *Admission to Hospital, Elective*.

3. Adequate preparation for hospitalization is essential for a satisfactory transition from home to hospital. See *Preparation for Hospitalization*.

4. Parent participation should be encouraged since it benefits both child and parents.
    a. The parents are most familiar with the child's needs and routines.
    b. Parental support will help the child cope with the many new experiences.
    c. Parents feel more useful when they can do something concrete to help the child.
    d. Parents who participate in care will be more comfortable in assuming the child's care at discharge.

5. Sources of anxiety for the child and the family include:
    a. Separation.
    b. Decreased mobility.
    c. Enforced dependence.
    d. Unfamiliar routines.
    e. Physical discomfort.
    f. Fears of the unknown.
    g. Concern for the child's recovery.
    h. Frightening equipment.
    i. Guilt for having allowed the child to become ill or not having recognized early symptoms.
    j. Concern about other family members.
    k. Financial burden of hospitalization.

6. The nurse should assume an advocacy role for the child and parents, since hospitalization is stressful for the entire family. See *Advocate*.

B. Nursing Management.
1. Meet the physical needs of the infant or child.
    a. Promote comfort.
       1. Prepare the child for procedures.
       2. Assess need for pain medication and administer as needed. See *Pain*.
    b. Provide good skin care since breakdown is more likely with the pediatric patient.
    c. Keep the child and the environment clean to decrease bacterial growth.
    c. Provide rest periods as well as activity periods.
    e. Meet the nutritional needs.
       1. Recognize that refusal to eat may be

one way the child can control the environment.

2. Obtain a history of what the child eats at home and any feeding routines and rituals.

3. Encourage parents to bring in foods or familiar feeding equipment from home.

4. Have someone stay with the child during mealtime or feed the child in a group with other children.

5. Avoid scheduling painful procedures around mealtime.

6. Allow the child as much autonomy as possible in feeding.

7. Meet with the dietician to provide sandwiches, soups, etc. that children prefer for lunch.

8. Provide food in small portions.

9. Offer nutritious snacks or juices if the child did not eat well at mealtime.

10. Encourage the parents to offer nutritious snacks when they visit if the child's intake has been poor.

f. Promote normal elimination.
   1. Follow home routines.
   2. Find out the child's terms for elimination.
   3. Encourage adequate fluids and bulk in diet.
   4. Provide privacy during elimination.
   5. Obtain an order for stool softener for the immobilized child.

g. Promote dental hygiene.
   1. Have the child brush teeth after meals and snacks.
   2. Encourage parents to bring fruits rather than candy.
   3. Provide mouth care for the child who is NPO.

2. Meet the emotional needs of the infant and young child.
   a. Prepare the child and parents for all procedures. See *Preparation for Procedures*.
   b. Encourage parent participation in care.
   c. Assign one staff member consistently for the child's care.
   d. Provide play opportunities especially for the child admitted as an emergency admission. See *Play* and *Play, Therapeutic*.
   e. Follow home routines and rituals whenever possible.
   f. Meet the child's increased need for security.
      1. Provide pacifier or security object.
      2. Offer physical comfort by rocking, holding, touching, etc.
      3. Have parents bring pictures or tape recordings of family members.

4. Tell parents to be honest with the child when they leave and to let the nurse know when they will return.

5. Have the parents leave a personal article with the child if they are unable to stay, e.g., scarf or handkerchief.

6. Let the child wear own clothing.

g. Promote mobility.
   1. Encourage child's cooperation to decrease need for restraints. See *Restraints*.
   2. Use wagons, wheelchairs, carts, to transport the child to other areas for stimulation.

h. Identify and support coping behaviors. See *Coping*.

i. Provide sensory stimulation, but avoid sensory bombardment. See *Stimulation*.

j. Discuss with the parents what care and comfort measures they want to provide for their child.

3. Meet the emotional needs of the older child and adolescent.
   a. Prepare the child and parents for all procedures. See *Preparation for Procedures*.
   b. Encourage parents to visit regularly.
   c. Assign one staff member consistently to the child's care.
   d. Provide the child with opportunities to express feelings about the illness and hospitalization.
   e. Identify and support coping behaviors. See *Coping*.
   f. Encourage the child to participate actively in health care procedures and in activities of daily living.
   g. Provide peer contact with visitors and other patients.
   h. Provide privacy and maintain confidentiality.
   i. Offer choices in procedures and daily activities whenever possible.
   j. Encourage the child to keep up with schoolwork.
   k. Allow the child to wear own clothing.
   l. Meet the child's food preferences when appropriate.
   m. Provide sensory stimulation, but avoid sensory bombardment. See *Stimulation*.

4. Meet the needs of the irritable child.
   a. Speak to the child in quiet, soothing tones.
   b. Explain what you plan to do before beginning the nursing activity.
   c. Plan nursing care in blocks so the child is not disturbed by physical care more frequently than necessary.
   d. Spend quiet time with the child sitting beside the child, holding hands, etc.

e. Keep noxious stimuli such as bright lights or loud noises to a minimum.

f. Indicate to parents that irritability is not uncommon in the sick child.

5. Explore alternatives with working parents so that the child's needs can be met while the parent maintains job security.

6. Support the parents if they are unable to stay with the child, but feel guilty about leaving.

7. Meet the needs of the parents.

a. Provide for the parent's physical comfort.

1. Orient the parents to the physical environment and routine.

2. Provide a cot or recliner chair for sleep.

3. Encourge the parent to get adequate rest and food.

4. Order meal trays or relieve the parents for meals.

5. Tell the parents what bathing facilities are available.

6. Provide a rocking chair or other comfortable chair.

b. Meet the parent's emotional needs.

1. Share information on the child's progress with the exception of specific medical data such as test results or initial diagnosis.

2. Encourage the parents' participation, but not responsibility for the child's care.

3. Discuss specific ways the parents can meet the child's comfort needs.

4. Provide opportunities for the parents to ask questions and discuss concerns and reduce their anxiety. See *Anxiety, Parental.*

8. Tell the parents how to reach the unit by phone if they are unable to stay.

9. Provide consistency in nursing care measures to reassure parents.

10. Plan intervention with the aggressive parent. See *Aggression, Parental.*

11. Arrange for an interpreter if language barriers are present.

12. Arrange for support of health team members as needed, e.g., chaplain, social worker, etc.

13. Prepare the parents for discharge. See *Discharge Planning.*

Hydrocephalus. Excess cerebrospinal fluid in the ventricle and subarachnoid spaces of the brain.

A. **General Considerations.**

1. There are two types of hydrocephalus.

a. Noncommunicating: blockage between the ventricular and subarachnoid systems caused by:

1. Congential lesions, particulary aqueductal stenosis.

2. Acquired lesions secondary to meningitis, trauma, spontaneous intracranial bleeding, and tumor.

b. Communicating: normal communication exists between the ventricular and subarachnoid space, but absorption of cerebrospinal fluid is prevented by:

1. Congenital lesions such as Arnold-Chiari malformation.

2. Acquired lesions secondary to infection, hemorrhage, or masses.

3. Overproduction of cerebrospinal fluid.

2. Symptoms of infantile hydrocephalus may be present at birth or become apparent by 3 months of age.

a. Tense, bulging fontanels.

b. Widening sutures.

c. Enlarged head diameter.

d. Taut, shiny scalp.

e. Prominent scalp veins.

f. Sunset eyes. (Sclera are visible above the iris.)

g. Irritability or lethargy.

h. High-pitched cry.

i. Frontal bossing (bulging of the brow).

3. Symptoms in older infants and children include:

a. Severe bifrontal headache.

b. Nausea and vomiting.

c. Irritability and listlessness.

d. Disturbances in reflexes and muscle tone.

e. Vision difficulties.

f. Gait difficulties.

g. "Cracked pot" sound on cranial percussion.

4. Diagnostic procedures include:

a. Computerized axial tomography (CAT or CT scan).

b. Ventriculogram.

c. Pneumoencephalogram (rare).

d. Ultrasound.

5. The purpose of surgical treatment is to bypass the point of obstruction and/or shunt the excess cerebrospinal fluid.

a. Ventriculoperitoneal (V-P): shunt from the lateral ventricle to the peritoneum.

b. Ventriculoatrial or ventriculojugular (V-J): shunt from the lateral ventricle through the internal jugular vein into the right atrium of the heart.

c. Direct cardiac: shunt from the lateral ventricle into the right atrium.

d. Ventriculopleural, ventriculocisternostomy, and lumbar-arachnoid shunts are used infrequently.

6. A one-way valve is inserted to allow cerebrospinal fluid to enter the circulation while preventing blood from flowing back to the ventricle.

7. Shunt revision due to mechanical obstruction, infection, or growth of the child is frequently necessary.

8. Many children with hydrocephalus have severe physical and/or neurological handicaps and few will be normal intellectually.

B. Nursing Management. See *Body Image.*

1. Support the child and parents during hospitalization. See *Hospitalization, Support During.*

2. Initiate discharge planning. See *Discharge Planning.*

3. Observe, record, and report symptoms of increased intracranial pressure. See *Increased Intracranial Pressure.*

4. Prepare the child and parents for diagnostic procedures. See *Preparation for Procedures.*

5. Measure the head circumference daily by passing the measuring tape just above the eyebrows and around the head's prominent posterior aspect.

6. Provide good skin care.
   a. Change the infant or child's position frequently.
   b. Place sheepskin under the head if enlarged.

7. Bathe the infant before feeding to decrease the likelihood of vomiting.

8. Support the head carefully when changing position or feeding the infant.
   a. Move the head and body together.
   b. Sit in a rocking chair with arm support.
   c. Place the baby on a pillow in the caregiver's arms if the head is enlarged.

9. Prepare the child and parents for surgery. See *Preoperative Care* and *Preparation for Surgery.*

10. Meet the needs of the infant/child postoperatively. See *Postoperative Care.*
    a. Observe, record, and report signs of increased intracranial pressure.
    b. Position infant/child flat or with head and shoulders elevated as ordered.
    c. Provide good skin care.
       1. Position on the unoperative side with the head flat or slightly elevated as ordered.
       2. Place cotton behind the ears and over the ears under the head dressing to prevent skin breakdown.
       3. Place sheepskin under the head.
    d. Irrigate the nasogastric tube and maintain NPO status if a ventriculoperitoneal shunt is performed.
    e. Pump the valve as ordered if ventriculotrial shunt is performed.
    f. Offer oral feedings in small amounts since vomiting increases intracranial pressure.
       1. Record successful techniques on the Kardex.
       2. Offer feedings on demand rather than on a schedule.
    g. Observe, record, and report symptoms of infection.
       1. Elevated vital signs.
       2. Poor feeding.
       3. Vomiting.
       4. Decreased responsiveness.
       5. Irritability.
       6. Seizures.
       7. Inflammation of incision sites.

11. Teach the child and parents home management.

    a. Assess the parent's ability to meet the child's physical needs and reinforce their knowledge as appropriate.
    b. Teach the child and parents the symptoms of increased intracranial pressure.
    c. Teach the child and parents the symptoms of dehydration.
       1. Cold extremities.
       2. Sunken eyes.
       3. Sunken fontanels in the infant.
       4. Thirst in the older child.
       5. Decreased urination.
    d. Demonstrate how to pump the shunt and discuss their feelings about this procedure.
    e. Encourage the parents to provide age-appropriate stimulation. See *Stimulation.*
    f. Initiate referrals for community health nurse follow-up, infant stimulation programs, etc. as needed.

Hyperalimentation. See *Total Parental Nutrition.*

Hyperglycemia. See *Diabetes Mellitus.*

Hypertension. Average of three consecutive readings of systolic and/or diastolic blood pressures taken at three different times which are equal to, or greater then the 95th percentile for their age-sex-adjusted levels on the National Heart, Lung, and Blood Institute Task Force on Blood Pressure pediatric blood pressure grids (McCrory, 1982).

A. General Considerations.
1. Blood pressure values increase slowly as the child ages and are frequently labile, especially in the adolescent.

2. Hypertension in children may be:
   a. Essential: hypertension for which there is no discoverable cause.
   b. Secondary: hypertension due to:
      1. Disorders of the renal, endocrine, vascular, or neurological systems, e.g., acute glomerulonephritis, Wilm's tumor, neuroblastoma, coarcation of the aorta, leukemia, increased intracranial pressure, and anxiety.
      2. Metabolic disorders, e.g., diabetes mellitus, hypernatremia, hyperthyroidism.
      3. Drug therapy or ingestion, e.g., steroid therapy, amphetamine overdose.
      4. Miscellaneous causes, e.g., burns.
3. Essential hypertension is usually asymptomatic.
4. Signs and symptoms associated with secondary hypertension include:
   a. Headache.
   b. Dizziness.
   c. Blurred vision.
   d. Nausea.
   e. Vomiting.
   f. Retinal changes.
   g. Reduced renal function.
   h. Seizure activity.
5. Treatment is based on:
   a. The age of the child.
   b. The underlying cause of the hypertension, if known.
   c. Whether the blood pressure is elevated on a consistent or intermittent basis.
   d. The severity of the elevation.
6. Treatment may include:
   a. Reducing weight.
   b. Decreasing sodium intake.
   c. Decreasing environmental stress factors.
   d. Eliminating smoking.
   e. Increasing exercise except isometric activities which may raise the blood pressure significantly.
   f. Antihypertensive and diuretic drugs in cases of marked elevation.
   g. Avoiding the use of pressor drugs, e.g., oral contraceptives, over the counter drugs which contain sympathomimetics.
   h. Surgery, if the underlying cause is correctible by this means, e.g., coarcation of the aorta.
7. Long-term follow-up care is essential to prevent complications such as coronary heart disease, strokes, and renal damage.
8. The child may be hospitalized for initial evaluation of the hypertension and initiation of treatment but is managed on an outpatient basis.
9. The adolescent may have a particularly difficult time complying with the therapeutic regimen.

B. **Nursing Management**. See NUTRITION.
   1. Support the child and parents during hospitalization. See *Hospitalization, Support During*.
   2. Initiate discharge planning when the cause of hypertension is known. See *Discharge Planning*.
   3. Obtain accurate blood pressure readings.
      a. Use a Doppler device, if available, for an infant since this provides both systolic and diastolic readings.
      b. Have the infant/child in a quiet state while obtaining blood pressure to avoid high readings.
         1. Bottle feed or offer a pacifier to infant during the procedure.
         2. Explain the procedure and encourage the older child to handle equipment to decrease fear and anxiety. See *Preparation for Procedures*.
      c. Fully expose the upper arm.
      d. Use a cuff whose inner rubber bladder covers at least two-thirds of the length of the upper arm and encircles the extremity without overlapping.
      e. Wrap the cuff snuggly and have the lower edge above the antecubital space.
      f. Inflate the cuff rapidly to 30 mm Hg above the point where the radial pulse disappears.
      g. Lower the pressure in the inflated cuff at the rate of 3 to 5 mm Hg per second in order to prevent a false low reading.
      h. Use the fourth Korotkoff sound, when muffling occurs, as the diastolic reading.
      i. Do not use heavy pressure on the stethoscope, since this distorts Korotkoff sounds.
   4. Record all blood pressure measurements so any pattern of elevation can be detected; use blood pressure grids such as those developed by the National Heart, Lung, Blood Institutes Task Force of Blood Pressure.
   5. Observe, record, and report signs and symptoms of elevated blood pressure.
   6. Observe, record, and report the child's response to antihypertensive and/or diuretic drugs.
   7. Ensure adequate potassium intake in the child on diuretic therapy.
   8. Weigh the child accurately.
      a. Use the same scale.
      b. Weigh the child at the same time each day.
      c. Have the child nude or wearing the same clothing.

9. Teach the child and parents ongoing home management.
   a. Decrease weight if the child is obese. See *Obesity*.
   b. Reduce salt intake.
      1. Remove salt shaker from the table.
      2. Cook with a salt substitute added to the cooking water for improved taste.
      3. Limit or eliminate the use of processed foods high in salt, e.g., lunch meats, hot dogs, potato chips.
   c. Decrease stress in the child's environment.
      1. Explore the home situation to identify stress situations.
      2. Involve the teacher in evaluating and reducing school pressures.
      3. Discuss with the child ways in which he feels he could decrease his stress level.
   d. Encourage the child who smokes to quit. See *Smoking*.
   e. Plan an appropriate exercise program. See *Exercise*.
   f. Teach the parents how to take a blood pressure reading.
      1. Demonstrate the procedure.
      2. Have parents perform a return demonstration.

10. Support the child and parents in accepting long-term therapy if the child's condition requires. See *Chronic Illness*.
   a. Explain the rationale for long-term care.
   b. State what may occur if therapy is not followed. See *Administration of Medications, Parental.*
      1. Cardiac disease.
      2. Strokes.
      3. Renal damage.
   c. Encourage the child and parents to express their feelings about the presence of a chronic disorder.
   d. Initiate a referral for continued evaluation and care.

11. Support the adolescent with hypertension.
   a. Encourage the physician to develop the plan of care in conjunction with the adolescent.
   b. Recognize that there will be variability in the adolescent's compliance with treatment measures.
   c. Reinforce positive behaviors and avoid negative statements when lapses occur.
   d. Help the adolescent learn to identify high sodium foods that can be avoided so that those they feel they must have occasionally can be eaten.

12. Serve as an advocate for the family by encouraging other family members to have their blood pressure checked.

Hyperthyroidism (thyrotoxicosis, Graves' disease).

Disorder due to excessive thyroid hormone production.

1. The cause of the condition has not been completely established but the following have been implicated:
   a. Altered autoimmune response.
   b. Heredity.
   c. Infections.
   d. Disturbed pituitary function.
2. Signs and symptoms may develop slowly and include:
   a. Irritability.
   b. Emotional lability.
   c. Easy fatigability with insomnia.
   d. Weight loss despite excessive appetite.
   e. Nervousness and hand tremors.
   f. Heat intolerance.
   g. Increased pulse.
   h. Elevated systolic blood pressure.
   i. Exopthalmos.
   j. Smooth, enlarged, and visible thyroid.
   k. Accelerated skeletal maturation.
   l. Diarrhea.
3. Thyroid function lab studies will be elevated.
4. The course of the disease is variable and may terminate in spontaneous remission or progress rapidly.
5. Treatment may be either medical or surgical or surgery may be performed if medical treatment is not successful.
   a. Medical treatment may include the use of:
      1. Drugs, e.g., thyroid inhibitors, sedatives, tranquilizers and/or antihypertensives.
      2. Diet high in calories, carbohydrates and vitamins.
      3. Bedrest in severe cases.
   b. Surgical intervention.
      1. Includes the subtotal removal of the thyroid gland after preparation with drugs.
      2. May result in hypoparathyroidism, thyroid "storm," hypothyroidism, and paralysis of the recurrent laryngeal nerve.
6. Inhibition of thyroid function causes decreased white blood cell production and, therefore, the child is more prone to infection.
7. Administration of iodine prior to a thyroidectomy may dramatically decrease symptoms, but surgery is still required since iodine cannot be used for maintenance therapy.

B. **Nursing Management.**
   1. Support the child and parents during hospitalization. See *Hospitalization, Support During.*

2. Initiate discharge planning. See *Discharge Planning.*
3. Observe, record, and report signs and symptoms related to the diagnosis.
4. Prepare the child for possible diagnostic tests. See *Preparation for Procedures.*
   a. Serum levels of thyroid hormone.
   b. Radioiodine uptake studies.
   c. X-ray determination of skeletal maturation.
5. Observe, record, and report the child's response to drugs which inhibit thyroid function, since they may cause fever, sore throat, and headache, etc.
6. Observe, record, and report the child's response to sedatives, tranquilizers, and antihypertensive drugs if used.
7. Promote rest and relaxation.
   a. Reduce environmental stimuli.
      1. Place in quiet location on unit.
      2. Keep television and radio volume down.
      3. Limit the number of visitors at one time.
   b. Plan care in blocks to provide rest periods.
   c. Provide quiet age-appropriate activities.
   d. Develop a consistent schedule and record it on the Kardex.
8. Meet increased metabolic requirements.
   a. Offer favorite foods.
   b. Plan diet to include increased calories, carbohydrates, and vitamins, especially vitamin B.
   c. Schedule between meal and bedtime snacks.
9. Promote physical comfort, since increased metabolic rate causes diaphoresis.
   a. Provide extra gowns and pajamas.
   b. Change the bed as needed.
   c. Provide or dress the child in light weight absorbent clothing.
   d. Provide adequate room ventilation.
   e. Encourage fluid intake.
   f. Bathe frequently.
10. Prevent diarrhea due to increased hormone levels.
    a. Plan adequate time periods for meals to prevent rushing.
    b. Limit fluid intake during meals.
    c. Avoid excessive roughage in diet.
11. Meet the needs of the child with exopthalmos.
    a. Employ strict safety precautions, since the child may have blurred vision and loss of visual acuity.
    b. Administer artificial tears as ordered to prevent drying of the eye.
12. Meet the needs of the child preoperatively. See *Preoperative Care* and *Preparation for Surgery.*
    a. Promote rest.
    b. Administer sedation as ordered.

c. Provide high calorie diet.
d. Administer iodine and thyroid inhibitors to decrease thyroid function.
e. Discuss the child's fear of having the throat cut during surgery.
f. Prepare the child and parents for the possibility of an endotracheal tube and ICU care postoperatively.
13. Meet the needs of the child postoperatively. See *Postoperative Care.*
    a. Support the child's head to decrease tension on the suture line.
    b. Keep calcium lactate and a tracheotomy tray at the bedside.
    c. Observe, record, and report bleeding in the operative area.
14. Observe, record, and report signs of hypoparathyroidism which include:
    a. Tetany.
    b. Seizures.
    c. Muscle cramps.
    d. Twitching.
    e. Paresthesia.
    f. Laryngeal stridor.
15. Observe, record, and report signs and symptoms of recurrent laryngeal nerve paralysis.
    a. Stridor and airway obstruction if paralysis is bilateral.
    b. Abnormal speech sound if paralysis is unilateral.
16. Observe, record, and report signs and symptoms of thyroid "storm."
    a. High fever.
    b. Circulatory collapse.
    c. Coma.
17. Teach the child and parents home management of the child to be managed medically.
    a. Administer medications as instructed. See *Administration of Medications, Parental.*
    b. Report the following signs and symptoms to the physician.
       1. Increase in presenting symptoms.
       2. Infections.
    c. Provide adequate nutrition and rest. See *Nutrition.*
    d. Assist the parents to plan how they will handle the child's emotional outbursts.
       1. Decrease environmental stress.
       2. Decrease stimulation.
       3. Increase rest.
       4. Use relaxation techniques.
    e. Encourage the parents to discuss the child's hyperactivity and emotional lability with school teachers so that school activities can be modified appropriately.

Hyphema. See *Eye Injury.*

Hypospadias. A congenital anomaly in which the urethral opening is located on the ventral side of the penis.

    A. General Considerations.
1. The urethral opening may occur at any point from near the tip of the glans to the penoscrotal junction.
2. Hypospadias is often accompanied by chordee; a downward bowing of the penis caused by fibrous bands.
3. The chordee is usually released when the child is 12 to 24 months of age.
4. A minimal defect may be repaired at the same time as the chordee release: 12 to 24 months.
5. Other associated defects include:
   a. Cryptorchidism.
   b. Malformed testes.
   c. Bifid scrotum.
6. Circumcision should not be performed, since this tissue may be used in the plastic repair.
7. Meatotomy may be necessary if there is a small meatus.
8. Plastic repair of the defect may be done in one or more stages, usually when the child is 3 to 4 years of age.
9. No surgery may be necessary if the meatus is near the tip of the penis.

    B. Nursing Management.
1. Support the child and parents during hospitalization. See *Hospitalization, Support During.*
2. Initiate discharge planning. See *Discharge Planning.*
3. Find out what the child and parents have been told about the defect and record on the Kardex or clinic record.
4. Provide opportunities for the parents to discuss their concerns about the child's sexual orientation and reproductive ability.
5. Meet the needs of the child admitted for the repair of the chordee.
   a. Prepare the child for surgery. See *Preoperative Care* and *Preparation for Surgery.*
   b. Meet the postoperative needs of the child. See *Postoperative Care.*
6. Prepare the older child for the plastic repair.
   a. Clarify with the surgeon what the child and parents should expect postoperatively.
      1. Foley catheter.
      2. Suprapubic tube.
      3. Perineal urethrostomy.
   b. Reinforce the explanation that the penis will be fixed, not cut off.
   c. Explain that the surgery is not a punishment for anything he has done or thought; i.e., masturbation, sex play, erotic feelings, etc.
   d. Tell him that the nurse will be looking at his bandage frequently.
   e. Explain that he will have a catheter or catheters postoperatively for 10 to 14 days.
7. Meet the child's needs postoperatively. See *Postoperative Care.*
   a. Observe the pressure dressing and record the drainage, but do not change the dressing.
   b. Apply ice packs to decrease edema if ordered.
   c. Provide privacy for the child when observing the dressing.
   d. Observe the color and amount of urine draining from the catheter(s).
   e. Provide support when the catheter is removed.
   f. Observe, record, and report the child's voiding pattern after catheter removal.

Hypothyroidism. Condition due to an inadequate amount of thyroid hormone.

    A. General Considerations.
1. The condition may be:
   a. Congenital (cretinism) due to an absent or nonfunctioning thyroid gland.
   b. Acquired, which is usually due to atrophy of the thyroid gland from an unknown cause.
2. Signs and symptoms usually appear at 3 to 6 months of age in bottle-fed infants with congenital hypothroidism.
   a. Prolonged neonatal jaundice.
   b. Lethargy.
   c. Poor muscle tone.
   d. Umbilical hernia.
   e. Chronic constipation.
   f. Delayed central nervous system development, especially the brain.
   g. Hoarse cry.
   h. Poor feeding accompanied by choking spells.
   i. Pale, cool, dry, scaly skin.
   j. Thick tongue.
   k. Puffy face.
   l. Low temperature and slow pulse.
3. Symptoms may be delayed in the breast-fed infant.
4. Signs and symptoms seen in older children with acquired hypothyroidism include:
   a. Delayed growth and development with:
      1. Short arms and legs.
      2. Large head.
      3. Short, thick neck.
   b. Delayed dentition and increased dental caries.
   c. Obesity.
   d. Lethargy.
   e. Pale, cool, dry, scaly skin.

5. Laboratory tests used in the diagnosis and in the evaluation of the child's response to thyroid hormone replacement therapy include:
   a. Protein-bound iodine.
   b. T3 (serum triiodothyronine level).
   c. T4 (serum thyroxine level).
   d. ^{131}I (radioactive iodine uptake).
6. Neonatal screening for hypothyroidism is mandatory in most states.
7. Treatment requires the administration of exogenous thyroid hormone throughout life.
8. The infant with congenital hypothyroidism who receives replacement therapy before the age of 3 months has an increased chance of having normal intelligence.
9. Adequate treatment of the infant will result in:
   a. An accelerated growth rate with the deficit restored within 9 to 24 months.
   b. A slow disappearance of the thick tongue over a period of many months.
   c. Increased activity levels.
10. Adequate treatment of the older child will result in:
    a. Rapid weight loss.
    b. Excessive hair shedding.
    c. Increased activity levels.
11. Supplemental vitamins, especially vitamin D, are required to meet physiological demands during the "catch-up" period of growth.
12. Excessive thyroid replacement therapy will result in the development of hyperthyroidism.

B. Nursing Management. See EXCEPTIONAL CHILD.
1. Support the child and parents during hospitalization. See *Hospitalization, Support During.*
2. Initiate discharge planning. See *Discharge Planning.*
3. Administer thyroid hormone accurately.
   a. Give by oral route only.
   b. Give as a single dose at breakfast time, since the drug increases energy levels.
   c. Do not skip doses.

4. Observe, record, and report the child's response to thyroid replacement therapy.
5. Feed the infant slowly to avoid choking.
6. Provide an age-appropriate diet which meets the child's need for increased protein, enriched bread and cereals, and increased vitamin D. See *Nutrition.*
7. Limit sweets and carry out frequent mouth care to decrease dental caries. See *Dental Care.*
8. Promote activities suitable to the child's energy level and stage of development. See *Stimulation.*
9. Relieve dry skin.
   a. Use plain water to bathe the child.
   b. Apply lanolin or lotion after bath.
10. Explain to parents that
    a. The child will become more interested in his environment after treatment is initiated.
    b. Drug levels take time to build in the body, so improvement will not be immediate.
    c. Thyroid replacement therapy will not improve any mental retardation which occurred prior to treatment.
11. Teach parents home management.
    a. Teach parents how to administer hormone replacement. See *Administration of Medications, Parental.*
    b. Teach parents how to count the child's pulse and to contact the physician if the pulse is above a value determined by the physician.
    c. Tell parents to report signs and symptoms of excess thyroid hormone.
       1. Tachycardia.
       2. Nervousness.
       3. Disturbed sleep.
       4. Irritability.
    d. Support the parents whose child is likely to be retarded. See *Mental Retardation.*
12. Support parents in caring for the child who exhibits mental retardation. See *Mentally Retarded Child.*
13. Support the child and parents in coping with altered body image after replacement therapy produces "catch-up" growth.

I

Identity. See *Appendix v.*

Ileal loop diversion. See *Spina Bifida.*

Ileostomy. See *Hirschsprung's Disease.*

Immobilized child. Physical restraint of the child to insure completion of therapeutic measures.

   A. General Considerations.
1. Immobilization may be of short duration for I.V. therapy, nasogastric tube placement, etc. or of longer duration for treatment of fractures, congenital anomalies, burns, etc.
2. Mobility is an important aspect of the development of children and serves a variety of purposes.
   a. Source of pleasure.
   b. Supports differentiation between self and nonself.
   c. Form of communication.
   d. Release of aggression.
   e. Protective function.
   f. Autonomy.
3. Immobilization may interfere with the interpersonal relationships necessary to learn social skills.
4. Articulation problems and speech delay may occur in older infants who are immobilized for longer than a month (Sibinga and Friedman, 1971).
5. Children have fewer physiological problems than adults as a result of immobilization.
   a. Constipation.
   b. Skin breakdown.
   c. Osteoporosis with prolonged immobilization.
   d. Hypercalcemia.
   e. Inadequate nutrition.
   f. Decreased vital capacity.
   g. Urinary retention.
   h. Renal calculi.
6. Infants may not physically protest restraint until they have learned to stand and/or walk.
7. The infant may forget to use the immobilized part after immobilization has been discontinued.
8. The peak of aggressive mobility is around $2\frac{1}{2}$ years.

9. The toddler may respond to restraint by:
   a. Attempts to tear off the restraint.
   b. Verbal protest.
   c. Withdrawal or depression.
10. The preschooler who believes illness is a punishment may feel that cooperating with immobilization will magically restore normal function.
11. The schoolchild and adolescent will be deprived of:
    a. The pleasure of independent activity.
    b. The number of adaptive devices for release of aggression.
    c. Communication with peers.
12. The older child who is immobilized as a result of an accident or emergency surgery will have more anxiety because of lack of time to mobilize his coping mechanisms.
13. Children's responses to the discontinuation of immobilization vary.
    a. Hyperactivity.
    b. Using the limb more than permitted.
    c. Oversensitivity to the slightest restraint.
    d. Expectation of immediate and perfect restoration of function.

   B. Nursing Management. See *Restraints.*
1. Meet the physical needs of the child.
   a. Prevent skin breakdown.
      1. Change the position every 2 hours.
      2. Use sheepskin or a pressure mattress.
   b. Prevent constipation.
      1. Encourage fluids, particulary juices.
      2. Increase fruit, raw vegetables, whole grain cereals in the diet.
      3. Obtain an order for a stool softener if needed.
   c. Prevent osteoporosis and hypercalcemia.
      1. Position upright as much as possible.
      2. Handle extremities carefully when turning and positioning.
      3. Maintain adequate fluid intake. See *Forcing Fluids.*
      4. Acidify urine.
      5. Administer medications, e.g., calcium mobilizer or antibiotics for urinary tract infections as ordered.
   d. Prevent inadequate nutrition.
      1. Encourage small, frequent feedings.
      2. Feed in upright position if possible.
      3. Offer favorite foods.
      4. Create a pleasant mealtime environment.

e. Prevent decreased vital capacity.
 1. Assure proper body alignment.
 2. Place in sitting position at least T.I.D. if possible.
 3. Avoid restriction of chest movement by restraints.
 4. Administer chest physiotherapy or observe the child's response if performed by others.
 5. Use devices such as rocking bed, circolectric bed, incentive spirometers as needed.

2. Meet the age-specific needs of the infant.
 a. Provide stimulation.
 b. Encourage the parents and other caregivers to talk to the infant and to provide frequent physical contact.

3. Meet the age-specific needs of the toddler.
 a. Provide activities that allow the child to release aggression.
 1. Pounding board.
 2. Throwing balloons or bean bags.
 3. Tearing paper or magazines.
 b. Provide activities that allow him to explore his environment.
 1. Stroller.
 2. Wheelchair.
 3. Wagon.
 4. Change the location of the crib in the child's room or move it to the playroom or corridor.
 c. Provide activities that give him information about his body.
 1. Water play.
 2. Body games (e.g., "this little piggy").
 3. Mirrors.
 d. Provide physical contact.

4. Meet the age-specific needs of the preschooler.
 a. Tell the child that his extremity or body part is still under the cast or bandage.
 1. A bandaged or casted part may seem larger than normal.
 2. The child's interest in the body part is magnified by the interest of adults in the body part.
 b. Recognize that all the child's energy is used to cope with immobilization and minor traumas such as injections may cause rage and intolerance.
 c. Provide activities that allow the child to release aggression.
 1. Punching bag.
 2. Throwing bean bags or jar rings at a target.
 3. Play kit.
 4. Drawings.
 d. Explain to parents that active behavior is healthy and rest and quiet games should not be the child's only outlets.

5. Meet the age-specific needs of the schoolchild and adolescent.
 a. Help the child identify new ways to deal with his frustrations.
 1. Ask him how he usually handles problems.
 2. Ask him what he thinks can help.
 3. Let him know the nurses will help him control his aggressive impulses.
 4. Plan with him ways he can use his capabilities.
 5. Communicate the plan to other staff via Kardex notations.
 b. Meet privacy needs.
 c. Allow him as much independence as possible.
 d. Discuss with the physician the possibility of outdoor walks or use of the physical therapy department.
 e. Expect the child to have some regression in his ability to cope with immobilization.
 f. Discuss the child's needs for and response to hospitalization with his parents.

Immunization. The use of specific biological preparations to provide active or passive artificial immunity against specific diseases or toxins.

A. General Considerations.
 1. Types of immunity include:
 a. Natural: present from time of birth.
 b. Naturally acquired active: gained from having had the disease.
 c. Naturally acquired passive: obtained via placental transfer and breast milk; decreases slowly and disappears at about 15 months of age.
 d. Artificially acquired active: use of live, attenuated or dead organism or its toxin (toxoid) to stimulate immune system to produce antibodies which may last for years or a lifetime, e.g., all immunizations.
 e. Artificially acquired passive: prophylactic protection against a disease by use of injected antibodies, does not involve immune system and steadily decreases, e.g., gamma globulin.
 2. The diseases for which active natural immunizations are commonly given include (See *Appendix vi*):
 a. Rubeola (measles).
 b. Mumps.
 c. Rubella (German measles).
 d. Diptheria.
 e. Tetanus.
 f. Pertussis (whooping cough).
 g. Polio.

3. Use of immunization preparation is contraindicated when the child:
   a. Has an acute febrile illness (101°F or more).
   b. Is receiving immunosuppressive therapy, e.g., steroid and/or antineoplastic drugs.
   c. Has received an injection of immune serum globulin in the past 8 to 12 weeks.
   d. Has received plasma or whole blood within the previous 8 weeks.
   e. Has an immunodeficiency disorder.
   f. Has had a previous allergic response to the same vaccine or a related one.
   g. Has active, untreated tuberculosis.
   h. Is pregnant.
   i. Has eczema.

4. Immunizations are not contraindicated if a child has a mild, nonfebrile infection, e.g., common cold.

5. Children allergic to eggs, chickens, ducks, and feathers:
   a. May receive the measles, mumps, and rubella vaccine.
   b. Should not be given the other vaccines used for immunizations.

6. The live attenuated viruses of measles, mumps, rubella, and polio cross the placental barrier.

7. Children whose mothers are pregnant can receive rubella vaccine.

8. A skin test for tuberculosis should be performed prior to use of the measles vaccine because the vaccine may stimulate the development of systemic tuberculosis.

9. Interruption of the schedule does not interfere with final immunity and does not ever require starting over with the series.

10. Side effects from immunizations include:
    a. Mild reactions which are fairly common.
       1. Swelling or induration at the point of injection.
       2. Tenderness.
       3. Low grade fever.
       4. Malaise.
    b. Serum sickness.
    c. Severe reactions, which are rare, and cause:
       1. High fever.
       2. Convulsions.
       3. Encephalitis.
       4. Anaphylaxis.

11. Epinephrine 1:1000, tourniquets, O₂, and an airway should be available where immunizations are given.

12. Parents or guardians must sign a consent form prior to the administration of an immunization.

13. Booster shots of some vaccines are given to maintain antibody levels.

14. Proper storage and administration of vaccines is critical to successful immunization.

15. Preferred sites for both intramuscular and subcutaneous administration of vaccines are the anterolateral aspect of upper thigh in children and the thigh or deltoid muscle in adolescents.

16. Household contacts of immunosuppressed children should not receive the oral polio virus vaccine because the virus can be transmitted; they can receive the measles, mumps, and rubella vaccine.

17. Postexposure immunization to measles may be given since the vaccine has a shorter incubation period than natural measles.

B. Nursing Management.
   1. Assess for current or recent illnesses, immunization status to date and presence of any allergies (the ability to eat a whole egg without a reaction indicates the child can receive vaccines).
   2. Store vaccines on the middle shelf of the refrigerator, not on the door shelves since temperature here varies and may affect the vaccines.
   3. Read the manufacturer's drug insert for dose, route, and side effects.
   4. Inform the child and parents about what immunization(s) is/are to be given.
   5. Explain to parents the benefits and risks involved with immunizations but stress benefits far outweigh risks.
   6. Have parent or guardian sign consent form.
   7. Prepare the child for the injection. See *Preparation for Procedures.*
   8. Use the lateral thigh or deltoid for injection, depending on the child's age. See *Appendix iii, Table 4.*
   9. Restrain the child as needed for safety. See *Restraints.*
   10. Record the immunization given and the site used since sites should be rotated.
   11. Observe, record, and report adverse reactions.
   12. Administer epinephrine 1:1000 as ordered if anaphylaxis occurs.
   13. Record immunization and booster shots on parents' record.
   14. Teach parents to:
       a. Handle mild reactions as ordered, e.g., antipyretic for fever, warm compresses for swelling. See *Administration of Medications, Parental.*
       b. Call the physician or bring the child to emergency room for more severe reactions.
       c. Keep record up to date to have for school entrance or activities.
       d. See that the child receives all necessary immunizations. See *Appendix vi.*

Immunotherapy. Stimulation of the body's immune response system as a means of treating cancer.

A. **General Considerations.**
1. Immunotherapy is used as an adjunct to surgery, chemotherapy and/or radiation therapy.
2. The body's immune response is mediated by B cell and T cell lymphocytes (Koren and Hermann, 1981).
   a. T cell lymphocytes are responsible for cell-mediated immunity which, in addition to other functions, can destroy tumor cells by producing chemicals which cross cell membranes.
   b. B cell lymphocytes are responsible for antibody-mediated (humoral) immunity.
   c. Both types can return to the lymphoid system as memory cells and respond rapidly to previously encountered antigens.
3. T lymphocytes are the ones involved in the destruction of malignant cells.
4. Immune response will be decreased in the presence of:
   a. Immunodeficiency disease.
   b. Stress.
   c. Chemotherapy.
   d. Radiation therapy.
   e. Cancer.
   f. Pregnancy.
5. In order to be considered for immunotherapy the child should:
   a. Be capable of demonstrating an immune response (assessed by skin tests).
   b. Have a localized tumor.
6. Immunotherapy is employed after the number of tumor cells has been decreased by surgery, chemotherapy, and/or radiation therapy to a level that the body's immune system can handle.
7. Goals of immunotherapy include (Koren and Hermann, 1981):
   a. Stimulation of the body's own immune responses.
   b. Prevention or reversal of natural or therapy induced immunosuppression.
   c. Countering disease associated immunodeficiency.
   d. Increasing immunocompetency.
8. Three methods of immunotherapy that are used include:
   a. Active immunotherapy used to stimulate the body's own responses which includes:
      1. Active nonspecific: use of antigens, e.g., BCG vaccine.
      2. Active specific: use of small doses of irradiated tumor cells or live tumor cells.
   b. Passive immunotherapy which uses antibodies or other immune factors, often from another donor who is in remission from a related cancer.
   c. Adoptive immunotherapy: transfer of live immune lymphocytes from a compatible donor.
9. Methods by which immunotherapy may be given vary.
10. Reactions to immunotherapeutic agents vary according to the method by which they were given.
    a. Allergic responses that may be immediate or delayed and which may be mild or life-threatening.
    b. Fever.
    c. Malaise.
    d. Tissue ulceration.
    e. Lymph node enlargement in the region of the treatment site.
    f. Drainage from the injection site.

B. **Nursing Management.**
1. Obtain knowledge relevant to the specific immunotherapeutic substance being used in order to provide safe care including:
   a. Type of material being used.
   b. Method of administration.
   c. Expected response.
   d. Treatment measures for side effects or toxic reactions.
   e. Possibility of any threat to the health of any family members with an intercurrent illness.
2. Find out if the child has a history of any allergies.
3. Make sure that a statement of informed consent has been signed if this is required, e.g., substance being used may be part of a research study.
4. Explain the method of administration to be used to the child and parents. See *Preparation for Procedures.*
5. Support the child during the administration procedure.
6. Observe, record, and report the child's response to the procedure.
7. Tell the child and parents that lymph node enlargement may occur so they do not think it is another tumor (McCalla, 1976).
8. Teach the child and parents to:
   a. Keep skin sites used for immunotherapy clean and dry.
   b. Force fluids and take antipyretics as instructed for fever. See *Fever Reduction* and *Forcing Fluids.*
   c. Schedule rest periods to prevent fatigue.
   d. Call the physician if:
      1. Fever does not respond to antipyretics and fluid.
      2. Signs of secondary infection occur.

Impetigo. Superficial skin infection usually caused by beta hemolytic streptococcus or possible staphylococcus organisms.

A. **General Considerations.**
1. Impetigo is autoinoculable and contagious because it is transmitted by direct contact.
    a. Several children in a family may be infected.
    b. Infection reflects the presence of organisms in the child's total environment rather than the child's hygiene (Pillitteri, 1977).
2. Areas most commonly affected are the face, extremities, and trunk.
3. Insect bites and pierced ears may be sites of secondary infection.
4. The infection begins with vesicles which become purulent, ooze, and form honey-colored crusts.
5. Lymphadenopathy may occur when the offending organism is streptococcus.
6. Treatment includes:
    a. Softening crusts with 1:20 Burow's solution compresses followed by careful removal.
    b. Topical application of bacteriocidal ointment.
    c. Systemic antibiotics in severe or extensive cases.
7. The child with an untreated or inadequately treated case may develop acute glomerulonephritis or rheumatic fever.
8. Scarring can occur if the lesions are deep and extensive.
9. The hospitalized child who has impetigo requires isolation.

B. **Nursing Management.**
1. Discuss the administration of the antibiotic(s) with the child and parents. See *Administration of Medications, Parental.*
2. Teach the older child or parents to remove the crust twice a day.
    a. Removal of the crust leaves a moist surface from which bacteria may be spread to other areas.
        1. Avoid vigorous scrubbing.
        2. Use cotton for cleansing and dispose of in a paper bag.
    b. The child should use his own towels, washcloth, and toilet articles until all lesions have cleared.
3. Prevent spread of infection.
    a. Keep the child's nails clipped and clean.
    b. Use elbow restraints or mitts with the infant or young child if necessary.

Imperforate anus. See *Anorectal Malformations.*

Incest. See *Sexual Abuse.*

Increased intracranial pressure (ICP). A rise in pressure due to an increase in the volume of cranial contents.

A. **General Considerations.**
1. Causes of increased intracranial pressure include:
    a. Cerebral edema.
    b. Bleeding.
    c. Increased CSF production.
    d. Decreased CSF absorption.
    e. Space-occupying lesion.
    f. Ventricular obstruction.
2. The signs of increased ICP result from cellular hypoxia and brain shift or distortion.
3. Signs and symptoms that result in seeking medical attention include:
    a. Infants and young children.
        1. Enlarged head.
        2. Vomiting.
        3. Lethargy.
        4. Irritability.
        5. Frequent grabbing or shaking of the head.
        6. Poor feeding.
        7. High pitched cry.
        8. Tense, bulging fontanel.
    b. Older children.
        1. Headaches.
        2. Vomiting.
        3. Behavioral or personality changes.
        4. Diplopia.
4. Classic signs and symptoms of ICP occur relatively late.
    a. Decreased level of consciousness.
    b. Change in pupil size and equality.
    c. Widening pulse pressure.
    d. Decreasing pulse rate.
    e. Irregular or decreasing respiratory rate.
    f. Seizures.
5. Activities that increase ICP in the individual patient can be identified if equipment for continuous monitoring of intraventricular pressure is available.
6. Barbiturate coma may be used to treat ICP.

B. **Nursing Management.**
1. Obtain thorough history of the child's preillness behavior as a baseline for recognizing behavioral changes.
    a. Is he a restless sleeper?
    b. Does he have nightmares or cry out during sleep?
    c. Is he difficult to rouse from sleep?
    d. Does he have nervous habits such as twisting a lock of hair, picking at stuffed toys?
2. Ask the parents for information which will assist in evaluating the child's orientation, e.g., Does the child know that he is in the hospital? Is the child called by a nickname?

I

3. Support the child and parents during hospitalization. See *Hospitalization, Support During.*
4. Initiate discharge planning. See *Discharge Planning.*
5. Observe, record, and report early signs and symptoms of increased ICP.
   a. Headache.
   b. Restlessness.
   c. Forced breathing.
   d. Purposeless movements, e.g., picking at bedclothes.
   e. Mental cloudiness, e.g., forgot what he was told or asked to do within an hour or so or asks the same question repetitively.
6. Describe behavior rather than a level of consciousness, e.g., state that the patient is drowsy and arousable only with repeated verbal stimuli rather than state he is stuporous.
7. Assess the child's motor function.
   a. Observe, record, and report spontaneous movement of the extremities.
   b. Evaluate voluntary movement by simple commands.
      1. Have the child squeeze your index and middle fingers with his right, and then with his left hand ask him to squeeze a ball.
      2. Ask him to pretend he is pedaling a bicycle, tricycle, etc.
      3. Avoid asking the child to push his feet against your hand since this increases ICP.
8. Assess the child's response to sensory stimulation.
   a. Apply light stroking or touch to each extremity.
   b. Use pressure to evoke a response if touch or stroking is ineffective.
9. Assess pupillary response.
   a. Darken the room.
   b. Have the child focus on a distant object.
   c. Shine the penlight first in one eye, then in the other eye.
   d. Approach the eye from the side with the penlight.
   e. Observe the pupil size and speed of pupillary constriction.
10. Providing nursing care which prevents a sudden rise in intracranial pressure (Hausman, 1981).
    a. Maintain a patent airway.
    b. Maintain adequate ventilation.
       1. Monitor blood gases.
       2. Auscultate chest.
       3. Limit suctioning to 15 seconds.
       4. Elevate the head 15 to 30 degrees.
    d. Prevent Valsalva's manuever. (Hold breath and strain.)

1. Encourage diet high in bulk.
2. Administer stool softeners.
3. Instruct the child to exhale while turning or moving in bed.
4. Discourage the child from pushing against the siderail or against the foot of the bed.
5. Assist the child to move up in bed.
    e. Position the child carefully.
       1. Avoid extreme head, neck, and hip flexion.
       2. Elevate head of bed 30 to 40 degrees.
       3. Avoid restraints or restrain minimally if absolutely necessary.
    f. Perform passive range of motion.
    g. Plan nursing care measures to allow rest periods between actions which may precipitate increased ICP.
    h. Avoid making comments in the child's hearing which might be upsetting and result in increased ICP.
11. Teach the child and parents home management if the child has chronic increased intracranial pressure from hydrocephalus, brain tumor, etc.
    a. Review symptoms of increased pressure.
    b. Discuss measures to prevent increased ICP (see above).

Industry. See *Appendix v.*

Infant. Child in the stage of development between 1 month and 1 year of life.

A. General Considerations.
1. Developmental tasks for the infant are a continuation of and an expansion of the developmental tasks for the neonate and include learning to (Duvall, 1977):
   a. Adjust physiologically.
   b. Take in food.
   c. Begin to express feelings.
   d. Adjust to other people in the environment.
   e. Begin to communicate with others.
   f. Love and be loved.
2. The time at which tasks are accomplished varies among infants.
3. The presence of a consistent, loving, caregiver is essential to the well-being of the infant.
4. The infant's growth rate is very rapid.
5. Physiological differences between the infant and the older child decrease during the year but must be considered when planning care.
6. Passive immunity received from the mother via placental transfer diminishes during infancy.
7. Illness in the infant tends to be generalized

rather than localized due to an immature immune system.

8. Mother has normal concerns for new infant and need for physiologic restoration.

B. Nursing Management.

1. Support the parents in meeting their infant's needs, since they are the most important people to him. See *Parenting*.

2. Consider physiological differences in the infant as you plan care.

   a. Maintain hydration and feed the infant on demand, since the rapid metabolic rate predisposes to fluid and electrolyte imbalance and hypoglycemia.

   b. Protect the infant from extremes in temperature, since the temperature regulating mechanism is still immature.

   c. Protect the skin from injury and infection, since it is still thin.

   d. Suction the congested infant prior to feeding, since infants are obligatory nose breathers.

   e. Provide postural drainage if necessary, since the infant is unable to cough up secretions.

   f. Be prepared to change diapers frequently, because the gastrocolic reflex may cause frequent stools, possibly with each feeding, and a small bladder capacity and rapid water turnover causes frequent urination.

   g. Protect from infection, since the immune system matures slowly during the first year of life.

   h. Prevent aspiration of regurgitated milk that may still occur after feeding due to immature development of the cardiac sphincter of the stomach.

   i. Observe the infant carefully for reactions to medications since immature body systems affect infant's responses (Bindler, Howry, Tso, 1981)

      1. Drug absorption from gastrointestinal tract, while complete, is slower, therefore adverse reactions may be later in appearing.

      2. Passage of eye drops through lacrimal duct may produce systemic effects.

      3. Increased permeability of the skin increases possibility of skin and systemic reactions.

      4. Decreased plasma protein available in early infancy means less drug binding and more circulating drug, increasing possibility of toxic reactions.

      5. Changing nature of cardiovascular dynamics alters uptake and distribution of drugs.

      6. Blood-brain barrier is immature and central nervous system may be affected by some drugs, e.g., chloramphenicol produces "gray baby" syndrome.

      7. Renal system immaturity contributes to increasing the half-life of many drugs.

3. Meet the daily physical needs of the infant.

   a. Bathe.

      1. Use warm, not hot, water.

      2. Use a mild soap.

      3. Use a soft washcloth.

      4. Prevent cradle cap by washing the head, including the areas over the fontanels.

      5. Wash the eyes from the inner canthus outward.

      6. Clean the outer ear gently using a washcloth wrapped around the index finger.

      7. Do not use cotton-tipped applicators to clean the ear canal.

      8. Wash in all the creases.

      9. Dry thoroughly.

   b. Change the diapers as often as needed and provide skin care.

      1. Wash the perineal area with each diaper change, since ammonia builds up on the skin.

      2. Dry the area completely.

      3. Expose the perineal area to the air for 10 minutes two to three times a day if the area is reddened. See *Dermatitis, Diaper*.

      4. Apply a protective coating of vaseline or A and D ointment as needed.

      5. Apply lotion or powder to the perineum but do not use both together since this clogs pores.

   c. Trim nails as needed to prevent scratching.

      1. Use blunt infant nail scissors.

      2. Cut the nails straight across.

   d. Dress the infant.

      1. In a shirt and diaper while in crib.

      2. Put on socks and shoes when the infant is out of the crib and walking.

   e. Feed on demand. See *Nutrition*.

      1. Hold the infant for feeding until old enough for a high chair or feeding table.

      2. Hold for bottle feedings.

      3. Do not prop the baby's bottle!

      4. Place the infant who cannot turn over on his stomach or side after feeding to prevent aspiration.

      5. Record how much the infant eats.

      6. Let the 7- to 8-month-old finger feed himself and/or have a spoon while you spoon feed him.

      7. Feed the older infant before his bath so you will not have rebathe him after he feeds himself.

      8. Offer a variety of foods with different tastes and textures.

   f. Provide for rest and sleep routines. See *Sleep*.

g. Protect from infection.
1. Do not care for the child if you have an infectious illness.
2. Do not hold the infant close to your face or kiss him.
3. Keep a gown in the infant's bedside table to wear while you care for him in order to prevent cross contamination.
4. Wash your hands before giving care and after each diaper change.
5. Discard remaining formula after feeding to prevent bacterial growth.

h. Protect from injury. See *Accident Prevention*.
1. Keep the side rails all the way up unless someone is with the infant.
2. Check that the crib sides are locked in place after they are raised.
3. Do not leave unattended in stroller, infant seat, high chair, or feeding table.
4. Keep the crib free of loose linens and free of toys with sharp edges and/or small parts.
5. Close safety pins and keep out of reach.
6. Do not allow cords to drape or dangle over the crib.

i. Provide for exercise. See *Exercise*.

4. Weigh daily.
a. On the same scale.
b. At the same time.
c. Nude.

5. Take vital signs in the following order.
a. Count respirations first, since the infant is likely to be quieter.
b. Take an apical pulse.
c. Take a rectal temperature last, since this:
1. Is an intrusive procedure and the infant may respond with crying and increased activity.
2. May cause a reflex bowel movement to occur.

6. Observe, record, and report signs and symptoms which may indicate illness.
a. Poor feeding.
b. Weight loss.
c. Diarrhea.
d. Vomiting.
e. Temperature instability, e.g., elevated or subnormal.
f. Irritability.
g. Lethargy.

7. Meet the emotional needs of the infant.
a. Involve the parents in the care of their infant as much as possible.
1. Encourage parents to give care.
2. Teach parents to do procedures that they indicate they would like to learn.
b. Encourage a parent to room-in with the infant if possible.

c. Respond consistently as soon as possible to the infant's needs.
d. Limit the number of caregivers to whom the infant must adjust.
e. Provide age-appropriate toys to stimulate the infant's physical, emotional, and cognitive development. See *Stimulation*.
f. Spend time with the infant solely for the purpose of social interaction.
g. Place the infant in a playpen by the nurse's station or in the playroom to provide stimulation.
h. Comfort the infant when his parents must leave if he is experiencing separation anxiety.
i. Make sure the infant has his security object with him, e.g., blanket, stuffed animal.

8. Approach the parents in a positive manner when discussing topics related to health care.
a. Reinforce appropriate parenting skills.
b. Do not act as an authority.
c. Teach the parents what they want to know first, then teach them what you have assessed that they need to learn.

9. Provide information as needed in relation to the following areas.
a. Growth and development norms. See *Appendix v*.
b. Nutrition. See *Nutrition* and *Appendix vii*.
c. Safety. See *Accidents*.
d. Teething. See *Teething* and *Dental Care*.
e. Provision for ongoing health care. See *Well-child Care, Immunizations,* and *Appendix vi*.
f. Signs and symptoms that may indicate illness.
g. Activities which will foster development.
h. The importance of establishing a flexible routine for daily activities such as eating, sleeping, and playing.

Infectious mononucleosis. Acute, self-limiting infectious disease caused by the Epstein-Barr virus (EBV).

A. **General Considerations.**
1. The disease is characterized by increased numbers of atypical lymphocytes and monocytes in the peripheral blood.
2. Signs and symptoms include:
a. Fever.
b. Sore throat.
c. Exudative tonsillitis.
d. Malaise.
e. Lymphadenopathy.
f. Splenomegaly.
g. Jaundice.
h. Abdominal pain.

3. Diagnosis is made by the Monospot screening test followed by a heterophile antibody test for confirmation.
4. The prognosis is good although weakness and fatigability may persist in the older adolescent.
5. Complications include:
    a. Chronic hepatitis.
    b. Ruptured spleen.
    c. Myocarditis.
    d. Secondary bacterial infection.
    e. Severe dysphagia.
6. Treatment is symptomatic.
    a. Bedrest during the acute febrile stage.
    b. Gradual activity increase based on adolescent's temperature and fatigability.
    c. Aspirin or aspirin substitutes for headaches, fever, and malaise.
    d. Penicillin may be ordered if sore throat is due to beta hemolytic streptococci.
    e. Corticosteroids may be used in severe cases for high fever and sore throat.
7. Hospitalization for I.V. therapy may be necessary if the adolescent becomes dehydrated.

B. **Nursing Management.**
1. Assist the adolescent to cope with bedrest. See *Home Management of Minor Illnesses.*
2. Initiate fever reduction measures. See *Fever Reduction.*
3. Observe for symptoms of secondary infection.
4. Encourage an adequate fluid intake. See *Forcing Fluids.*
    a. Offer cold, bland fluids.
    b. Administer analgesics 20 to 30 minutes prior to mealtimes.
5. Monitor I.V. accurately in the hospitalized adolescent.
6. Administer steroids as ordered if the adolescent has complications.
7. Involve the adolescent in planning for increased activity as he improves.
8. Help the adolescent keep up with schoolwork.
    a. Arrange for a tutor or home-bound teacher.
    b. Have his parents or a friend obtain homework assignments.
    c. Plan time for homework to be completed.
9. Teach the adolescent and parents home management.
    a. Explain to the adolescent that activity restrictions are temporary and encourage him to take the responsibility for establishing his own rest periods.
    b. Help the adolescent plan a schedule with appropriate rest periods.
    c. Discuss how to maintain an adequate intake.
    d. Explain measures to prevent secondary infection.
    d. Discuss measures for fever reduction.

Influenza. See *Home Management of Minor Illnesses.*

Ingestion of harmful products. See *Poisoning.*

Inguinal hernia. See *Hernia, Inguinal.*

Initiative. See *Appendix v.*

Injections, intramuscular. See *Administration of Medications.*

Insect bites. See *Home Management of Minor Emergencies.*

Interview. See *History Taking.*

Intravenous therapy. See *Fluid and Electrolyte Imbalance.*

Intussusception. Invagination of one portion of the intestine into another resulting in intestinal obstruction.

A. **General Considerations.**
1. The cause of the obstruction is unknown although predisposing factors can include:
    a. Diarrhea or constipation.
    b. Intestinal polyps.
    c. Meckel's diverticulum.
    d. Parasites.
    e. Foreign bodies.
    f. Cystic fibrosis.
2. Signs and symptoms occur suddenly.
    a. Periodic abdominal pain with drawing up of knees.
    b. Vomiting.
    c. "Current jelly" stools after 12 hours, followed by absence of stools.
    d. Restlessness followed by severe prostration.
    e. High fever.
    f. Sausage-shaped mass in the upper abdomen.
3. Older children may have chronic intussusception characterized by periodic diarrhea, constipation, vomiting, and sudden attacks of abdominal pain that subside spontaneously.
4. The diagnostic procedure of a barium enema under fluoroscopy will reduce the intussusception by hydrostatic pressure in most children.

5. Surgery will be necessary if the obstruction is not reduced by the barium enema or if shock or perforation contraindicate the barium enema.
   a. Manual reduction in simple cases.
   b. Resection of the involved segment if gangrene or irreducible mass is present.

B. **Nursing Management.**
1. Support the child and parents during hospitalization. See *Hospitalization, Support During.*
2. Initiate discharge planning. See *Discharge Planning.*
3. Prepare the child and parent for both the barium enema procedure and for surgery since the child may go directly to the OR if the first procedure is unsuccessful.
4. Meet the needs of the child preoperatively. See *Preoperative Care* and *Preparation for Surgery.*
   a. Administer a narcotic I.M. as ordered prior to the barium enema.
   b. Maintain NPO status.
   c. Monitor I.V. accurately.
   d. Irrigate nasogastric tube as ordered.
   e. Administer antibiotics as ordered.
   f. Administer mouth care frequently.
   g. Meet the child's comfort needs by holding, rocking, or giving a pacifier.
   h. Change the child's position frequently.
5. Meet the needs of the child postoperatively. See *Postoperative Care.*
   a. Observe for passage of barium.
   b. Observe for stool pattern, since the intussusception may recur in the first 36 hours postreduction.
6. Teach the child and parents home management.
   a. Have the parents demonstrate wound care.
   b. Review methods of preventing infection.
      1. Frequent handwashing.
      2. Adequate rest.
      3. Adequate nutrition.
   c. Discuss activity restrictions as stated by the surgeon, e.g., tricycle riding.

Iron deficiency anemia. See *Anemia, Iron Deficiency.*

Isolated child. The child who is separated from his peers.

A. **General Considerations.**
1. The child may be isolated.
   a. If an infectious disease is suspected or diagnosed, e.g., mumps, meningitis, chicken pox.
   b. To limit exposure to others who may have an infectious disease, e.g., the burned child, the child with a malignancy.

2. The most commonly used guidelines for isolation procedures are those recommended by the Center for Disease Control (CDC).
3. The rationale for isolation must be explained carefully to the child and the parents.
4. The child may interpret separation from his peers as punishment.
5. Providing age-appropriate stimulation should be a priority nursing intervention. See *Stimulation.*
6. Printed instructions for family members will make it easier for them to understand and remember isolation procedures.
7. It may be possible to arrange for the long-term isolated child (e.g., the burned child who is stabilized) to be taken outside if protected adequately.
8. The psychological effects of isolation on the young child whose family cannot room-in is of major concern.
9. Self-stimulation activities such as rocking, head-banging, or masturbation may be intensified in the isolated child who is unsupported and/or understimulated by parents and staff.
10. Stimuli that help the child and parents maintain orientation to time, place and person should be provided during the period of isolation.
11. The parents may feel very frustrated in their attempts to comfort the child, particularly if gloves must be worn.

B. **Nursing Management.**
1. Review the hospital's policy and procedure about isolation techiques.
   a. Explain and/or clarify the child's and parent's understanding of the isolation procedure.
   b. Organize the nursing care to minimize trips in and out of the room.
2. Encourage the parents to arrange care of siblings, transportation, etc. so that a family member is available to stay with the child.
3. Tell the child in terms he can relate to, when you will return to care for him, e.g., when it's time for medicine; when the cartoons are over.
4. Spend time interacting with the child when nursing interventions are not necessary.
5. Explain to the older child and to the parents the reason for wearing gloves.
6. Tell the young child that people can smile under their masks and draw a picture to illustrate this.
7. Provide auditory stimuli by using an intercom, radio, record player, television or phone calls to family or friends.
8. Provide visual stimulation.
   a. Place the child's bed by the window.
   b. Plant seeds or vegetable rootings.

c. Obtain fish or an ant farm.

d. Have parents bring in family snapshots.

e. Help the child create a mobile or collage.

f. Arrange for an outdoor visit if the child's conditions permits.

9. Provide toys which are disposable, washable, or which can be gas sterilized. See *Toys.*

10. Provide opportunities for therapeutic play to help the young child cope with the additional stress of isolation. See *Play, Therapeutic.*

11. Help the older child keep up with schoolwork.

12. Encourage the older child or adolescent to create intriguing signs for the door such as "Enter at your own risk" or "Many have entered, but few have left" (Whaley and Wong, 1983).

13. Arrange for several reliable peers to be ori-ented to isolation technique so they can visit the isolated teenager.

14. Have the adolescent's parents purchase inexpensive posters to decorate the isolation room since they are disposable.

15. Be sure that the parent who is rooming-in is able to meet his/her own physical and emotional needs.

a. Adequate rest.

b. Proper nutrition.

c. General hygiene.

d. Relief from constant contact with the sick child.

e. Exercise.

f. Diversionary activities.

g. Communication with other adults.

h. Opportunities to verbalize feelings.

Jaundice. See *Hepatitis, Viral* and *Neonate.*

Jock itch. See *Tinea.*

Ketoacidosis. See *Diabetes Mellitus.*

Ketogenic diet. See *Seizures.*

Kirschner's wires. See *Traction, Care of Child.*

Kawasaki's disease (mucocutaneous lymph node syndrome). Nonspecific inflammatory vasculitis of unknown etiology which initially involves microvasculature of all parts of the body.

A. **General Considerations.**

1. Confirmation of the diagnosis is dependent on the presence of at least five of the six major criteria.

a. Unexplained fever of at least 5 days duration.

b. Bilateral conjunctival injection.

c. Truncal rash.

d. Changes in extremities: palmar erythema, indurative edema of hands and feet, refusal to use extremities, marked peeling of extremities 2 to 3 weeks after diagnosis.

e. Erythema of mucous membranes; injected pharynx, dry, fissured lips, strawberry tongue.

f. Lymphadenopathy.

2. Additional findings include: arthralgia, diarrhea, photophobia, and tympanitis.

3. The clinical course typically occurs in three stages.

a. Acute febrile—1 to 10 days duration. Abrupt onset of fever followed in 1 to 3 days by other symptoms.

b. Subacute—19 to 25 days duration characterized by persistent irritability, anorexia, thrombocytosis, desquamation.

c. Convalescent—25 days to 6 to 8 weeks.

4. Complications include:

a. Coronary arteritis.
b. Carditis.
c. Gallbladder hydrops.
d. Necrosis of liver, duodenum, jejunum.
e. Coronary artery thrombosis.

5. Treatment is aimed at controlling fever, maintaining hydration, and minimizing cardiac complications.
   a. Steroids alone or in combination with warfarin or aspirin.
   b. Aspirin in very high doses.
   c. Surgical correction of complications of gallbladder obstruction or bowel involvement.
   d. Supportive measures.

6. Hospitalization is recommended to confirm the diagnosis and to monitor cardiac status.

7. Moderately and acutely ill children usually require intravenous therapy and continuous nursing care.

8. The prognosis is generally good, but cardiac complications are the most serious concern and good follow-up after the illness is essential.

B. Nursing Management.

1. Support the child and parents during hospitalization. See *Admission to Hospital, Emergency,* and *Hospitalization, Support During.*

2. Initiate discharge planning. See *Discharge Planning.*

3. Observe, record, and report the following:
   a. Symptoms of fluid and electrolyte imbalance. See *Fluid and Electrolyte Imbalance.*
   b. Appearance and location of rash. See *Rash.*
   c. Appearance and location of edema.
   d. Response to medication.
   e. Level of irritability.
   f. Intake and output.

4. Prepare the child for procedures used to rule out other disorders or to monitor condition. See *Preparation for Procedures.*
   a. CBC and differential, sedimentation rate, SGOT, SGPT, LDH, serum protein electrophoresis, platelet count, bilirubin, serum aspirin levels.
   b. Urinalysis.
   c. Cultures of blood, throat, and urine.
   d. Chest x-ray.
   e. EKG.
   f. Echocardiogram.
   g. Angiogram and/or technetium scan if echocardiogram abnormal.

5. Institute measures to lower temperature. See *Fever Reduction.*

6. Administer aspirin as ordered.
   a. Validate high dosages with physician.
   b. Document specific administration time if peak and trough levels are being monitored.
   c. Observe for signs and symptoms of toxicity.
   d. Decrease gastric irritation by administering with liquids or food if not buffered.

7. Administer sedatives, anticonvulsants, or antidiarrheal medications as ordered. See *Seizures* and *Diarrhea.*

8. Observe, record, and report signs and symptoms of complications.
   a. Arrhythmia.
   b. Altered blood pressure.
   c. Increased pulse.
   d. Chest pain.
   e. Altered respirations.
   f. Cyanosis.

9. Promote comfort (Lynch and Gray, 1982).
   a. Explain to parent that extreme irritability is typical with this disease.
   b. Use nontactile comfort measures until child's condition has improved.
      1. Soft music.
      2. Dim lighting.
      3. Parent/nurse presence in room.
      4. Soft toys.
   c. Promote skin integrity with sheepskin, soft night clothes.
   d. Elevate edematous extremities if tolerated.
   e. Promote rest by organizing nursing care activities in blocks of time.
   g. Relieve eye discomfort with cool washcloths, artificial tears, sunglasses for the older child.

10. Meet nutritional needs. See *Nutrition.*

11. Increase the child's activities as condition improves. See *Stimulation.*

12. Discuss follow-up care with parents.
    a. Child may need periodic EKG and/or echocardiograms to monitor cardiac status.
    b. Tell parents to notify physician of the following:
       1. Change in color.
       2. Shortness of breath.
       3. Chest pain.
       4. Lethargy.
       5. Behavior changes.

Language development.
The acquisition of verbal communication skills.

A. General Considerations.
1. Language development parallels the child's cognitive development.
2. Girls learn to talk before boys.
3. Language development follows a predictable pattern.
   a. Birth—crying.
   b. 2 months—cooing.
   c. 6 months—babbling (one syllable at a time).
   d. 6 to 10 months—syllabic babbling (repetition of a syllable).
   e. 9 months—imitation of simple sounds.
   f. 12 to 14 months—first word.
   g. 18 months—3 to 50 words, usually nouns.
   h. 24 months—50 words or more and two-word phrases.
   i. 36 months—1,000 words and short sentences with a subject, verb, and object; use of plurals.
   j. Preschool—use of language in a symbolic way to communicate with others.
   k. Schoolage—use of words as vehicle of expression; language rules learned.
4. The child learns speech by naming objects, repeating words, experimenting with language forms, and asking questions.
5. The child's first adjectives are usually "good" and "bad" because parents use them frequently.
6. Adverbs are learned in the early preschool years followed by pronouns.
7. Delays in language development may be related to:
   a. Lack of verbal stimulation.
   b. Meeting the child's needs when he points to objects so that he has no need to talk.
   c. Hearing loss.
   d. Low intelligence.
   e. Extended hospitalization.
8. Children from deprived backgrounds frequently have poor verbal development because of limited language experience.
9. The use of "baby talk" by adults when speaking to children may interfere with language development.
10. Children who do not speak by the age of 2 years should be evaluated to determine the cause of the delay.
11. Language development in the young child hospitalized for extended periods may be delayed because there is no consistency in word stimulation.

B. Nursing Management.
See IMMOBILIZED CHILD and STIMULATION.
1. Teach parents to encourage language development in the infant and toddler.
   a. Talk to the baby.
   b. Encourage repetition of sounds.
   c. Teach appropriate word forms such as bye and dog rather than bye-bye or doggie.
   d. Teach body parts during bath and other care activities.
   e. Name objects in picture books.
   f. Make up stories about familiar objects.
   g. Combine rhymes and tactile stimulation as a means of word play.
2. Discuss ways to improve language skills of the preschooler.
   a. Listen to what the child has to say and consider it important.
   b. Help the child to use the right word.
   c. Answer the child's questions with short and simple responses.
   d. Read to the child.
   e. Involve the child in storytelling.
   f. Provide experiences the child can talk about.
   g. Encourage verbalization of feelings.
   h. Encourage the child to listen.
3. Discuss ways to improve the language skills of the older child (see above).
   a. Have parents serve as role models by reading themselves.
   b. Encourage the child to read.
   c. Encourage the child to learn a new word each day.
   d. Define words that the child hears in conversation or through news media.
   e. Help the child work simple crossword puzzles.
   f. Play board games such as *Scrabble* or create new word games.
   g. Use flash cards to increase vocabulary.
4. Plan specific nursing care to promote language development in the infant or young child who is hospitalized for an extended period.
   a. Have staff agree on the sequence of words to be taught to the child, e.g., ball, light, truck.

b. Provide verbal stimulation through books, storybook records, radio, television, as well as personal contact.

c. Expose the child to a wide variety of stimuli by arranging walks outside the hospital, peer contact, elevator rides, water play, etc.

d. Implement the same measures to stimulate language that parents would use at home (see above).

Laryngotracheobronchitis (LBT) (viral croup).
Viral infection in which there is acute inspiratory obstruction occurring below the level of the vocal cords.

A. **General Considerations.**
1. Must be differentiated from acute spasmodic croup and epiglottitis which are also present with inspiratory stidor and altogether comprise the croup syndrome (Lipow, 1977).
2. Signs and symptoms include:
    a. Increasing inspiratory stridor.
    b. Hoarseness.
    c. Barking, metallic sounding cough.
    d. Supraclavicular and sternal retractions.
    e. Low grade fever.
    f. Mildly red pharynx with some swelling of epiglottis.
    g. Scattered rales and rhonchi.
3. The onset of symptoms is usually gradual and often occurs during the course of an upper respiratory infection.
4. Treatment is directed at reduction of the laryngeal spasm, edema, and liquefaction of secretions by increasing the humidity.
    a. Cool mist.
    b. Oxygen.
    c. Rest.
    d. Hydration.
    e. Intermittent positive pressure aerosol of racemic epinephrine for severe cases.
5. Complete airway obstruction is rare but may occur, requiring tracheotomy or endotracheal intubation.
6. Arterial pH and blood gas measurement may be monitored to help guide treatment. See *Appendix ii.*
7. Suctioning of oropharyngeal secretions is avoided since stimulation may cause reflex laryngeal and bronchial constriction (Tooley, Lipow, 1979).

B. **Nursing Management.**
1. Support the child and parents during hospitalization. See *Hospitalization, Support During.*
2. Initiate discharge planning. See *Discharge Planning.*

3. Increase environmental humidity by using a:
    a. Cool steam vaporizer at the bedside.
    b. Mist tent. See *Mist Tent.*
4. Promote hydration to liquify secretions. See *Forcing Fluids.*
    a. Encourage oral fluids.
    b. Avoid cold fluids which may cause spasm of laryngeal muscles.
5. Promote rest to decrease respiratory effort.
    a. Decrease environmental stimuli.
    b. Give the child a favorite toy to hold.
    c. Disturb the child as little as possible when giving care.
6. Provide someone to stay with the child to decrease anxiety, since stress may increase the symptoms.
7. Observe, record, and report.
    a. Rising temperature.
    b. Fatigue due to respiratory effort.
    c. Increasing stridor.
    d. Increasing retractions.
    e. Restlessness due to air hunger.
    f. Increasing pulse and respiratory rate.
    g. Cyanosis and/or circumoral pallor.
8. Change damp clothes and bedding frequently so child does not become chilled.
9. Decrease parental concerns by explaining:
    a. Cool mist will help rather than cause further symptoms.
    b. Antibiotics are ineffective against a virus.
    c. Sedation is not given for restlessness, since it may mask increasing respiratory distress.
    d. A hacking cough may persist for a week or two after the child is well.
10. Teach parents home management.
    a. Increase environmental humidity.
        1. Run hot shower in bathroom with door closed.
        2. Use cool mist vaporizer at bedside.
        3. Place sheet over crib while running vaporizer to create a "mist tent."
    b. Promote hydration.
    c. Advise parents of signs that indicate the child should be seen by a physician.
        1. Stridor which persists even when the child is not crying or coughing.
        2. Increasing fever.
        3. Difficulty in swallowing.

Lead poisoning (plumbism). Increased lead absorption and clinical evidence of toxicity.

A. **General Considerations.**
1. Sources of lead that may result in toxic levels include:
    a. Chips of lead paint from walls, window sills,

furniture, or toys if painted with lead-based paint.

b. Fluids stored in lead-glazed earthenware, more common in the Southwest.

c. Vegetables grown in soil contaminated with lead paint, more common in urban renewal areas.

d. Colored ink used in newspapers, candy and popsicle wrappers, and gift wrap.

e. Fumes from burning storage batteries.

f. Fruit tree sprays.

g. Gasoline fumes.

2. The nurse should be alert for lead poisoning in stressed, disorganized families since the child may ingest lead-containing items when he lacks parental attention or stimulation.

3. Signs and symptoms vary with the severity and duration of the poisoning.
   a. Mild or chronic.
      1. Anorexia.
      2. Vomiting.
      3. Irritability.
      4. Changes in normal behavior.
      5. Clumsiness.
      6. Ataxia.
      7. Anemia.
   b. Acute.
      1. Cerebral edema.
      2. Stupor.
      3. Coma.
      4. Convulsions.
      5. Joint pains.

4. Clinical manifestations appear after 3 to 6 months of steady ingestion.

5. Diagnostic tests include:
   a. Urine lead levels.
   b. Blood lead levels.
   c. X-rays may reveal "lead lines" near the epiphyseal lines of long bones or lead deposits in the alimentary tract.

6. Treatment of acute lead poisoning includes:
   a. Gastric lavage followed by a saline cathartic.
   b. Administration of chelating agents that combine with the metal ions in the blood and tissues to prevent them from entering the cells.
      1. D-Penicillamine.
      2. BAL (British Anti-Lewisite).
      3. EDTA (ethylenediamine tetra-acidic acid).
   c. Anticonvulsants.
   d. Oxygen therapy.
   e. Enemas to remove lead from the G.I. tract.

7. Treatment for chronic lead poisoning includes:
   a. Removing the child from the source of exposure.
   b. Chelating agents.

c. Large doses of vitamin D to remove lead from the blood and deposit it in the bones.

d. Anticonvulsants to terminate or prevent convulsions.

e. Hemodialysis if renal shutdown has occurred.

8. The prognosis varies.
   a. Acute encephalopathy is associated with a high mortality and children who do survive are often retarded.
   b. Children with mild cases may have deficits in fine motor function and behavior.
   c. Late symptoms of retardation may appear 3 to 9 years after treatment.

9. Prevention is aimed toward:
   a. Laws preventing the use of lead paint on articles designed for children.
   b. Informing parents about environmental hazards.
   c. Screening high risk children.
      1. Blood lead determination.
      2. FEP (free erythrocyte protoporphrin) test.

B. Nursing Management.

1. Meet the needs of the child hospitalized for lead poisoning.
   a. Support the child and parents during hospitalization. See *Hospitalization, Support During.*
   b. Initiate discharge planning. See *Discharge Planning.*
   c. Assist with the collection of the 24-hour urine sample.
   d. Prepare the child for the numerous I.M. injections of chelating agent(s). See *Preparation for Procedures* and *Apendix iii, Table 4.*
   e. Plan a rotation schedule for injections.
   f. Provide a diet high in calcium and phosphorus, since this removes lead from the blood and deposits it in the bones.
   g. Apply warm soaks to injection sites to relieve discomfort.
   h. Observe, record, and report symptoms of encephalopathy.
      1. Headache.
      2. Vomiting.
      3. Altered mental state.
      4. Change in vital signs.
   i. Monitor hydration.
      1. Monitor I.V. fluid if ordered.
      2. Force fluids. See *Forcing Fluids.*
      3. Measure intake and output.

2. Meet the special nursing needs of the child who has developed encephalopathy.
   a. Restrict fluids.
   b. Observe, record, and report signs of increased cerebral involvement.

L

1. Convulsions.
2. Loss of consciousness.
3. Increased blood pressure and decreased pulse.
c. Keep emergency equipment at bedside or place child in a room near nurses' station.
d. Monitor the I.V. accurately to prevent increased cerebral edema.
e. Keep an anticonvulsant at the bedside if ordered.
f. Observe, record and report the child's response to antihypertensive medication.
g. Provide safe care during seizure activity. See *Seizures*.
h. Assist with the lumbar puncture if performed to decrease intracranial pressure. See *Increased Intracranial Pressure*.
i. Administer oxygen for respiratory depression.
j. Catheterize for urinary retention.
3. Teach the child and parents home management.
a. Inform parents in high risk housing to observe for and report symptoms of lead poisoning.
b. Discuss measures to prevent the child from ingesting lead paint chips.
1. Cover walls to a height of 3 feet with paneling, masonite, or plastic-covered contact paper.
2. Keep the child's crib away from walls.
3. Place furniture in front of window sills to prevent the toddler from reaching them.
c. Identify public agencies which could help the parents if the landlord is uncooperative in efforts to protect the child from lead exposure.
d. Inform the parents of clinics where screening procedures can be performed.
e. Encourage parents to maintain follow-up so that development testing can be used to plan for the child's schooling.
f. Initiate referrals to community health nurse and other agencies for family counseling, infant stimulation programs, parenting classes, alternate housing, etc.

Learning disabilities. See *Minimal Brain Dysfunction*.

Legg-Perthes disease (osteochondritis). Aseptic necrosis of the femoral head of unknown etiology.

A. General Considerations.
1. The pathophysiology of the disease is divided into three stages each lasting 9 to 12 months.
a. Early necrosis and avascularity—spontaneous interruption of blood supply to the upper femoral epiphysis.
b. Revascularization—new blood supply arises, old bone is reabsorbed, and new bone is deposited.
c. Healing—new bone is ossified.
2. Some patients suffer residual deformity that leads to degenerative disease in later life.
3. Signs and symptoms begin in stage 2.
a. Hip pain.
b. Pain referred to the knee or inner thigh.
c. Protective limp.
d. Limited movement of the hip joint.
4. In general, the younger the child at the time of diagnosis, the better the treatment results.
5. An arthrogram may be done to confirm the diagnosis since hip x-rays may be equivocal.
6. Treatment is aimed at preventing abnormal forces on the femoral head and maintaining the femoral head in the acetabulum.
a. Bedrest and traction are used initially for several weeks.
b. Abduction casts or braces will be applied when full range of motion has been accomplished. (Casts and braces may be worn for 2 years or more.)
c. A Sam Browne belt which holds the affected leg suspended with the knee flexed may be used instead of a cast or braces.
d. A surgical reconstruction and containment procedure may be performed on the older child who is considered "at risk" for poor results from conservative treatment.
7. The advantage of surgical treatment is the decrease in long-term activity restriction.

B. Nursing Management. See *Chronic Illness* and *Immobilized Child*.
1. Support the child and parents during hospitalization. See *Hospitalization, Support During*.
2. Initiate discharge planning. See *Discharge Planning*.
3. Prepare the child and parents for all procedures. See *Preparation for Procedures*.
4. Meet the needs of the child in traction. See *Traction, Care of Child*.
5. Provide sensory stimulation for the child. See *Stimulation*.
6. Initiate referral to the public health nurse or other commuity agency as needed.
7. Discuss how the child will explain his illness to peers.
8. Help the parents find ways to stimulate development.
a. Encourage visits to the circus, museums, sporting events, etc.
1. Call facility in advance to make arrangements.

L

2. Borrow a wheelchair from a community agency.
d. Identify activities such as scorekeeper or mascot which allows the child to participate in peer group activities.
c. Encourage swimming if approved by the physician.
d. Arrange for continued schooling.
  1. Plan transportation.
  2. Discuss the child's needs with the school nurse.
9. Teach the child and parents home management of the casts. See *Cast Care.*
10. Teach the child and parents home management of braces.
  a. Check the skin daily for areas of irritation by the braces.
  b. Apply alcohol to bony prominences to toughen the skin.
  c. Clean the plastic molds of the braces daily with soap and water.
  d. Cleanse the leather cuffs with leather rubbing compound.
  e. Check daily for indications that the braces need adjustments.
    1. Tight cuff.
    2. Brace joints are no longer aligned with the child's joints.
  f. Review the swing-through gait for crutch walking.
  g. Check the crutches daily for loose screws and worn crutch tips.
  h. Keep the floor free of hazards such as toys or scatter rugs.
  i. Review exercise routine if needed.
  j. Keep the child on bedrest if braces need repair.
11. Meet the needs of the child requiring surgery. See *Preoperative Care, Preparation for Surgery,* and *Postoperative Care.*

Leukemia, acute lymphoblastic. Malignant disease in which the normal bone marrow elements are replaced by abnormal accumulations of leukocytes and their precursors.

A. **General Considerations.**
  1. Children with acute lymphoblastic leukemia commonly present with the following signs and symptoms:
    a. Fever.
    b. Pallor.
    c. Petechiae.
    d. Ecchymoses.
    e. Lymphadenopathy.
    f. Hepatosplenomegaly.
    g. Bone pain.
    h. Anemia.
    i. Malaise
    j. Infection
    k. Abdominal pain
    l. Anorexia
  2. There are two major forms of childhood leukemia and they are classified according to the predominating white blood cell (Greene and Bloomquist, 1979).
    a. ALL—acute lymphoblastic or lymphocytic leukemia 85% of cases.
    b. AML—acute myelocytic or myeloblastic leukemia 15% of cases.
  3. Differential diagnosis of early ALL includes
    a. Leukemoid reactions.
    b. Idiopathic thrombocytopenic purpura.
    c. Aplastic anemia.
    d. Infectious mononucleosis.
    e. Infectious lymphocytosis.
    f. Rheumatoid arthritis.
    g. Rheumatic fever.
    h. Other malignancies.
  4. Diagnostic studies to determine the presence of leukemia cells include:
    a. Complete blood count (CBC).
    b. Peripheral blood smear.
    c. Lumbar puncture.
    d. Bone marrow aspiration usually using the posterior iliac crest.
  5. In addition to bone marrow invasion there may be leukemic infiltration of any other organ system in the body, e.g., central nervous system, lungs, kidneys, bones, etc.
  6. Signs and symptoms of central nervous system involvement include:
    a. Nausea.
    b. Vomiting.
    c. Headache.
    d. Lethargy.
  7. Treatment includes the use of chemotherapy and central nervous system prophylaxis and is divided into three parts:
    a. Induction of remission by the use of combinations of drugs.
    b. Irradiation of the brain and the use of intrathecal methotrexate to prevent central nervous system involvement, since chemotherapeutic drugs do not cross the physiological blood-brain barrier.
    c. Maintenance of remission by the continued use of chemotherapy.
  8. Cranial irradiation may cause:
    a. Postradiation somnolence syndrome.
    b. Learning disability.
    c. Mental retardation.
    d. Psychological problems.
  9. Terms related to treatment that are important to know include:
    a. Induction—use of chemotherapeutic drugs

L

to reduce the number of leukemic cells to the point where remission is attained.

b. Remission—state in which the child:

1. Is free of signs and symptoms.

2. Has adequate bone marrow function.

3. Has less than 5 percent abnormal blast cells and 40 percent lymphocytes in the bone marrow.

4. Has a normal CBC and cerebrospinal fluid.

c. Maintenance—use of chemotherapy to continue a remission.

d. Relapse—reappearance of abnormal cells.

10. The length of time the leukemia has been present prior to starting therapy does not appear to affect the response to treatment (Fochtman, 1976).

11. The course of the disease will be followed by the use of repeated bone marrow aspirations and lumbar punctures.

12. Relapse may occur in the following sites and treatment includes:

a. Central nervous system:

1. Cranial irradiation.

2. Intrathecal methotrexate.

3. Intraventricular methotrexate via the insertion of an Ommaya reservoir.

b. Testicles: irradiation.

c. Bone marrow: chemotherapy.

13. Remission may be reinduced following relapses, but each remission is usually shorter in duration.

14. Chemotherapy used in treatment can produce the same physiological problems as the disease, e.g., cellular breakdown leading to increased uric acid formation that affects kidney function.

15. Complications include:

a. Infection.

b. Hemorrhage.

c. Leukemic invasion of one or more organ systems.

16. Specific factors have been identified which influence the prognosis and are used in making decisions about treatment protocols (Stockman, 1982).

a. Factors associated with a favorable prognosis include:

1. Child between 2 and 8 years of age.

2. White blood count less than 30,000.

3. Cell type: common ALL.

4. No mediastinal mass.

5. Race: white.

6. No central nervous system disease.

7. Sex: female.

8. Cell morphology: L_1.

b. Factors associated with an unfavorable prognosis include:

1. Child less than 2 or greater than 8 years of age.

2. White blood cell count greater than 30,000.

3. Cell type: T cell or B cell.

4. Mediastinal mass.

5. Race: black.

6. Central nervous system disease.

7. Sex: male.

8. Morphology: L_3.

17. The prognosis for the child with leukemia is better if he:

a. Has ALL.

b. Has a white blood count less than 10,000 per mm³.

c. Is between 2 and 10 years of age.

d. Has no significant body organ involvement.

18. Children in remission feel well and should be able to carry out normal age-appropriate activities.

19. Children with leukemia will be immunosuppressed.

20. Administration of allopurinol prevents hyperuricemia that results from rapid cell breakdown.

B. **Nursing Management.**

1. Support the child and parents during hospitalization. See *Hospitalization, Support During.*

a. Record on the Kardex what the child and parents have been told about the disease and treatment.

b. Repeat information as needed, since the anxiety produced by the life-threatening nature of this illness may reduce comprehension.

c. Provide a private, quiet place for conferences with parents.

d. Plan extra time to sit and talk with the child and parents.

e. Facilitate the child and parents' adjustment to the diagnosis. See *Crisis Intervention.*

2. Initiate discharge planning. See *Discharge Planning.*

3. Prepare the child and parents for diagnostic tests. See *Preparation for Procedures.*

a. Explain the positioning required for a lumbar puncture and a bone marrow aspiration.

b. Tell the child that someone will be with him to help him hold still in the correct position.

c. Tell the child that he will experience some brief pain when the periosteum is penetrated and bone marrow aspirated.

L

4. Carry out nursing measures to relieve or prevent physiological problems related to the leukemic process.

   a. Reduce fatigue caused by anemia.

      1. Plan care in blocks to provide rest periods.

      2. Reduce environmental noise.

      3. Provide activities appropriate to the child's age and energy level.

      4. Administer packed red blood cells as ordered to reduce anemia.

   b. Prevent bleeding due to decreased platelets.

      1. Handle the child gently.

      2. Take an axillary temperature.

      3. Do not give I.M. injections unless absolutely essential.

      4. Apply pressure for 5 minutes over venipuncture sites.

      5. Provide gentle oral hygiene using cotton swabs or sponges.

      6. Do not give aspirin without discussing with the physician, since it may increase bleeding.

      7. Protect the child from accidents such as falls or from playing with sharp toys.

      8. Administer platelets as ordered.

   c. Prevent infection.

      1. Maintain skin integrity, e.g., lotion applied to dry skin, turning to prevent pressure sores, vaseline applied to dry lips.

      2. Care for any skin breaks immediately using aseptic technique.

      3. Wash hands thoroughly.

      4. Prevent contact with people who have infections.

      5. Use protective isolation technique as ordered.

      6. Prep the skin twice with alcohol and betadine before venipuncture, lumbar puncture, and bone marrow aspiration.

      7. Provide frequent oral hygiene.

   d. Promote good nutrition to combat anorexia and anemia caused by the disease process. See *Nutrition.*

   e. Promote hydration.

      1. Offer fluids frequently.

      2. Leave a pitcher of a favorite fluid at the bedside.

      3. Provide cool, bland fluids.

   f. Decrease bone and/or joint pain.

      1. Maintain body alignment.

      2. Support extremities with pillows, rolled towels, or sand bags.

      3. Carry out range of motion exercises in a gentle manner to maintain optimal mobility.

      4. Apply heat as ordered.

      5. Administer analgesics as ordered.

   g. Relieve pressure due to organomegaly.

      1. Change the child's position every 2 hours if he is not moving.

      2. Turn the child on his side to relieve downward pressure of the abdominal organs.

      3. Place the bed in a semi-Fowler's position.

   h. Prevent uric acid build-up due to cell breakdown.

      1. Administer allopurinol as ordered to decrease uric acid formation.

      2. Force fluids. See *Forcing Fluids.*

5. Observe, record, and report the child's response to chemotherapy.

6. Carry out nursing measures to relieve or prevent physiological problems related to chemotherapy. See *Chemotherapy.*

7. Observe, record, and report signs and symptoms related to the disease and/or treatment.

   a. Infection.

   b. Bleeding.

   c. Decreased urinary output.

   d. Increased urine specific gravity.

   e. Anorexia.

   f. Nausea.

   g. Vomiting.

   h. Diarrhea.

   i. Weight gain or loss.

   j. Ulcers of the mouth, anus, and/or skin.

   k. Personality changes.

8. Observe, record, and report signs and symptoms of central nervous system involvement.

   a. Nausea.

   b. Vomiting.

   c. Lethargy.

   d. Headache.

   e. Irritability.

9. Prepare the child and parents for central nervous system irradiation. See *Radiation Therapy.*

   a. Find out what the child and parents have been told and record on the Kardex.

   b. Answer questions and clarify concerns.

   c. Have someone from radiation therapy meet with the child and parents.

   d. Explain that radiation therapy to the head will cause hair loss but that it will grow back in a couple of months, although the color and texture may change.

   e. Tell the child and parents that from 5 to 8 weeks after CNS irradiation the child may experience somnolence possibly accompanied by fever, anorexia, nausea, and vomiting for a period of 3 days to 2 weeks (Stagner and Wood, 1976).

10. Support the child and parents in coping with the disease on an ongoing, outpatient basis.
    a. Establish who will be the health professional who coordinates the child's care and make sure the parents know how to reach that person.
    b. Demonstrate care used to treat side effects of the disease and/or treatment and allow for a return demonstration, e.g., oral hygiene.
    c. Discuss the importance of:
       1. Preventing infection since the child will be immunosuppressed.
       2. Maintaining optimal nutrition, since this helps the child tolerate treatment and resist infection.
    d. Make sure the parents understand:
       1. The drugs they are to give. See *Administration of Medications, Parental.*
       2. When and where they are to bring the child for further treatment.
    e. Tell parents to call physician if the child:
       1. Develops an infection or ulcers.
       2. Bleeds.
       3. Develops a rash or is exposed to a contagious disease.
       4. Has nausea and vomiting that does not respond to medication.
       5. Has diarrhea for more than 8 to 10 hours (less if the child is under a year and/or is vomiting).
    f. Encourage the child and parents to lead as normal a life style as possible. See *Life-Threatening Illness.*
       1. Attend school.
       2. Become involved in peer group activities.
       3. Carry out assigned household tasks.
11. Support the child and parents during relapses and during the terminal course of the disease. See *Dying Child, Care of.*

Lice. See *Pediculosis.*

Life-threatening illness. The presence of a condition that may cause the death of the child.

A. **General Considerations.** See DEATH, CONCEPT DEVELOPMENT.
   1. Life-threatening illnesses include:
      a. Acute emergency situations, such as burns and automobile accidents.
      b. Congenital defects such as diaphragmatic hernia and transportation of the great vessels of the heart.
      c. Chronic conditions such as cystic fibrosis and leukemia.
   2. The child, his family, and all persons involved in his care pass through a series of stages as they adapt to a life-threatening situation. See *Crisis Intervention.*
   3. The stages of adaptation include (Benoliel, 1979):
      a. Denial, which is characterized by an inability to believe that death could actually occur.
      b. Anger, which is characterized by an "it is not fair" reaction.
      c. Bargaining, which is characterized by conscious or unconscious attempts to make promises or strike bargains in return for postponement of death.
      d. Depression, which is characterized by quiet, withdrawn, detached behavior as the child/parents become more aware of the death being inevitable.
      e. Acceptance, which is characterized by resolution of the grieving and incorporation of the changes taking place.
   4. Individuals vary in the rate at which they work through each stage, and some remain at one of the earlier stages either because they are unable to move or because the child's condition does not change.
   5. The longer the life-threatening condition exists the more likely it is that those involved will work through the stages.
   6. In a condition characterized by remissions the child and family may need to start working through the stages all over again each time a relapse occurs, e.g., leukemia.
   7. How the child reacts to a life-threatening situation will depend on his age and what and how he is told. See *Coping.*
   8. Somatic symptoms such as headaches, chest pain, palpitations, etc. may occur in family members causing them to fear for their own lives.
   9. Parents of children who survive a life-threatening condition may have difficulty accepting the fact that their child is no longer in danger and may not be able to let him live a normal life.
   10. Anticipatory mourning, in which emotional attachment to the child is relinquished over a period of time, often occurs when the course of the illness has been long.
   11. Problems develop when parents work through their grief and relinquish their attachment to the child before he actually dies.
   12. Parents will vary in their ability to participate in the care of their child.
   13. In addition to all other feelings they may have, parents generally experience tremendous guilt, especially if the child's life is threatened by an accident.

14. Siblings, grandparents, peers, teachers, and others who are involved with the child must be considered when care is planned.
15. The child with a life-threatening illness who returns to the community may have difficulty with his:
    a. Parents.
    b. Siblings.
    c. Peers.
    d. Classmates.
    e. Teachers.
    f. Other relatives.
    g. Neighbors.
16. Children who are dying:
    a. Are usually aware of the life-threatening illness, although they may be too young to verbalize their understanding.
    b. Can cope very effectively with honest answers about their condition if given support.
    c. Who are given honest answers show a decreased amount of anxiety.
17. The adolescent with a life-threatening illness experiences extreme stress because it (Waechter, 1979):
    a. Becomes a major threat to independence and/or body image.
    b. Interferes with development of an individual identity.
    c. Alters the ability to function sexually.
    d. Interrupts planning for future goals.
18. The type of nursing care required will depend on the nature of the life-threatening illness, e.g., intensive care nursing will be required for the child whose life is threatened by burns.
19. The cultural and religious practices and beliefs of a family must be considered when care is planned. See *Cultural Aspects of Health Care* and *Religious Aspects of Health Care.*
20. The complex nature of care given to many children with life-threatening illnesses requires the adjustment to a number of caregivers.

B. **Nursing Management.** See ANXIETY, CHILD and ANXIETY, PARENTAL.
   1. Read about the specific life-threatening illness in order to plan appropriate nursing care.
   2. Meet the physical needs of the child in acute distress.
       a. Maintain the child's:
           1. Airway.
           2. Breathing.
           3. Circulation.
       b. Monitor vital signs as ordered and report and record all changes.
       c. Administer fluids as ordered.
       d. Assist with procedures and/or diagnostic tests.
       e. Suction as needed.
       f. Obtain and/or set up necessary equipment, e.g., apnea monitor.
       g. Observe, record, and report the child's response to all medications.
       h. Keep the child as comfortable as possible.
           1. Administer pain medication as ordered.
           2. Position for comfort, if possible.
           3. Remove all drainage promptly.
       i. Carry out additional care related to the child's diagnosis.
   3. Meet the emotional needs of the child in acute distress. See *Admission to the Hospital, Emergency.*
       a. Continue to talk to the child while you provide care.
       b. Explain, in a calm manner, what you are doing or what is happening.
       c. Answer his questions honestly.
       d. Let the parents stay with the child or have someone in the room just to support the child.
       e. Attempt to carry out care in as calm a manner as possible.
       f. Limit the number of staff interacting with the child.
       g. Do not allow a stream of observers.
       h. Consolidate interruptions, e.g., do all blood tests at one time.
   4. Meet the emotional needs of the parents of the child with an acute life-threatening illness.
       a. Keep the parents informed about what is happening.
       b. Designate someone to be a liaison with the parents.
       c. Answer questions honestly.
       d. Let the parents participate in the child's care as they indicate a desire, if feasible.
       e. Assign someone to stay with the parents while the child is being treated or call someone for them, e.g., friend, relative, clergyman.
       f. Be nonjudgmental of parental reactions.
       g. Repeat information as needed, since anxiety reduces the ability to retain information.
       h. Accept parental expressions of guilt but point out where the situation was taken out of their control.
       i. Provide for religious and/or cultural practices.
   5. Meet the physical needs of the child with a chronic life-threatening illness as they arise.
   6. Meet the emotional needs of the child with a chronic life-threatening illness. See *Chronic Illness.*
       a. Find out what the child knows or wants to know about his illness and record the information.

L

b. Answer questions as honestly as possible.

c. Discuss with the parents providing information about the illness to the child who has not been told but indicates an awareness of his condition and/or asks questions.

d. Permit siblings and peers to visit.

e. Support the child in returning to his community. See *Discharge Planning.*

   1. Discuss what and how he will tell siblings, peers, classmates, teachers, etc. about his illness.

   2. Explain or demonstrate how he can cope with the effects of illness on body image, e.g., wig to cover hair.

   3. Teach him how he can handle altered body functions.

   4. Give him the name and phone number of someone he can call to discuss his concerns.

   5. Make a referral to a community health nurse for follow-up care as appropriate

7. Meet the emotional needs of the adolescent with a life-threatening illness. See *Adolescent.*

a. Provide an environment which maintains contact with others and supports open communication.

b. Accept challenges to authority in calm manner and do not become hostile.

c. Act as an advocate for the adolescent to participate in decisions made about treatment.

d. Set firm, realistic limits on behavior until the adolescent can assume control in a situation.

e. Support developmental needs, e.g., have friends visit, permit wearing of personal clothing, protect privacy.

f. Listen to the adolescent and protect confidentiality.

8. Meet the emotional needs of the parents of a child with a chronic life-threatening illness.

a. Provide privacy and time to talk with the parents about their concerns.

b. Answer questions honestly and repeat information as needed.

c. Encourage parents to meet their own ongoing needs, since they may feel guilty in doing so.

d. Encourage, but do not force, parents to remain involved with their child.

e. Accept anticipatory mourning which may occur.

f. Discuss referral to a community agency which might offer help, e.g., Cancer Care.

g. Explain that the child still needs specific limits in order to feel secure. See *Discipline.*

h. Accept the fact that each time the child is readmitted the parents may start the grieving process all over again.

9. Support parents in dealing with other children in the family.

a. Explain that the siblings of the child may:

   1. Exhibit a variety of behaviors, e.g., fear, anger, regression, guilt.

   2. Need help in discussing the child's illness with peers, classmates, teachers, etc.

   3. Worry that the same illness will occur in them.

   4. Need to visit the hospital, clinic, physician etc. when the child goes in order for them to incorporate the experience into their lives.

   5. Desire to participate in the child's care and should be permitted to do so when possible.

b. Encourage parents to be as open and honest about the child's condition as they can be.

c. Use knowledge about the child's development of a concept of death to help parents decide what they might tell other children.

d. Encourage parents to remain involved in the lives of the children at home.

10. Support the parents in dealing with grandparents if this becomes a problem.

a. Help them to understand that the grandparents grieve both for their child and grandchild.

b. Expain that grandparents often feel helpless, since they are not involved in the direct care of the child.

c. Discuss ways in which grandparents might be allowed to help.

11. Discuss with parents ways in which they might help their child readjust to the community.

a. Visit with the child's teacher.

   1. Help plan for the needs of the child in the classroom, e.g., limit-setting, adjustment of work assignments, decreased physical activity.

   2. Discuss with the teacher what the children in the class should be told to prepare them for the child's return.

b. Meet with the school nurse.

   1. Explain the child's illness.

   2. Tell her what medications the child is receiving.

c. Encourage the child to do as much for himself as he can.

d. Set consistent limits which provides a sense of security for the child.

12. Recognize the needs of health care professionals who work with children with life-threatening illnesses.

a. Accept the fact that this is emotionally draining work.
b. Arrange for someone to talk to or hold group discussions to deal with feelings.
c. Involve yourself in activities outside your work.

Limit-setting. See *Discipline*.

Lip, cleft. See *Cleft Lip*.

Lipid pneumonia. See *Pneumonia*.

Lipoid nephrosis. See *Nephrotic Syndrome*.

Maintenance of health. See *Health Promotion and Maintenance* and *Well-child Care*.

Malnutrition. See *Nutrition*.

Malrotation of intestines. See *Volvulus*.

Masturbation. See *Sex Education*.

Measles, German. See *Rubella*.

Measles, red. See *Rubeola*.

Meckel's diverticulum. An outpouching of the terminal ileum resulting from incomplete obliteration of the yolk stalk in fetal life.

A. **General Considerations.**
1. The abnormality is often asymptomatic and is discovered accidentally during treatment for another illness.
2. Signs and symptoms result from irritation by secretions of the gastric mucosal lining of the diverticulum.
   a. Painless rectal bleeding.
   b. Shock from massive untreated bleeding.
   c. Chronic iron deficiency anemia with mild recurrent bleeding.
   d. Abdominal pain which may be acute and due to diverticulitis, or vague and recurrent.

3. The diverticulum may cause:
   a. Peritoneal bleeding secondary to perforation of an ulcer in the diverticulum.
   b. Intussusception secondary to inverson of the diverticulum.
   c. Intestinal obstruction as a result of herniation of a loop of bowel.
4. A scan with the radioactive substance ^{99m}Technetium Pertechnetate may be helpful since standard x-ray techniques are not usually diagnostic.
5. Treatment is surgical excision of the diverticulum and anastomosis of the remaining bowel segments.
6. The prognosis is good.

B. **Nursing Management.**
1. Support the child and parents during hospitalization. See *Hospitalization, Support During*.
2. Initiate discharge planning. See *Discharge Planning*.
3. Prepare the child and parents for the diagnostic procedures. See *Preparation for Procedures*.
4. Meet the needs of the child preoperatively. See *Preoperative Care* and *Preparation for Surgery*.
   a. Reassure child and parents that blood loss is less than they perceive and will be corrected by transfusion if necessary.
   b. Test all stools for the presence of occult blood.
   c. Observe, record, and report.
      1. Pallor.
      2. Decreased pulse or blood pressure.
      3. Positive tests for blood in stools.
   d. Administer blood transfusion as ordered. See *Fluid and Electrolyte Imbalance*.
5. Meet the needs of the child postoperatively. See *Postoperative Care*.

Medications. See *Administration of Medications*.

Megacolon. See *Hirschsprung's Disease*.

Meningitis, aseptic (viral). Inflammation of the menges caused by a virus.

    A. General Considerations.
      1. The onset may be abrupt or gradual and signs and symptoms include:
        a. Headache.
        b. Fever.
        c. Malaise.
        d. Anorexia.
        e. Nausea.
        f. Abdominal pain.
        g. Vomiting.
        h. Stiff neck and/or back.
      2. A child may occasionally exhibit additional signs and symptoms.
        a. Sore throat.
        b. Chest pain.
        c. Generalized muscular aching.
        d. Maculopapular rash.
      3. Aseptic meningitis is a benign disease which lasts from 3 to 10 days and has no sequelae.
      4. Lab studies that will be done to differentiate aseptic meningitis from bacterial meningitis include:
        a. Lumbar puncture for cerebrospinal fluid which shows the following:
          1. Clear color.
          2. Normal or slightly elevated WBC count with lymphocytes predominant.
          3. Normal or elevated glucose level (70 to 90 mg/dl).
          4. Normal or slightly elevated protein level (newborn to 1 month 20 to 120 mg/dl; infant/child 15 to 45 mg/dl).
          5. Normal cerebrospinal fluid lactate dehydrogenase.
        b. Cultures of:
          1. Cerebrospinal fluid.
          2. Blood.
          3. Nasopharynx.
      5. Treatment is symptomatic but antibiotics may be given and isolation enforced until bacterial meningitis is ruled out (Whaley and Wong, 1979).

    B. Nursing Management.
      1. Support the child and parents during hospitalization. See *Hospitalization, Support During*.
      2. Initiate discharge planning. See *Discharge Planning*.
      3. Maintain isolation as ordered until bacterial meningitis is ruled out. See *Isolated Child*.

        a. Follow hospital procedure for isolation.
        b. Explain the rationale for isolation to the child and parents.
      4. Initiate fever reduction measures as ordered. See *Administration of Medications, Parental* and *Fever Reduction*.
      5. Reduce discomfort of muscle aches as ordered.
        a. Administer analgesics.
        b. Apply warm, moist heat.
        c. Position for comfort but make sure the child turns.
      6. Provide age-appropriate diversional activities. See *Play*.
      7. Teach the parents to carry out comfort measures as needed when the child is discharged.

Meningitis, bacterial. Inflammation of the meninges caused by a bacterium.

    A. General Considerations.
      1. Early symptoms in the infant/young child tend to be nonspecific.
        a. Poor feeding.
        b. Irritability.
        c. Labile temperature.
        d. Vomiting and/or diarrhea.
        e. Crying, especially when the legs are elevated to change diapers. (Langner and Schott, 1977).
      2. Early signs and symptoms in the older child include:
        a. Upper respiratory infection.
        b. Irritability.
        c. Fever greater than 101°F.
        d. Vomiting.
        e. Headache.
      3. Later signs and symptoms in the infant/young child include:
        a. Symptoms of increased intracranial pressure with a bulging fontanel the most significant sign in the infant.
        b. Nuchal rigidity (stiff neck) may or may not be present.
      4. Kernig's sign (pain produced when the leg is extended at the knee with the thigh flexed) and Brudzinski's sign (passive flexion of the head produces flexion of both thighs and legs) are difficult to elicit and evaluate in children under 2 years.
      5. Later signs in older children are more specific and include:
        a. Positive Brudzinski's and Kernig's signs.
        b. Nuchal rigidity.
        c. Signs and symptoms of increased intracranial pressure.
        d. Opisthotonos (backward arching of the body due to muscle spasm).
        e. Seizures.

f. Petecial rash found in meningococcal meningitis.

6. Vascular dissemination of bacteria from an infection elsewhere in the body is the most common form of infection.

7. Lab studies done to establish a diagnosis include:
   a. Lumbar puncture for cerebrospinal fluid which shows the following:
      1. Cloudy, turbid, or frankly purulent appearance.
      2. Markedly elevated WBC count with polymorphonuclear leukocytes predominant.
      3. Elevated protein.
      4. Decreased or absent glucose.
      5. Visualization of bacteria on a Gram-stained smear.
   b. Cultures of:
      1. Cerebrospinal fluid.
      2. Blood.
      3. Nasopharynx.

8. Counterimmunoelectrophoresis (CIE) and Limulus lysate assay tests may be used when bacterial meningitis is suspected but previous antibiotic therapy has produced a negative Gram-stain.

9. Chemoprophylaxis may be recommended for individuals living with children who have meningococcal or *H. influenzae* meningitis and includes use of:
   a. Rifampin for meningococcal meningitis and *H. influenzae*.
   b. Vaccine as adjunctive therapy to rifampin if the meningococcal serotype is A or C.

10. Emergency hospitalization will be required and the child and parents are likely to be frightened. See *Admission to Hospital, Emergency*.

11. Treatment consists of:
    a. Isolation for 24 hours.
    b. Antibiotics.
    c. Maintenance of optimal hydration.
    d. Reduction of increased intracranial pressure.
    e. Fever reduction.
    f. Management of shock.
    g. Control of seizures.
    h. Supportive nursing care.

12. Early complications include:
    a. Septic shock, rapidly fatal if untreated.
    b. Inappropriate antidiuretic hormone secretion causing fluid retention.
    c. Cerebral edema.
    d. Disseminated intravascular coagulation.

13. Later complications include:
    a. Subdural effusion.
    b. Noncommunicating hydrocephalus.

c. Septic arthritis with *H. influenzae* and meningococcal meningitis.
    d. Seizures.
    e. Developmental delays.
    f. Deafness.
    g. Mental retardation.

14. Early diagnosis and adequate treatment contribute to an improved prognosis.

B. Nursing Management.
   1. Support the child and parents during hospitalization. See *Hospitalization, Support During*.
   2. Initiate discharge planning as the child's condition improves. See *Discharge Planning*.
   3. Weigh the child accurately as a basis for drug and fluid therapy on admission and daily.
      a. Use same scale.
      b. Weigh at same time each day.
      c. Weigh child nude.
   4. Maintain isolation technique for the first 24 hours of antibiotic therapy to prevent spread of infection. See *Isolated Child*.
   5. Observe, record, and report the child's response to antibiotic therapy.
   6. Monitor I.V. and oral fluids accurately to prevent cerebral edema.
      a. Record all intake and output.
      b. Do not exceed fluid limits.
   7. Initiate fever reduction measures. See *Fever Reduction*.
      a. Use hypothermia mattress as ordered.
      b. Give cool liquids within the limits of fluid restriction.
   8. Observe, record, and report neurological status.
      a. Vital signs.
      b. Neurological signs.
      c. Level of consciousness.
      d. Behavior.
   9. Promote rest.
      a. Decrease environmental stimulation.
         1. Limit visitors.
         2. Dim lights, pull shades.
         3. Avoid loud talking, television, or radio.
      b. Handle gently and avoid overhandling.
      c. Schedule care in blocks to increase rest periods.
   10. Measure and record head circumference daily.
   11. Initiate seizure precautions as indicated by the child's condition. See *Seizures*.
   12. Maintain skin integrity.
       a. Change the child's position when giving care.
       b. Use lanolin rich skin cream on pressure points.
   13. Provide mouth care.
   14. Observe, record, and report signs indicative of complications.

a. Increasing irritability.
b. Decreasing level of consciousness.
c. Alterations in vital signs.
   1. Rising temperature.
   2. Rising blood pressure.
   3. Decreasing pulse.
   4. Irregular respirations.
d. Weight gain or loss.
e. Urinary retention.
f. Increasing head circumference.
g. Inability to move the arms and/or legs.
h. Decreased hearing.
15. Meet the psychological needs of the child during the acute stage when stimulation is decreased.
   a. Sit quietly by the bed to provide companionship.
   b. Talk softly to the child.
16. Promote optimal nutrition to aid recovery as the child's diet is progressed. See *Nutrition.*
17. Provide age-appropriate play activities during the convalescent period. See *Play* and *Play, Therapeutic.*
18. Provide age-appropriate stimulation if developmental lags are noted during convalescence. See *Stimulation.*
19. Teach parents home care.
   a. Administer medications as instructed, e.g., anticonvulsants, antibiotics. See *Administration of Medications, Parental.*
   b. Provide instruction as to how parents can stimulate development in the child with residual neurological damage.
   c. Tell them to call the physician if they note:
      1. Temperature elevation.
      2. Irritability.
      3. Poor feeding.
      4. Decreased hearing.

Meningocele. See *Spina Bifida.*

Meningomyelocele. See *Spina Bifida.*

Menstruation (menses). Period of uterine bleeding accompanied by shedding of the endometrium.

A. **General Considerations.**
1. Menstruation.
   a. Is regulated by hormonal control.
   b. Normally begins between the 10th and 17th year of life.
   c. Lasts an average of 3 to 6 days.
   d. Is accompanied by a blood loss of from 3 to 6 tablespoons.
   e. Occurs on an average of every 21 to 35 days with the first day of bleeding counted as day 1 of each cycle.
2. The menstrual cycle consists of four phases.
   a. Menstruation—period of uterine bleeding.
   b. Proliferative phase—accompanied by:
      1. Restoration of the uterine epithelium.
      2. Thickening of the endometrium.
      3. Estrogen secretion.
      4. Ovulation.
   c. Secretory phase—accompanied by:
      1. Secretion of progesterone by the corpus luteum.
      2. Continued thickening of the endometrium.
   d. Premenstrual phase—accompanied by:
      1. Constriction of the blood vessels of the endometrium.
      2. Involution of the corpus luteum.
3. Adolescent girls frequently experience variability in the:
   a. Length of the menstrual cycle and skipping of periods is common.
   b. Number of days the flow lasts.
   c. Amount of blood lost.
4. Early menstrual periods are frequently anovulatory and painless, since it is the secretion of progesterone that leads to discomfort.
5. Common problems of the menstrual cycle and their signs and symptoms include:
   a. Mittleschmerz—low abdominal pain occurring at the time of ovulation.
   b. Premenstrual tension—headache, irritability, breast tenderness, depression, and weight gain due to water and sodium retention.
   c. Dysmenorrhea—cramping, abdominal pain, backache, and leg ache severe enough to interfere with activities of daily living.
   d. Dysfunctional uterine bleeding—irregular, long, or excessive bleeding not associated with organic disease.
6. Treatment varies according to the problem and its severity.
   a. Mittleschmerz—mild analgesics.
   b. Premenstrual tension—decreased salt intake, analgesics, and possible mild diuretics.
   c. Dysmenorrhea—mild analgesics, exercise, and possibly cyclic estrogen therapy to prevent ovulation, and prostaglandin inhibitors given at the onset of each period.
   d. Dysfunctional uterine bleeding—reassurance and promotion of good health; possible dilatation and curettage if bleeding is excessive.
7. Physiological adjustment and appropriate education to promote emotional acceptance of menstruation often bring a rapid reduction in the number and/or severity of problems.

8. Toxic shock syndrome (TSS), associated with *Staphylococcus aureas* infection, has been linked to the use of tampons.

B. Nursing Management.
1. Provide accurate information about menstruation and the menstrual cycle.
    a. Explain the phases of the cycle.
    b. Give information about the common variations found among adolescents concerning menstruation and the menstrual cycle.
    c. Assist the parents in providing appropriate information to their daughter. See *Sex Education.*
2. Encourage the child and parents to view menstruation in a positive manner and to see it as representing the achievement of a developmental milestone.
3. Discuss areas of health promotion that foster physical and psychological adjustment to menstruation.
    a. Eating a balanced diet high in protein and iron. See *Nutrition.*
    b. Getting adequate sleep. See *Sleep.*
    c. Participating in moderate exercise. See *Exercise.*
    d. Practicing good posture.
    e. Maintaining appropriate personal hygiene, e.g., bathing, washing hair, changing sanitary pad.
4. Teach ways of reducing the threat of toxic shock syndrome:
    a. Do not use tampons.
    b. Wear pads at night and use tampons during the day; change them every 4 hours.
5. Teach the adolescent and parents methods of reducing discomfort.
    a. Administer analgesics and/or diuretics as instructed. See *Administration of Medications, Parental.*
    b. Carry out specific exercises.
        1. Assume a knee-chest position several times a day for 10 to 15 minutes.
        2. Do pelvic rocking. Lie on floor and tilt the pelvis down until the small of the back is flat against the floor, repeat several times.
    c. Take warm baths or showers.
    d. Apply a heating pad on low or moderate heat.
    e. Limit salt intake in the diet the week before a menstrual period is due.
6. Teach the administration of iron preparations if ordered for anemia due to blood loss. See *Anemia, Iron Deficiency.*
7. Teach the adolescent and parents about the use of estrogen preparations for treatment of dysmenorrhea if this is ordered.
8. Support the adolescent during a pelvic exam if this is necessary to rule out an organic cause of persistent discomfort. See *Preparation for Procedures.*
9. Support the adolescent and parents if dilatation and curettage is required to control excessive dysfunctional bleeding.
10. Meet the needs of the hospitalized adolescent who is menstruating.
    a. Provide sanitary napkins or tampons as needed.
    b. Make the physician aware that the girl is menstruating.
    c. Discuss ways of relieving cramps if they occur, e.g., pelvic rocking, mild analgesics.
    d. Provide privacy.

Mentally retarded child.
A child with limited intellectual functioning and deficient adaptive behavior for chronological age.

A. General Considerations.
1. Mentally retarded children can be classified into four groups.
    a. The borderline child:
        1. Is usually called a slow learner.
        2. Requires educational assistance to succeed in the regular classroom.
        3. May need outside support to cope with major crises or stresses.
        4. Should be able to complete high school, hold a job, support a family.
    b. The educable child:
        1. Is mildly retarded.
        2. Reaches a mental age of 8 to 12 years.
        3. Can learn self-care.
        4. Can perform simple manual services or trades.
    c. The trainable child:
        1. Is moderately retarded.
        2. Reaches a mental age of 3 to 7 years.
        3. Can communicate at a simple level.
        4. Can learn activities of daily living.
        5. Can perform a simple task for a brief period of time.
    d. The profoundly retarded child:
        1. Is dependent on others for care.
        2. Reaches a mental age of 0 to 2 years.
        3. May never learn to speak or to walk.
        4. Usually requires institutionalization.
2. Causes of mental retardation include:
    a. Infection and intoxication during the prenatal period.
    b. Trauma, anoxia, or exposure to radiation prenatally or at birth.
    c. Metabolic or nutritional disorders.
    d. Gross postnatal brain disease.
    e. Gestational disorders.
    f. Congenital disorders.

g. Psychiatric disorders.

h. Suboptimal environment during child-hood.

i. Chromosomal abnormalities.

3. The mentally retarded child may have had neurological damage at birth as indicated by a low Apgar score.

4. The mentally retarded child has the same needs as other children of the same mental age.

5. The retarded child goes through the same developmental stages as normal children until the child reaches his developmental limits.

6. The retarded child has difficulty with paying attention to relevant cues, short-term memory, and understanding abstract concepts.

7. The retarded child frequently has lowered resistance to infection and a higher incidence of congenital anomalies.

8. Parents require support for the decision they make about home care or institutional care.

9. Plans for the child's care and educational opportunities should involve the parents as active members of the team.

10. The availability of community resources will be a major factor influencing home care versus placement of the child.

11. Nurses must deal with their own feelings about the retarded child before they can be effective in caring for the child.

12. Hospitalization is a stressful time for the retarded child whose comprehension of the event is limited and whose need for structure is great.

B. Nursing Management. See EXCEPTIONAL CHILD and GENETIC COUNSELING.

1. Support the child and parents during hospitalization. See *Hospitalization, Support During.*

2. Initiate discharge planning. See *Discharge Planning.*

3. Assess the child's level of development as the basis for planning nursing care.

4. Obtain information about the child's usual routines from the parents or institutional caretaker and record on the Kardex and place the information at the child's bedside to encourage consistency.

5. Prepare the child for all procedures and for surgery according to developmental level rather than chronological age. See *Preparation for Procedures* and *Preparation for Surgery.*

a. Use demonstration rather than verbal explanations since the child is more successful with the concrete rather than the abstract.

b. Use colors and singing words or instructions to increase cues for learning.

c. Emphasize the procedure, rather than the rationale for performing it.

d. Provide generous positive reinforcement for cooperation and small successes.

6. Provide supervision to prevent self-injury, but do not use restraints as a substitute for nursing care.

7. Contact the occupational or physical therapy departments for feeding utensils with built-up handles if the child cannot grasp a regular spoon.

8. Make behavioral expectations clear and reinforce appropriate behavior. See *Discipline.*

9. Support the child's continued development.

a. Observe for signs of readiness to learn a new task, e.g., reaching for the spoon or cup; indicating that he knows diaper is wet.

b. Break tasks into their component behaviors and teach the child each behavior in sequence, e.g., grasping spoon, inserting spoon into bowl, bringing spoon to mouth, etc.

c. Offer opportunities for repetition of behaviors.

d. Provide verbal reward for successful learning.

10. Provide the child with toys and play activities which are developmentally appropriate, but also stimulating. See *Play, Stimulation,* and *Toys.*

a. Lengthening of attention span.

b. Accepting limitations.

c. Peer group interactions.

11. Expose the child to experiences that widen his or her horizon.

a. Take to the playroom.

b. Take for rides in a wheelchair.

c. Arrange for outdoor walks or rides if possible.

d. Take for rides on the elevator.

e. Provide frequent physical contact.

12. Facilitate parent involvement in care.

a. Encourage the parents of the older child to room-in, since the child's needs are those of a younger child in regard to development.

b. Ask parents to demonstrate feeding and toileting techniques and medication administration so that consistency can be provided by staff.

c. Comment positively about how parents handle the child, since they need reinforcement too.

d. Refer the parents to as many community resources as possible for assistance. See page 321.

1. Association for Retarded Citizens.

2. Developmental Disabilities Council.
3. College or university infant/child stimulation programs or development centers.
4. Printed material such as the Washington Guide to Promoting Development in the Young Child or Teaching Children with Developmental Problems: A Family Care Approach.

13. Support the parents' decision to continue home care of the severely retarded child.
   a. Inform them of day care facilities in the community if they are unaware.
   b. Discuss sharing of responsibilities at home so that each parent can meet his or her individual needs.
   c. Share information about parent discussion groups available in the community.

14. Support the parents who have institutionalized their child.
   a. Provide opportunities for them to verbalize their feelings.
   b. Share information about the child's hospital response so they will "know" their child.

Metabolic acidosis. See *Fluid and Electrolyte Imbalance.*

Metabolic alkalosis. See *Fluid and Electrolyte Imbalance.*

Milwaukee brace. See *Scoliosis.*

Minimal brain dysfunction (MBD). Syndrome in which children with near average, average, or above average intelligence experience mild to severe behavioral and/or learning disabilities due to functional deviations in the central nervous system.

A. **General Considerations.**
   1. The specific cause of MBD is unknown but it has been linked to:
      a. Hypoxic episodes before, during, and/or shortly after birth.
      b. Illnesses or injuries affecting the brain.
      c. Genetic factors.
      d. The ingestion of foods with additives, e.g., food coloring.
   2. MBD may manifest itself primarily in a hyperkinetic form or in a specific learning disability form (SLD), or it may occur in a mixed form.

3. The term specific learning disability (SLD) is an educational term applied to the child with MBD who has difficulty with one or more of the processes involved in using and/or understanding spoken or written language.
4. Signs and symptoms associated with the hyperkinetic form include:
   a. Hyperactivity.
   b. Decreased attention span.
   c. Constant repetition of actions.
   d. Impulsiveness.
   e. Labile emotions.
   f. Distractibility.
   g. Poor coordination of both fine and gross motor movements.
   h. School problems related to performing tasks in a hasty manner.
5. Signs and symptoms associated with the specific learning disabilities form include:
   a. Decreased activity level.
   b. Perceptual disorders in which they confuse concepts related to time, space, sound, and/or sequence.
   c. Disorders of language and symbol development such as reading (dyslexia), writing, arithmetic, and/or spelling.
   d. Short attention span.
6. Children with a mixed form of MBD may exhibit any combination of signs and symptoms.
7. Normal children exhibit the same signs and symptoms, but the child with MBD exhibits them:
   a. In greater numbers.
   b. With much more intensity.
   c. For much longer time periods.
8. The diagnosis of MBD will be based on the overall results of the following, since there is no specific diagnostic test or criterion.
   a. History of delayed developmental milestones and presence of signs and symptoms listed above.
   b. Complete physical assessment and neurological evaluation for the presence of "soft signs" of impairment such as hyperactive tendon reflexes, motor awkwardness, and difficulty differentiating right from left.
   c. Evaluation of vision and hearing.
   d. Performance on one or more tests such as the following:
      1. Denver Developmental Screening Test (DDST) which identifies developmental delays.
      2. Wechsler Intelligence Scale for Children—Revised (WISC-R) which evaluates cognitive abilities.
      3. Bender-Gestaldt Test that evaluates sensory motor deficits related to perceptual learning skills.

9. Treatment involves the use of one or more of the following:
   a. Family education and counseling.
   b. Medications, especially central nervous system stimulants which produce a paradoxical effect and calm the child.
   c. Remedial education.
   d. Psychotherapy, possibly for the whole family, but particularly for the child, since the child's self-esteem may be severely damaged by the negative response he has received from his environment.
   e. Special diet that excludes a number of food additives.
10. Treatment takes time, the child will have good and bad days, and the response to treatment varies.
11. A team approach which involves the child, parents, physician, nurse, counselor/therapist, and teacher(s) will provide the best results.
12. Federal law PL-142 requires free and appropriate education related services in a manner which best meets the child's needs.

B. Nursing Management.
1. Assist in collecting data that help to identify MBD.
   a. Record observations of the child's behavior.
   b. Administer or assist with administering tests.
   c. Obtain a nursing history. See *History Taking*.
2. Support the child and parents in dealing with the diagnosis.
   a. State that no one is to blame for the condition.
   b. Be nonjudgmental of behaviors exhibited.
   c. Accept parental expressions of guilt, frustration, anger, and hostility which the condition may cause.
   d. Tell them that help is available.
   e. Reinforce all positive parenting behaviors. See *Parenting*.
3. Teach parents to carry out home management.
   a. Explain to parents the use of, and expected response to, stimulant drugs. See *Administration of Medications, Parental*.
      1. Tell them that the child will be calmer.
      2. Explain that addiction does not occur.
      3. Advise them that the drug(s) may cause a decrease in appetite, stomach distress, and/or insomnia which are reduced by dosage alterations by the physician.

4. Tell them not to alter the dosage without consulting the physician.
5. Tell them not to expect a miracle, since the child's behavior will still exhibit variability.
   b. Support the child and parents in adhering to diet modifications.
   c. Teach parents to manage the hyperactive child.
      1. Accept the child's limitations.
      2. Provide activities to release energy, e.g., daily outdoor activities, indoor room where he can do what he wants within reasonable limits.
      3. Keep siblings from provoking the child.
      4. Establish and follow a home routine, e.g., meals, bedtimes, etc.
      5. Prevent fatigue by scheduling adequate rest.
      6. Avoid situations where the child must behave, e.g., church, restaurants.
      7. Set consistent limits on behavior. See *Discipline*.
      8. Enforce limits with nonphysical punishment, e.g., "time out" from activity, placement in a "quiet room."
      9. Reward positive behavior and ignore hyperactive behavior.
   d. Encourage parents to focus on the positive aspects of the child's behavior and personality in order to build self-esteem.
   e. Support the parents in discussing their child's condition with the school in order to:
      1. Obtain remedial help if needed.
      2. Promote consistency in limiting setting.
      3. Improve relationships with the teacher and peers which enhance self-esteem.
   f. Tell parents that it is a good idea for them to take a break from the child's care in order to meet their own needs.
   g. Encourage parents to keep in mind the ongoing needs of their other children.
4. Meet the needs of the hospitalized child with MBD.
   a. Limit the amount of time the child must spend in any one place or activity.
   b. Provide concrete demonstrations of all tests and procedures. See *Preparation for Procedures*.
   c. Give short, simple explanations but do not "talk down" to the child.
   d. Involve the child in deciding what rules must be followed (Cochran, 1972).
      1. Limit the list to a number that is reasonable, e.g., 5 to 7.
      2. Print them on a card.

3. Tape the card to the bed.

4. Draw pictures if the child cannot read.

5. Make the rules positive, e.g., "Stay on the bed for rest period."

e. Reward good behavior and ignore negative behavior, e.g., place stars on the card over the child's bed.

Mist tent. Equipment designed to provide increased humidity and/or oxygen.

A. **General Considerations.**

1. Increased humidity liquifies secretions in the bronchioles, decreases swelling, and makes coughing less distressful.

2. Mist in the tent makes it difficult to assess the child accurately.

3. Enclosure in a tent is very frightening to the young child.

4. Parents are often frightened because they assume the child is in the tent because he needs oxygen rather than cool mist.

5. Opening the tent frequently for procedures, monitoring the child, etc. lowers the oxygen and/or humidity concentration.

6. Using excess linen or hanging a towel inside the tent to catch drips will absorb the moisture that the child needs to ease breathing.

7. The mist tent may be powered by oxygen or an air compressor depending on the child's need.

8. Other equipment may be used in conjunction with the mist tent to increase oxygen or humidity.

9. Inadequate cleaning of equipment can result in noxious fumes from residues of cleaning solutions or in cross infection to the next child to use the equipment.

B. **Nursing Management.**

1. Explain the purpose and procedure of care to the child and his parents.

a. Place your head inside the tent to show there is nothing to fear.

b. Tell the young child it is like a "little house" or "rocket ship for an astronaut," etc.

c. Show the parents how they can reach inside to comfort the child while minimizing the loss of oxygen and humidity.

d. Tell the child the nurse will come to see him frequently.

2. Prepare the tent for use.

a. Check the canopy for tears.

b. Check the functioning of the zippers.

c. Add distilled water to the humidifier bottle.

d. Attach the call bell to the outside of the tent if oxygen is in use to prevent an electrical spark from coming in contact with the oxygen.

e. Add ice to the chamber at the back of the croupette.

f. Flood the tent with condensation before placing the child inside.

g. Tuck the sides of the canopy under the mattress.

3. Check to see that rails are up, since there is a tendency to feel the child is safe once the canopy is closed.

4. Maintain the oxygen and humidity level.

a. Coordinate nursing procedures to minimize opening of the tent.

b. Tuck in the sides of the canopy.

c. Keep zippers closed.

d. Clean the filter frequently.

e. Refill the humidity jar as needed.

f. Maintain ice level.

5. Open the tent to assess the child's condition, since mist makes it difficult to see the child.

6. Observe, record, and report the child's response to therapy.

a. Color.

b. Nature of respirations.

c. Degree of restlessness.

7. Record the oxygen concentration if appropriate.

8. Change the child's linen and pajamas frequently to prevent chilling.

Moniliasis. See *Candida albicans*.

Mononucleosis. See *Infectious Mononucleosis*.

Mothering. See *Parenting*.

Mourning. See *Life-threatening Illness*.

Mumps (parotitis). Acute viral disease characterized by painful salivary gland enlargement.

A. **General Considerations.**

1. The submandibular and sublingual glands may also be involved.

2. Signs and symptoms include:

a. Mild fever.

b. Headache.

c. Malaise.

d. "Earache(s)" aggravated by chewing.

e. Pain and swelling of parotid gland(s).

f. Redness and edema at the orifice of Stensen's duct.

3. Glandular swelling caused by mumps occurs primarily above the jaw line.

4. Treatment is symptomatic.
5. Complications include:
   a. Meningoencephalitis.
   b. Epididymo-orchitis or oopharitis.
   c. Postinfectious encephalitis.
   d. Arthritis.
   e. Myocarditis.
   f. Hepatitis.
6. Sterility following mumps orchitis would require extensive atrophy of both testes, which is rare.
7. The disease is prevented by immunization. See *Immunization.*
8. Subclinical cases are common in unvaccinated individuals.
9. One attack confers life-long immunity.

B. **Nursing Management.** See *Home Management of Minor Illnesses.*
1. Isolate the child from other children and susceptible adults until the swelling has resolved. See *Isolated Child.*
2. Adjust the diet to the child's needs.
   a. Avoid citrus fruits, tomatoes, pickles, and highly seasoned foods.
   b. Avoid foods that require chewing.
3. Promote comfort.
   a. Ice collar or moist heat.
   b. Frequent sponge baths.
   c. Mouth care.
   d. Administration of analgesics as instructed.

See *Administration of Medications, Parental.*
   e. Fever reduction. See *Fever Reduction.*
4. Teach the child and parents to report symptoms of meningoencephalitis.
   a. Sudden fever.
   b. Headache.
   c. Vomiting.
   d. Neck stiffness.
   e. Convulsions.
5. Teach the older male child and parents to report symptoms of orchitis.
   a. Sudden fever.
   b. Chills.
   c. Headache.
   d. Nausea.
   e. Lower abdominal pain.
6. Provide comfort for the child with orchitis.
   a. Maintain bedrest.
   b. Provide testicular support with tight-fitting underpants or stretch bathing suit.
   c. Administer analgesics.
7. Teach the older female child to report symptoms of oopharitis.
   a. Pelvic pain.
   b. Pelvic tenderness.

Mutilation, fear of. See *Fears.*

Myelomeningocele. See *Spina Bifida.*

Nasopharyngitis. See *Colds* and *Pharyngitis, Viral.*

Necrotizing enterocolitis (NEC). Interstitial mucosal injury secondary to ischemia, particularly to the small intestine.

A. **General Considerations.**
1. Ischemia may be related to a variety of causes including sepsis, hypoxemia, hypothermia, hyperviscosity, or patent ductus arteriosis (Chang and Lilly, 1982).
2. Necrotizing enterocolitis classically occurs in stressed premature newborns of less than 10 days of age.
3. Older infants, children, and adolescents may exhibit the same symptoms following apnea,

heart failure, arrhythmia, severe and/or extensive burns.
4. Gas-forming bacteria invade the damaged mucosa causing the symptomatology.
5. Signs and symptoms include:
   a. Distended, shining abdomen.
   b. Gastric retention.
   c. Blood in stools or vomitus.
   d. Lethargy.
   e. Poor feeding.
   f. Unstable vital signs.
   g. Bile-stained vomitus.
   h. Apnea.
6. Diagnostic studies include:
   a. CBC and differential.
   b. Serum protein level.

c. X-rays of the G.I. tract repeated at intervals of several hours.

d. Radioisotope scanning.

7. Pneumatosis cystoides intestinales, air in the submucosal or subserosal surfaces of the colon, is a consistent and diagnostic x-ray finding.

8. Treatment is medical initially.
   a. Oral feedings withheld.
   b. Continuous gastric suction.
   c. Parenteral alimentation. See *Total Parenteral Nutrition.*
   d. Antibiotic therapy, I.V., oral, or through nasogastric tube.

9. Complications may occur immediately or several months after treatment.
   a. Perforation.
   b. Sepsis.
   c. Disseminated intravascular coagulation.
   d. Renal cortical necrosis.
   e. Fluid and electrolyte imbalance.
   f. Small bowel or colonic stricture. (Late.)
   g. Lactose intolerance. (Late.)

10. Surgical resection and anastomosis, ileostomy, or colostomy will be required if intestinal necrosis occurs.

11. Surgery may also be needed to correct stenotic areas.

B. **Nursing Management.**
1. Support the child and parents during hospitalization. See *Hospitalization, Support During.*
2. Initiate discharge planning. See *Discharge Planning.*
3. Observe, record, and report symptoms of complications.
   a. Abdominal distention.
   b. Change in vital signs. See *Sepsis.*
   c. Decreased output. See *Fluid and Electrolyte Imbalance.*
4. Take axillary temperatures to avoid rectal perforation.
5. Monitor nasogastric suction.
   a. Observe, record, and report amount and character of secretions.
   b. Irrigate tube as ordered.
   c. Position tape so that nostril is not eroded.
   d. Provide mouth care every 4 hours.
6. Meet nutritional needs:
   a. Monitor hyperalimentation fluids.
   b. Reinstitute oral feedings in 7 to 10 days as ordered.
      1. Water or electrolyte solution for several feedings.
      2. Progress to diluted breast milk, then full strength in increasing volume.
7. Meet the needs of the infant/child requiring surgery.

a. Prepare the child and parent for surgery. See *Preoperative Care* and *Preparation for Surgery.*
b. Meet postoperative needs. See *Postoperative Care* and *Play, Therapeutic.*

8. Prepare the parents for home management.
   a. Be sure the parents are comfortable with feeding techniques since the infant's problems began when oral feedings were initiated.
   b. Teach care of ileostomy or colostomy if appropriate. See *Hirschsprung's Disease.*
   c. Tell parents to maintain medical follow-up since a barium enema may be done in 1 month postdischarge to evaluate progress.

Neglect. See *Abused Child* and *Failure to Thrive.*

Neonate. Infant in the period of development between birth and 1 month of age.

A. **General Considerations.**
1. Developmental tasks for the neonate include learning to (Duvall, 1977):
   a. Adapt physiologically to extrauterine life.
   b. Take in food.
   c. Adjust to other people in the environment, especially the mother.
2. These tasks continue in infancy and the time at which they are accomplished varies.
3. The neonatal period is one of rapid growth and development.
4. The neonate requires a consistent, loving caregiver for optimal growth and development to occur.
5. There are multiple physiological adaptations in this period which must be considered in planning care.
6. Illnesses occurring during this period tend to be generalized rather than localized.
7. The neonate possesses passive immunity received from the mother that provides protection against some illnesses.
8. From birth, the child is a unique individual and all care should be planned on this basis.
9. The first month is a period of great adjustment for both the neonate and the parents, and it will take time to develop daily routines.
10. The first 6 weeks of life are crucial to the establishment of the maternal–infant bonding process.

B. **Nursing Management.** See DISCHARGE PLANNING and PARENTING.
1. Promote maternal–infant bonding which is essential to optimal development of the child and his family.

a. Allow the mother to give as much care as possible to her infant.

b. Emphasize the positive characteristics of the infant.

c. Praise the mother for appropriate parenting skills.

d. Provide for periods of uninterrupted contact between mother and infant.

e. Encourage the mother to room-in if possible.

2. Consider the physiology of the neonate as you develop a care plan.

a. Maintain adequate hydration and nutrition because the:

1. Rapid metabolic rate predisposes the neonate to fluid and electrolyte imbalance and hypoglycemia, e.g., the stomach empties in 3 to 4 hours.

2. Fluid reserve is low.

3. Optimal development of organs, especially the brain, is dependent on adequate nutrition.

b. Maintain warmth because the:

1. Neonate raises his body temperature by increasing his respiratory rate (nonshivering thermogenesis) and this becomes a stressor.

2. Skin is thin and superficial capillaries do not contract adequately to maintain body heat.

c. Prevent overheating since sweating does not occur yet to lower body temperature.

d. Suction the nose with a bulb syringe prior to feeding if there is congestion, since the neonate is an obligatory nose breather.

e. Provide postural drainage to clear the respiratory tract if needed, since the neonate cannot cough up secretions.

f. Protect from infection since the skin is thin, the immune system is immature, and the umbilicus is a major portal of entry until the cord has dried and fallen off.

g. Position the neonate on his abdomen or prop on his right side after feeding to prevent aspiration of regurgitated milk which often occurs because the cardiac sphincter of the stomach is not fully developed.

h. Change diapers frequently since the gastrocolic reflex causes frequent intestinal emptying, and a small bladder capacity causes frequent urination.

3. Meet the daily physical needs of the neonate.

a. Bathe.

1. Use warm, not hot, water.

2. Use a mild soap.

3. Wash the head including the area over the fontanels to prevent cradle cap.

4. Wash the eyes from the inner canthus out.

5. Clean the outer ear with a washcloth wrapped around the index finger.

6. Do not use cotton tipped applicators in the ears, as this may lead to injury.

7. Wash in all the creases.

8. Dry thoroughly.

b. Provide care until the umbilical cord stump dries and drops off and the area heals.

1. Clean the area with cotton balls moistened with alcohol to promote drying and prevent infection.

2. Give a sponge bath instead of a tub bath.

c. Dress the neonate in a shirt and diaper and cover with one or two blankets to provide adequate warmth.

d. Provide skin care when the diaper is changed.

1. Keep the diaper folded below the umbilicus until healing occurs.

2. Keep vaseline gauze over the glans penis of the circumcised male until the area heals to prevent irritation.

3. Wash the perineal area with each change, since ammonia builds up on the skin.

4. Dry the area completely.

5. Expose the diaper area to the air two to three times a day for 10 to 20 minutes if redness occurs. See *Dermatitis, Diaper.*

6. Apply white petroleum jelly or an ointment to protect from moisture.

7. Use lotion or powder to the diaper area but do not use the two together.

e. Prevent scratching of the face by:

1. Cutting long, rough nails straight across using blunt baby nail scissors.

2. Folding cuffs of long sleeve shirts over hands while sleeping.

f. Feed on demand. See *Nutrition.*

1. Hold the neonate for all feedings.

2. Do not prop the bottle!

3. Make sure the nipple allows a smooth, steady stream of milk to flow when the neonate sucks.

4. Let the neonate set the pace of the feeding.

5. Do not have the baby wrapped too warmly, since he may go off to sleep again before he is full.

6. Burp after every ounce.

7. Record the time the neonate was fed and how much he took.

8. Place the neonate on his abdomen or side after feeding to prevent aspiration of regurgitated feeding.

g. Provide for rest and sleep periods. See *Sleep.*

h. Protect from infection.
1. Wash your hands before touching the neonate and after diaper changes.
2. Do not care for the neonate if you have an infectious illness.
3. Do not hold the neonate close to your face or kiss him.
4. Wear a gown over your uniform when giving direct care.
5. Discard formula which is left after a feeding to prevent bacterial growth.
i. Prevent injuries. See *Accident Prevention.*
1. Keep the crib side rails all the way up.
2. Do not leave loose linens lying in the crib.
3. Do not use a pillow in the crib.
4. Keep one hand on the neonate when on the scale or the crib rails are down, since even the smallest infant may wiggle around.

4. Weigh daily.
1. On the same scale.
2. At the same time.
3. Nude.
4. Prior to feeding.

5. Take and record vital signs as ordered.
a. Count the respirations and pulse for a full minute.
b. Take an apical pulse.
c. Take an axillary temperature as ordered or lubricate a rectal thermometer and insert just past the anal sphincter to avoid tissue trauma.

6. Observe, record, and report signs and symptoms that may indicate illness.
a. Poor feeding.
b. Weight loss.
c. Diarrhea.
d. Vomiting.
e. Temperature instability, e.g., elevated or subnormal.
f. Irritability.
g. Tremors.
h. Lethargy.

7. Meet the emotional needs of the neonate.
a. Involve the parents in the care of their child as much as possible.
b. Respond consistently and as soon as possible to the neonate's needs.
c. Limit the number of caregivers.
d. Provide age-appropriate stimulation. See *Stimulation.*

8. Approach the parents in a positive manner when discussing topics related to health care.
a. Reinforce appropriate parenting skills.
b. Do not act as an authority.
c. Help parents to work out their own approaches in giving care and foster flexibility.

9. Provide information to parents as needed in relation to the following areas:
a. Growth and development norms. See *Appendix v.*
b. Common variations in the neonate, e.g., bluish black pigmented areas over the lower back and buttocks, mongolian spots, in the black infant.
c. Nutrition.
d. Safety.
e. Provision for ongoing health care. See *Well-child Care.*
f. Signs and symptoms that may indicate illness.
g. Ways to stimulate development.

Nephroblastoma. See *Wilm's Tumor.*

Nephrotic syndrome, primary. Syndrome affecting kidney function and characterized by proteinuria, hypoproteinemia, edema, and hyperlipidemia.

A. **General Considerations.**
1. Primary nephrotic syndrome is divided into subcategories on the basis of histopathology (Travis, 1982).
a. Minimal change nephrotic syndrome (MCNS).
b. Focal segmental sclerosis (FSS).
c. Membranoproliferative glomerulonephritis (MPGN).
d. Mesangial proliferative glomerulonephritis (MPN).
e. Membranoglomerulonephritis (MGN).
f. Other lesions.
2. Within the subcategories, MCNS accounts for 80 percent of the cases and FSS and MPGN account for an additional 16 percent.
3. The cause of primary nephrotic syndrome is unknown.
4. The major clinical signs and symptoms are the same for the subcategories and include:
a. Edema (periorbital in the morning progressing to dependent, often pitting, later in the day).
b. Anorexia.
c. Fatigue.
d. Irritability.
e. Abdominal discomfort.
f. Diarrhea: due to edema of the intestinal mucosa.
5. Additional signs and symptoms include:
a. Hematuria: occurs with varying frequency.
b. Hypertension: may represent a response to decreased plasma volume and varies in frequency and severity.

N

c. Azotemia.
6. Severe edema may cause:
   a. Respiratory distress.
   b. Decreased activity.
   c. Safety hazards since the center of gravity is altered.
   d. Skin breakdown due to stretching.
   e. Rectal prolapse and urethral obstruction.
   f. Umbilical and inguinal hernias.
7. Laboratory studies reveal:
   a. Proteinuria.
   b. Hypoalbuminemia.
   c. Hyperlipemia.
   d. Hypercholesterolemia.
   e. Elevated serum creatinine and blood urea nitrogen values.
8. Treatment includes (Travis, 1982):
   a. Steroids and, occasionally, immunosuppressive drugs for children with frequent relapses.
   b. Observation for and active treatment of any infection.
   c. Diuretics of the loop variety (less common) given alone by oral route, or with salt-poor albumin when given by I.V.
   d. Curtailment of dietary salt intake.
9. The specific action of steroids in bringing about termination of proteinuria is unknown.
10. Response of children with MCNS to steroid therapy varies (Travis, 1982).
    a. Nonresponders who have progressive renal involvement.
    b. Responders.
       1. 30 percent do not relapse and are considered cured.
       2. 25 percent have infrequent relapses.
       3. 45 percent have frequent relapses.
11. Treatment for FSS and MPGN varies and is often symptomatic in nature; the prognosis is poorer than with MCNS.
12. Complications include:
    a. Infections (especially viral).
    b. Ascites.
    c. Malnutrition.
    d. Thrombus formation due to the existing hypercoagulative state.
    e. Hypertension.
    f. Hematuria.
    g. Hypovolemic shock.
    h. Peritonitis.
13. The child with nephrosis generally feels well, although the edematous child may be irritable.
14. The nephrotic syndrome is a chronic disease requiring long-term follow-up care.
15. Immunizations:
    a. Are not given while child is on steroid or immunosuppressive therapy.
    b. May be withheld, for varying periods of time, after therapy is stopped, since they can cause a relapse in a child in remission.
16. Home management is usually possible after hospitalization in the acute phase.

B. Nursing Management.
1. Support the child and parents during hospitalization. See *Hospitalization, Support During.*
2. Initiate discharge planning. See *Discharge Planning.*
3. Place the edematous child in semi-Fowler's position to facilitate breathing.
4. Assess edema.
   a. Weigh daily and record.
      1. Use the same scale.
      2. Weigh at the same time, preferably before breakfast.
      3. Weigh nude or in underpants.
   b. Observe the child's entire body.
   c. Measure the abdomen daily at the umbilicus.
   d. Record intake and output.
   e. Test urine for specific gravity and albumin.
5. Prevent infection.
   a. Practice good hygienic technique.
   b. Teach the child good hygienic measures.
   c. Protect the child from contact with staff, other children on the unit and/or visitors with infections, especially upper respiratory infections.
   d. Provide meticulous skin care.
   e. Administer prophylactic antibiotics as ordered.
6. Prevent skin breakdown.
   a. Bathe as often as needed.
      1. Avoid the use of drying soaps.
      2. Be particularly careful to wash and dry all skin fold areas.
   b. Use lanolin rich lotion on pressure areas.
   c. Change the immobile child's position every 1 to 2 hours.
   d. Use nonallergenic powder or cornstarch on opposing skin surfaces.
   e. Support an edematous scrotum with a T-binder.
   f. Place absorbent cotton between skin folds.
   g. Place a pillow between the child's legs when he is lying on his side.
   h. Make sure the pajamas, shoes, and other clothing are nonbinding.
   i. Give medications by oral route if possible or use the deltoid muscle for injections, since edema in the lower extremities would reduce absorption of medications.
7. Care for breaks in the skin immediately.
   a. Clean the area completely.

N

b. Dry the area thoroughly.

c. Expose the area to the air.

d. Use a heat lamp, as ordered, to promote healing.

    1. Use a 25-watt bulb.

    2. Keep the light 18 inches from the skin.

    3. Use for only 15 to 20 minutes 3 to 4 times a day.

8. Monitor TPR and blood pressure every 4 hours.

a. Compare to the child's usual values.

b. Report deviations.

9. Observe, record, and report signs and symptoms of complications.

a. Increasing weight.

b. Increasing abdominal circumference.

c. Rising or falling blood pressure.

d. Increasing pulse rate.

e. Elevated temperature.

f. Difficulty breathing.

g. Hematuria.

h. Decreased urinary output.

i. Diarrhea.

10. Observe, record, and report the child's response to medications.

11. Provide a regular diet with: See *Nutrition.*

a. Increased protein (2 to 3 g/kg/day).

b. Additional potassium if diuretics are being used, e.g., orange, grapefruit, or grape juice.

c. No added salt or excessively salty foods, e.g., potato chips, luncheon meats, or limited to 1 to 2 g/day during severe edema.

d. Unrestricted fluids unless otherwise ordered.

12. Encourage the anorexic child to eat.

a. Find out food preferences and record on the Kardex.

b. Let the child have some choice in foods.

c. Serve smaller, more frequent meals.

d. Serve foods in an attractive manner.

e. Permit parents to bring foods from home.

f. Provide company for the child at mealtimes.

13. Plan activities appropriate to the child's exercise tolerance. See *Play* and *Play, Therapeutic.*

a. Place on bed rest only if the child has an acute infection or is undergoing rapid diuresis.

b. Let the child pace himself, but stop activity before the child becomes fatigued.

c. Encourage socialization with people who do not have an infectious disease.

d. Promote ambulation to prevent osteoporosis due to steroid therapy.

14. Maintain a safe environment, since the edematous child has a shift in his center of gravity and edematous eyelids may impede vision.

15. Observe, record, and report signs and symptoms related to long-term steroid therapy.

a. Rounding of the face.

b. Increased appetite.

c. Abdominal distention.

d. Hirsutism.

e. Decreased growth.

f. Hypertension.

g. Abdominal pain, which may indicate a gastric ulcer.

h. Bone pain, which may indicate a pathological fracture.

16. Observe, record, and report signs and symptoms related to the use of immunosuppressive drugs if these are used, e.g., leukopenia, hair loss. See *Immunotherapy.*

17. Support the child and parents in coping with an altered body image. See *Body Image.*

a. Do not comment on the child's size.

b. Explain that the edema will decrease and the child will have a normal appearance again.

18. Support the child and parents in coping with a chronic illness. See *Chronic Illness.*

19. Teach the child and parents home management.

a. Teach how to:

    1. Test urine for protein.

    2. Administer medications. See *Administration of Medications, Parental.*

    3. Recognize a relapse, e.g., proteinuria, decreased urinary output.

    4. Recognize the side effects of steroid and immunosuppressive therapy.

b. Explain the need to protect the child from infection.

    1. Avoid large crowds.

    2. Get adequate rest.

    3. Avoid playmates with active infection.

c. Encourage the parents to have the child attend school on a regular basis except when the child is severely edematous and/or immunosuppressed.

d. Explain why immunization schedule will be altered.

e. Tell the parents to call the physician if the child:

    1. Shows evidence of a relapse.

    2. Develops an infection.

    3. Refuses to take medication as ordered.

f. Discuss the importance of:

    1. Following the prescribed drug regimen.

    2. Maintaining follow-up care.

    3. Providing as normal a life as possible for the child to support development.

g. Encourage parents to develop and/or maintain individual interests and contact with support persons since chronic nature of illness is draining.

N

Neuroblastoma. A malignant tumor which arises from the adrenal glands, retroperitoneal sympathetic chain, or sympathetic ganglia.

A. General Considerations.

1. At the time of diagnosis, the majority of children will have metastasis via the lymphatics or bloodstream to:
   a. Lymph nodes.
   b. Skeletal system, particularly the eye orbit.
   c. Bone marrow.
   d. Liver.
   e. Meninges.
2. Symptoms may be due to the metastatic lesion(s) rather than the primary tumor.
   a. Infants.
      1. Markedly distended abdomen.
      2. Subcutaneous nodules.
      3. Jaundice due to liver involvement.
      4. Feeding problems.
      5. Listlessness.
      6. Failure to thrive.
   b. Older children.
      1. Enlarged abdomen or abdominal mass.
      2. Bone pain.
      3. Bulging eye or bruising of the orbit.
      4. Anorexia.
      5. Weight loss.
      6. Diarrhea.
      7. Neurological signs ranging from sensory changes to total paralysis.
3. Many procedures will be used to diagnose neuroblastoma.
   a. X-ray of the abdomen and/or chest.
   b. 24-hour urine for catecholamines, particularly VMA (vanillylmandelic acid) and HVA (homovanillic acid).
   c. Intravenous pyelogram.
   d. Bone marrow aspiration.
   e. Ultrasound.
   f. Computerized axial tomography (CAT or CT scan).
   g. Skeletal survey and bone scan.

4. Neuroblastoma is usually classified into stages based on the extent of tumor involvement.
5. The treatment regimen is based on the clinical stage.
6. Treatment involves surgical removal of as much of the tumor as possible followed by chemotherapy and radiation therapy.
7. Large inoperable tumors may be biopsied initially and then excision attempted after chemotherapy and irradiation have reduced the tumor size.
8. Immunotherapy may be used in conjunction with chemotherapy. See *Immunotherapy.*

9. Chemotherapy and radiation therapy are frequently performed on an outpatient basis.
10. Determination of urine catecholamines, ultrasound, and CAT scan may be used to monitor response to treatment.
11. Prognosis is more dependent on the age of the patient at diagnosis and the extent of the disease than on the treatment used although age and stage of the disease are independent variables.
12. The child under 12 months of age at the time of diagnosis has a better prognosis whatever the stage of the disease.
13. Spontaneous remission or maturation of the cells of neuroblastoma sometimes occurs for unknown reasons.
14. Spinal deformity may be a complication of the disease or radiation therapy (Mayfield et al., 1981).

B. Nursing Management. See ANXIETY, CRISIS INTERVENTION, and LIFE-THREATENING ILLNESS.

1. Support the child and parents during hospitalization. See *Hospitalization, Support During.*
2. Initiate discharge planning. See *Discharge Planning.*
3. Provide consistency and continuity of care, since the child must endure so many painful diagnostic and therapeutic procedures.
4. Accompany the physician, if possible, when explanations are given to the child and parents so that consistent, accurate information is communicated.
   a. Anxiety interferes with the ability of the child and parents to comprehend information.
   b. The information should be recorded on the Kardex so that the same explanation can be given each time the child or parent asks.
      1. Answer all questions honestly.
      2. Use terminology the child understands.
   c. Arrange for uninterrupted periods of contact with the child and parents so supportive discussions can be held.
   d. Anticipate that the parents will have increased guilt feelings and anger if metastasis occurred before the diagnosis was made.
5. Meet the needs of the child preoperatively. See *Preoperative Care* and *Preparation for Procedures.*
6. Meet the needs of the child postoperatively. See *Postoperative Care.*
7. Meet the needs of the child receiving chemotherapy or radiation therapy. See *Chemotherapy* and *Radiation Therapy.*
8. Teach the child and parents home management.

a. Encourage the parents to help the child and the family to make home life as normal as possible.
 1. Have the child resume normal activities such as play groups or school.
 2. Encourage normal peer relationships.
 3. Maintain normal discipline. See *Discipline.*
 4. Encourage adequate rest and nutrition for all family members.
b. Help the child continue to work through feelings about intrusive procedures through therapeutic play, since chemotherapy may continue on an outpatient basis. See *Play, Therapeutic.*
9. Meet the needs of the child and parents if the child requires enucleation of the eye.
a. Provide opportunities for the child and parents to verbalize their concerns about disfigurement and loss of some vision.
 1. Prepare the child and parents through explanations and interviews.
 2. Anticipate that the child may handle his fears of disfigurement by becoming angry and irritable.
b. Provide information about the prosthesis.
 1. The prosthesis will be fitted when the edema subsides.
 2. The child will not be able to see with the new eye.
 3. The artificial eye can be attached to the eye muscles so that it moves in coordination with the real eye.
c. Meet the needs of the child preoperatively.
d. Meet the needs of the child postoperatively.
 1. Observe, record, and report hemorrhage, edema, or signs of infection of the orbit.
 2. Reinforce the dressing if necessary, but do not change unless ordered.
 3. Help the child cope with body image changes. See *Body Image.*
 4. Assist with fitting the prosthesis if done during hospitalization.
e. Teach care of the artificial eye.
 1. Review the physician's guidelines about whether the prosthesis should be removed for sleep or other specific instructions.
 2. Wash hands before beginning the procedure.
 3. Irrigate the socket with normal saline.
 4. Clean the socket and eye when excessive tearing or crusting occur.
 5. Wipe away the normal watery discharge with sterile, disposable tissues.
 6. Clean the prosthesis with soap and warm water only.
 7. Store a plastic prosthesis in a container with plain tap water.
 8. Store a glass prosthesis in its own case after drying.
f. Teach measures for eye safety.
 1. Wear safety glasses or goggles if prescribed as a method of protecting the normal eye.
 2. Do not carry sharp objects while walking or running.
 3. Avoid rubbing the eyes when a foreign body is present.
 4. Seek medical assistance promptly for any injuries or infections.
10. Meet the needs of the child who does not respond to therapy. See *Dying Child.*

Nocturnal emission ("wet dreams"). Ejaculation of semen during sleep.

A. **General Considerations.**
 1. Nocturnal emissions:
 a. Are a part of normal sexual maturation in the male; as the testes produce more spermatozoa, more seminal fluid is produced.
 b. Usually start between the ages of 13 to 15 years.
 c. May occur during the course of an erotic dream or result from pressure of a full bladder on the seminal vesicles.
 2. Boys who have not been prepared for this experience may worry that (Pellitteri, 1977):
 a. They have contracted a disease.
 b. They have a problem related to sexual function.
 c. Loss of seminal fluid will weaken them.
 3. Seminal fluid:
 a. Consists of secretions from the testes, epididymides, seminal vesicles, prostate gland, and the bulbourethral glands.
 b. Is milky white in color.
 c. Loss with each ejaculation is approximately 5 to 10 ml.
 d. Is constantly being produced.

B. **Nursing Management.**
 1. Provide accurate information.
 2. Encourage the child and parents to see the occurrence of nocturnal emissions as a positive experience. See *Sex Education.*
 3. Dispel myths by telling the boy that nocturnal emissions will not:
 a. Cause him to lose his strength.
 b. Impair his adult sexual functioning.

Nosebleed. See *Home Management of Minor Emergencies.*

Nursing bottle syndrome. Extensive caries and discoloration of the teeth in the toddler or preschooler.

A. General Considerations.
1. The affected child has a history of being put to bed at naptime or nighttime with a bottle of milk or juice or a sugar-coated pacifier.
2. The syndrome is completely preventable.
3. Saliva flow decreases during sleep, therefore, the milk or juice remains in contact with the teeth.
4. The child tends to hold fluid in his mouth during sleep.
5. The breakdown of the carbohydrate by bacterial enzymes forms acids that destroy tooth enamel.
6. The upper front teeth are the most severely affected by decay.
7. The lower front teeth are protected by the nipple and tongue.
8. Extensive decay may result in:
   a. Refusal to eat foods that require chewing.
   b. Herpetic stomatitis secondary to dehydrated and inflamed gingiva.
   c. Malpositioned permanent teeth.
   d. Increased susceptibility to decay after nursing ceases.
9. Restorative dentistry under general anesthesia may be necessary to fill caries, cap salvageable teeth, or extract unsalvageable teeth.
10. Extraction of a number of teeth may make eating impossible for the child or may cause emotional problems because of poor body image.
11. Expensive dental appliances may be necessary for eating and proper speech.
12. Serous otitis media secondary to pooling of milk around the eustachian tube is also a possible complication in the child who sleeps with a bottle.

B. Nursing Management.
1. Initiate teaching with expectant parents or parents of young children to prevent the problem.
   a. Feed the baby prior to putting to bed for a nap or for the night.
   b. Fill a bottle with water if the child needs fluid during sleep.
   c. Discourage use of juice in ready-to-feed bottles since this may prolong dependence on the bottle.
2. Examine the mouth carefully, including the back side of the front teeth if the nursing history reveals that the child goes to bed with a bottle.
3. Meet the needs of the child requiring dental repair under anesthesia.
   a. Support the child and parents during hospitalization. See *Hospitalization, Support During.*
   b. Initiate discharge planning. See *Discharge Planning.*
   c. Prepare the child and parents for surgery. See *Preparation for Procedures* and *Preparation for Surgery.*
   d. Meet the needs of the child postoperatively. See *Postoperative Care.*
      1. Position the child prone or on the side with support to the back.
      2. Provide frequent mouth care as ordered.
      3. Discuss dietary restrictions with the parents.
      4. Encourage dental follow-up with a private dentist or dentist in the public health department. See *Dental Care.*

Nutrition. The science of food and its relation to health.

A. General Considerations.
1. Nutrition is:
   a. Fundamental to the growth and development of the child.
   b. Essential to the quality of health and life.
   c. Influenced by factors that determine what foods are supplied to the body and how the body uses what is supplied.
      1. Economics.
      2. Culture.
      3. Education.
      4. Social role.
      5. Physical status.
2. Malnutrition occurs when:
   a. Proper nutrients are unavailable, e.g., lack of money to purchase them.
   b. The body is unable to metabolize nutrients, e.g., the child with cystic fibrosis has inadequate fat metabolism.
   c. Inappropriate, insufficient, or oversufficient nutrients are consumed, e.g., one whole food group is missing, obesity.
3. The major nutrition related problems are:
   a. Iron deficiency anemia. See *Anemia, Iron Deficiency.*
   b. Obesity. See *Obesity.*
   c. Dental caries. See *Dental Care.*
4. The required nutrients are the same for all people throughout life, but the required amounts will vary according to:
   a. Sex—an adolescent boy requires more than an adolescent girl.
   b. Activity level—an active child has greater needs than an inactive one.
   c. Body size—larger body size requires more nutrients.

d. Growth status—the child requires more during periods of rapid growth, e.g., infancy and adolescence.

e. State of health—the ill child has increased nutrient needs, but may have an impaired appetite or decreased ability to digest and absorb food.

5. Nutrition is related to the psychosocial development of the child.

a. Infant learns trust through the taking in of food in a caring relationship.

b. Toddler increases sense of autonomy through experience of self-feeding.

c. Preschooler increases sense of initiative through participation in the social aspects of feeding.

d. Schoolage child increases sense of industry in the selection and preparation of food.

e. Adolescent increases sense of identity through the acceptance or rejection of foods and eating practices accepted by the family.

6. The adequacy of nutrition may be assessed by:

a. Plotting height and weight on a graph. See *Well-child Care* and *Appendix v.*

b. Measurement of the head circumference. See *Well-child Care.*

c. Observation of clinical signs.
1. Activity level.
2. Condition of the skin, teeth, and hair.
3. Posture.
4. Nervous control.

7. The institution of sound nutrition following a period of undernutrition or illness often results in a period of "catch up" growth in which the child grows at a rate greater than expected for his age.

8. Severe malnutrition in the first 2 years of life and especially in the first 6 months may result in irreversible deficits in height, weight, and intellectual development.

9. The major necessary nutrients include:
a. Protein.
b. Minerals.
1. Calcium.
2. Iron.
c. Fat.
d. Carbohydrate.
e. Vitamins.
1. A.
2. B complex.
3. C.
4. D.
f. Water.

10. Caloric needs differ according to age group.
a. Infant:
1. 0 to 6 months: 120 cal/kg.
2. 6 months to 1 year: 110 cal/kg.
b. Toddler: 1300 cal/day.

c. Preschooler: 1800 cal/day.
d. Schoolchild: 2400 cal/day.
e. Adolescent:
1. Girls: 2400 cal/day.
2. Boys: 2800–3000 cal/day.

11. Water requirements differ according to age group.
a. Infant: 150 ml/kg.
b. Toddler: 120 ml/kg.
c. Preschooler: 100 ml/kg.
d. Schoolchild: 75 ml/kg.
e. Adolescent: 50–75 ml/kg.

12. The four food groups include See *Appendix vii.*
a. Meat.
b. Milk.
c. Vegetables, fruits.
d. Bread, cereals.

13. Foods, the amounts needed, and ways in which the needs can be met are different during the first year of life. See *Appendix vii.*

14. Nutritional supplements are required in some situations.

a. Iron—for 1 year for all infants whether they receive evaporated milk or a commercial formula (unless it is iron fortified) until their diet meets iron requirements.

b. Vitamin D—needed by breastfed infants.

c. Fluoride—needed by breastfed infants (fluoride is not excreted in breast milk) and infants on evaporated milk unless the water contains one part per million fluoride.

15. Additional vitamin supplementation is generally unnecessary unless the child:

a. Consumes a diet that does not contain the four food groups.

b. Experiences an illness that alters nutrition.

16. Solid foods are not needed until 4 to 6 months of age when infant iron stores are depleted.

17. Milk intake should be decreased as solid food intake is increased to avoid excessive weight gain.

18. Major parental concerns about nutrition include:

a. Differences in food intake at different ages.

b. Addition of solid foods to the infant's diet.

c. Weaning from breast or bottle.

d. Preparing infant foods at home versus buying commercial foods.

e. Finicky food habits of toddlers.

19. At all ages it is the quality of food rather than the quantity of food consumed that influences the nutritional status of an individual most directly.

20. Plant nitrates found in spinach, carrots, and beets can be converted, during home processing, to nitrites and cause methemoglobinemia

N

when consumed by infants (Howard and Herbold, 1982).

21. Cultural and religious beliefs and practices related to food may affect a child's nutrition and must be considered. See *Cultural Aspects of Health Care* and *Religious Aspects of Health Care.*

22. Children with chronic illnesses or handicapping conditions will require careful nutritional planning to meet special needs.

23. Consider cultural and religious practices when providing nutritional guidance.

B. **Nursing Management.** See FAILURE TO THRIVE, FEEDING PROBLEMS, OBESITY, ANEMIA, DENTAL CARE.

1. Assess the child's nutritional status.
   a. Measure height and weight and plot on a standardized growth chart.
   b. Measure and record head circumference in child under 2 years of age.
   c. Observe, record, and report:
      1. Activity level—energetic or listless.
      2. Hair—shiny or dull.
      3. Teeth—straight, clean, noncarious or malpositioned, mottled, or carious.
      4. Skin—smooth, moist, good turgor or rough, dry, scaly.
      5. Nervous control—good attention span, not irritable or inattentive and irritable.
   d. Obtain a nutrition history. See *Appendix vii.*
   e. Obtain a nursing history that may help identify nutrition-related problems, e.g., frequent illnesses. See *History Taking* and *Appendix v.*

2. Teach parents:
   a. Basic four food groups.
   b. Amounts and kinds of food required by the child at different ages.
   c. Sources for meeting food group requirements.
   d. Nutritional supplements that may be needed.
   e. Water requirements of the child.
   f. How nutrition is tied in with the psychosocial development of the child.
   g. To avoid excess sugar, sodium, and calories as a means of health promotion and maintenance.

3. Discuss nutritional concerns of parents as indicated.
   a. Differences in food intake at different ages.
      1. Infants and adolescents have the greatest needs because of their rapid growth.
      2. Toddlers have reduced food intake needs because their rate of growth has slowed.
      3. Preschool and schoolage children have erratic growth patterns marked by plateaus and spurts and therefore may consume larger quantities of food at one time than at others.
   b. Addition of solid foods after 4 to 6 months of age.
      1. Introduce the food when the infant is hungry.
      2. Use a small bowled spoon, e.g., long-handled infant spoon.
      3. Start with 1 to 2 tsp. of the food and increase gradually.
      4. Introduce only one food at a time and wait 4 to 7 days before starting another new food in order to detect any allergic reactions.
      5. Decrease the amount of milk as the amount of solid food is increased.
      6. Do not add food to the bottle or use an infant feeder.
   c. Weaning from the breast or bottle (Heimann, 1977).
      1. Do not begin weaning until 5 to 6 months of age.
      2. Progress slowly until infant is weaned completely at about 1 year of age.
      3. Eliminate one bottle or breastfeeding per month starting with the one at which the infant nurses least and ending with the favorite one.
      4. Start introducing the cup with meals at 6 months.
      5. Follow meals by offering the bottle or breast for as long as the infant wants. (Give a few sips before meals if infant is very hungry and requires a little milk to "settle down.")
      6. Substitute water in bottle of infant who takes bottle at night in crib. See *Nursing Bottle Syndrome.*
      7. Decrease amount of milk offered as infant grows. See *Appendix vii.*
   d. Preparing foods at home versus buying commercially prepared foods.
      1. Commercial foods can be used to meet the infant's nutritional needs, but may increase sugar and sodium intake.
      2. Commercial food labels should be checked, since contents are listed according to quantity of nutrients present and therefore excess sugar, sodium, and starch can be avoided.
      3. Commercial food should be heated in a separate container unless the whole jar is eaten to avoid reheating.
      4. Open jars should not be kept for more than 24 hours.
      5. Food, hands, and all utensils should be washed prior to preparation.

6. Foods prepared at home should be fresh, well cooked, and should not have any additional seasoning.

7. Foods prepared at home can be put through a food mill or blender, and the cooking fluid used in the food to increase liquid content.

8. Home prepared foods can be frozen in ice cube containers then stored in freezer bags.

9. Parents should avoid making home prepared beets, spinach, and carrots for infants.

e. Meeting the nutritional needs of the toddler.

1. Concentrate on the quality of the food rather than the quantity.

2. Offer finger foods which can be "eaten on the run" by the active toddler, e.g., vegetable and fruit slices, cheese cubes, pieces of hot dog.

3. Provide differences in texture, e.g., one soft, one crisp, one chewy food.

4. Avoid strongly flavored or mixed foods (onions or stew) or serve strong flavored vegetables raw since these are better accepted (Pipes, 1977).

5. Add color to food since this stimulates the toddler to eat.

6. Avoid battles over food intake, serve well-balanced meals in age-appropriate portions, and do not comment on uneaten food; when he gets hungry the toddler will eat.

7. Give only nutritious between meal snacks, e.g., cheese cubes, peanut butter crackers, fortified nonsugar coated dry cereal.

4. Meet the nutritional needs of the hospitalized infant.

a. Offer the bottle or cup on the infant's home schedule as much as possible.

b. Record how much the infant drinks and eats at each feeding so that:

1. A total calorie count can be kept, e.g., an infant took a total of 23 ounces/24 hours; total caloric intake equals 23 × 20 or 460 cal.

2. The next caregiver will know how much the infant took at the last feeding and when the feeding took place.

c. Allow for adequate sucking time but do not prolong the feeding for more than 20 to 30 minutes.

d. Offer age-appropriate solid foods.

1. Mix dry cereal with formula.

2. Do not add salt or sugar to the food.

3. Refeed solids which are pushed out over

lips by the tongue extrusion reflex if still present.

5. Meet the needs of the breastfeeding infant and mother.

a. Provide a comfortable chair for the mother.

b. Permit the breastfeeding mother who cannot stay with the infant to pump her breasts and leave milk on the unit to be fed to the infant.

c. Avoid giving formula to the breastfed infant if possible, since he

1. Is not used to it and may vomit.

2. Will have to use a different sucking approach with a bottle and this is confusing.

d. Remember that the breastfed infant usually nurses every 2 to 3 hours, since breast milk is digested more quickly than cow's milk.

e. Breastfed babies are less likely to overfeed and become obese.

f. Breast milk provides passive immunity to some illnesses.

g. Breast milk is a totally balanced diet except for iron, vitamin D, and fluoride.

h. Feeding problems and allergies are less common, e.g., colic, spitting, eczema.

i. Maternal–infant bonding is promoted.

6. Meet the nutritional needs of the hospitalized toddler, preschool, and schoolage child.

a. Find out daily nutritional needs for the age of the child. See *Appendix vii*.

b. Select, or help the child select, foods which are from all four food groups.

c. Find out the child's favorite foods and record on the Kardex.

d. Provide nutritious snacks midway between meals.

e. Provide age-appropriate finger foods.

f. Encourage the child and/or parents to limit the amount of refined sugar eaten, e.g., avoid sugar-coated cereals, cakes, pies, sodas, but do permit occasional treats.

g. Record how much the child eats and drinks.

7. Meet the nutritional needs of the hospitalized adolescent.

a. Provide increased:

1. Calories.

2. Protein.

3. Iron.

b. Provide nutritious snacks which the adolescent can get himself.

c. Allow for favorite foods such as hamburgers, pizza, and french fries when possible.

d. Encourage the adolescent to select well-balanced meals by tying nutritional education to improved body image.

8. Work with a nutritionist to meet the needs of the child and family.

Obesity. Excessive accumulations of body fat.

A. General Considerations.

1. Excessive fat cells that develop in infancy can be reduced in size as the child grows, but the number of fat cells remains the same throughout life.
2. Eating habits are:
   a. Learned in infancy.
   b. Modeled for the child by his parents.
   c. Influenced by the family's cultural identification.
   d. Extremely difficult to alter once they become established.
3. Obesity contributes to the development of:
   a. Coronary artery disease.
   b. Hypertension.
   c. Diabetes.
   d. Orthopedic problems, e.g., slipped femoral epiphysis.
   e. Psychological problems, e.g., decreased self-esteem, difficulty achieving role identity.
4. Hormonal imbalance rarely causes obesity.
5. Treatment measures include:
   a. Dietary changes for the:
      1. Child as an individual.
      2. Family as a group.
   b. Increasing exercise.
   c. Behavior modification.
   d. Treating underlying psychological problems.
6. Drugs are not recommended for treatment.
7. Low protein diets should not be used, since they may result in negative nitrogen balance that causes growth retardation.
8. Everyone who feeds the obese child must cooperate in helping him lose weight if a plan is to be successful.
9. Group weight loss programs may be of value in helping the obese adolescent lose weight.
10. Solid foods are not necessary in an infant's diet until the age of 4 to 6 months and contribute to excessive weight gain.
11. A child may be overweight (weight greater than average for height and body build) without being obese.
12. Weight reduction should be limited to a pound a week in the older child and younger children should have weight stabilized until they grow into it (Pipes, 1981).
13. No food should be forbidden; moderation in intake and compensation for calories at another meal contribute to the child/adolescent developing a sense of control.

B. Nursing Management.

1. Assess the following areas (Pipes, 1977):
   a. What foods are regularly eaten at home?
   b. How has the child's pattern of obesity been achieved? e.g., sudden development or long-standing problem.
   c. How does the family feel about the obese child?
   d. Is the child rewarded for eating? e.g., given special privileges for eating all the food on the plate.
   e. How active is the child?
   f. What type of snacking pattern has developed?
2. Work with the child and/or parents to develop a treatment plan which:
   a. The child and/or parents are motivated to follow.
   b. Fits their life style, culture, and economic status.
3. Consult with a nutritionist to help you plan and/or refer the child and parents to the nutritionist.
4. Assist parents of infants who are obese.
   a. Explain that an infant does not need to be fat to be healthy.
   b. Plot the infant's height and weight on a growth chart to help them see the relationship between height and weight.
   c. Reinforce parenting skills which are not related to feeding, e.g., "Talking to your baby, like you do, helps him learn."
   d. Help parents recognize signs of satiation in their infant, e.g., decreased sucking, closing of eyes, turning the head away.
   e. Teach parents types of nutrients and quantities of each that the infant requires at different ages. See *Nutrition.*
   f. Teach parents methods of decreasing caloric intake.
      1. Do not prop the bottle so the infant does not take in extra calories.
      2. Use a spoon to feed solids instead of an infant feeder.
      3. Offer water or diluted juice in place of some milk feedings.
      4. Employ comforting techniques other than feeding when the infant is crying, e.g., rocking.

5. Assist parents of obese toddlers and preschoolers.
   a. Explain the decreased growth rate seen in the toddler and preschooler age periods.
   b. Give the parents a sample menu for their child's age group and discuss the types and amounts of foods the child requires. See *Appendix vii.*
   c. Reinforce parenting skills which are not related to feeding, e.g., reading to the child.
   d. Encourage parents to provide opportunities for exercise. See *Exercise.*
   e. Teach parents how to decrease caloric intake.
      1. Do not use food as a reward.
      2. Do not put the child to bed with a bottle.
      3. Use a smaller size and/or lower calorie version of sweets, e.g., vanilla wafer instead of cream filled cookie.
      4. Make less seem like more, e.g., five jelly beans instead of one chocolate bar.
      5. Substitute skim milk for whole milk for drinking and cooking.
      6. Provide low calorie snacks, e.g., fruit slices, vegetable sticks.
      7. Increase portions of meat, fruit and vegetables; decrease portions of bread, potatoes, sweets, etc.
6. Assist the obese schoolchild and parents.
   a. Provide a sample menu and discuss the types and amounts of foods the child requires. See *Nutrition.*
   b. Reinforce parenting skills that are not related to feeding, e.g., playing with the child. See *Parenting.*
   c. Involve the child in the planning of the meals. See *Nutrition* and *Appendix vii.*
   d. Discuss the developing of a contract for weight loss that takes into consideration the schoolchild's desire for achievement.
   e. Help the child and parents develop an age-appropriate exercise plan. See *Exercise.*
   f. Tell parents to prepare plates at the kitchen counter rather than the table so additional food is not available.
   g. Encourage the parents to keep nutritious snacks readily available, e.g., vegetable sticks, fruit cubes, peanut butter crackers.
   h. Explain ways in which a diet may be incorporated into the school day and peer activities.
      1. Take a lunch to school rather than buying lunch.
      2. Save some calories allowed for the day and use for an after school snack.
      3. Allow a limited amount of a favorite caloric food, e.g., fill a glass full of ice and then add coke to decrease amount.

4. Help the child learn to select lower calorie foods from a menu, e.g., baked or broiled foods instead of fried, white meat rather than dark meat chicken.
   i. Discuss ways in which the child's self-esteem can be improved.
      1. Praise success with adherence to the diet and ignore failures.
      2. Select clothing which is slimming in appearance, e.g., one-piece dresses, shirts with up and down stripes, small prints, soft or dark colors.
      3. Provide good grooming tips.
   j. Prepare the child and parents for plateaus that develop in a weight loss pattern and encourage the child to stay with the diet so weight loss will continue.
7. Assist the obese adolescent.
   a. Support the adolescent's developmental level by helping him to:
      1. Identify problem areas that lead to overeating.
      2. Set a realistic weight loss goal.
      3. Develop a plan to achieve the goal.
      4. Recognize assistance which may be needed in achieving the goal.
   b. Discuss with parents how they can support the adolescent.
      1. Buy and prepare foods that are lower in calories.
      2. Support success with adherence to the diet and ignore failures.
      3. Avoid comments about the adolescent's weight.
   c. Give the adolescent and/or parents a sample menu and discuss types and amounts of foods required at this age. See *Nutrition.*
   d. Teach the adolescent ways of decreasing caloric intake.
      1. Break old habits, e.g., make only one sandwich at a time instead of two.
      2. Use a smaller plate so the quantity looks bigger.
      3. Remove junk food from the house.
      4. Make a meal and put the food away to avoid making seconds.
      5. Do nothing else while you eat, e.g., turn television off, put book away.
   e. Encourage participation in school sports activities to increase activity. See *Exercise.*
   f. Explain ways in which a diet may be incorporated into the school day and peer activities. See above.
   g. Teach good grooming techniques and selection of clothes that promote a slimmer appearance. See above.
   h. Discuss possible participation in a teenage weight reduction program.

O

i. Support the adolescent in coping with a new body image which may create new social situations, e.g., dating, attention from peers.

Only child. The single child in a family.

A. General Considerations.
1. Each first-born child is an only child until the second child is born.
2. Parents who do not plan to enlarge their family treat the only child differently from parents who plan to have an additional child.
3. Single-child parents need assistance with the unfamiliar aspects of child care.
4. The parents of the only child tend to:
   a. Have more difficulty letting the child enjoy age-appropriate independence, e.g., spending the night at a friend's house.
   b. Expect the child to behave in a more mature way in every situation, e.g., expect adult table manners at every meal.
5. Only children are more likely to have imaginary companions.
6. The adolescent who is an only child will turn to peers and other adults for support just as other adolescents do.
7. The child who is considerably younger than his siblings may be treated by his parents the same way the only child is treated.

B. Nursing Management.
1. Provide the parents with anticipatory guidance about growth and development norms, safety needs, nutrition, etc., since the parent's experience may be limited.
2. Explore ways in which the parents can encourage age-appropriate independence.
   a. Overnight trips with friends or relatives.
   b. Deciding how to spend his allowance.
3. Help parents identify alternatives for peer contact if there are no children in the neighborhood.
   a. The child needs contact with other children; younger, same age, and older.
   b. The child needs friends to help him get to know and understand himself.
4. Discuss how the parents can help the child begin to play with other children if he has had limited peer exposure (Hawke and Knox, 1977).
   a. Have the parent introduce the child to other children.
   b. Invite other children into the child's own home where he is comfortable.
   c. Invite another child to join an outing to a park, movie, museum, etc.
5. Discuss with parents how they can cope with the child's desire for a sibling.

a. Explore with the child why the parents have decided that one child is the best for their family.
b. Reassure the child that the decision not to have another child is not because of dissatisfaction with him.
6. Encourage the parents to develop and maintain their own interests.
7. Assist the parents to view the older child's or teenager's friends as valuable to the child.

Orchiopexy. See *Cryptorchidism.*

Osteochondrosis. See *Legg-Perthes Disease.*

Osteomyelitis. Infection of the bone, usually caused by staphylococci, streptococci, or salmonella.

A. General Considerations.
1. Exogenous osteomyelitis occurs as a result of a penetrating wound or fracture.
   a. Involves one bone and does not metastasize from bone to bone or from bone to another area.
   b. Diagnosis is based on the appearance of the wound.
   c. Antibiotic therapy is necessary.
   d. Adequate wound management will prevent the disease.
2. Hematogenous osteomyelitis is caused by bacteria which enter the bloodstream through skin infections or through the mucous membranes after a nose or throat infection.
   a. The metaphysis of the bone is usually the primary site.
   b. Bone which has been traumatized is more susceptible to infection.
   c. Without treatment, septicemia develops and carries the infection to other bones.
3. Signs and symptoms of the hematogenous type vary with age.
   a. Infant.
      1. Little or no fever.
      2. Irritability.
      3. Reluctance to use the affected limb.
      4. Tenderness.
      5. Swelling.
   b. Children.
      1. Pain at the site.
      2. Refusal to use the limb or to stand.
      3. Septicemia (malaise, fever, anorexia).
      4. Soft-tissue swelling.
      5. Redness and warmth at the site.
4. Pressure from pus formation may cause interference with the blood supply resulting in bone necrosis.

5. A sequestrum may develop when a piece of necrotic bone separates from living bone.
6. X-rays are not helpful until bone destruction has occurred in 5 to 10 days.
7. Bone scans and tomography reveal bone changes at an early stage.
8. Parenteral antibiotic therapy is begun as soon as cultures are obtained by venipuncture or surgical aspiration at the involved site.
9. Parenteral antibiotic therapy may be necessary for as long as 2 to 3 months.
10. After parenteral antibiotic therapy is completed and oral therapy begun, serial blood levels will be drawn until appropriate dosage is determined.
11. Additional treatment measures may include the use of removable splints or traction to reduce pain, to prevent movement which could spread the infection, and to prevent soft tissue contractures.
12. Surgical debridement followed by irrigation of the area may be indicated in some cases.
13. Inappropriate or inadequate treatment and sequestrum development may lead to chronic osteomyelitis.

B. Nursing Management.
1. Support the child and parents during hospitalization. See *Hospitalization, Support During*.
2. Initiate discharge planning. See *Discharge Planning*.
3. Observe, record, and report symptoms that could aid in diagnosis.
4. Prepare the child and parents for procedures. See *Preparation for Procedures*.
   a. Blood and/or wound culture.
   b. Surgical aspiration of fluid for culture.
   c. I.V. therapy.
   d. X-rays.
   e. Bone scan.
   f. Application of splints, traction, or cast. See *Cast Care* and *Traction, Care of Child*.
   g. Surgical drainage.
5. Observe, record, and report the child's response to therapy.
6. Assess the neurovascular status of the limb if the child is immobilized. See *Immobilized Child*.
7. Assess the child's need for pain medication. See *Pain*.
8. Monitor the administration of wound irrigation fluid if ordered.
9. Provide wound care.
   a. Observe, record, and report amount and character of drainage, swelling, heat, and tenderness.
   b. Monitor wound irrigation fluid.

   c. Cleanse, apply ointment, pack and/or dress as ordered.
10. Follow isolation procedures according to hospital policy. See *Isolated Child*.
11. Encourage good nutrition to aid healing. See *Nutrition*.
12. Provide age-appropriate stimulation and diversion. See *Play* and *Stimulation*.
13. Teach the child and parents home management.
    a. Review the administration of oral antibiotics.
    b. Have the parent demonstrate dressing change technique if needed.
    c. Evaluate the older child's ability to use crutches.
    d. Initiate contact with community resources if indicated.
    e. Discuss the need for medical follow-up.

Osteosarcoma (osteogenic sarcoma).
Malignant tumor which affects the metaphyses of a long bone; more common in adolescents.

A. General Considerations.
1. The most common sites are the lower end of the femur, upper end of the tibia, and upper end of the humerus.
2. Symptoms include:
   a. Pain that progresses from intermittent to intense and continuous.
   b. Limitation of joint function as the tumor enlarges.
   c. Warmth and swelling over the tumor site.
   d. Dilatation of veins overlying the tumor site.
3. Diagnostic procedures include bone scan and tomography of the affected bone and the lungs since pulmonary metastasis is common.
4. Pathological fractures may occur as a result of bone invasion by malignant cells.
5. Metastasis may also occur in the other organs and bones.
6. Treatment may include surgical excision of the primary tumor, amputation of the involved extremity, and chemotherapy.
   a. Chemotherapy may involve high doses of methotrexate followed by citrovorum factor rescue.
      1. Side effects from this regimen can be serious or even lethal.
      2. Chemotherapy may be used preoperatively and/or postoperatively.
   b. Femur replacement may be possible if chemotherapy is effective in destroying malignant cells in the affected bone.

7. The adolescent may react to the information that he will undergo amputation by (Ritchie, 1980):
   a. Protesting with anger and denial.
   b. Expecting the stump to be ugly.
   c. Wanting the artificial limb to be identical to his own leg in appearance and function.
   d. Loss of self-esteem and fear of rejection by others.
8. After amputation the adolescent may respond with (Ritchie, 1980):
   a. Grieving over the loss of the limb.
   b. Depression and withdrawal.
   c. Wishing the limb would be returned.
   d. Somatic symptoms of fever, nausea and vomiting, and pain of unknown origin.
   e. Phantom limb pain and other sensations where the limb used to be.

B. Nursing Management. See ADOLESCENT.
1. Support the adolescent and parents during hospitalization. See *Hospitalization, Support During.*
2. Initiate discharge planning. See *Discharge Planning.*
3. Prepare the adolescent and parents for the biopsy of the bone lesion. See *Preparation for Procedures.*
4. Support the adolescent and parents when the diagnosis is made.
   a. Find out what the adolescent and parents have been told about the diagnosis and treatment and record on the Kardex.
   b. Answer all questions honestly.
   c. Use terminology which the adolescent understands.
   d. Arrange for uninterrupted periods of contact with the adolescent and his parents so supportive discussions can be held.
5. Observe, record, and report symptoms of lung metastasis.
   a. Chest pain.
   b. Coughing.
   c. Expectoration of blood.
6. Move the patient carefully to prevent pain and pathological fractures.
7. Supervise the adolescent when ambulating.
   a. Protect from falls.
   b. Report symptoms of a fracture if the adolescent does fall.
8. Meet the needs of the adolescent receiving chemotherapy. See *Chemotherapy.*
9. Meet the needs of the adolescent who requires amputation.
   a. Provide preoperative care. See *Preoperative Care* and *Preparation for Surgery.*
      1. Prepare the adolescent and parents through explanations and interviews.
      2. Provide the adolescent with opportunities to talk with the nurse or doctor when parents are not present.
      3. Anticipate that the adolescent may handle his fears of disfigurement by becoming hostile and uncooperative with the staff.
      4. Involve the adolescent in the decision to amputate.
      5. Tell the adolescent and his parents that a temporary prosthesis will be fitted soon after surgery and the permanent prosthesis will be fitted in 6 to 8 weeks.
   b. Provide postoperative care. See *Postoperative Care.*
      1. Check the stump for bleeding as ordered.
      2. Elevate the stump for the first 24 hours.
      3. Position on the abdomen to prevent hip contractures.
      4. Wrap the stump with a figure 8 bandage as ordered.
      5. Turn the patient frequently without causing indentations on the cast or disturbing the compression bandage depending on which is used.
      6. Administer pain medication as ordered, since the adolescent's phantom pain is indeed a normal phenomenon.
      7. Treat the stump matter-of-factly in order to help the adolescent accept it.
      8. Encourage the adolescent to examine the stump for irritation and breakdown and to bathe it with soap and water daily.
      9. Support the adolescent in exercises for muscle strengthening.
      10. Discuss with the adolescent and his parents how the adolescent will modify clothing, maneuver at school, etc. after discharge.
      11. Teach the adolescent how to use crutches.
10. Meet the needs of the adolescent who requires femur replacement (Staudt, 1975).
    a. Provide preoperative care. See *Preoperative Care* and *Preparation for Surgery.*
       1. Prepare the adolescent and parents through explanations and interviews.
       2. Provide the adolescent with opportunities to talk with the nurse or doctor when parents are not present.
       3. Show the adolescent how to use the trapeze and demonstrate how the linens will be changed postoperatively.
       4. Help the adolescent adjust to the long leg brace that will also be worn after surgery.

b. Provide postoperative care. See *Postoperative Care.*
   1. Maintain the adolescent supine in Trendelenburg position as ordered.
   2. Irrigate the wound with antibiotic solution as ordered.
   3. Maintain the leg in proper alignment, e.g., 30 degree hip rotation and elevated at 45 degrees.
   4. Support the adolescent if exercises are ordered.
   5. Observe for symptoms of fluid loss, e.g., decreased central venous pressure, decreased output, increased urine specific gravity, decreased blood pressure, and increased pulse.
   6. Use sterile technique for wound care as ordered.
   7. Maintain skin integrity.
   8. Help the patient cope with the prolonged immobilization.
   9. Encourage the adolescent to keep up with schoolwork during the recovery period.
11. Help the adolescent cope with body image changes. See *Body Image.*
12. Teach the adolescent and parents home management.
   a. Give written and verbal instructions for medications to be administered at home. See *Administration of Medications, Parental.*
   b. Emphasize the importance of following instructions for outpatient chemotherapy (Rose-Williamson and Rathbun, 1981).
   c. Encourage the parents to make the home life as normal as possible.
      1. Have the adolescent resume normal activities.
      2. Encourage normal peer relationships.
      3. Maintain normal discipline. See *Discipline.*
      4. Encourage adequate rest and nutrition for all family members.
   d. Help the adolescent continue to work through feelings about intrusive procedures, since chemotherapy will continue on an outpatient basis.
13. Assist the adolescent and family to cope with failure to respond to therapy when this happens. See *Dying Child.*

Otitis externa. Inflammation of the skin lining of the ear canals.

   A. **General Considerations.**
      1. Signs and symptoms include:
         a. Pain, especially with movement of the pinna or tragus.
         b. Itching in the ear.
         c. Moist or dry crusting exudate.
         d. Swelling of the ear canal.
         e. Epithelial debris in ear canal.
         f. Bleeding of tissues in ear canal.
      2. Predisposing factors include:
         a. Accumulation of water in the ear from swimming or showers.
         b. Trauma to the ear canal from use of cotton-tipped applicators.
         c. Contact dermatitis as a result of using hair spray, eardrops, and drainage from a ruptured eardrum.
         d. Skin disorders such as seborrhea, eczema, or psoriasis.
      3. Superimposed infection may occur.
      4. Treatment consists of:
         a. Removal of epithelial debris and cerumen.
         b. Use of combined antibiotic-corticosteroid eardrops.
         c. Oral antibiotics for any superimposed infection.
         d. Analgesics until the swelling decreases.
         e. Avoiding swimming until the condition clears up.
      5. Instillation of two to three drops of 1:1 solution of white vinegar/70 percent ethyl alcohol in the child's ear prior to swimming may prevent the condition (Schmitt, 1978).
      6. The child should be examined when swelling decreases to make sure the eardrum is intact.

   B. **Nursing Management.** See *Cerumen.*
      1. Assist with the removal of accumulated ear canal debris.
      2. Teach the child and parents home management.
         a. Administration of eardrops, antibiotics, and analgesics as instructed. See *Administration of Medications, Parental.*
         b. Have the child wear a shower cap in the shower.
         c. Avoid swimming until the condition clears up.
         d. Instill 1:1 drops of white vinegar/70 percent ethyl alcohol as instructed.
         e. Use commercial eardrops, recommended for prevention of otitis externa, after swimming as instructed.
      3. Explain the importance of returning for an examination of the eardrum when the swelling and pain are gone.

Otitis media, acute (suppurative otitis media). Bacterial or viral infection of the middle ear.

   A. **General Considerations.**
      1. The signs and symptoms may be absent or nonspecific and vary among age groups.

2. Signs and symptoms in infants include:
   a. Vomiting.
   b. Diarrhea.
   c. Anorexia.
   d. Irritability.
   e. Cough.
   f. Nasal congestion.
   g. Fever
   h. Red, bulging tympanic membrane.
   i. Sleeping disturbances.
   j. Pulling at ears or tilting of head.
3. Signs and symptoms in the older child include:
   a. Earache.
   b. Fever.
   c. Cough.
   d. Congestion.
   e. Rupture of the eardrum.
   f. Temporary decrease in hearing acuity.
   g. Red, bulging tympanic membrane.
4. Diagnosis may be made on the basis of:
   a. Decreased mobility of the tympanic membrane in response to a pneumatic otoscope, since redness of the eardrum can occur in other conditions.
   b. A flat tympanogram.
   c. Tympanocentesis with culture and sensitivity when:
      1. An infant is under 8 months of age.
      2. A child is immunosuppressed.
      3. Antibiotics are already being given for another infection.
5. Otitis media often occurs as a complication of:
   a. Upper respiratory infections.
   b. Respiratory allergies.
   c. Adenoiditis.
   d. Unrepaired cleft palate.
6. Children are predisposed to otitis media due to:
   a. Short, straight eustachian tubes which lie in a relatively horizontal position.
   b. Obstruction of the opening of the eustachian tube because of the amount of lymphoid tissue in the area.
   c. Their immature immune response.
   d. Pooling of milk in the pharyngeal area when the infant drinks a bottle lying down.
7. Treatment measures include:
   a. Antibiotics for 10 days to 2 weeks.
   b. Comfort measures for fever and pain.
8. Eardrops promote comfort but may not be used, because they prevent a clear view of the eardrum (Whaley and Wong, 1979).
9. Repeated episodes of otitis media may lead to chronic otitis media and serous otitis media. See *Otitis Media, Serous*.
10. Complications include:
    a. Hearing loss.
    b. Mastoiditis (rare).
    c. Meningitis, especially under 4 months of age.
11. The child should be reexamined at the end of antibiotic therapy to assess the:
    a. Response to antibiotics.
    b. Function and appearance of the eardrum.
12. The infant may be hospitalized; the older child is usually managed at home.
13. Myringotomy may be needed in severe and/or unresponsive cases.

B. **Nursing Management.**
1. Support the child and parents during hospitalization. See *Hospitalization, Support During*.
2. Initiate discharge planning. See *Discharge Planning*.
3. Employ comfort measures.
   a. Administer antipyretics and/or analgesics as ordered. See *Fever Reduction*.
   b. Apply heat to ear.
      1. Use a warm water bottle (120°F) wrapped in a towel.
      2. Use a heating pad set on low.
      3. Have the child lie with the affected ear down to facilitate drainage.
   c. Use a covered ice bag if the child prefers, since this reduces edema and pressure.
4. Administer antibiotics as ordered and record response.
5. Provide care for a draining ear.
   a. Wash hands thoroughly.
   b. Use hydrogen peroxide on small cotton balls to remove caked drainage from the external ear.
   c. Insert small wicks of cotton to promote absorption.
      1. Pull the earlobe down and back in the child under age 2.
      2. Pull the earlobe up and back in the child over age 2.
   d. Promote free drainage.
      1. Do not pack ear.
      2. Position the child on side with affected ear down.
   e. Prevent excoriation from drainage by coating the external ear with petroleum jelly or zinc oxide ointment.
6. Observe, record, and report:
   a. Pain behind the ear.
   b. Increased fever.
   c. Increased irritability.
   d. Lethargy.
   e. Stiff neck.
7. Teach parents home management of the child who is not hospitalized. See *Home Management of Minor Illnesses*.
   a. Employ comfort measures.
   b. Clean drainage from ear.

c. Give medications as ordered. See *Administration of Medications, Parental.*

d. Explain the importance of giving all the medication even though the child usually seems better in 24 to 48 hours after therapy is begun.

e. Teach parents to call the physician promptly if the child does not respond to therapy within 48 hours, e.g., still has fever, pain, and/or purulent drainage.

f. Schedule follow-up examination to determine if infection has responded to therapy and prevent the development of serous otitis media.

Otitis media, serous. A sterile effusion which develops as a result of failure of the eustachian tube to open and close normally in order to equalize middle ear and external barometric pressure.

A. General Considerations.
1. Signs and symptoms include:
   a. Feeling of "fullness" in the ear.
   b. Popping sensation in the ear when swallowing.
   c. Sensation of movement in the ear if air is present above the fluid level.
   d. Decreased hearing.
2. Severe pain, fever, and an appearance of illness are absent.
3. Diagnosis is made on the basis of:
   a. Decreased mobility of the eardrum in response to testing with a pneumatic otoscope.
   b. The dull gray appearance of the eardrum.
   c. A visible fluid level behind the drum if air is present above the fluid.

4. The following conditions predispose the child to abnormal eustachian tube function.
   a. Acute otitis media.
   b. Allergic exudate.
   c. Adenoidal enlargement.
   d. Propping the baby's bottle. See *Nursing Bottle Syndrome.*
   e. Cleft palate.
   f. Cystic fibrosis.
5. Treatment is aimed at restoring aeration of the middle ear and may be done by the use of:
   a. Conservative measures.
      1. Teaching the older child to "pop" his ears to promote autoinflation of the eustachian tube.
      2. Having the child chew chewing gum (sugarless) to promote equalization of pressure.
      3. A trial of antihistamines and/or decongestants may be used but is often ineffective.
   b. Surgical procedures.
      1. Adenoidectomy if the adenoids are markedly enlarged.
      2. Myringotomy with the insertion of polyethylene tubes to promote aeration and drainage.
   c. Desensitization program for the allergic child.
6. Conservative measures will be tried for varying lengths of time before myringotomy is done.
7. Many children show spontaneous improvement.
8. The fluid may become very thick and opaque; this condition is referred to as "glue ear."
9. Periodic hearing screening should be done since hearing loss may occur.

Pain. Uncomfortable sensations resulting from stimulation of nerve endings.

A. General Considerations.
1. The child often has difficulty in localizing and/or describing pain.
2. It is possible that pain perception begins in the neonate even if myelinization is incomplete.
3. Nursing observations and accurate descrip-

tions of pain may be helpful in diagnosing illness.
4. Nurses should not hesitate to administer pain medication even to the infant or young child if an adult would be medicated in the same circumstances.
5. Anger, fear, loneliness, and anxiety are factors that influence pain and affect the child's behavioral response to pain.
6. The child may cry and express pain when par-

ents arrive because he now feels it is safe to tell them it hurts (McGuire and Dizard, 1982).

7. Fear of abandonment, separation, death, or the unknown may be interpreted as pain by the child.

8. The child's perception of pain is influenced by degree of fatigue, environmental stress, and his developmental level.

9. The child who observes adult role models overreact to pain may also be hypersensitive to pain.

10. Boys may try to appear "brave" and complain less about pain because some parents and society expect the male child to repress emotion.

11. The older schoolchild may exaggerate pain while boasting of scratches and bruises.

12. Cultural and ethnic background will influence the intensity with which the child expresses pain.

13. The older child who chronically complains of pain may be signalling that he is under severe environmental stress, needs parental attention, or cannot cope with his problems.

14. Adolescents may develop functional pain in response to developmental stresses.
    a. Descriptions of pain are vague.
    b. Associated or precipitating events are not identified.
    c. Descriptions of severity of the pain are inconsistent with the teenager's participation in school and peer activities.
    d. Information that the problem is not serious and diagnostic tests are not required does not reassure the adolescent.

15. Children with chronic pain may not be taken seriously until behavior and school performance are adversely affected.

16. Relaxation techniques or behavioral modification may be effective even in the young child.

17. Treatment for chronic pain may include:
    a. Psychotropic drugs to decrease pain, induce sleep, and relieve depression.
    b. Neuroaugmentation with transcutaneous stimulator (TENS unit) to stimulate normal nerve or nerve pathways and to prevent painful signals from reaching the conscious level.
    c. Stimulation of peripheral nerves through a needle electrode placed through the skin.

B. **Nursing Management.** See HOSPITALIZATION, SUPPORT DURING.
    1. Observe, record, and report nonverbal cues that the child is in pain so other personnel will recognize the reason for his behavior.
        a. Crying.
        b. Restlessness.
        c. Irritability.
        d. Anorexia.
        e. Insomnia.
        f. Perspiration.
        g. Shallow respirations.
        h. Refusal to move.
        i. Rigid body movements.
        j. Grimaces.
        k. Refusal to talk.
        l. Aggressive behavior.
        m. Dependent behavior.
    2. Use an assessment tool to help the young child communicate the presence of pain (Eland, 1983).
        a. Have the child indicate on a body outline where it hurts.
        b. Give the child four different colored objects, tell which color indicates a little hurt, more hurt, yet more hurt, and the most hurt.
        c. Have the child choose whichever color(s) he needs to indicate his hurt.
    3. Reduce fear that may intensify the child's perception of pain. See *Fears*.
        a. Encourage parents or parent-substitute to participate actively in the child's care.
        b. Explain all procedures at the child's developmental level. See *Preparation for Procedures*.
        c. Reassure the preschool child that illness is not a punishment for behavior.
        d. Provide as much consistency as possible in assignment of personnel.
        e. Follow home routines as much as possible.
        f. Provide the young child with opportunities for therapeutic play. See *Play, Therapeutic*.
        g. Help the schoolchild and adolescent to maintain control while supporting expression of feelings and concerns.
    4. Discuss with the parents how the child usually indicates pain and record on the Kardex.
    5. Elicit a description and location of the pain if the child is old enough to verbalize this information.
    6. Observe touching, rubbing, or guarding of a body part that may indicate the site of the child's pain.
    7. Let the child know you can and will relieve the pain.
    8. Consider other causative factors as well as pain when assessing the need to administer medication.
        a. Has the child just been left alone by parents or other visitors?
        b. Does the child need to void?
        c. Is the child frightened by events in the room or on the unit?
        d. Is the child tired?

e. Is the child bored?

9. Medicate the child early once you have observed the child's pain and tell the child that the medication will help him feel better.

10. Request an order for oral medication, if possible, since the child may fear injections so much that pain is denied.

11. Do not let the child talk you out of giving an I.M. medication when you have assessed that he needs pain relief. See *Appendix iii, Table 4.*

12. Provide other nondrug methods of pain relief.
    a. Offer toys and activities for distraction. See *Play* and *Toys.*
    b. Provide a massage of the painful area, if appropriate.
    c. Apply a warm or cool cloth to the forehead or affected body part if appropriate.
    d. Reposition the child.
    e. Help the child relax (McCaffrey, 1977).
       1. Demonstrate to the child how to take a deep breath and go limp as he exhales.
       2. Ask the child to yawn.
       3. Repeat the request until the child relaxes.

13. Ask the older child what will make him or her more comfortable.

14. Verbalize for the schoolage child and adolescent that you think he is in pain and offer support and pain relief.

15. Make the environment conducive to rest by turning off lights, darkening the room, etc.

16. Teach rhythmic breathing to the child for relaxation (McCaffrey, 1977).
    a. Have the child take a breath and say "ha" on exhalation.
    b. Have the child take another breath and say "who" on exhalation.
    c. Decrease or increase the rate of the breathing according to the intensity of the pain.
    d. Add rhythmic rubbing of the body part to the breathing to increase relaxation.

17. Teach more complex relaxation techniques to the older child with chronic pain (McCaffrey, 1977).
    a. Position the child with a pillow under the neck and a pillow under the knees to prevent hyperextension during relaxation.
    b. Have the child stare at an object or imagine a pleasant scene.
    c. Tell the child to deep breathe, tense the muscles, exhale, and then go limp.
    d. Test the body parts for relaxation by moving the extremities slowly and gently at the joints.

18. Help the child cope with painful procedures which must be implemented frequently and/or over a prolonged period of time (desensitization) (McCaffrey, 1977).
    a. Rank each aspect of the procedure from the least anxiety producing to the most anxiety producing.
    b. Provide a pleasant environment for the child.
    c. Discuss and/or demonstrate the least frightening aspect of the procedure to the child.
    d. Continue to introduce additional stimuli until the child begins to show fear.
    e. Reintroduce the nonfearful stimuli.
    f. Repeat the process the next day or so according to the child's tolerance.

19. Use the "fade-in" technique if desensitization is ineffective (McCaffrey, 1977).
    a. Provide a pleasant environment for the child.
    b. Discuss the painful procedure with the child.
    c. Place the equipment used in the procedure outside the room, but within the child's sight or on the opposite side of the room from the child.
    d. Move the equipment closer and closer until the child becomes frightened.
    e. Later reintroduce the equipment moving it slowly closer until the child is able to handle the equipment beginning with the least threatening object.

20. Encourage the child to participate in activities of daily living and peer relationships so he or she feels more positive about being "well."

21. Reinforce instructions for the child with chronic pain and his parents when a TENS (transcutaneous electrical nerve stimulator) is prescribed (Meyer, 1982).
    a. Place electrodes correctly.
    b. Use appropriate coupling agent.
    c. Adjust setting as instructed.
    d. Replace batteries as needed.
    e. Observe for and treat skin irritations.

Palate, cleft. See *Cleft Palate.*

Palsy, cerebral. See *Cerebral Palsy.*

Parenteral nutrition. See *Total Parenteral Nutrition.*

Parenting. The use of specific skills and behaviors in supporting the child's development. See ADOPTION, SINGLE-PARENT FAMILIES, and WORKING MOTHER.

A. General Considerations.
   1. Successful achievement of parental tasks is

more likely if the parents understand their own:
   a. Values.
   b. Problems.
   c. Conflicts.
   d. Patterns of adaptation.
2. Developmental tasks for parents correspond to the different developmental levels of the child.
   a. Parents of the infant must learn their child's cues, how to respond appropriately to these cues, and how to provide age-appropriate developmental stimulation.
   b. Parents of the toddler must learn how to accept and support the child's independent behavior, promote training habits, encourage speech, and promote socialization.
   c. Parents of the preschooler must learn to separate themselves from the child, set limits which foster security, and continue to foster learning.
   d. Parents of the schoolchild must learn how to support their child's sense of industry, provide a role model for appropriate behavior, help the child adjust to the larger world, and support the development of more complex cognitive skills.
   e. Parents of the adolescent must learn to restructure their lives independent of the child, provide support to the child in achieving his or her own personal identity, set limits and standards, and remember how difficult it is for adolescents to establish their own identity.
3. Parenting skills associated with the developmental tasks include:
   a. Interpreting the child's cues correctly.
   b. Responding to the child's needs.
      1. As they arise.
      2. In an appropriate manner.
      3. On a consistent basis.
   c. Meeting the child's physical needs for:
      1. Food. See *Nutrition*.
      2. Rest and exercise. See *Exercise* and *Sleep*.
      3. Safety. See *Accident Prevention*.
      4. Hygienic care.
      5. Shelter.
   d. Meeting the child's psychological needs for:
      1. Love.
      2. Security.
      3. Self-esteem.
      4. Stimulation. See *Stimulation*.
   e. Meeting the child's need for health promotion and maintenance. See *Dental Care, Health Promotion and Maintenance, Immunization, Well-child Care*.
4. The bond between parents and child, especially the mother and child, is established in the first couple of months of life, and failure to bond with the child interferes with the later parent–child relationship.
5. Parenting behaviors tend to be learned from one's own parents, since society provides little formal education for parenting
6. Tradition, rather than rational planning, tends to determine how parents fulfill their roles.
7. There are three major parenting styles (Whaley and Wong, 1983).
   a. Authoritarian or dictatorial parents demand unquestioning obedience and specific behaviors.
   b. Laissez-faire or permissive parents exert little or no control over the child and have few expectations.
   c. Authoritative or democratic parents set consistent limits for the child, expect the child to behave, and employ discipline but also respect the child's individuality and include the child in family decision making.
8. Most families exhibit characteristics of more than one of the parenting styles, but the authoritative/democratic form is considered most conducive to a good parent–child relationship.
9. Families in which both parents have the same or similar parenting styles tend to have less parent–child conflict.
10. The parent–child relationship is greatly influenced by the:
   a. Birth order of the child in the family.
   b. Sex of the child.
   c. Overall acceptance of the child.
   d. Disciplinary orientation of the parents, e.g., parents may expect more from an oldest child or permit a youngest child to remain a "baby" longer.
11. Inadequate parenting may lead to failure to thrive or child abuse. Signs include (See *Child Abuse* and *Failure to Thrive*):
   a. Failure to claim the child as one's own, e.g., not naming, refusal to hold.
   b. Seeing the child as a disappointment, e.g., wrong sex, or revolting, e.g., bad smelling.
   c. Failure to protect the child from injury.
   d. A mechanical approach to care in which the mother does not smile, talk to, or make eye contact with the child.
   e. Hygienic neglect, e.g., crusted hair, dirty skin.
   f. Inability to set any limits on the child's behavior.
   g. Too early and/or inappropriate discipline measures, e.g., using a paddle on a young infant.
   h. Too little or too much stimulation, e.g., parent never plays with the child; parent

P

continues to bounce, tickle, etc. child long after child asks to stop.

12. Parents whose own needs are being met will be better able to meet the needs of their child.

13. Adolescents who become parents are often in the midst of completing the developmental tasks associated with this period and may be overwhelmed by the demands of parenthood.

B. Nursing Management.

1. Discuss the concept of parental development tasks with parents, since many parents are unaware that these tasks exist.

2. Reinforce positive parenting skills and behaviors by telling parents that they are doing a good job.

3. Support the development of parent–child bonding in the newborn period.
   a. Encourage the parents to be involved in the care of their child.
   b. Point out positive aspects of the infant.
   c. Provide assistance as needed but do not act as an authority figure.

4. Give parents some examples of specific things they can do in order to master their development tasks when their child is a(an):
   a. Infant.
      1. Listen to the infant's cry and begin to associate it with being hungry, sleepy, etc.
      2. Provide appropriate physical care. See *Infant* and *Neonate.*
      3. Provide appropriate psychological care.
      4. Respond quickly to the infant's needs so the child develops a sense of trust.
   b. Toddler.
      1. Give the child an opportunity to make simple choices, e.g., Do you want a peanut butter or cheese sandwich?
      2. Provide the child with a safe, explorable environment. See *Accident Prevention.*
      3. Respond to temper tantrums appropriately. See *Discipline* and *Temper Tantrums.*
      4. Provide appropriate physical and psychological care. See *Toddler.*
   c. Preschooler.
      1. Permit increasing freedom of choice and opportunities to learn about the environment.
      2. Provide appropriate physical and psychological care. See *Preschooler.*
      3. Employ consistent limit setting. See *Discipline.*
   d. Schoolchild.
      1. Provide the child with tasks that can be completed.
      2. Praise the child for accomplishments.

3. Provide appropriate physical and psychological care. See *Schoolchild.*
   e. Adolescent.
      1. Permit the adolescent to have privacy.
      2. Support the adolescent in developing personal goals.
      3. Accept the adolescent's desire for peer rather than family activities.
      4. Develop more individual or couple activities with other adults so that they have their own lives separate from their child's.

5. Support parents in meeting their own needs so that they will be more able to meet the needs of their children.
   a. Adequate rest.
   b. Proper nutrition.
   c. Exercise.
   d. Diversionary activities.
   e. Contact with other adults.
   f. Opportunities to verbalize their feelings.
   g. Opportunities to pursue personal goals.

6. Observe the parent–child relationship for signs of conflict and intervene appropriately.
   a. Do not side with either the parents or the child.
   b. Be willing to serve as a neutral sounding board for thoughts of both parents and child.
   c. Discuss with the parents and child developmental tasks for the specific age period.
   d. Discuss with the parents that conflict is reduced by:
      1. Use of the authoritative or democratic style of parenting.
      2. The use of a consistent approach by both parents.
   e. Initiate a referral for counseling as indicated.

7. Assess for signs of inadequate parenting and intervene appropriately.
   a. Avoid making judgmental statements or comparing the parents to other parents in an unfavorable manner.
   b. Teach or refer parents of infants to classes on parenting given by such groups as the YMCA/YWCA, churches, or United Way Organization in the town.
   c. Initiate a referral to a social service worker for follow-up care.

8. Meet the special needs of adolescent parents (Mercer, 1979):
   a. Provide support in helping them achieve their own developmental tasks. See *Adolescent.*
   b. Support them in recognizing responses to parenting that are common to all parents, e.g., fatigue, disorganization.
   c. Assist them in identifying experiences they

P

have had that contribute to developing parenting skills, e.g., coping with a younger sibling, babysitting.

d. Help them locate resource persons and groups, e.g., parenting classes at YMCA/YWCA, college or university child development centers. See *National Resources* (p. 321).

e. Identify individuals who can serve as role models for adolescent parents and involve them in an interdisciplinary approach to care, e.g., teacher, clinic nurse, social worker.

f. Support them in meeting their own and their infant's health care needs (the adolescent should be seen by a separate health care provider).

g. Serve as an advocate for the child; do not take sides in conflicts between the adolescent parents and their parents.

Parotitis. See *Mumps.*

Patent ductus arteriosus. See *Congenital Heart Disease.*

Pediculosis. Disease caused by infestation of lice.

A. General Considerations.
1. Lice may infest the head (pediculosis capitas), the body (pediculosis corporis), and/or pubic hair (pediculosis pubis).
2. Signs and symptoms include:
   a. Pinpoint erythematous lesions at feeding sites.
   b. Itching.
   c. Excoriated skin and bloody crusts due to scratching.
   d. Swollen lymph nodes near infestation sites.
   e. Small, white, tenacious flecks along hair shafts which are the ova (nits).
3. Lice are easily spread from person to person and fomite spread is possible.
4. Body lice frequently live in clothing seams, moving to the body only to feed.
5. Secondary infection from scratching is a common complication (impetigo is most common).
6. Treatment includes the use of medicated shampoos, creams, or body lotion; removal of nits by combing with a fine tooth comb; and washing in washing machine set on hot cycle or dry cleaning of personal items such as combs, brushes, hats, bedclothes, etc.
7. Treatment medications include one of the following substances:
   a. Lindane: safe if used only once or twice; is absorbed through the skin and may cause nausea, vomiting, or blood dyscrasias.

b. Malathion: may cause mild scalp irritation.
c. Pyrethrin: may cause allergic reactions and dermatitis.

B. Nursing Management.
1. Be nonjudgmental in your approach, since anyone may develop pediculosis.
2. Teach child and parents.
   a. Use medicated shampoo, cream, or lotion as instructed.
   b. Comb hair with fine tooth comb to remove nits.
   c. Launder all personal items.
   d. Iron clothing seams on child's clothing.
   e. Use a lice control spray on carpets, mattresses, and other nonwashable items, and air the room before reoccupying.
   f. Keep the child out of school until treated.
   g. Use a soothing lotion to reduce itching.
3. Prevent the transmission of lice.
   a. Teach the child not to exchange personal items such as towels, combs, or hats with other children.
   b. Wear gloves or use tongue depressors to inspect child for lice since they are easily picked up under the fingernails.
4. Tell the parents to call the physician if the child shows signs of a secondary infection.

Perthe's disease. See *Legg–Perthe's Disease.*

Petit mal seizures. See *Seizures.*

Pharyngitis, streptococcal (strep throat). Group A beta hemolytic streptococcal infection of the pharynx.

A. General Considerations.
1. Signs and symptoms include:
   a. Sore throat, possibly accompanied by difficulty swallowing.
   b. Nausea.
   c. Vomiting.
   d. Abdominal pain.
   e. Headache.
   f. Bright red, enlarged tonsils that develop white or yellow exudate.
   g. Enlarged cervical lymph nodes.
   h. A scarlatinaform rash which feels like sandpaper and peels in 1 week.
2. Positive diagnosis is difficult (Sloane, 1982).
   a. A positive culture may occur in a child who is a carrier and whose symptoms are the result of other causes.
   b. False negative cultures may result from poor culture plating procedures.

3. Throat cultures can be read after 24 hours (provisional reading) and 48 hours (final report).
4. Complications from the spread of infection include:
   a. Peritonsillar abscess.
   b. Otitis media.
   c. Sinusitis.
   d. Cervical adenitis.
5. Rheumatic fever or acute glomerulonephritis may result from an altered immune response to certain strains of group A beta hemolytic streptococci.
6. Treatment with penicillin, or erythromycin if the child is allergic to penicillin, for at least 10 days eliminates streptococci and prevents rheumatic fever and acute glomerulonephritis.

B. **Nursing Management.**
1. Obtain throat culture as ordered.
   a. Explain the procedure to the child and parents. See *Preparation for Procedures.*
   b. Collect culture specimen.
      1. Have child stick out tongue and pant in order to expose posterior pharynx.
      2. Use sterile swab and rub posterior pharynx, tonsillar area, and exudative spots.
   c. Streak the plate as directed.
2. Teach child and parents home management.
   a. Adhere to the medication regimen.
      1. Teach parents administration of medication. See *Administration of Medications, Parental.*
      2. Explain possible consequences if full course of medication is not given.
   b. Teach comfort measures for sore throat.
      1. Use warm saline gargles.
      2. Apply warm or cold compresses to the neck.
      3. Run cold mist vaporizer.
      4. Give aspirin as ordered. See *Administration of Medications, Parental.*
      5. Have the child chew gum, since swallowing increases circulation which promotes healing.
      6. Give cold, bland liquids to drink.
      7. Do not give citrus juices.
   c. Encourage bedrest or quiet activities during acute stage.
      1. Read to the child or play records.
      2. Fill cardboard box with variety of small toys to be used in bed.
      3. Play board games with the child, e.g., checkers, Scrabble.
   d. Call the physician if the following occur:
      1. Increasing difficulty swallowing.
      2. Severe ear pain.
      3. Marked swelling of the cervical lymph nodes.
      4. Sudden increase in temperature.

3. Manage child in hospital who has a strep throat.
   a. Isolate from other children on unit. See *Isolated Child.*
   b. Employ good handwashing technique.
   c. Dispose of waste contaminated with respiratory secretions in appropriate manner.

Pharyngitis, viral. Sore throat due to a viral infection.

A. **General Considerations.**
1. Usually occurs during the course of a cold. See *Colds.*
2. Signs and symptoms include:
   a. Localized soreness in throat.
   b. Rhinorrhea.
   c. Low grade fever.
   d. Increased pink color of throat on observation.
   e. Vesicles and/or ulcerations on throat.
   f. Pain on swallowing.
   g. Tender cervical lymph nodes.
3. It can be difficult to differentiate a viral from a streptococcal sore throat and a throat culture may be necessary.
4. Treatment is completely symptomatic and can be managed at home.
5. Antibiotics are ineffective in treating a viral sore throat.

B. **Nursing Management.** See *Home Management of Minor Illnesses.*
1. Teach parents.
   a. Soothe sore throat.
      1. Offer cool, clear liquids.
      2. Do not give citrus juices.
      3. Have older child use salt water gargles.
      4. Give younger child hard candy to suck.
      5. Administer analgesic as ordered. See *Administration of Medications, Parental.*
   b. Give antipyretic as ordered for temperature elevation.
   c. Provide quiet diversional activities for the child to promote rest.
2. Tell parents to call physician if there is:
   a. Sudden rise in temperature.
   b. Increased soreness in throat.
   c. Vomiting.

Phobia, school. See *School Phobia.*

Pica. Eating of any unnatural material.

A. **General Considerations.**
1. Pica must be differentiated from the normal characteristic of infants and young children to explore objects with their mouths.

P

2. Pica is more commonly found in:
   a. Mentally retarded children who may be unable to differentiate edible and inedible materials.
   b. Maternally deprived children who need increased oral gratification.
   c. Children whose diets are deficient in iron and vitamin C.
   d. Pregnant adolescents.
   e. Children whose families are experiencing acute or chronic stress.
3. Pica may result in problems for the child.
   a. Lead poisoning.
   b. Visceral larval migrans (infection with the larvae of cat or dog roundworms).

B. **Nursing Management.** See ACCIDENT PREVENTION and LEAD POISONING.
   1. Provide the older infant and toddler with finger foods such as crackers, cooked carrots, or pieces of cheese to meet the child's need for biting and chewing.
   2. Observe the parent–child interaction. See *Parenting.*
      a. Does the parent use formula or food as the only comfort measure?
      b. Does the parent stimulate the infant/child by talking, touching or providing toys? See *Stimulation.*
   3. Provide anticipatory guidance for the parent about normal growth and development, safety, and nutrition as needed.
   4. Assess the child's nutrition intake if height and weight are below normal.
      a. Discuss how the parent can provide the child with an adequate diet within budget restraints.
      b. Refer to community agencies for financial assistance if needed.
   5. Discuss the safety precautions necessary for the protection of the retarded child, e.g., empty ashtrays, remove plants from tables, supervise use of crayons, etc.
   6. Explore the pregnant adolescent's knowledge of what foods are essential to her own health and that of the baby.
   7. Talk with parents about the hazards of lead painted objects and animal feces.
   8. Refer to community health nurse or other agency for assistance with problems creating family stress, e.g., housing, inadequate food, birth of a sibling, etc.

P

Pigeon-toe. Toeing-in.

A. **General Considerations.**
   1. Causes include:
      a. Adduction of the forefoot (metatarsus adductus).
      b. Bowing of the tibia (inward tibial torsion).
      c. Bowing of the femur (femoral torsion).
   2. Bowing of the tibia requires no treatment.
   3. Bowing of the femur occasionally requires surgery for cosmetic purposes.
   4. The foot cannot be passively placed in a normal position if adduction of the forefoot is present.
   5. Treatment of adduction of the forefoot should begin when the child starts to walk.
      a. Passive stretching exercises.
      b. Corrective shoes.
      c. Denis-Browne splints.
      d. Casting.
   6. Adduction of the forefoot may be associated with congenital hip dysplasia.
   7. The prognosis is excellent.

B. **Nursing Management.**
   1. Reassure the parents that bowing of the tibia will correct itself spontaneously with growth.
   2. Discuss with the parents that bowing of the femur usually will be compensated for by outward tibial torsion as the child grows.
   3. Teach the parents home management of adduction of the forefoot.
      a. Have the parents return the demonstration of the stretching exercises.
      b. Explain the use of the Denis–Browne splints.
         1. Apply the splints for sleep only, unless instructed otherwise by the physician.
         2. Protect the infant's feet with socks.
         3. Observe the feet for swelling, irritation, or discoloration.
         4. Instruct the parents not to reposition the shoes on the bar.
         5. Show the parents how to tighten the shoes against the bar with a splint key.
      c. Teach the parents to care for the child in a cast. See *Cast Care.*
         1. Report coldness, blueness, or pallor in the toes.
         2. Use the open palms to move the wet cast, since finger indentations cause pressure points.
         3. Petal the edges of the cast with waterproof adhesive.
         4. Sponge bathe the child daily.
         5. Encourage the parents to provide age-appropriate stimulation. See *Stimulation.*

Pink eye. See *Conjunctivitis.*

Pinworm. See *Worms.*

Play. Activity in which the child is free to do what he or she wants because he or she enjoys doing it.

A. **General Considerations.**
  1. Play is important in promoting all aspects of the child's development.
  2. Play behavior tends to change in fairly predictable patterns.
    a. Infant play is primarily exploratory as the baby learns about his body and about his environment.
      1. Exploring fingers and toes.
      2. Manipulation of objects.
      3. Interactions with parents and other people.
    b. Toddler play is exploratory in a more diverse and complex way.
      1. Exploring the home environment.
      2. Exploring materials such as water, sand, and clay that appeal to the senses.
      3. Separation from parents and independent exploration.
      4. Controlling the environment by destruction of block towers, sand castles, etc.
      5. Practicing motor skills.
    c. Preschool play moves toward socially oriented activities, imitation of adult activities, and refinement of motor and intellectual skills.
      1. Use of play materials alone or with groups of children.
      2. Playing grown-up roles.
      3. Large muscle activities such as climbing or riding wheeled toys.
      4. Small muscle activities such as puzzles or crayons.
      5. Activities that involve discrimination of shape, form, color, texture, etc.
    d. Schoolage play is characterized by increased physical activity, games with rules, and gang play.
      1. Advanced motor activities such as roller skating, rope skipping, and team sports.
      2. Cooperative games such as hide and seek, tag, and hopscotch.
      3. "Secret" clubs or organizations with same-sex peers.
    e. Adolescents move toward recreational activities and hobbies with peers of both sexes.
  3. Solitary play in which the toddler or young preschool child uses materials alone is sometimes interpreted as a less mature form of play.
  4. Solitary play that is educational or goal-directed in nature may, in fact, be more mature than parallel play which involves playing with another child.
  5. The child moves from parallel and/or solitary play to associative play in which there is sharing of toys.

  6. Cooperative play is characteristic of older preschool children who are given specific "tasks" by one or more leaders of the play group.
  7. Dramatic play is also characteristic of older preschoolers who reenact adult roles in home, job, and recreation.
  8. The number of props, e.g., cowboy hat and guns, the child needs to play a role is greater in the young preschooler.
  9. The young schoolchild has difficulty accepting rules and may want to change the guidelines during the course of the game or activity.
  10. Play is important for the hospitalized child because it is a normal part of the child's life.
    a. Play keeps the child from becoming bored.
    b. Play allows the child to cope with the stress and trauma of hospitalization.
    c. The child can learn about nursing and medical procedures through play.
  11. The child needs a balance between passive play such as watching television, reading, etc. and active play that involves motor activity.
  12. The child who is extremely anxious may not be able to play.
  13. Play activities should be part of the planned nursing care for every hospitalized child.
  14. A playroom or cart with play materials is an essential part of the pediatric unit.
  15. The child will be inhibited in play if the emphasis is on keeping the playroom neat and clean.
  16. Observation of the child's play can be helpful in understanding his perception of what is happening to him.

B. **Nursing Management.**
  1. Plan play activities which consider the child's:
    a. Age.
    b. Developmental level.
    c. Interests.
    d. Diagnosis.
    e. Limitations caused by stress and illness.
    f. Safety.
  2. Encourage the parents to bring in toys and play materials from home if the hospital supplies are inappropriate or inadequate for the child's needs.
  3. Play for the child who is unable to play for physical reasons, e.g., the burned child.
  4. Let the child know in advance when the play period will end.
  5. Arrange for peers to participate in activities with the child if possible.
  6. Provide activities that facilitate expressions of feelings and creativity.
    a. Art media, e.g., fingerpaints, clay, play dough.
    b. Music.
    c. Puppets.

d. Aggressive toys, e.g., pounding boards, bean bags.

7. Provide activities that use large muscles.
   a. Riding tricycles, wagons, and carts.
   b. Exercises in the physical therapy department.
   c. Walks outside the hospital.

8. Provide activities that use small muscles.
   a. Making jig-saw puzzles.
   b. Beads to string.
   c. Blocks.
   d. Art work.
   e. Craft activities.

9. Provide board games and short-term projects for the schoolchild and adolescent.
   a. Alter the rules as necessary to involve children of varying intellectual and/or physical skills.
   b. Emphasize the benefits of playing the game rather than winning.
   c. Provide arts and craft activities which the child can give to others.

10. Use the play kit when preparing the child for a procedure or allowing the child to work through his feelings about a procedure. See *Play, Therapeutic.*

11. Observe, record, and report the child's response to play.
    a. Can the child use the opportunities to play or is the anxiety level too high?
    b. Does the child play with younger, same age, or older children?
    c. Does the child select activities or toys that are developmentally appropriate?
    d. Is the child relaxed and at ease during play?
    e. Is the child's play different from that described by parents or noted earlier during hospitalization?

12. Discuss with parents how they can facilitate the child's play at home.
    a. Provide indoor and outdoor space for play even though this may necessitate some changes in the "neat" appearance of the home.
    b. Arrange for peer contact for the child of toddler age or older.
    c. Provide play activities and toys that are appropriate to the child's developmental level and that allow the child to be creative.
    d. Provide a selection of less expensive play materials rather than a limited amount of costly materials, since the young child needs variety.
    e. Alternate periods of active outdoor and quieter indoor play.
    f. Allow the child to decide how he or she wants to use the play materials even if this

differs from the instructions or the adult's expectations.

g. Recognize that the child may knock down the tower of blocks or paint streaks on the newest picture just to experience the sensation.

h. Join the child's play, but avoid competing, since the adult is able to color better, make better clay figures, etc., and this lowers the child's self-esteem.

i. Give the child advance notice that play time will soon end because of meals, bedtime, etc.

j. Provide the child with a balance between educationally oriented and "free" play time.

Play, therapeutic. Provision of toys and materials that help the child work through feelings concerning hospitalization experiences.

A. **General Considerations.**

1. Therapeutic play helps the nurse to understand the child's fears and concerns so the nursing care plan can be revised appropriately.

2. The role of the nurse is to provide the play materials for the child and to observe the child's behavior, but not to interpret the behavior to the child.

3. Therapeutic play is used primarily with preschoolers, but some schoolchildren will be willing to overcome their resistance to playing with "dolls" and use the play kit constructively.

4. The ideal situation is the availability of a play kit and a quiet room off the unit for the child and the nurse.

5. The play kit should consist of a variety of toys and materials.
   a. Aggressive toys—guns, drum.
   b. Regressive toys—stuffed animals, baby bottle.
   c. Family dolls or puppets—parent and child figures appropriate to the child's family and racial characteristics.
   d. Hospital dolls or puppets—doctor and nurse dolls.
   e. Hospital equipment—syringes, bandages, I.V. tubing, etc., appropriate to the child's condition.
   f. Safe materials—paper, crayons, finger paints, toy telephone.

6. The child will feel more free to express his concerns and feelings if parents are not present during the play sessions.

7. The child may be so anxious initially that he

or she is unable to play with hospital equipment or the nurse and doctor dolls.

8. The toddler may use pretend telephone conversations to describe concerns that he or she could not express directly to the nurse.

9. Drawings, storytelling, and story completion can also be useful ways for the preschooler or schoolchild to express feelings.

10. Providing the child with toys and materials from the play kit list to help express feelings is valuable even if a "play kit" does not exist.

11. Therapeutic play can also be used with groups of children and parents in a playroom situation to:
    a. Teach the child about procedures or surgery.
    b. Clarify the child's misunderstandings about procedures and surgery.
    c. Give parents the same information the child receives.

12. Therapeutic play must be distinguished from play therapy that is a psychiatric technique used with emotionally disturbed children to help them gain insight into their behavior.

B. Nursing Management.

1. Explain to the parents that playing with the toys and materials in the play kit will help the child cope with what is happening in the hospital.

2. Tell the child you have some special toys that he or she can play with.

3. Provide as much privacy for the child as possible during the play session, e.g., pull the curtain or shut the door if the child's room is used.

4. Allow the child to select those toys or materials with which he or she feels able to play.

5. Permit the child to use the toys or materials in a way which is not physically harmful to the child or to the nurse.

6. Observe the toys or materials the child selects and how he or she chooses to play with them.

7. Comment on the child's play only if he or she indicates the need by asking a question or telling something.

8. Participate in the child's play only if asked to manipulate one of the dolls or puppets; do not ask if he or she wants you to do so.

9. Record the child's needs for new or corrected information on the Kardex.

10. Observe the child's behavior at other times to see if there is consistency in the expressed interests or concerns.

11. Plan a later time to explain gaps or misunderstandings in the child's information about hospitalization, procedures, and/or surgery.

12. Continue to observe and record the child's behavior as a method of evaluating the effectiveness of the play in reducing the child's anxiety.

13. Initiate referrals to other health professionals if the child's play indicates intense death and/or mutilation fears that cannot be relieved through play sessions or giving the child additional information.

Pneumonia. Inflammation of the pulmonary tissue including small airways and alveoli.

A. General Considerations.

1. The inflammation may be:
   a. Localized in a specific segment of the lung or it may be diffuse.
   b. Caused by a variety of agents including:
      1. Viruses (most common).
      2. Bacteria (frequently follows a viral upper respiratory infection that disturbs natural defense mechanisms).
      3. Aspiration of food (nuts, popcorn), fluids, and rarely, hydrocarbons, lipids, and powder.
   c. Acute or a long-term smoldering process.

2. Signs and symptoms are similar in viral and bacterial pneumonia and include:
   a. Cough, which may be productive in the older child.
   b. Fever.
   c. Dyspnea.
   d. Tachypnea.
   e. Grunting, in the younger child.
   f. Rales.
   g. Decreased breath sounds.
   h. Pain in abdomen and/or chest.
   i. Vomiting and diarrhea, especially in the young child.

3. Differential diagnosis between viral and bacterial pneumonia is difficult because clinical and laboratory findings are similar (Denny, 1983).

4. Treatment measures include:
   a. Rest.
   b. Hydration.
   c. Antipyretics.
   d. Postural drainage and percussion.
   e. Oxygen therapy for respiratory distress.
   f. Antibiotics for identified bacterial infections.

5. Treatment for aspiration pneumonia will vary according to the causative factor.

6. Complications of viral pneumonia include otitis media and secondary bacterial infection (rare).

7. Thoracentesis may be necessary to drain fluid or pus that may develop as a complication.

8. Oil-based nasal or oral medications should be

P

administered carefully to avoid aspiration pneumonia.

9. Young children are unable to cough up secretions because of immature respiratory tract muscle development.

10. Cough suppressants are not used since it is important that secretions be loosened.

11. Home management is usually possible if the condition is detected and treatment begun early in the course of the disease; infants and severely ill children will be hospitalized.

B. Nursing Management. See HOME MANAGEMENT OF MINOR ILLNESSES.

1. Support the child and parents during hospitalization. See *Hospitalization, Support During*.

2. Initiate discharge planning. See *Discharge Planning*.

3. Initiate isolation precautions as ordered.

4. Facilitate adequate respiratory function.
   a. Position the child in a semi-Fowler's, prone, or side lying position with the affected lung down.
   b. Change the child's position every 2 hours to prevent pooling of secretions.
   c. Provide increased humidity.
   d. Encourage coughing, turning, and deep breathing, e.g., use incentive spirometry as ordered, have child blow a pinwheel.
   e. Suction as needed.
   f. Administer oxygen as ordered.
   g. Carry out percussion and vibration as ordered.
   h. Ease respiratory efforts by promoting rest and decreasing anxiety.

5. Promote rest.
   a. Plan care in blocks to decrease number of times the child must be disturbed.
   b. Do not stimulate excessive coughing.
   c. Limit the number of visitors.
   d. Provide quiet diversional activities, e.g., coloring books, board games.
   e. Decrease anxiety-producing situations.
      1. Encourage parents to stay with the child.
      2. Have someone stay with the child at all times during periods of acute respiratory distress.
      3. Employ restraints only when needed. See *Restraint*.

6. Initiate fever reduction measures as ordered. See *Fever Reduction*.

7. Promote hydration and liquefacation of secretions.
   a. Monitor I.V. fluid accurately if I.V. fluids are used.
   b. Encourage oral fluid intake; give slowly to reduce the chances of stimulating the cough reflex and causing aspiration. See *Forcing Fluids*.
   c. Use mist tent as ordered. See *Mist Tent*.

8. Observe, record, and report the child's response to antibiotic therapy.

9. Monitor vital signs.

10. Promote optimal nutrition to support the body's natural defenses. See *Nutrition*.
    a. Record favorite foods on the Kardex.
    b. Feed the child smaller, more frequent feedings.
    c. Schedule postural drainage between meals.
    d. Provide mouth care prior to eating.

11. Observe, record, and report indications of respiratory status.
    a. Rate.
    b. Rhythm.
    c. Associated sounds, e.g., cough, wheeze.
    d. Presence of nasal flaring, retractions.
    e. Alterations in skin color, e.g., pallor, cyanosis.

12. Observe, record, and report signs and symptoms related to complications.
    a. Decreased respiratory function.
    b. Increased fever.
    c. Chest pain.
    d. Abdominal pain.

13. Teach the child and parents home management.
    a. Continue to administer antibiotics as instructed. See *Administration of Medications, Parental*.
    b. Limit activities which might fatigue the child and initiate coughing, e.g., running.
    c. Call the physician if the child:
       1. Runs a fever.
       2. Develops respiratory problems.
       3. Develops chest pain.

Poison ivy. See *Dermatitis, Contact*.

Poisoning. Ingestion of harmful substances.

A. General Considerations. See *Child Abuse*.

1. Poisoning in infants may occur as an overdose of a therapeutic agent, e.g., aspirin, or as child abuse when drugs or alcohol are administered to quiet the child.

2. Toddlers and young preschoolers are at risk for poisoning because they are actively exploring their environment and because they imitate adult behavior.

3. Toddlers and preschoolers are more likely to ingest:
   a. Liquids, since they do not interpret these as hazardous.

b. Products which are attractively advertised in the media.

c. When they are hungry and/or thirsty.

d. When adults are using a product, not when the product is stored.

4. Syrup of Ipecac and activated charcoal powder should be available in the home if there are young children.

5. Poisoning is more likely to occur in time of stress.

a. Moving from one home to another.

b. When a family member is ill.

c. Death in the family.

d. Preparing for a vacation.

e. Marital difficulties.

f. When parent is preparing meals or getting ready for work.

6. Toxic agents which may result in poisoning include:

a. Drugs.

b. Household products.

c. Plants.

d. Solvents, insecticides, etc. which can be inhaled.

e. Dyes that can be absorbed through the skin.

7. Common clinical symptoms include:

a. Abdominal pain.

b. Vomiting.

c. Diarrhea.

d. Shock.

e. Cyanosis.

f. Coma.

g. Convulsions.

8. Treatment for poisoning may include:

a. Induced vomiting unless the substance is a corrosive or alkali or if the child is comatose or convulsing. (Induced vomiting is controversial with ingestion of hydrocarbons because of the danger of aspiration pneumonia.)

b. Gastric lavage if vomiting is ineffective.

c. Activated charcoal or a chemical neutralizer when vomiting is completed.

d. Alkaline cathartic if the poison has already left the stomach.

e. A specific antidote, if available.

f. Peritoneal dialysis or hemodialysis.

g. Exchange transfusion.

9. Acetaminophen poisoning occurs as accidental ingestion or an acute overdose of the drug administered therapeutically.

a. Hepatic damage due to drug metabolites is of primary concern.

b. Signs and symptoms of toxicity include:

1. Profuse sweating.

2. Nausea and vomiting.

3. Cyanosis.

4. Slow, weak pulse.

5. Depressed respirations.

6. Hypothermia.

7. Circulatory collapse.

8. Coma.

c. Diagnosis is confirmed by the serum acetaminophen level.

d. Treatment includes:

1. Induction of emesis or gastric lavage.

2. Oral or nasogastric administration of acetylcistine (Mucomist) mixed with cola or fruit juice.

3. Monitoring of cardiac function.

4. Monitoring of renal and hepatic function.

10. Salicylate intoxication may occur as an overdose of aspirin used therapeutically or as an accidental ingestion.

a. Toxicity can occur with as little as two times the normal dose for the child's weight.

b. Signs and symptoms of acute toxicity include:

1. Hyperventilation.

2. Anorexia.

3. Vomiting.

4. Dehydration.

5. Fever secondary to increased metabolism.

6. Coma.

7. Convulsions.

8. Anuria.

c. Salicylates affect the respiratory system and cause hyperventilation that results in respiratory alkalosis.

d. Salicylates also interfere with normal fat and carbohydrate metabolism and cause accumulation of ketones and other organic acids resulting in metabolic acidosis.

e. Diagnosis is confirmed by determination of the serum salicylate level.

f. Treatment includes:

1. Induction of emesis or gastric lavage.

2. I.V. therapy to correct acidosis and dehydration.

3. Sodium bicarbonate.

4. Potassium citrate.

5. Potassium chloride.

6. Peritoneal dialysis or hemodialysis for severe cases.

11. Iron poisoning occurs when the child ingests an iron preparation prescribed for a family member, particularly the prenatal mother.

a. Signs and symptoms include:

1. Vomiting.

2. Profuse diarrhea, often bloody.

3. Dehydration.

4. Pallor.

5. Shock.

6. Convulsions.

P

7. Coma.

b. Diagnosis is confirmed by determination of the serum iron level.

c. Treatment includes:
1. Gastric lavage using sodium bicarbonate or disodium phosphate duohydrate.
2. Saline cathartics since many iron preparations are enteric coated.
3. Rectal lavage with the same neutralizing solution to prevent damage to rectosigmoid mucosa by iron fragments.
4. I.V. therapy to correct acidosis, dehydration and maintain urinary function.
5. Blood or plasma to prevent peripheral vascular collapse.
6. Deferoxamine (a chelating agent which binds the iron for urinary excretion) intravenously in severe cases.
7. Peritoneal dialysis or hemodialysis or exchange transfusion if renal function is inadequate.

B. Nursing Management.

1. Obtain information from the parent who calls to report the child has ingested a harmful product.
   a. What product, when, and how much the child ingested.
   b. The ingredients of the product.

2. Give information to the parent about home management.
   a. Do not induce vomiting if the child:
      1. Is comatose.
      2. Is convulsing.
      3. Has lost the gag reflex.
      4. Has ingested a strong base or alkali.
      5. Has ingested a hydrocarbon.
   b. Administer syrup of Ipecac 1 tablespoon (15 ml) to the child over 1 year of age.
      1. Encourage the child to drink water and other liquids.
      2. Keep the child ambulatory.
      3. Repeat the Ipecac once in 20 minutes if necessary.
   c. Stimulate vomiting in the infant or in the older child if Ipecac is ineffective by tickling the back of the throat with a spoon.
   d. Save any vomitus for chemical analysis.
   e. Administer activated charcoal when the child stops vomiting.
      1. Mix 1 to 2 tbs. in 8 ounces of water.
      2. Do not add ice cream or milk to make the mixture more palatable.
      3. Be positive and firm when persuading the child to drink it.
   f. Give water (1 or 2 glasses) to the child who has swallowed a strong base or alkali.
   g. Prevent shock by elevating head and legs to heart level and providing warmth.

3. Meet the needs of the child brought to the emergency room or physician's office.
   a. Observe, record, and report:
      1. Level of consciousness, including behavioral changes.
      2. Vital signs, including Kussmaul or Cheyne-Stoke's breathing.
      3. Pupil size and reaction.
      4. Presence of burns, excessive salivation, or dryness of oral mucosa.
      5. Presence of ataxia, nystagmus, paralysis, drowsiness, or convulsions.
      6. Color and temperature of skin, lips, and mucous membranes.
      7. Specific odor of breath or vomitus.
   b. Administer syrup of Ipecac as ordered if parents have not done so.
   c. Initiate or assist with gastric lavage if ordered.
      1. Explain the procedure to the child and parents. See *Preparation for Procedures.*
      2. Apply a mummy restraint and position the child on the side with head down to prevent aspiration.
      3. Pass the appropriate size tube.
      4. Inject and then aspirate small amounts of irrigating solution until all traces of poison are removed.
      5. Record the amount of solution instilled and removed.
   d. Administer activated charcoal as ordered after emesis or lavage is completed.
   e. Obtain a urine specimen for chemical analysis.
   f. Observe, record, and report the child's response to medication, e.g., antidote, anticonvulsant, narcotic antagonist.

4. Meet the needs of the child hospitalized for ingestion.
   a. Support the child and parents during hospitalization. See *Hospitalization, Support During.*
   b. Initiate discharge planning. See *Discharge Planning.*
   c. Promote hydration.
      1. Monitor I.V. accurately.
      2. Encourage oral fluids. See *Forcing Fluids.*
   d. Maintain strict I and O records.
   e. Assist with peritoneal dialysis, hemodialysis, or exchange transfusion according to hospital policy.

5. Meet the specific needs of the child with acetaminophen poisoning.
   a. Assist with lavage as ordered.
   b. Monitor I.V. accurately.
   c. Administer acetylcistine as ordered.
   d. Initiate EKG monitoring.

P

e. Measure intake and output.

f. Monitor vital signs frequently.

6. Meet the specific needs of the child with salicylate poisoning.

a. Initiate fever reduction measures as ordered. See *Fever Reduction.*

b. Do not add potassium chloride to the I.V. until the child has voided, since it is excreted by the kidney.

c. Administer vitamin K as ordered to prevent bleeding.

d. Observe, record, and report signs and symptoms of complications.

1. Increased fever.

2. Dehydration, e.g., poor skin turgor, decreased urine output, dry mucous membranes.

3. Coma.

4. Seizures. See *Seizures.*

7. Meet the specific needs of the child with iron poisoning.

a. Monitor central venous pressure (CVP) line if appropriate.

b. Observe, record, and report the child's response to I.V. deferoxamine.

1. A urine color change to light pink indicates iron excretion.

2. Lack of urine output indicates that the therapy will be ineffective.

c. Prepare the child and parents for an upper gastrointestinal series if ordered to assess residual damage. See *Preparation for Procedures.*

8. Teach the parents measures to prevent poisoning.

a. Plan specifically for child supervision during times of stress, e.g., father care for child when mother preparing dinner or vice versa.

b. Anticipate the child's developmental progress and childproof the environment. See *Accident Prevention.*

c. Keep all potentially harmful products locked out of reach.

d. Put safety caps on containers of potentially hazardous products.

e. Do not remove products from their original containers and store in containers which the child might associate with food, e.g., soft drink bottles.

f. Affix labels to harmful products to warn the child, e.g., "Mister Yuk" stickers.

g. Do not leave a product where the child can reach it when answering the phone or doorbell.

h. Read and follow instructions with all medications.

i. Do not refer to medicine as candy.

j. Encourage adult family members to take medications out of the child's sight.

k. Remove all poisonous houseplants.

l. Teach the child to ask permission before eating anything.

9. Review with parents how to manage poisons at home.

a. Discuss administration of syrup of Ipecac and activated charcoal.

1. Keep two doses of syrup of Ipecac on hand, since the dose may need to be repeated.

2. Do not purchase an Ipecac preparation other than the syrup.

b. Review how to induce vomiting using a spoon.

c. Memorize the phone number of the poison control center and/or place it on the telephone.

d. Put safety caps on all jars/bottles which contain inedible products.

e. Discuss the contraindications to inducing vomiting.

Postoperative care. Meeting the special needs of the child after surgery.

A. General Considerations.

1. Suffocation as a result of aspiration of foreign materials such as blood is the most common cause of postoperative death in pediatric surgery.

2. The pulse rate is not a reliable indicator of blood loss in infants and young children.

a. Norms for pulse vary with age.

b. Accurate determination of pulse rate is difficult in the restless or crying patient.

3. Additional moisture via vaporizer or croupette may be needed because the child's narrow glottis and trachea increase the possibility of respiratory difficulty.

4. Problems with fluid and electrolyte imbalance are more frequent in pediatric patients. See *Fluid and Electrolyte Imbalance.*

5. A nasogastric tube will be inserted for the child who needs gastric decompression, e.g., abdominal surgery.

6. A Foley catheter is frequently inserted during surgery if the procedure is expected to last more than 90 minutes.

a. The catheter may be removed before the child leaves the operating room.

b. The catheter may be left in place for 12 to 24 hours or more.

7. An I.V. will be inserted before or during induction of anesthesia.

a. Discontinuing the I.V. may be done in the

P

recovery room if the solution is totally absorbed.

   b. The I.V. may be continued on the pediatric unit until the child is taking and retaining fluid satisfactorily.

8. Behavioral regression should be expected as a normal response to the stress of hospitalization and surgery.

9. Anxiety will be greater for the child and parents if the surgical procedure were an emergency one.

B. Nursing Management.

1. Meet the needs of the child during recovery from anesthesia.

   a. Tell the child where he or she is and that the operation is over.

     1. Call the child by a nickname if appropriate.

     2. Tell the child that he or she is in the "wake-up" room.

     3. Tell the child where the parents are if known.

     4. Tell the child that he or she has an I.V., bandage, tube, etc., if appropriate.

   b. Take vital signs every 15 minutes as ordered.

   c. Reposition the child every 30 minutes.

   d. Observe, record, and report signs and symptoms of respiratory distress.

     1. Weak cry.

     2. Increased respiratory rate.

     3. Tense, anxious facial appearance.

     4. Restlessness.

     5. Retracting.

     6. Nasal flaring.

     7. Cyanosis.

   e. Observe, record, and report signs and symptoms of hemorrhage.

     1. Pale conjunctiva.

     2. Hypotension.

     3. Excessive blood on dressing or linen.

     4. Pallor.

   f. Observe for shock due to hypovolemia or hemorrhage.

     1. Cyanosis.

     2. Increased pulse.

     3. Increased respirations.

     4. Decreased blood pressure.

   g. Administer treatment for shock as ordered.

     1. Warmth.

     2. Oxygen.

     3. Respiratory assistance.

     4. Sodium bicarbonate.

     5. Blood replacement.

     6. Pain medication.

   h. Provide warmth, particularly for the infant, since exposure during surgery may lower body temperature drastically.

   i. Provide increased moisture via croupette or vaporizer as ordered.

   j. Monitor the I.V. rate accurately, since circulatory overload or dehydration occur more rapidly and are more serious in the pediatric patient.

   k. Administer pain medication as ordered. See *Pain.*

   l. Observe urinary drainage if a Foley catheter is in place.

   m. Restrain the child as necessary. See *Restraints.*

   n. Observe for complications specific to the surgical procedure.

2. Meet the needs of the child in the immediate postoperative period.

   a. Prepare the room with necessary equipment before the child returns from the recovery room.

   b. Initiate action when the child returns from the recovery room.

     1. Receive report from the recovery room staff.

     2. Review postoperative orders.

     3. Obtain vital signs.

     4. Check dressing, tube, catheter, etc.

     5. Begin I.V. flow sheet and I and O sheet if necessary.

     6. Change I.V. tubing or volutrol to pediatric drip if necessary.

   c. Observe, record, and report signs and symptoms of respiratory distress, hemorrhage and shock as listed above.

   d. Discontinue I.V. as ordered.

   e. Observe, record, and report first postoperative voiding, since this indicates adequacy of blood flow.

     1. Note burning, irritation, etc.

     2. Notify physician if the child is unable to void within 12 hours.

   f. Initiate measures to stimulate voiding.

     1. Turn on the water faucet.

     2. Place a warm cloth or pour warm water on the perineum.

     3. Place the child in a tub with a few inches of warm water unless contraindicated.

   g. Explain treatment measures such as I.V. restraints, tubes, etc. in age-appropriate terms.

   h. Tell the parents how they can comfort the child and assist in his recovery.

     1. When and how the child can be held.

     2. What he can drink and eat.

     3. When and how he can be ambulated.

   i. Begin ice chips or small amounts of clear liquids as ordered to prevent dehydration and hypoglycemia.

     1. Fill a small medicine cup or fill a regular cup half full.

2. Give a spoon and ice chips.

j. Meet the needs of the child who vomits.
   1. Administer medication as ordered.
   2. Withhold fluids for 1 hour.
   3. Resume oral fluids slowly.

k. Reposition the child every 2 hours to prevent skin breakdown and orthostatic pneumonia.

l. Have the child cough and deep breathe using feathers, pinwheel, or straw if needed.

m. Reinforce or change the dressing as ordered.

n. Irrigate the Foley catheter according to hospital policy and procedure.

o. Irrigate the nasogastric tube as ordered to insure patency.
   1. Do not aspirate the solution after gastric surgery.
   2. Observe, record, and report the amount and appearance of drainage.

p. Meet the needs of the child who is NPO.
   1. Offer mouth care frequently.
   2. Provide a pacifier or hold the infant.
   3. Provide diversion for the older child when other children are eating.

q. Observe for potential complications.
   1. Infection.
   2. Paralytic ileus.
   3. Pneumonia.
   4. Constipation.

3. Meet the needs of the child who is recuperating.
   a. Encourage a high fluid intake if appropriate. See *Forcing Fluids.*
   b. Provide a diet high in protein and vitamin C to promote healing. See *Nutrition.*
   c. Provide opportunities for the child to express feelings about the surgery, particularly if the procedure was an emergency one.
      1. Therapeutic play for the young child. See *Play, Therapeutic.*
      2. Drawings.
      3. Stories.
      4. Discussions.
   d. Provide opportunities for the parents to discuss their feelings about the child's surgery.
   e. Help the child cope with changes in body image. See *Body Image.*
   f. Encourage the child to assume responsibility for self-care as condition improves.
   g. Provide sensory stimulation. See *Stimulation.*
   h. Begin ambulation when ordered.
      1. Dangle feet at bedside.
      2. Assist and support as needed.
      3. Let the child know in advance how far he is expected to ambulate.

4. Praise the child for his attempt to ambulate even if the goal could not be reached.

   i. Provide substitutes for mobility if ambulation is not appropriate. See *Immobilized Child.*
   j. Plan rest periods as well as activity periods.
   k. Encourage the older child to resume schoolwork.
   l. Support the young child who is having sutures removed, since he will be afraid his insides will fall out.

4. Prepare the child and family for discharge. See *Discharge Planning.*
   a. Demonstrate the use of equipment and techniques for home care as appropriate.
   b. Review activity limitations.
      1. Bathing.
      2. School attendance.
      3. Physical activities.
   c. Stress the importance of follow-up visits.
   d. Review medication instructions. See *Administration of Medications, Parental.*

Preoperative care. Meeting the special needs of the child before surgery.

A. **General Considerations.**
   1. Psychological preparation for surgery is as essential as physical care.
      a. Fears have no relation to the magnitude of surgery.
      b. Preparation should begin at home for the child 4 years of age and older.
   2. The nurse should not assume that parents have told the child what to expect.
   3. Emotional preparation for surgery must take into consideration the following facts about the child.
      a. Age.
      b. Level of maturity.
      c. Anxiety level.
      d. Past experiences.
      e. Parental support.
      f. Operative procedure planned.
   4. Children, as a whole, have fears that affect their response to surgery. See *Fears.*
      a. Separation and abandonment (infant and young child).
      b. Intrusive procedures.
      c. Mutilation of body parts.
      d. Pain.
      e. Loss of life (older child).
   5. Children become dehydrated rapidly necessitating a shorter NPO period prior to surgery.
      a. Birth to 6 months—no solids or formula

P

after midnight; clear liquids until 4 hours before surgery.
  b. Six months to 3 years—NPO after midnight, except offer clear liquids at 2:00 A.M. if surgery is scheduled at 8:00 A.M.
  c. Over 3 years—NPO after midnight for 8:00 A.M. surgery.
  d. Afternoon surgery—sweetened clear liquids until 4 hours before surgery.
6. Preoperative medication dosage should be based on weight, not age.
  a. Atropine can cause a blotchy rash and heat retention which is frightening to the child and parents.
  b. Some children may have excitement secondary to barbiturates and this may frighten other children in the room.
  c. A hypnotic agent may be given 1½ hours preoperatively to decrease the trauma of the injection of a belladonna agent and a narcotic.
7. Children scheduled for elective surgery have difficulty understanding why surgery is necessary when they feel so well.

B. Nursing Management.
1. Discuss what preparation was started prior to admission.
  a. Determine what the child and parents understand about the procedure.
  b. Find out what terms were used to describe the surgery.
  c. Ask about the child's usual reactions to examinations, treatments, etc.
  d. Explore any specific concerns of the child or parents.
  e. Clarify any misconceptions of the child or parents.
2. Prevent intercurrent infections.
  a. Assign the child to a room with a noninfectious child.
  b. Wash hands thoroughly.
  c. Prevent exposure to staff or visitors who are infectious.
3. Prepare the child psychologically according to age and individual experience. See *Preparation for Procedures.*
4. Provide instruction on the day before surgery. See *Preparation for Surgery.*
  a. Explain what is meant by NPO.
  b. Explain the preoperative bath if this will be given.
  c. Describe or show the child how he or she will be transported to the operating room.
  d. Describe the appearance of the operating room (OR) personnel.
  e. Tell the child he or she will be given a special sleep by the doctor and will not feel the operation or remember it.

  f. Orient the older child to the Recovery Room or Intensive Care Unit if appropriate.
  g. Tell the child where the parents will be during surgery if possible.
  h. Have the child practice coughing and deep breathing.
    1. Use pinwheels, feathers, straws, etc., with the young child.
    2. Demonstrate the splinting technique.
  i. Tell the child of preschool age or older that a preoperative medication will be given.
  j. Tell the child and parents the kind and degree of postoperative pain to be expected and that medication will be given if the child needs it.
5. Encourage the parents to be present when the child leaves for the OR.
6. Review the events that are about to happen on the morning of surgery.
7. Prepare the preoperative medication.
  a. Bring the medication to the child's room and place it out of sight.
  b. Tell the child it is time for medication.
  c. Administer the medication immediately.
    1. Have another staff member, not the parent, restrain the child if needed.
    2. Avoid delays that increase the anxiety of the child and the nurse.
  d. Follow hospital policy in relation to clothing, loose teeth, signing off the chart, and positive identification of the child.
8. Allow the young child to take his security object to the OR. (Attach an identification band to the object.)
9. Accompany the child to the operating room if possible.
  a. Describe what is happening if the child is awake.
  b. Introduce him to the operating room personnel.
10. Provide support until the child is anesthetized.
  a. Have parents stay if hospital policy permits.
  b. Stay with the child if parents cannot.
11. Tell the parents where to wait during the operation.

Preparation for hospitalization. Measures to prepare the child for admission to the hospital.

A. General Considerations.
1. Information about hospitalization may need to be repeated or clarified for parents, since they are often upset when told hospitalization is necessary.

2. Many parents do not tell the child that hospitalization will be necessary because they:
   a. Are unaware preparation is important to the child.
   b. Do not know when or how to prepare the child.
   c. Feel it would be more upsetting to the child than not knowing.
3. Parents need specific information about the pediatric unit where the child will be admitted through printed material, telephone call, or a personal visit.
   a. Items to bring, e.g., pajamas, shoes or slippers, toothbrush.
   b. Facilities for parents.
   c. Routines and procedures.
4. The nurse may be involved by sharing information with the parents so they can prepare the child or by preparing the child directly.
5. The child's developmental level should determine the amount and complexity of preparatory information which is given.
   a. The similarity of activities between home and hospital should be described as well as the differences.
   b. Parents should use the same kind of approach they employ when preparing the child for other new experiences.
   c. The younger child will be primarily concerned about whether the parents will be there and how he or she will feel during the hospitalization. See *Fears*.
   d. The older child will need more specifics about the routines and procedures. See *Preparation for Procedures*.

B. **Nursing Management.** See COPING and HOSPITALIZATION, RESPONSE TO.
1. Have the child and parents participate in a hospital preadmission program, if possible.
   a. Visit the pediatric unit, admitting area, laboratory, x-ray department, and recovery room, or ICU if appropriate.
   b. Participate in a preoperative program if appropriate.
   c. Meet the nursing staff.
2. Prepare the child in advance according to his age.
   a. Tell the toddler 2 to 3 days in advance.
   b. Tell the preschooler 4 to 5 days in advance.
   c. Tell the schoolchild 1 to 2 weeks in advance.
   d. Tell the adolescent as soon as the admission is scheduled.
3. Provide materials for the young child to cope with the experience through play. See *Play, Therapeutic*.
   a. Doctor or nurse kit.
   b. Books about hospitalization, e.g., *Pop-Up*

Going to the Hospital, Curious George Goes to the Hospital. See *Appendix iii*.
   c. Replicas of hospital equipment for dramatic play.
4. Encourage the older child to ask questions and discuss hospitalization.
5. Drive by the hospital so the child will know what it looks like, then drive directly home to assure the child that the parents can find the way.
6. Have the child select the toys and personal articles to take to the hospital.
7. Let the child pack the suitcase for hospitalization.

Preparation for procedures.
Providing information to the parent and child about a diagnostic or therapeutic activity.

A. **General Considerations.**
1. Children who are not given accurate information about procedures will fantasize about the event, perhaps to a greatly exaggerated degree.
2. The nurse must have accurate data about the procedure to be performed.
3. The nurse must know what the parents understand about the procedure and what they have told the child.
4. Parents need to be included in the preparation.
   a. Some parents may prefer to give all the information to the child.
   b. Some parents prefer the nurse to share the information with them and the child at the same time.
   c. Other parents prefer the nurse to assume the total responsibility for preparing the child.
5. Decision on how long in advance of the procedure to prepare the child should be determined by the child's age and the parents' description of how the child copes with new situations.
6. Preparing the parents of the infant and young toddler will reduce the anxiety that parents may transmit to the child.
7. The preparation should be done in a quiet room that is free from distractions.
8. Telling the child what will happen and how he or she can help allow the child to cope in a positive manner.
9. Information should be presented at a level consistent with the child's development.
10. Information should be presented in small amounts over time.
11. Information about what the child will feel,

taste, see and/or smell is more helpful than information on the procedure itself.

12. The child should always be encouraged to ask questions during the preparation.

13. The child should not be offered a choice about a painful procedure if there is no choice, e.g., "Are you ready for your shot?"

14. When a painful procedure is to be performed, the nurse should proceed as soon as possible, since anxiety will increase if the procedure is delayed.

15. Distracting the child during a procedure may be successful if the child is not acutely anxious.

16. Preparation of the adolescent should begin with the rationale for treatment, since the adolescent can deal with abstract concepts.

B. Nursing Management.

1. Prepare the older toddler and preschooler for procedures.
   a. Find out what the child believes will happen during the procedure and clarify any misconceptions.
   b. Tell the child just before a traumatic procedure which will be of short duration, e.g., finger prick or injection.
   c. Tell the child the day before a traumatic procedure which will be of longer duration, e.g., cast, I.V., intrusive x-ray.
   d. Provide the child with actual equipment or replicas to familiarize him with what to expect, since he can deal better with the concrete than the abstract. See *Play, Therapeutic.*
   e. Use dolls, puppets, or body outlines during preparation, since the child needs visual, motor, tactile, and auditory images as well as words (Pidgeon, 1977).
   f. Tell how the child can cooperate, e.g., holding still, handing a band-aid.
   g. Tell the child it is all right to cry if the procedure hurts or squeeze the nurse's hands hard.
   h. Record on the Kardex and in the nurses' notes what preparation the child has received.
   i. Let the child play with the equipment, particularly needles and syringes, again after the procedure to work through feelings.

2. Prepare the schoolchild for procedures.
   a. Find out what the child believes will happen during the procedure and clarify any misconceptions.
   b. Use medical or scientific terminology during preparation.
   c. Teach concrete aspects of the procedure before teaching the abstract, e.g., how to

do a Clinitest, then the interpretation of results (Pidgeon, 1977).
   d. Use diagrams or body outlines as a basis for explaining procedures.
   e. Use a teaching doll if the child is unable to conceptualize the procedure from the outlines.
   f. Prepare the schoolchild as soon as the procedure is scheduled.
   g. Record on the Kardex and in the nurses' notes what preparation the child has received.

3. Prepare the adolescent for procedures.
   a. Find out what the adolescent believes will happen during the procedure and clarify any misconceptions.
   b. Use medical or scientific terminology during preparation.
   c. Use body diagrams or models as a basis for explaining the procedure.
   d. Give the scientific rationale for the procedure, then describe the procedure (Pidgeon, 1977).
   e. Prepare the adolescent separately from the parents.
   f. Discuss the future implications of the results of the procedure.
   g. Record on the Kardex and in the nurses' notes what preparation the adolescent has received.

Preparation for surgery. Providing information for the parents and child about an operative procedure.

A. General Considerations.

1. Preparation should begin before the child enters the hospital.
   a. The child under 4 should be told several days in advance.
   b. The preschool and young schoolchild can be told from 1 to 2 weeks in advance.
   c. The older schoolchild and adolescent can be told as soon as the surgery is scheduled.

2. The nurse should not assume that the child has been prepared by the parents.

3. The child who has been prepared at home needs opportunities in the hospital setting to talk about surgery so that misconceptions can be clarified.

4. All children need to be prepared for routine admission x-ray and laboratory procedures.

5. The young child often interprets surgery as punishment so he or she needs reassurance that he or she did not cause the condition.

6. Visits by staff from anesthesia, recovery room, or ICU will introduce the child to people by whom he or she will be cared for in those areas.

P

B. **Nursing Management.** See PREPARATION FOR PROCEDURES.

1. Prepare the mature toddler and preschooler for surgery.
   a. Use less threatening words such as opening and drainage rather than cut and bleeding.
   b. Avoid trying to cover too much content in one teaching session.
      1. Plan two or three short sessions with play time in between.
      2. Focus on information that is essential if time is limited, e.g., what will be fixed, where the parents will be, bandages or cast.
   c. Encourage the child to practice coughing and deep breathing, repositioning, use of respiratory therapy equipment, or any other special equipment which will be used postoperatively.
   d. Present material in a sequence which introduces frightening information such as preoperative medications and pain medication last.
   e. Show the child the stretcher or gurney if this is how the child will be transported to the operating room.
   f. Explain that the doctor is going to fix the affected body part, since the child may be more anxious if told the part will be removed.
   g. Explain that the surgeon will fix only the affected body part and no other, since the child may have fears of castration or mutilation.
   h. Tell the child he will not have anything to drink before the surgery, since food and drink might make the stomach sick.
   i. Use a doll or stuffed animal to demonstrate sutures, casts, bandages, and injections.
   j. Use a replica of the operating room if possible or describe its appearance.
      1. People dressed in green or blue and wearing masks.
      2. Anesthesia equipment.
      3. Other equipment appropriate to the procedure.
      4. Bright lights.
   k. Tell the child that the doctor will give a "special sleep" and he or she will not feel the operation, but will wake up.
   l. Describe the "wake-up" room and what will happen there.
      1. Other people will be in the room.
      2. Nurses will ask the child's name and location.
      3. The parents will not be in this room, but will be waiting. (If you know this is true.)
   m. Prepare the child for what should be expected postoperatively.
      1. Dressings, bandages, cast, traction, or I.V.
      2. Where the child might be sore and what can be done about it.
      3. When the child can expect to have fluids.
   n. Discuss the sutures.
      1. Sutures will keep the child's insides where they belong.
      2. The sutures will not break when the child moves around or walks.
   o. Record on the Kardex and in the nurses' notes how the child was prepared.

2. Prepare the schoolchild and adolescent for surgery.
   a. Tell the schoolchild that the anesthesia is a "special sleep."
   b. Reassure the adolescent that there will be a nurse or doctor whose job it is to see that the patient does not wake up during the operation.
   c. Prepare the child for what to expect postoperatively.
      1. Dressings, bandages, cast, traction, or I.V.
      2. Pain and its relief.
      3. Positioning.
      4. Special equipment and/or appliances.
      5. Fluid or food restrictions.
   d. Take the child on tour of the recovery room or ICU if possible.
   e. Provide opportunities for the child to discuss the effect of surgery on his body image. See *Body Image*.
   f. Encourage the adolescent to discuss the future implications of the surgery.
   g. Record on the Kardex and in the nurses' notes how the child was prepared.

Preparation for well-child visits. Measures to help the child cope with a clinic or office visit.

A. **General Considerations.**
   1. Parents may not prepare the child for a well-child visit because they do not recognize the importance or because they do not know how to prepare the child.
   2. Children can mobilize their coping behaviors when they know what is going to happen. See *Coping*.
   3. The young child may become anxious if told in advance about immunization injections, but any questions should be answered honestly.

B. **Nursing Management.**
   1. Schedule the visit for a time which does not interfere with the child's usual nap time or mealtime.
   2. Tell the child in advance about the clinic or office visit.

a. Tell the toddler the day before or morning of the visit.

b. Tell the preschooler 2 to 4 days in advance.

c. Tell the schoolchild 1 to 2 weeks in advance.

3. Read a book to the young child about a visit as a way to introduce and/or discuss the topic, e.g., *Mister Rogers Talks About* or *The Clinic.*

4. Describe the appearance of the waiting room and the equipment in the examining room.

5. Discuss with the child the kinds of examination procedures that will take place, e.g., the nurse/doctor will look in your mouth and nose. See *Preparation for Procedures.*

6. Provide the young child with play materials before and after the visit so he can work through feelings about the intrusive parts of the examination. See *Play, Therapeutic.*

Preschooler. Child in the period of development between 3 and 6 years of age.

A. **General Considerations.**

1. The preschooler is faced with the following developmental tasks (Duvall, 1977).

a. Adjusting to healthy daily routines.

b. Mastering physical skills that require large and small muscle coordination.

c. Becoming a participating member of the family.

d. Conforming to the expectations of others.

e. Learning to express emotions.

f. Learning to communicate effectively.

g. Learning to use initiative.

h. Laying the foundation for understanding the meaning of life.

2. The rate at which each child masters these tasks will vary.

3. The rate of growth remains slow during the preschool period.

4. The family remains the most important social group for the preschooler, but he is ready and eager for socialization with other adults and children.

5. Learning how to do things is the major development task and play is the way by which preschoolers learn about themselves and their world.

6. "Why" and "how" are the favorite words of the preschooler who asks questions constantly.

7. The preschooler has a vivid imagination which not only helps him learn but also contributes to the development of fears and the stretching of reality when describing experiences.

8. The psychosexual development of preschoolers leads them to develop a strong attachment to the opposite sex parent and castration fears are common.

B. **Nursing Management.**

1. Support the parents in meeting the child's needs. See *Parenting.*

2. Support the preschooler's adjustment to hospitalization. (See *Hospitalization, Support During.*)

a. Find out what the daily home routine has been, record it on the Kardex, and follow it as much as possible.

b. Find out the preschooler's usual means of coping and any known fears. See *Coping* and *Fears.*

c. Use knowledge of the preschooler's response to hospitalization to plan care. See *Hospitalization, Response to.*

3. Meet the daily physical needs of the preschooler.

a. Bathe.

1. Give a bedbath if the child is on bedrest; otherwise supervise the preschooler in taking a tub bath.

2. Wash hair as needed.

3. Teach the child how to clean the outer ear.

b. Provide mouth care.

1. See that the child has a tooth brush.

2. Allow the child to brush his or her own teeth.

3. Supervise tooth brushing as needed to make sure the child brushes all teeth.

c. Promote adequate nutrition. See *Nutrition.*

d. Provide for rest and sleep routines. See *Sleep.*

1. Schedule quiet times but do not force the preschooler to nap.

2. Provide a pillow.

3. Make the bed with top covers like an adult's.

e. Meet elimination needs.

1. Make sure the child knows where bathrooms are located.

2. Show the child how the toilet and sink work if hospital ones are different from home.

3. Provide the child on bedrest with a call light or bell so he or she can get assistance.

4. Remember that bed wetting may still occur; do not scold the child.

5. Record all stools.

6. Keep I and O records as ordered.

f. Protect from injury.

1. Know where the child is at all times.

2. Keep the crib sides all the way up when the child is unattended if he or she is still in a crib.

3. Keep the bed in the lowest position so the child in a regular bed can get in and out easily.

4. Remove all unnecessary equipment from the bedside table, room, and halls.
5. Do not leave equipment cords across traffic areas.
g. Prevent infection.
1. Practice good hygienic techniques when giving care.
2. Teach appropriate hygienic practices to the child.
3. Do not care for the child if you have an infectious illness.
4. Prevent contact with other children on the unit who have infectious illnesses.
h. Provide for exercise. See *Exercise.*

4. Consider the developmental level of the preschooler when:
a. Taking vital signs. See *Preparation for Procedures.*
1. Let the child examine all equipment.
2. Take an oral temperature when possible to avoid an intrusive procedure.
b. Administering medications. See *Administration of Medications* and *Appendix iii.*

5. Meet the emotional needs of the preschooler.
a. Involve the parents in the care of the preschooler.
b. Follow home routines.
c. Place with other children of the same age if possible.
d. Involve the child in his own care and teach him what he can do in relation to his care.
e. Explain all procedures honestly, clearly, and repeat as needed for reassurance.
f. Encourage the child to be as independent as possible.
g. Do not belittle the child's fears, e.g., provide a night light if the child fears the dark.
h. Provide play experiences that meet the preschooler's need.
1. Take to the playroom.
2. Bring play materials to the child on bedrest.
3. Supply play materials which can be used in imaginative ways, e.g., clay, blocks.
i. Accept the preschooler's constant questioning about everything and everyone.
j. Accept regression that may occur.

6. Provide anticipatory guidance to parents related to the following areas as indicated on the basis of an assessment.
a. Growth and development norms.
b. Common problems, e.g., fears, tale telling. See *Fears.*
c. Nutritional needs and habits. See *Nutrition.*
d. Dental care. See *Dental Care.*
e. Safety. See *Accident Prevention.*
f. Need for peer group contact. See *Day Care Center.*

g. Need for play to learn and to work through situations. See *Play* and *Play, Therapeutic.*
h. Ways to stimulate development. See *Stimulation.*
i. Provision for ongoing health care. See *Well-child Care.*
j. Sex education. See *Sex Education.*

Prickly heat (miliaria). Transient, inflammatory rash seen primarily in infancy.

A. **General Considerations.**
1. Predisposing factors include:
a. Warm, humid weather.
b. Overdressing the baby.
c. Overheated bedroom.
2. Symptoms include pinpoint papules with occasional vesicles and pustules surrounded by erythema.
3. Affected areas are the neck, cheeks, trunk, and perineum.

B. **Nursing Management.**
1. Bathe the infant twice a day in tepid water.
a. Add ½ cup of baking soda, starch, or oatmeal to ½ tub of water.
b. Pat dry.
2. Dress the infant in soft, lightweight clothing, preferably cotton.
3. Lower the room temperature.

Pulmonic stenosis. See *Congenital Heart Disease.*

Punishment See *Discipline.*

Pyelonephritis. See *Urinary Tract Infection.*

Pyloric stenosis. Condition in the infant in which there is hypertrophy of the muscle around the pylorus resulting in constriction.

A. **General Considerations.**
1. The cause of the hypertrophy is unknown.
2. Signs and symptoms include:
a. Vomitus which becomes projectile and may be blood streaked.
b. Constipation.
c. Fretfulness.
d. Weight loss.
e. Visible peristaltic waves in the upper abdomen from left to right.
f. Palpable olive-sized mass in the right upper quadrant.
g. Dehydration.

3. Metabolic alkalosis and potassium depletion may result from the vomiting and will require correction preoperatively through I.V. therapy. See *Fluid and Electrolyte Imbalance.*
4. Surgical treatment is the usual choice (pyloromyotomy).
5. Medical treatment may be attempted with:
   a. Antispasmodic drugs.
   b. Thickened feedings.
   c. Changes in feeding technique.
6. Feedings are gradually increased in strength and amount postoperatively.
7. The prognosis is excellent.

B. **Nursing Management.**
1. Support the child and parents during hospitalization. See *Hospitalization, Support During.*
2. Initiate discharge planning. See *Discharge Planning.*
3. Meet the infant's needs preoperatively. See *Preoperative Care* and *Preparation for Surgery.*
   a. Maintain NPO status.
   b. Monitor I.V. accurately.
   c. Irrigate nasogastric tube as ordered.
4. Meet the infant's needs postoperatively. See *Postoperative Care.*
   a. Begin oral feedings carefully.
      1. Hold the infant in a more upright position.
      2. Use a nipple that does not allow formula to flow too fast.
      3. Burp the infant frequently.
      4. Position the infant on the right side, abdomen, or in an infant seat after feeding.
      5. Chart the infant's response to feeding and any vomiting.
   b. Involve the mother in feeding.
      1. Recognize that the mother may feel incompetent due to the infant's vomiting.
      2. Reassure the mother that some vomiting may occur postoperatively.
   c. Clarify with the surgeon about using a pacifier, since this increases the amount of air the baby swallows.
   d. Obtain an accurate weight.
      1. Weigh at the same time each day.
      2. Use the same scales.
      3. Weigh nude.
   e. Protect incision site by pinning the diaper low or using a pediatric urine collecting (PUC) bag.
5. Teach the parents home management.
   a. Assess the mother's ability to feed and make suggestions as needed.
   b. Teach the parents to protect the wound site.
      1. Demonstrate dressing change if appropriate.
      2. Pin diaper low.
      3. Give a sponge bath daily until the incision heals.

Radiation therapy. Therapeutic use of ionized radiation.

A. **General Considerations.**
1. Radiation therapy is frequently used in conjunction with chemotherapy and/or surgery in the treatment of childhood malignancies.
2. The radiation dose will depend on the (Fernandez and Sutow, 1975):
   a. Child's age—the younger the child the smaller the dose.
   b. Tissue tolerance—tissues in different parts of the body vary in their tolerance to radiation, and a child has less tolerance than an adult.
   c. Concurrent use of chemotherapy—since both depress bone marrow function the dose will be lower. See *Chemotherapy.*
3. Children have fewer general side effects from radiation therapy than do adults, but they are more significant because the child's homeostatic balance is more precarious than the adult's (Williams, 1975).
4. Early side effects vary according to the dose given and the site irradiated and include (Whaley and Wong, 1983):
   a. Skin—alopecia (occurring in approximately 2 weeks) and peeling.
   b. Head—nausea, vomiting, alopecia, postradiation somnolence in 4 to 6 weeks.
   c. Neck—loss of taste, inflammation of the parotid gland.
   d. Eyes—none.
   e. Ears—possible otitis media.
   f. Lungs—possible pneumonitis.
   g. Heart—possible pericarditis.

h. Kidneys—possible nephritis.

i. Bladder—possible cystitis (rare).

j. Gastrointestinal tract—nausea, vomiting, anorexia, diarrhea, ulceration.

k. Bones—none.

l. Bone marrow—suppression.

m. Endocrine glands—none.

n. Testes—none.

o. Ovaries—possible delay or absence of secondary sex characteristics.

p. Central nervous system—fatigue.

5. Late side effects are rarer, depend on the site irradiated and dose given, and include (Whaley and Wong, 1983):

a. Skin: hyperpigmentation, permanent hair loss.

b. Head: possible intellectual deficits in young children, dental caries or loss of teeth.

c. Eyes: cataract formation.

d. Ears: decreased hearing.

e. Lungs: fibrotic changes.

f. Heart: myocardial infarctions, endocardial or myocardial fibrosis.

g. Kidneys: chronic nephritis.

h. Bladder: possible fibrosis.

i. Gastrointestinal tract: esophageal stricture, gastric or small bowel ulceration.

j. Bones: linear growth retardation, spinal deformities, asymmetric growth, pathological fractures.

k. Bone marrow: long-term anemia, leukemia.

l. Endocrine glands: potential for cancer of thyroid, delayed growth, retarded pubertal changes.

m. Testes: sterility, testicular hypertrophy.

n. Ovaries: potential for sterility, premature menopause, chromosomal damage to germ cells.

6. Radiation therapy may be used as palliative rather than curative treatment to:

a. Decrease pain.

b. Relieve pressure from large tumor masses.

c. Shrink disfiguring tumor masses.

7. The development of high speed, high energy equipment permits better delivery of a specific amount of radiation to a particular site and decreases the amount of scatter radiation to other tissues.

8. Radiation therapy is usually carried out on an outpatient basis, although it may be begun during hospitalization.

9. Helping the infant and young child learn to remain still during therapy and to accept separation from parents is a major task for the nurse and parents.

10. Some children may require sedation prior to treatments.

11. The peeling of skin following radiation therapy should not be referred to as a "burn."

B. Nursing Management.

1. Prepare the child and parents for radiation therapy. See *Preparation for Procedures.*

a. Orient the child and parents to the radiation therapy department, e.g., what machines look and sound like.

b. Introduce the child and parents to the people in the department.

c. Teach parents how to prepare the toddler and preschool child at home through the use of practice sessions (Tealey, 1977).

1. Limit the length of the session to a half hour.

2. Use the kitchen table.

3. Practice immobilizing the child for increasing periods of time in the position he will have to assume.

4. Use a camera or small box for the x-ray machine.

5. Provide the child with a table, doll, and toy camera in order to play out the situation. See *Play, Therapeutic.*

6. Praise the child for all attempts to cooperate and ignore any failure.

d. Explain to parents of infants that the infant can often be distracted during treatment by giving a pacifier after the infant has been immobilized.

e. Tell parents that children over 7 years of age can be given explanations similar to those of an adult because of their developmental level.

f. Explain that sedation may be ordered prior to each treatment in order to assist the child in remaining still.

g. Teach parents not to remove skin markings.

2. Teach parents what they can do to help the child experiencing:

a. Anorexia.

1. Offer favorite foods and fluids.

2. Supply major calories at breakfast, since anorexia often increases as the day passes (Rose, 1978).

3. Have the child help select diet to increase interest.

4. Serve food in different ways or settings to stimulate the child to eat, e.g., hold an indoor "picnic" on a blanket.

b. Nausea.

1. Provide foods such as saltine crackers, baked potatoes, and cooked cereals that are bulky and bland.

2. Eliminate unpleasant environmental odors if possible.

3. Encourage clear fluid intake.

R

4. Give medications as instructed.
c. Vomiting.
  1. Give medications as instructed.
  2. Offer clear, noncarbonated or "flat" carbonated beverages.
  3. Provide mouth care.
d. Mouth ulcers.
  1. Do not use tooth brush.
  2. Use toothettes.
  3. Rinse mouth frequently with half-strength peroxide, half-strength mouthwash, or cool water.
  4. Use viscous Xylocaine before meals as instructed.
  5. Serve foods at room or cool temperature.
  6. Chop foods, or blend them, if chewing is difficult.
  7. Avoid foods with high acid content, e.g., tomatoes, citrus juices.
e. Diarrhea.
  1. Keep perineal area clean and dry.
  2. Give medications as instructed.
  3. Do not give fresh fruits, fruit juices, or vegetables high in cellulose.
  4. Decrease or eliminate milk since lactose intolerance may develop.
f. Alopecia.
  1. Cut hair short.
  2. Have the child wear a cap to bed so hair falling on pillow does not get in the mouth, ears, and eyes.
  3. Provide wig, cap, or scarf for daytime wear.
  4. Wash hair frequently to prevent cradle cap.
  5. Remove dead skin with lotions or lubricants.
  6. Cover the head in cool weather to prevent heat loss.
g. Peeling of skin.
  1. Keep skin clean.
  2. Wash daily in tepid water.
  3. Dry gently.
  4. Use bland, nonperfumed powder if desired.
  5. Avoid exposure to the sun.
h. Fatigue or somnolence.
  1. Provide for rest periods during the day.
  2. Promote age-appropriate quiet activities.
  3. Make sure the child changes position frequently if he stays in bed.
i. Dryness of the mucous membranes.
  1. Provide frequent mouth care.
  2. Offer fluids frequently.
3. Tell the parents to call the physician if:
  a. Nausea and vomiting are not controlled by medication.

b. The child shows signs and symptoms of dehydration.
c. The child runs a fever.
d. Mouth and rectal ulcers develop.
e. Bleeding occurs.
f. Signs and symptoms of the following develop:
  1. Nephritis—headache, malaise, hematuria, edema.
  2. Pneumonitis—cough, chest pain.
  3. Pericarditis—chest pain.
4. Support the child and parents in dealing with alterations in body image. See *Body Image.*
5. Meet the needs of the hospitalized child receiving radiation therapy as outlined above.

Rash (exanthem). Lesions of the skin.

A. **General Considerations.**
  1. Rashes are frequently a sign of common childhood diseases.
  2. Terms used in the description of rashes include:
    a. Macules—flat lesions of varying size and color.
    b. Maculopapules—slightly raised macules.
    c. Papules—lesions that are elevated from the skin, but contain no fluid.
    d. Vesicles—papules filled with clear, serous fluid.
    e. Pustules—vesicles filled with purulent exudate.
    f. Nodules—solid papules.
    g. Bullae—vesicles filled with serous or seropurulent fluid.
    h. Wheals (urticaria)—edematous flat elevations.
    i. Discrete lesions—lesions separated by areas of normal skin.
    j. Coalesced lesions—lesions that have fused together.
  3. Most, but not all, rashes itch.

B. **Nursing Management.**
  1. Observe, record, and report appearance and location of the rash.
    a. Avoid comparative statements, e.g., "rash looks better than yesterday."
    b. Use lay description if unsure of exact terminology, e.g., "beefy red, raised rash the size of a quarter on the left forearm."
  2. Promote comfort.
    a. Administer antihistamines, if ordered, or analgesics such as aspirin to relieve pain.
    b. Bathe the child in tepid water with 1 cup of starch, baking soda, or oatmeal per half-tub of water.
    c. Pat, rather than rub dry.
    d. Avoid overheating the child with clothing or excess blankets.

R

e. Apply antihistamine lotion with a patting motion.

3. Reduce fever if present. See *Fever Reduction* and *Forcing Fluids*.

4. Prevent secondary infection.
   a. Encourage frequent handwashing.
   b. Keep the child's fingernails short and clean.
   c. Apply mitts, gloves, or elbow restraints to prevent scratching.

5. Provide diversional activities that occupy the hands.
   a. Puzzles.
   b. Modular toys.
   c. Sewing.
   d. Coloring.

Regression. Behavioral response to illness characterized by return to earlier level of development.

A. **General Considerations.**
   1. Regression is a normal occurrence in ill children of all ages.
   2. Regression occurs more rapidly and more intensely in the young child.
   3. The most recently acquired motor skill is the first to be lost in the infant or toddler.
   4. Toddlers regress in the areas of toileting, self-feeding, verbal communication, and dependency on thumbsucking or security objects.
   5. Regression allows the preschooler to return to a more dependent state so the child can cope with the demands of illness.
   6. Regression may be frightening to the school-child or adolescent who cannot accept the need to become more dependent.
   7. The child who must be isolated is very likely to regress because of separation from supportive people and because of lack of stimulation. See *Isolated Child.*
   8. Regressive behavior will usually diminish as the child's health improves if his or her needs have been met by parents and nurses.

B. **Nursing Management.**
   1. Encourage parental participation in care so they can support the child's coping.
   2. Use the nursing history to obtain data on what the child can accomplish in self-care. See *History Taking.*
      a. Include this information on the Kardex care plan so that nursing personnel do not put diapers on the toilet-trained child, etc.
      b. Follow the home routines so the child is more likely to be successful in self-care.
      c. Revise the care plan to list areas in which the child needs assistance if he regresses.
   3. Discuss with parents that regression is a normal developmental response to illness so they will not feel frustrated or embarrassed by the child's dependent behavior.
   4. Verbalize to the young child that his regressive behavior is accepted and that you will help the child regain independence, e.g., tell him you realize he is upset about wetting his pants and you will move the potty chair where he can reach it easier next time.
   5. Provide regressive toys such as stuffed animals or baby bottles as well as aggressive and expressive toys in the playroom.
   6. Allow the older child to regress during threatening and traumatic situations while supporting the goal of independence.
   7. Provide support for the schoolchild and adolescent in subtle ways, e.g., "I have some free time now and since you don't have any visitors right now, would it be all right if I talk with you for a while?"

Religious aspects of health care. Religious beliefs and practices which influence the delivery of health care.

A. **General Considerations.** See *Cultural Aspects of Health Care.*
   1. Religion is an integral part of many cultural beliefs and practices.
   2. Providing effective nursing care requires an awareness of the child's and parents' religious:
      a. Beliefs.
      b. Practices.
      c. Taboos.
   3. Members of the same religious group may differ widely in their personal religious beliefs and practices.
   4. The religious beliefs of the parents may be in conflict with what the physician orders for the child, e.g., an order for a blood transfusion would be opposed by parents adhering to the Jehovah's Witnesses' prohibition against giving and/or receiving blood.
   5. Modern science and religion may be seen as being incompatible by some religious groups.
   6. The young child may have little understanding of his family's religious beliefs and practices but still be strongly influenced by them because of parental behaviors.
   7. The adolescent's developmental task of establishing a personal identity may cause him to reject parental religious beliefs and practices.
   8. Illness often leads to intensification of religious concerns, beliefs, and/or practices.
   9. Some religious groups believe illness is a punishment sent from God.
   10. A nurse need not hold a particular belief in order to carry out a required religious practice

R

for a child, e.g., anyone can, and should baptize an unbaptized Roman Catholic child in danger of death.

B. Nursing Management.
1. Examine your own religious beliefs and practices and your willingness to provide care for persons with different beliefs and practices.
2. Include the following areas related to religious beliefs and practices in your nursing assessment and record on the Kardex:
   a. Religious preferences related to diet, dress, practice of certain rituals, etc., e.g., Kosher food for Jews, special undergarment worn by Mormons, anointing of the sick by Roman Catholics.
   b. Religious taboos, e.g., body of deceased Muslim to be prepared by someone of same sex.
   c. Adherence of the child and family to the stated beliefs of their religious group since individual practices vary.
3. Find out and record on the Kardex, as appropriate, the child's and/or parents' wishes related to:
   a. Birth, e.g., baptism, circumcision.
   b. A health crisis, e.g., administration of medications, blood transfusions, surgical procedures.
   c. Death, e.g., preparation of the body, last rites, autopsy.
4. Use knowledge of growth and development to help parents understand a child's response to their religious beliefs and practices, e.g., young child does not have capability for abstract thought or adolescent testing own beliefs.
5. Serve as an advocate for the child and parents. See *Advocate*.
   a. Permit verbalization of personal beliefs.
   b. Do not seek to alter religious beliefs of others.
   c. Provide for visits of appropriate clergy as requested.
   d. Involve the child and/or parents in planning care that takes into account religious beliefs and practices.
   e. Provide for attendance at religious services if available.

Restraint. Use of materials and/or equipment to prevent the movement of an extremity or extremities.

A. General Considerations.
1. The primary function of restraint is to ensure the child's safety.
2. Restraint should never be used as a substitute for good nursing care.

3. The child's need for emotional support and for stimulation increases with restraint.
4. The older child frequently needs restraint only during sleep, since he can understand the reasons for not dislodging the I.V. tubes, etc.
5. Restraining all four extremities in a spread eagle position should be used only as a last resort.
6. Parents may be hesitant to interact with the child who is restrained, since they know the I.V. dressing, etc. should not be dislodged.
7. Restraints used for infants and children include:
   a. Extremity restraints made of strips of gauze, muslin or Kerlex, or commercial devices.
   b. Elbow restraints may be jacket or cuff type with tongue depressors or strips of masonite inserted into pockets.
   c. Mummy restraints involve wrapping the child securely in a blanket or sheet so the head or neck area can be examined or treated.
   d. Jackets and belts are used to keep the child from falling out of a chair, wheelchair, or stroller.

B. Nursing Management. See IMMOBILIZED CHILD.
1. Prepare the child and parents by telling them how and why the child will be restrained.
2. Discuss with the parents when and how they can remove the restraints safely to interact with the child.
3. Use the minimal restraint necessary to accomplish the purpose. (e.g., An elbow restraint is less restrictive, but will prevent the child from touching his mouth, face, eye, etc.)
4. Apply the restraint gently and slowly while talking to the child.
   a. Pad the wrist or ankle before applying an extremity restraint.
   b. Secure an extremity restraint with a clove hitch rather than a slip knot to prevent the restraint from tightening when the child moves.
   c. Check the restrained extremity for discoloration, coolness, or irritation.
   d. Dress the child in a long sleeve shirt before applying an elbow restraint.
   e. Tie the jacket or belt restraint in the back where the child cannot reach and untie it.
   f. Position the belt restraint so it cannot slip and compromise respirations.
5. Restrain the infant or young child so he can comfort himself by sucking his thumb, rubbing his special blanket, etc.
6. Remove the restraints at least every 4 hours.
   a. Remove one arm restraint at a time if the child is too young to cooperate and not touch the I.V. site, dressing, etc.

b. Provide passive or active range of motion while supervising the child.

c. Remove the restraint whenever the parent or nurse is available to supervise the child.

7. Change the child's position before reapplying the restraint.

8. Provide age-appropriate stimulation. See *Stimulation.*

Retinoblastoma. Congenital, highly malignant tumor of the eye.

A. **General Considerations.**

1. About 75 percent of affected children will have involvement of one eye only.

2. Symptoms include:
   a. White spot in the pupil.
   b. Strabismus.
   c. Glaucoma with steamy cornea and red eye.
   d. Painful red eye if the tumor bursts through the globe.
   e. Loss of or limited vision.

3. The tumor may affect a small section of the eye or the entire eye.

4. Retinoblastoma may be transmitted as an autosomal dominant trait.
   a. Patients who survive retinoblastoma have a 50 percent chance of transmitting the disease to their children.
   b. Other cases may occur as a germinal mutation in a nonaffected parent.

5. Diagnostic tests include.
   a. Indirect opthalmoscopy under general anesthesia.
   b. Assay of urinary excretion of VMA (vanillylmandelic acid) or HVA (homovanillic acid).
   c. Transillumination of the retina.
   d. Fluorescein angiography.
   e. Ultrasonography.

6. Retinoblastoma may extend down the optic nerve into the subarachnoid space and the brain.

7. Metastasis may also occur via the bloodstream to the skull, ribs, and humerus.

8. Extension of the tumor via the optic nerve is a grave prognostic sign.

9. Treatment varies with the degree of involvement.
   a. Small discrete unilateral tumors may be treated with:
      1. Surgical implantation of cobalt plaque applicators.
      2. Light coagulation via laser beam.
      3. Cryotherapy.
   b. Larger unilateral retinoblastoma will be enucleated with as much optic nerve as possible.

c. Bilateral retinoblastoma necessitates enucleation of the more involved eye and radiation and chemotherapy of the opposite eye.

d. Bilateral enucleation may be performed if radiation therapy would be ineffective in saving vision.

10. Prompt enucleation of a small unilateral retinoblastoma results in a survival rate of 90 percent.

11. The opposite eye should be examined every 1 to 3 months throughout childhood.

B. **Nursing Management.**

1. Support the child and parents during hospitalization. See *Hospitalization, Support During.*

2. Initiate discharge planning. See *Discharge Planning.*

3. Support the child and parents when the diagnosis is made.
   a. Be present when the child and parents are told the diagnosis or find out what they have been told and record on the Kardex.
   b. Answer all questions honestly.
   c. Use terminology which the child understands.
   d. Arrange for uninterrupted periods of contact with the child and parents so supportive discussions can be held.

4. Provide consistency and continuity of care, since the child must endure so many painful diagnostic and therapeutic procedures. See *Preparation for Procedures.*

5. Meet the needs of the child and parents preoperatively. See *Preoperative Care* and *Preparation for Surgery.*
   a. Provide opportunities for the child and parents to verbalize their concerns about disfigurement and loss of vision if enucleation is necessary.
      1. Prepare the child and parents through explanations and interviews.
      2. Support the parents who must make a decision about bilateral enucleation, since this will result in blindness.
      3. Anticipate that the child may handle his fears about disfigurement by becoming angry and irritable.
   b. Provide information about the prosthesis.
      1. The prosthesis will be fitted when the edema subsides.
      2. The artificial eye may be attached to the eye muscles so that it moves in coordination with the real eye.
      3. The child will not be able to see out of the artificial eye.

6. Meet the needs of the child and parents postoperatively. See *Postoperative Care.*

R

a. Observe, record, and report hemorrhage, edema, and signs of infection.
b. Reinforce the dressing as necessary, but do not change unless ordered.
c. Help the child cope with the body image changes. See *Body Image.*
d. Provide opportunities for the child to express his feelings through play. See *Play, Therapeutic.*
e. Assist with fitting of the prosthesis if done during hospitalization.
f. Provide measures to meet the needs of the child who requires bilateral enucleation and becomes blind. See *Blindness.*
   1. Encourage a family member to stay with the child if possible, since the child will be very frightened.
   2. Explain new sounds, since the child will lack visual cues.
   3. Let the child handle all materials/equipment that will be used in his care.
   4. Place items the child will use in same place, record the location on the Kardex, and place a diagram at the bedside.
7. Meet the needs of the child who requires radiation therapy or chemotherapy. See *Chemotherapy* and *Radiation Therapy.*
8. Teach the child and parents home management.
   a. Encourage the parents to make the home life as normal as possible.
      1. Have the child resume normal activities such as play groups or school.
      2. Encourage normal peer relationships.
      3. Maintain normal discipline. See *Discipline.*
      4. Encourage adequate rest and nutrition for all family members.
   b. Reinforce the explanation for frequent examination of the uninvolved eye.
   c. Encourage the parents to receive genetic counseling about additional children and to plan for the child to receive counseling when he reaches puberty. See *Genetic Counseling.*
   d. Teach care of the artificial eye.
      1. Review the physician's guidelines about whether the prosthesis should be removed for sleep or other specific instructions.
      2. Wash hands before beginning the procedure.
      3. Irrigate the socket with normal saline.
      4. Clean the socket and eye when excessive tearing or crusting occurs.
      5. Wipe away the normal watery discharge with sterile, disposable tissues.
      6. Clean the prosthesis with soap and warm water only.
      7. Store a plastic prosthesis in a container with plain tap water.
      8. Store a glass prosthesis in its own case after drying.
   e. Teach measures for eye safety.
      1. Wear safety glasses or goggles if prescribed as a method of protecting the normal eye.
      2. Do not carry sharp objects while walking or running.
      3. Avoid rubbing the eyes when a foreign body is present.
      4. Seek medical assistance promptly for any injuries or infections.

Reye's syndrome. Acute, noninflammatory encephalopathy with fatty degenerative changes of the viscera following a viral-like illness.

A. **General Considerations.**
1. The etiology of the disease is unknown although research has linked the illness with chemical toxins, salicylates, acetaminophen, and antiemetic drugs.
2. Three types of antecedent illnesses are most frequently associated with Reye's syndrome:
   a. Respiratory.
   b. Varicella.
   c. Gastrointestinal.
3. Signs and symptoms include:
   a. Persistent vomiting and diarrhea in the recovery phase of an acute viral illness.
   b. Alterations in level of consciousness from combative and hyperexcitable to lethargy and coma.
4. Laboratory procedures which are part of the diagnostic evaluation are:
   a. Liver function tests: SGOT, SGPT, LDH.
   b. Ammonia levels.
   c. Blood glucose.
   d. Serum electrolytes.
   e. BUN.
   f. Osmolality.
   g. Blood gases.
5. Treatment is directed toward correction of metabolic imbalance and prevention of increased intracranial pressure. See *Increased Intracranial Pressure.*
   a. Adequate oxygenation via ventilator, if necessary.
   b. Hydration with 10 percent dextrose to prevent fat deposits in the liver.
   c. Thermoregulation via cooling blanket.
   d. Coma induced by curare, pancuronium bromide, barbiturates, etc.
   e. Barbiturate therapy.
   f. Intracranial pressure monitoring.
   g. Sedation.

h. Osmotic diuretics.

i. Dexamethasone, vitamin K, and neomycin may be ordered if blood ammonia levels are excessive.

j. Monitoring liver function, fluid and electrolyte balance, and kidney function.

6. Staging criteria established by Lovejoy may be used to initiate treatment or to determine progress:

   a. Stage I: Vomiting, lethargy, abnormal lab values, evidence of liver dysfunction, type 1 EEG.

   b. Stage II: Disorientation, combativeness, hyperventilation, hyperreflexia, abnormal lab values, evidence of liver dysfunction, type 2 EEG.

   c. Stage III: Coma, decorticate posturing, hyperventilation, abnormal lab values, evidence of liver dysfunction, type 2 EEG.

   d. Stage IV: Deeper coma, decerebrate posturing, loss of oculocephalic and pupillary reflexes, minimal evidence of liver dysfunction, evidence of brainstem impairment, type 3 or 4 EEG.

   e. Stage V: Seizures, absence of deep tendon reflexes, muscular flaccidity, respiratory arrest, type 4 EEG.

7. Patients in Stages I and II will usually have treatment which is anticipatory and noninvasive with emphasis on observation and hydration.

8. Patients in Stage III or greater on admission will have more aggressive treatment.

B. **Nursing Management.**

1. Support the child and parent during hospitalization. See *Hospitalization, Support During.*

2. Initiate discharge planning. See *Discharge Planning.*

3. Observe, record, and report neurological and cardiovascular status as ordered.

4. Prepare the child and parents for procedures. See *Preparation for Procedures.*

   a. Cardiac monitoring.

   b. Apnea monitoring.

   c. I.V. initiation.

5. Assist with invasive monitoring equipment as condition warrants.

   a. Foley catheter.

   b. Arterial, central venous pressure, or pulmonary capillary wedge pressure lines.

   c. Intracranial pressure monitor.

   d. Nasogastric tube.

   e. Endotracheal intubation.

   f. Hypothermia blanket.

6. Assess level of consciousness, alertness, and responsiveness every hour.

   a. Check pupillary size, position, light response.

b. Note verbalization, motor response to command or pain.

   c. If unconscious, note spontaneous movement and pain responses.

7. Monitor intake and output strictly.

   a. Fluid may be restricted to two-thirds of maintenance to treat increased ICP.

   b. Dehydrating agents may be used to induce diuresis.

8. Discontinue hypothermia if shivering or cardiac arrythmia occurs.

9. Observe, record, and report side effects of all medications.

10. Meet needs of the immobilized child (Miller and Arsenault, 1983). See *Immobilized Child.*

    a. Elevated head of bed 30 degrees.

    b. Keep head and neck aligned.

    c. Provide range of motion at least once a shift.

    d. Provide frequent turning, suctioning, but postural drainage is contraindicated.

    e. Use mattress or bed designed to prevent pressure on bony prominences, but which does not require frequent repositioning of the child.

11. Support the parents in dealing with an acutely ill child. See *Crisis Intervention* and *Life-threatening Illness.*

12. Begin reorientation to person, time, and place as soon as the child awakens from the comatose state.

13. Provide appropriate play activities as the child's condition improves since the ICU experience is very traumatic to the young child. See *Play, Therapeutic* and *Stimulation.*

14. Refer to community health nurse or other agencies as needed.

Rhabdomyosarcoma. Malignant soft tissue neoplasm involving striated muscle.

A. **General Considerations.**

1. Rhabdomyosarcoma can be found almost anywhere in the body.

   a. Head and neck area, particularly orbit and nasopharynx.

   b. Genitourinary tract.

   c. Extremities.

   d. Trunk.

2. The tumor may occur as a solid mass or as grapelike lesions.

3. The tumor is rarely painful and produces few symptoms except a palpable mass.

   a. Orbital tumors cause proptosis and diplopia.

   b. Nasopharyngeal tumors cause respiratory obstruction, epistaxis, or discharge.

R

c. Vaginal tumors cause bleeding and tissue passes through the vagina.

d. Bladder or prostate tumors cause urinary retention.

4. Metastasis occurs early by lymphatic and hematogenous routes, particularly to the bone, liver, lymph nodes, and lungs.

5. Diagnostic studies may be numerous in order to determine the extent of tumor involvement.

a. Chest x-ray.

b. Tomograms of the facial bones, skull, and pharynx.

c. Lymphangiograms.

d. Intravenous pyelogram.

e. Liver scan.

f. Bone scan.

g. CAT scan (computerized axial tomography).

h. Bone marrow aspiration.

i. Renal function studies.

j. Liver function studies.

6. Rhabdomyosarcoma is usually classified into stages based on the extent of tumor involvement so that treatment can be planned.

7. The primary tumor will be treated with surgical excision and/or radiation therapy unless the surgery would be too mutilating, e.g., orbital tumor.

8. Radiation therapy or chemotherapy may be used preoperatively to shrink a large tumor mass.

9. Chemotherapy with multiple drugs is used in all cases.

10. The survival rate may reach 80 to 100 percent if the child has localized disease that is treated aggressively.

11. Prognosis is poorer when the tumor cannot be totally excised surgically or when metastasis has occurred prior to diagnosis.

B. **Nursing Management.** See CRISIS INTERVENTION and LIFE-THREATENING ILLNESS.

1. Support the child and parents during hospitalization. See *Hospitalization, Support During.*

2. Initiate discharge planning. See *Discharge Planning.*

3. Provide consistency and continuity of care, since the child must endure so many painful diagnostic and therapeutic procedures. See *Preparation for Procedures.*

4. Accompany the physician, if possible, when explanations are given to the child and parents so that consistent, accurate information is communicated.

a. Anxiety interferes with the ability of the child and the parents to comprehend information.

b. The information should be recorded on the Kardex so that the same explanation can be given each time the child or parents ask.

1. Answer all questions honestly.

2. Use terminology the child understands.

c. Arrange for uninterrupted periods of contact with the child and parents so supportive discussions can be held.

5. Meet the needs of the child and parents preoperatively. See *Preoperative Care* and *Preparation for Surgery.*

6. Meet the needs of the child and parents postoperatively. See *Postoperative Care.*

7. Meet the needs of the child receiving chemotherapy or radiation therapy. See *Chemotherapy* and *Radiation Therapy.*

8. Teach the child and parents home management.

a. Encourage the parents to make home life as normal as possible.

1. Have the child resume normal activities such as play groups or school.

2. Encourage normal peer relationships.

3. Maintain normal discipline. See *Discipline.*

4. Encourage adequate rest and nutrition for all family members.

b. Encourage therapeutic play to help the child work through feelings about intrusive procedures, since chemotherapy and radiation therapy will continue on an outpatient basis. See *Play, Therapeutic.*

9. Meet the needs of the child who does not respond to therapy. See *Dying Child.*

Rheumatic fever. An inflammatory process that affects the heart, joints, central nervous system, and subcutaneous tissues.

A. **General Considerations.**

1. The disease usually develops 2 to 6 weeks after a group A beta hemolytic streptococcal upper respiratory infection, e.g., streptococcal pharyngitis.

2. The exact pathogenic mechanism is unknown but is felt to be an altered immune response to the organism or its products.

3. Acute rheumatic fever does not occur following streptococcal skin infections (Kaplan, 1978).

4. Diagnosis is difficult since there are no specific diagnostic lab tests, and similar signs and symptoms may occur with other illnesses, e.g., juvenile rheumatoid arthritis, erythema nodosum.

5. The revised Jones criteria are used to establish the diagnosis and include:

a. Major criteria:

1. Polyarthritis—migratory arthritis,

particularly of the large joints of the extremities presenting with heat, redness, swelling, pain, and tenderness.

2. Carditis—pericarditis, myocarditis, and endocarditis.

3. Erythema marginatum—thin wavy red lines surrounding an area of normal skin on the trunk and/or proximal parts of the extremities.

4. Subcutaneous nodules—small, hard, painless, freely moveable swellings found on the extensor surface of joints.

5. Sydenham's chorea—involuntary, purposeless movements affecting all parts of the body which may occur weeks or months after the initial infection.

  b. Minor criteria:
1. Previous rheumatic fever.
2. Arthralgia.
3. Fever.
4. Acute phase reaction—elevated ESR, C-reactive protein, leukocytosis.
5. Prolonged P-R interval on an electrocardiogram.

  c. Other manifestations include abdominal pain, epistaxis, vomiting, malaise, and weight loss.

6. The presence of two major or one major and two minor Jones criteria plus evidence of a recent streptococcal infection (elevated ASO titer, positive throat culture, scarlet fever) is considered diagnostic.

7. Treatment measures include (Hoffmann, 1983):

  a. Antibiotics.
1. Used initially to eradicate all streptococcal organisms.
2. Continued indefinitely if heart disease present or for approximately 10 years if no heart involvement.

  b. Salicylates—for arthritis and mild carditis.

  c. Steroids—for severe carditis.

  d. Bed rest—for carditis and chorea.

  e. Activity restrictions—for residual rheumatic heart disease.

  f. No specific treatment is available for Sydenham's chorea.

8. Antibiotics used:

  a. For initial attack include one of the following:
1. Benzathine penicillin G intramuscularly (one dose only).
2. Procaine penicillin G intramuscularly for 10 days.
3. Erythromycin orally for 10 days for child allergic to penicillin.

  b. For long-term prophylaxis include one of the following:

1. Benzathine penicillin G intramuscularly once a month.
2. Penicillin orally twice a day.
3. Sulfadiazine orally once a day.

9. The child who has had rheumatic fever is prone to recurrences following streptococcal infections.

10. Cardiac complications of rheumatic fever include:

  a. Valvular damage: mitral (most common) and aortic; other valves are less commonly affected.

  b. Pericardial effusion.

  c. Congestive heart failure.

11. Patients with heart valve damage are at increased risk for endocarditis following dental procedures and gastrointestinal and genitourinary surgery and require increased antibiotic prophylaxis (Fitzmaurice, 1980).

12. The characteristic heart lesions of rheumatic fever are called Ashoff bodies.

13. Treatment will not stop the rheumatic process but will decrease the chance of complications and alleviate symptoms.

14. Return of the sleeping pulse to normal range is a good guide to improvement.

15. The child may be hospitalized initially but the trend is toward home management.

B. Nursing Management. See CHRONIC ILLNESS.

1. Support the child and parents during hospitalization. See *Hospitalization, Support During.*

2. Initiate discharge planning. See *Discharge Planning.*

3. Meet the ongoing needs of the child according to his age and developmental level, e.g., hygienic care, nutrition.

4. Meet the needs of the child with carditis.

  a. Carry out bed rest regimen as ordered. See *Immobilized Child.*
1. Teach the child and parents why bed rest is necessary.
2. Position the child in correct alignment.
3. Use a semi-Fowler's position to facilitate breathing.
4. Use a footboard to prevent footdrop.
5. Plan care to provide frequent rest periods.
6. Provide age-appropriate activities that give the child some sense of mastery to decrease boredom and promote compliance with staying in bed.
7. Arrange for continuation of education as child's condition permits.

  b. Observe, record, and report the child's response to medications which may be ordered:

R

1. Antibiotics: rash, gastrointestinal upset.
2. Salicylates: increased bleeding tendency, salicylate poisoning (uncommon with usual dosage schedule).
3. Steroids: fluid retention, moon face, striae, acne; will depend on the length of treatment.

c. Monitor vital signs accurately; take an apical pulse for a full minute.
d. Take and record a sleeping pulse each night.
e. Observe, record, and report signs and symptoms of congestive heart failure.
   1. Tachypnea.
   2. Tachycardia.
   3. Weight gain.
   4. Dyspnea.
   5. Easy fatigability.
   6. Restlessness.
   7. Orthopnea.
   8. Neck vein distention.
   9. Cyanosis.
f. Administer oxygen as ordered to decrease the heart's workload.
g. Record intake, output, and daily weight.
h. Offer smaller, more frequent feedings.
i. Perform passive range of motion exercises.
j. Provide meticulous skin care to prevent skin breakdown due to inactivity.

5. Meet the needs of the child with arthralgia.
   a. Observe, record, and report the child's response to salicylates.
   b. Move the child gently.
   c. Support affected joints.
   d. Promote joint movement that the child can tolerate, to decrease threat of contractures.
   e. Tell the child and parents that inflammation will subside and no residual joint damage will occur.

6. Meet the needs of the child with Sydenham's chorea (St. Vitus' dance).
   a. Promote bed rest to prevent injury and reduce energy needs.
   b. Pad the bed to prevent injury.
   c. Observe, record, and report the child's response to sedatives or tranquilizers that may be ordered.
   d. Provide the child with a private room or one in which there is minimal noise and activity.
   e. Give the child soft toys that do not require fine motor coordination.
   f. Provide a light, nourishing diet that is high in protein.
   g. Feed the child if he cannot feed himself.
   h. Approach the child in a calm, pleasant manner, since tension increases symptoms.
   i. Respond to the child's needs in a prompt, consistent manner to decrease stress.
   j. Tell the child and parents that symptoms will eventually go away and the child will not have residual damage.
   k. Assist the child who is ambulatory.
   l. Prevent falls by restraining the child who is out of bed.
   m. Provide support during the convalescent period.
      1. Encourage increasing muscle control by giving the child large muscle tasks and progressing to small muscle activities.
      2. Encourage gradual return to schoolwork, e.g., home tutor followed by shortened school day, etc.

7. Prepare the child and parents for long-term antibiotic therapy.
   a. Find out which drug and route of administration is planned.
   b. Discuss the rationale for long-term antibiotic therapy, e.g., prevent rheumatic heart disease.
   c. Discuss ways in which the older child may be helped to cope with monthly injections if these are planned. See *Coping*.
      1. Offer a choice of site to be used.
      2. Keep record of site used previously.
      3. Praise for cooperating.
   d. Explain the administration of oral antibiotics by parents if this is planned. See *Administration of Medications, Parental.*
   e. Explore family's beliefs and practices that may interfere with compliance with the long-term therapy. See *Cultural Aspects of Health Care* and *Religious Aspects of Health Care.*
   f. Support the adolescent, who may rebel against long-term therapy, in the development of an acceptable form of long-term management.

8. Assist the child and parents in developing a plan for home management.
   a. Provide opportunities for the child and parents to discuss their feelings about the long-term nature of care, since this promotes acceptance of the situation and compliance with the plan.
   b. Promote rest.
      1. Give the child a room or bed of his own.
      2. Make sure the child and parents understand exact activity limitations.
      3. Involve the child in the plan to promote compliance.
      4. Incorporate the child's usual schedule into the plan as much as possible, e.g.,

schoolwork periods, television watching, meals.

   c. Minimize feelings of boredom and isolation.

     1. Involve all family members in child's care.

     2. Encourage contact with peers via phone, cards, or short visits.

     3. Provide age-appropriate activities. See *Stimulation*.

   d. Promote comfort.

     1. Administer medications for joint pain.

     2. Keep bedclothes off joints by use of bedcradle.

     3. Handle carefully.

     4. Support extremities.

   e. Promote nutrition. See *Nutrition*.

9. Teach parents care measures for child with chorea (see above).

10. Plan for a resumption of schoolwork.

   a. Find out what physician plans.

   b. Help parents plan for a tutor.

   c. Support parents in contacting the child's teacher to discuss assignments, when the child may be returning to school and ways in which the child can be included in schoolwork, e.g., carry out a part of a larger class project.

11. Teach parents to call the physician if the child:

   a. Develops signs of congestive heart failure.

   b. Experiences an increase in any associated minor criteria, e.g., fever, arthalgia.

   c. Develops an upper respiratory infection.

12. Initiate a referral to a community health nurse.

Rocky Mountain spotted fever.

A noncommunicable acute febrile illness caused by *Rickettsia rickettsii* and transmitted by ticks.

A. General Considerations.

1. Signs and symptoms develop suddenly 3 to 10 days after attachment of, or exposure to, a disease-carrying tick.

   a. High fever.

   b. Severe headache.

   c. Muscle aching.

   d. Vomiting.

   e. Anorexia.

   f. Abdominal pain.

2. One to 5 days after the onset of fever a rose-red macular or maculopapular rash develops that:

   a. Starts on extremities and involves palm, wrists, soles, and ankles and blanches on pressure.

   b. Spreads inward toward trunk and involves the face.

   c. May become petechial after 2 to 3 days and no longer blanches.

   d. Does not itch.

3. Rocky Mountain spotted fever must be differentiated from other conditions which present with similar signs and symptoms, e.g., meningococcemia, atypical measles, rubella, thrombotic thrombocytopenic purpura.

4. Confirmation of the diagnosis is made by:

   a. Complement fixation: requires 14 to 21 days for antibody titer to rise.

   b. Indirect fluorescent antibody test of punch biopsy of rash: permits early positive diagnosis.

5. Prompt treatment with the antibiotics tetracycline, chloramphenicol, and/or doxycycline with rifampin is necessary to prevent complications.

6. Complications caused by rickettsial invasion include:

   a. Central nervous system symptoms, e.g., delirium, stupor, coma.

   b. Thrombocytopenia.

   c. Pneumonia.

   d. Peripheral circulatory collapse.

B. Nursing Management.

1. Support the child and parents during hospitalization. See *Hospitalization, Support During*.

2. Initiate discharge planning. See *Discharge Planning*.

3. Administer antibiotics as ordered and observe, record, and report the child's response.

4. Reduce fever. See *Fever Reduction*.

5. Encourage fluids. See *Forcing Fluids*.

6. Administer analgesics as ordered.

7. Observe, record, and report signs and symptoms of fluid and electrolyte imbalance. See *Fluid and Electrolyte Imbalance*.

8. Monitor I.V. accurately.

9. Observe, record, and report:

   a. Alterations in level of consciousness.

   b. Increasing temperature, pulse, and/or respirations.

   c. Falling blood pressure.

   d. Coughing.

   e. Skin breakdown in hemorrhagic rash areas.

10. Promote nutrition. See *Nutrition*.

11. Teach the parents to administer all the medication as prescribed. See *Administration of Medications, Parental*.

12. Teach the child and parents who live in tick infested areas:

   a. Dress appropriately to avoid tick bites.

     1. Wear long pants and tuck them into socks or boots.

     2. Keep shirt or blouse buttoned and shirt-tail tucked into pants.

R

b. Check for ticks on clothing and skin, and in hair and ears after being in the woods or long grass.

c. Remove tick promptly and handle appropriately.

   1. Use tweezers or cover fingers.

   2. Grasp close to point of attachment and pull steadily to dislodge.

   3. Wash area and apply antiseptic.

d. Call physician immediately if signs and symptoms develop.

Roseola (exanthem subitum).
Childhood disease affecting the child from 6 months to 3 years of age.

A. General Considerations.

1. The cause is suspected to be a virus.
2. Signs and symptoms include:
   a. High fever.
   b. Irritability.
   c. Anorexia.
   d. Lymphadenopathy.
3. The fever drops in 3 to 5 days.
4. A rose-pink macular rash appears after the drop in fever.
5. The rash appears on the trunk then spreads to other parts of the body.
6. The child remains alert and playful in spite of the high fever.
7. Febrile convulsion can be a complication. See *Seizures, Febrile.*
8. Treatment is symptomatic although an antibiotic may be prescribed if the pharynx is inflamed.
9. Prophylactic use of phenobarbital after a febrile convulsion is controversial.
10. One attack confers life-long immunity.

B. Nursing Management.

1. Reduce fever. See *Fever Reduction* and *Forcing Fluids.*
2. Administer antibiotic as instructed and observe the child's response to the medication. See *Administration of Medications, Parental.*
3. Provide comfort measures for the rash. See *Rash.*

Rubella (German measles).
A contagious viral disease of childhood.

A. General Considerations.

1. The child may or may not have prodromal symptoms 1 to 5 days before the rash.
   a. Mild fever.
   b. Coughing.
   c. Sneezing.
   d. Nasal congestion.

e. Enlargement of posterior cervical, suboccipital, and postauricular nodes.
2. A pink, discrete macular eruption begins on the face and spreads rapidly to the trunk and proximal extremities.
3. The rash fades in 2 days in the same order in which it appeared.
4. The total duration of the rash (exanthem) is about 3 days.
5. Complications are rare.
   a. Encephalitis.
   b. Arthritis.
   c. Thrombocytopenic purpura.
6. Treatment is symptomatic.
7. The prognosis is excellent.
8. The major importance of the rubella virus is its teratogenic effects on the fetus of the susceptible woman during the first trimester.
   a. Growth retardation.
   b. Cardiac anomalies, e.g., patent ductus arteriosis, ventricular septal defect, branch stenosis of the pulmonary arteries.
   c. Eye defects, e.g., congenital glaucoma, cataracts, microphthalmia.
   d. Deafness.
   e. Thrombocytopenia.
   f. CNS defects, e.g., mental retardation, learning disability, behavioral disorders.
9. The infant with congenital rubella may shed the virus in the blood or urine for 12 to 18 months.
10. Prevention can be obtained by immunization with live attenuated rubella virus vaccine. See *Immunizations.*

B. Nursing Management.

1. Keep the child on bed rest when febrile or if the complication of arthritis occurs. See *Home Management of Minor Illnesses.*
2. Initiate fever reduction measures if needed. See *Fever Reduction* and *Forcing Fluids.*
3. Administer aspirin as instructed for joint pain if arthritis occurs. See *Administration of Medications, Parental.*
4. Provide comfort measures for the rash. See *Rash.*
5. Isolate the child with rubella who is hospitalized. See *Isolated Child.*

Rubeola (measles, red measles).
A highly contagious infection caused by the rubeola virus.

A. General Considerations.

1. Signs and symptoms include:
   a. Fever.
   b. Malaise.
   c. Sneezing.
   d. Nasal congestion.
   e. Brassy cough.

R

f. Conjunctivitis.

g. Koplick's spots on the buccal mucosa.

h. Photophobia.

i. Erythematous, maculopapular rash.

2. The child feels most ill on the 4th or 5th day.

3. The fever drops and symptoms improve considerably on the 5th or 6th day.

4. A branny desquamation of the skin occurs after the rash fades.

5. The administration of immune serum globulin after exposure may reduce the intensity and duration of the illness.

6. Treatment is supportive.

7. Antibiotic therapy may be necessary if complications occur.

   a. Otitis media.

   b. Pneumonia.

   c. Postinfectious encephalitis.

   d. Sensorineural deafness.

   e. Arthritis.

   f. Hepatitis.

8. Live attenuated vaccine should be given to children over 1 year of age. See *Immunizations*.

B. **Nursing Management.**

1. Reduce fever. See *Fever Reduction* and *Forcing Fluids*.

2. Promote comfort. See *Home Management of Minor Illnesses*.

   a. Keep the child on bed rest.

   b. Relieve the discomfort of the rash. See *Rash*.

   c. Administer a cough suppressant.

   d. Increase the room humidity to decrease cough.

   e. Dim the room light since the child is photophobic.

   f. Irrigate the eyes with normal saline or apply moist compresses to relieve itching.

3. Isolate the child from others until 5 days after the rash appears.

4. Observe, and report signs and symptoms of complications.

   a. Prolonged fever.

   b. Increased lethargy.

   c. Respiratory difficulty.

   d. Pulling at the ears.

   e. Stiff neck.

   f. Vomiting.

   g. Hearing difficulty.

   h. Joint pain.

   i. Jaundice.

Safety. See *Accident Prevention*.

St. Vitus dance. See *Rheumatic Fever*.

Salicylate poisoning. See *Poisoning*.

Sarcoma, Ewing's. See *Ewing's Sarcoma*.

Sarcoma, osteogenic. See *Osteosarcoma*.

Scabies. Communicable skin infestation caused by the female itch mite *Sarcoptes scabiei*.

A. **General Considerations.**

1. Transmission of the disease occurs through:

   a. Close physical contact with infected person.

   b. Contact with contaminated clothing or linens (less common).

2. Signs and symptoms include:

   a. Burrows made by the mature female which may appear as:

      1. Papular erythematous lines.

      2. Black-colored lines (less common).

   b. Erythematous round papules caused by intracutaneous invasion of larvae.

   c. Intense itching, which is worse at night, after 2 to 3 weeks as a result of host sensitization.

3. Diagnosis is confirmed by finding the mite or ova in skin scrapings.

4. Areas commonly infected include the:

   a. Areas between fingers and toes.

   b. Palms.

   c. Axillae.

   d. Genitalia.

   e. Buttocks.

   f. Periumbilical area.

   g. Periareolar area of female breasts.

5. Treatment of the child, family members, and, if the patient is a sexually active adolescent, sexual partner should be carried out simultaneously using one of the following scabicides:
   a. 1 percent gamma benzene hexachloride cream or lotion (Kwell, Lindane).
   b. 12.5 to 25 percent benzyl benzoate.
   c. 10 percent crotamiton cream or lotion (Eurax).
6. Crotamiton cream or lotion should be used with infants, young children, and during pregnancy since use of gamma benzene hexachloride has been linked with neurotoxicity (Wittner, 1982).
7. One thorough application of scabicide should eliminate the disease; if retreatment is necessary it can be repeated in 1 week to kill mites which hatched after the initial treatment.
8. Clothing and bedding should be washed in a washing machine and ironed or dry cleaned.
9. Pruritus may continue for several days to a few weeks as a result of the hypersensitivity, and secondary infection may occur as a result of scratching.
10. Topical corticosteroids may be prescribed to reduce itching.

B. **Nursing Management.**
1. Be nonjudgmental in your approach to care; anyone can catch scabies.
2. Care for the hospitalized child who has scabies.
   a. Place child on wound/skin precautions for 24 hours after treatment (Wachtel, 1979).
   b. Wash hands thoroughly after contact to prevent infection or wear gloves during contact.
   c. Reduce holding time until treatment is carried out.
   d. Apply scabicide as ordered.
   e. Use soothing ointment for pruritus.
   f. Double bag all linens and mark for isolation while child is on isolation precautions.
3. Teach older child and parents correct application of gamma benzene hexachloride.
   a. Bathe thoroughly and wash hair at bedtime; allow skin to dry completely.
   b. Start at the neck and work down using gauze pads or a soft paint brush to apply cream or lotion; cover all skin.
   c. Wait 10 to 15 minutes for skin to dry, then dress in clean pajamas.
   d. Shower the following morning to remove scabicide.
4. Teach younger child and parents correct application of crotamiton.
   a. Bathe child and wash hair; allow skin to dry completely.
   b. Rub cream over entire skin surface and allow to dry.
   c. Repeat application in 24 hours.
   d. Wash thoroughly after 48 hours.
5. Teach the child and parents.
   a. Treat all family members at the same time.
   b. Wash clothes and bedlinens in washing machine/boiling water or dry clean.
   c. Reduce itching.
      1. Use ½ box of baking soda in a tub of tepid water to relieve itching.
      2. Apply lotion.
      3. Apply corticosteroid cream as ordered.
   d. Prevent secondary infection from scratching by cutting the child's fingernails short and keeping them clean.
   e. Use only own personal clothes and bath linens.
6. Tell the parents to call the physician if:
   a. The medication does not clear the condition.
   b. Signs of secondary infection occur.

Scarlet fever (scarlatina). An infection caused by erythrogenic toxin-producing group A streptococci.

A. **General Considerations.**
1. The primary site of infection is the pharynx. See *Pharyngitis, Streptococcal.*
2. Signs and symptoms include:
   a. High fever.
   b. Vomiting.
   c. Sore throat.
   d. Chills.
   e. Malaise.
   f. Edematous, enlarged tonsils covered with patches of exudate.
   g. Edematous and beefy red pharynx.
   h. Erythematous lesions and petechiae on the soft palate and uvula.
3. The tongue appears like a white strawberry for the first day or two, then becomes bright red by the 4th or 5th day.
4. A characteristic rash occurs 12 to 72 hours after the disease onset.
   a. The rash begins as a diffuse, erythematous papular rash at the base of the neck, axillae, groin, and trunk.
   b. The rash has a "sandpaper" feel.
   c. The rash covers the body within 24 hours.
   d. Circumoral pallor occurs because the cheeks are red and flushed.
   e. The rash begins to peel beginning with the neck at the end of the 1st week.
   f. The entire rash peels by the 3rd week.
5. Penicillin or other antibiotics are administered to prevent secondary infections of rheumatic fever or acute glomerulonephritis.

6. Other complications include cervical adentitis, otitis media, sinusitis, and bronchopneumonia.

B. Nursing Management.

1. Keep the child on bed rest during the febrile period. See *Home Management of Minor Illnesses.*
2. Initiate fever reduction measures. See *Fever Reduction.*
3. Observe the child's response to antibiotic therapy.
4. Promote comfort.
   a. Administer aspirin or analgesics as instructed. See *Administration of Medications, Parental.*
   b. Have the older child gargle with warm saline.
   c. Keep a cool mist vaporizer at the bedside.
   d. Provide comfort measures for the rash if needed. See *Rash.*
   e. Provide mouth care frequently.
   f. Apply hot or cold compresses to the cervical nodes if tender.
5. Encourage clear fluids during the febrile period. See *Forcing Fluids.*
6. Offer soft, bland foods such as ice cream, sherbet, and soups when the fever subsides.
7. Begin quiet play activities as the child's condition improves. See *Play.*
8. Prevent infection of family members.
   a. Wash all the child's eating utensils, clothing, and linen separately.
   b. Clean and air the child's room thoroughly after the illness.
9. Report continued or recurrent fever to physician.
10. Report any symptoms of scarlet fever in other family members so a throat culture can be done.
11. Isolate the child with scarlet fever if hospitalization is necessary. See *Isolated Child.*

School phobia. Extreme reluctance to attend school.

A. General Considerations.

1. The child's basic fear is that of separating from home rather than fear of going to school.
2. The school-phobic child may have physical symptoms that resolve as soon as the parent states the child can remain at home.
   a. Vomiting.
   b. Diarrhea.
   c. Headache.
   d. Abdominal pain.
   e. Dizziness.
   f. Pain in an extremity.
3. Several causes have been identified.

a. A fear of separating from the mother with whom the child has a strong, mutually dependent relationship is characteristic.
   1. The mother is as unwilling to have the child leave as the child is unwilling to leave.
   2. The extreme dependency may be precipitated by an event which intensified the mother–child relationship, e.g., illness, birth of a sibling.
   3. If the parent has threatened to leave him, the child may fear this will happen while he attends school.
b. Problems within the school environment may be a cause.
   1. Overcritical, sarcastic teacher.
   2. Fear of academic failure.
   3. Fear of physical harm by peers.
   4. Actual or imagined discrimination by peers.
4. The child who has school-phobia differs from the child who is a truant.
   a. The school-phobic child does well in school; the truant does not.
   b. The school-phobic child stays at home; the truant does not go home when not at school.
   c. The school-phobic child is out of school for long continuous periods; the truant skips school intermittently.
   d. The school-phobic's parents know of school absences; the truant's parents may not be aware of school absence.
5. Young children usually respond better to treatment than older children in whom the phobia may be a symptom of a serious emotional problem.
6. Treatment is usually aimed at getting the child back into school as soon as possible.
   a. The child can be helped to cope with a specific fear such as oral class presentation or peer relationship.
   b. Gradual return to full school attendance (desensitization) may be necessary in some cases.
   c. Counseling or psychotherapy may be required for the family if desensitization is ineffective.

B. Nursing Management. See ADOLESCENT and SCHOOLCHILD.

1. Obtain additional data about family relationships and the child's attitude toward school if the nursing history indicates problems in school attendance. See *Nursing History.*
2. Prepare the child and parents if diagnostic procedures are done to rule out organic disease. See *Preparation for Procedures.*
3. Reinforce the expectation that the child can return to school if support is given by the par-

S

ents, health professionals, and school authorities.

4. Initiate a referral to the school nurse to share nursing approaches to the child and family.

5. Review the plans to return the child to school, e.g., parent(s) accompanying the child, half-day attendance, etc.

6. Assist both the child and parents in coping with referral to the psychiatrist or psychologist by reminding them that referrals are frequently made to other specialists such as ophthalmologists, orthopedic surgeon, etc.

School, preparation for. Measures to help the child adjust to the school experience.

A. General Considerations.

1. Most young children look forward to entering kindergarten or first grade because it signifies being a "big kid."

2. The child must adjust to certain changes at whatever age he begins formal schooling.
   a. Separation from parents or primary caregivers.
   b. Supervision by different adults.
   c. Having safety and satisfaction needs met by new people.
   d. Responsibility for self-care, e.g., putting on coat and boots.
   e. Competition with other children for adult attention and assistance.
   f. Cooperation with others.

3. The child must learn the code of behavior expected at school in general and in his particular classroom.

4. The greater the gap between the kind of behavior expected at home and that expected at school, the more difficult the child's school adjustment will be.

5. The child's ability to cope with new experiences and developmental level will also affect his school adjustment.

B. Nursing Management.

1. Provide opportunities for the parents, particularly the mother, to express feelings about the child's separation from home and family.
   a. The child will perceive the parents' nonverbal feelings of anxiety and uncertainty.
   b. Parents frequently have ambivalent feelings of wanting to hold on to the child, yet wanting the child to be independent.

2. Suggest to parents that they obtain information about school routines, class size, and lunch and recess times so they can help the child know what to expect.

3. Encourage the parents to arrange a visit to the school so the child has a concrete idea of what a "school" is.

   a. The child who copes well with new experiences and/or has had nursery school experience may enjoy a visit when school is in session so the activities can be observed.
   b. The child who is hesitant in new experiences and/or has not had nursery school experience may cope better if shown the building when school is not in session and therefore the environment is less active.

4. Show the child the route from home to school and back, even if he will ride a school bus.

5. Suggest that the child participate in the purchase of pencils, notebook, etc., and selection of clothes to wear the first day.

6. Encourage the parent to accompany the child (without bringing younger siblings) the first day and to tell the child, in advance, how long the parent will stay.

7. Encourage the mother to tell the child what her activities will be during the day.
   a. The child may be concerned about missing out on special activities.
   b. The child may be jealous about a younger sibling having more of the mother's attention.

8. Discuss with the parents the importance of planning time each day for the child to share school activities so that the positive experiences can be reinforced and negative experiences dealt with immediately.

Schoolchild. Child in the period of development between the ages of 6 years and puberty.

A. General Considerations.

1. The schoolchild is faced with the following development tasks (Duvall, 1977):
   a. Decreasing dependence on family and gaining satisfaction from relationships with others.
   b. Increasing neuromuscular skills.
   c. Learning basic adult concepts and facts that prepare him for daily living.
   d. Becoming a more active family member.
   e. Earning money and saving it for later purchases.
   f. Learning to handle strong emotions appropriately.
   g. Accepting a changing body image and accepting a masculine or feminine social role.
   h. Developing a positive attitude toward his or her own attitudes and beliefs and the beliefs and attitudes of others.

2. Accomplishment of these developmental tasks is spread over a long time period.

3. Care must be individualized for each child.

4. Learning how to do things well occupies a great deal of the schoolchild's time, and the child en-

joys being involved in projects he or she can complete alone.

5. Growth is steady for both boys and girls during this time period.

6. School and peer group relationships become increasingly important during the schoolage period.

7. The schoolchild becomes increasingly aware of his or her body and desires to learn about how the body functions.

B. **Nursing Management.**

1. Support the parents in meeting the child's needs but assist them in accepting increasing independence. See *Parenting*.

2. Meet the daily physical needs of the schoolchild.
   a. Provide for hygienic care.
      1. Promote self-care.
      2. Assist as needed and/or requested.
      3. Let the older schoolchild take a shower if desired and available.
      4. Make sure that the child has a toothbrush and toothpaste and uses them.
      5. Wash hair as needed.
      6. Provide nail care as needed.
   b. Promote adequate nutrition. See *Nutrition*.
   c. Provide for rest and sleep routines. See *Sleep*.
   d. Protect from injury.
      1. Keep the bed in low position.
      2. Allow to ambulate freely but set limits as to where the child is allowed to go.
      3. Inform the child what the limits are, e.g., no wheelchair races or running in the halls.
   e. Protect from infection.
      1. Practice good hygienic techniques when giving care.
      2. Teach appropriate hygienic practices to the child.
      3. Prevent contact with others who have an infectious illness.
   f. Provide for exercise. See *Exercise*.

3. Meet the emotional needs of the schoolchild.
   a. Involve the child in planning and carrying out care.
   b. Accept regression which may occur but encourage as much independence as possible.
   c. Explain all procedures carefully and give the child adequate time for emotional preparation. See *Preparation for Procedures*.
   d. Provide age-appropriate group activities. See *Play*.
   e. Provide privacy for the child.
   f. Give the child some responsibility for his or her room and belongings.
   g. Help the child maintain contact with friends and classmates.

4. Meet the educational needs of the schoolchild who is able to do schoolwork while hospitalized.
   a. See that books and homework are brought to child.
   b. Schedule study time into child's care.
   c. Encourage the child to carry out assignments.
   d. Make arrangements for a hospital/homebound teacher, if the child will be absent from school for several weeks.

5. Provide anticipatory guidance to the child and parents related to the following areas on the basis of an assessment.
   a. Growth and development norms. See *Appendix v*.
   b. Common problems.
   c. Nutritional needs and habits. See *Nutrition*.
   d. Dental care. See *Dental Care*.
   e. Safety. See *Accident Prevention*.
   f. The importance of peer group relationships.
   g. Provision for ongoing health care. See *Well-child Care*.
   h. Sex education. See *Sex Education*.

Scoliosis, idiopathic. Lateral, S-shaped curvature of the spine, the cause of which is unknown.

A. **General Considerations.**

1. Scoliosis is asymptomatic.

2. Signs of scoliosis are frequently missed because it occurs most commonly in adolescence which is a healthy life period and because teenagers are seldom observed nude by their parents.
   a. Prominence of one hip.
   b. Deformity of the rib cage.
   c. Prominence of one scapula.
   d. Difference in shoulder or scapular height.
   e. Curve in the vertebral spinous process alignment.
   f. Breasts appear unequal in size.

3. Severe rib cage deformity may compromise respirations, but straightening the spine will not restore respiratory function.

4. Diagnosis is confirmed by x-rays.

5. Screening for scoliosis should be routine for all children beginning in second grade and above, but this does not always occur.

6. Screening for scoliosis includes:
   a. Observation of the anterior, lateral, and posterior appearance of the child who is nude from the waist up.
   b. Observation of the child's back while bending over and reaching his toes with arms loose and palms facing each other.

7. Treatment varies with the severity of the curvature.

S

a. Curves of less than 30 degrees are treated by exercises and are followed with serial x-rays.

b. Curves of less than 40 degrees may be treated with electrical stimulation of the muscles (Scolitron) if the adolescent has at least 2 or more years of skeletal growth remaining and no previous treatment.

c. Curves of 30 to 60 degrees are treated conservatively with a Milwaukee brace or T.L.S.O. (thoracic-lumbar-sacral orthosis) brace.

1. The brace may be worn from 6 months to 3 years until the curve is corrected or growth has ceased.

2. Weaning from the brace requires a year.

d. Curves over 60 degrees, rapidly progressing curves, or cervicothoracic curves with marked cosmetic defect usually require surgery.

1. Moderate curvatures may be corrected by plaster casts or traction before surgery, followed by spinal fusion and immobilization in a cast.

2. Severe curvatures may be corrected with a Harrington or Leuke rod or other instrumentation, followed by spinal fusion and immobilization in a cast.

8. The prognosis is better when the curvature is mild and when the curvature begins at an older age and less growth remains.

9. The Risser localizer cast extends from the cervical area to the pelvis.

a. Used to maintain traction and lateral compression to correct curvature or to stop progression of curvature.

b. May be applied preoperatively when the child requires spinal fusion.

10. Halo traction involves skeletal traction extending from pins in the head to either the femurs or the pelvic bones.

11. Halo traction is sometimes incorporated into a body cast, and the child can be ambulatory.

12. Harrington rods or Dwyer or Zielke instrumentation provides firm reduction of the curvature and support for the fused spine.

a. The rods or instruments are placed on each side of the spine.

b. The rods or instruments are left in place unless irritation occurs at a later time.

c. Evoked potential monitoring may be used during surgery to prevent compression of the spinal cord and/or nerves.

13. Spinal fusion of affected vertebrae is usually supplemented by an autogenous bone graft from the posterior iliac crest.

14. Instrumentation and spinal fusion may be a one- or two-stage procedure depending on the instrumentation used.

15. Postoperative ambulation is usually allowed after 2 weeks if instrumentation is used and after 3 months if fusion alone was performed.

16. The child with scoliosis will need help coping with body image changes during and after treatment.

17. The child and family will need to participate actively in decisions about treatment options, since they must assume responsibility for long-term management of the treatment selected.

B. Nursing Management.

1. Support the child and parents during hospitalization. See *Hospitalization, Support During*.

2. Initiate discharge planning. See *Discharge Planning*.

3. Provide opportunities for the teenager and the parents to verbalize their feelings about the length of time required for treatment, body image concerns, and the possibility of surgery if bracing is ineffective or inappropriate.

4. Teach the child and parents about the brace.

a. Wear the brace 24 hours a day, 7 days a week.

1. Remove for hygiene and/or swimming for a total of 1 hour per day.

2. Lie beside the pool when not swimming.

b. Apply alcohol, not lotions or powders, to pressure points in order to toughen the skin.

c. Keep the skin clean to prevent pustules and pimples.

d. Cover the throat mold of the Milwaukee brace with silk, linen, nylon, or dacron-cotton blend if sweating or irritation occur.

e. Choose loose and comfortable clothing.

f. Follow the exercise routine daily as instructed.

g. Continue physical activity except use of the trampoline, violent gymnastics, skateboards, diving, and contact sports.

h. Check the brace daily and tighten any loose screws.

i. Clean according to the instructions of the orthotist.

j. Tighten the straps if needed, but see the physician or orthotist for all adjustments.

k. Use a drafting table or portable easel to maintain good posture while doing schoolwork.

l. Use prism glasses to make reading possible in a prone position.

5. Meet the needs of the child in a Risser localizer cast.

a. Explain the procedure or have a child who

has experienced the cast tell the child about it.

1. Stockinette will be applied to the body.
2. Felt padding will be applied to bony prominences.
3. Head and pelvic traction will be applied to attain the best alignment possible.
4. A localizer pad will be applied over the apex of the curve.
5. The cast will be molded to the body.

b. Reassure the female adolescent that breast development will not be altered by the cast.

c. Explain that the teenager may feel that he or she is losing his or her balance while suspended for the cast application.

d. Remove excess plaster with a warm washcloth.

e. Provide skin care with alcohol around cast edges four times a day.

f. Assess neurovascular status every 4 hours.

1. Color.
2. Temperature.
3. Capillary filling.
4. Presence or absence of edema.
5. Sensation.
6. Motion.

g. Petal the cast when dry.

h. Turn every 2 hours.

i. Observe for signs of the cast syndrome.

1. Nausea and vomiting.
2. Severe abdominal pain.
3. Abdominal distention.

j. Discuss home care with the child and parents.

1. Have parents demonstrate the ability to turn the child.
2. Use a firm mattress.
3. Review cast care. See *Cast Care*.
4. Arrange for a tutor, home-bound teacher, or communication link-up if the child cannot return to school.
5. Maintain peer activities.
6. Emphasize need for follow-up for cast change to accomplish further correction and to accommodate growth.
7. Encourage exercises to maintain muscle tonicity.

6. Meet the needs of the child in halo traction.

a. Prepare the child by showing pictures of the apparatus or having a child who has had the traction applied talk to him.

1. The hair will be shampooed or the head shaved as necessary.
2. Local anesthesia will be used to insert four pins into the external cortex of the cranium and to insert Steinman pins into the distal end of the femur.

3. The child will be placed on a flotation pad, frame, or hoop to facilitate nursing care.
4. Weights will be added gradually.

b. Observe, record, and report the child's response to analgesics for pain at the pin sites or generalized headache.

c. Shampoo the hair frequently.

d. Provide pin care as ordered.

e. Check the pins daily to be sure they are tight.

f. Avoid bumping against the halo, since sounds are magnified by the halo.

g. Observe, record, and report signs and symptoms of complications.

1. Cyanosis.
2. Respiratory distress.
3. Diplopia
4. Pupil irregularity.
5. Numbness of hands or feet.
6. Inability to void.
7. Paralysis of lower extremities.

h. Observe, record, and report signs of infection at the pin site.

1. Irritation.
2. Swelling.
3. Drainage.
4. Pain or tenderness.

i. Check to see that all ropes and weights are hanging free.

j. Prevent skin breakdown.

1. Turn the child at least every 2 hours.
2. Use alcohol for skin care every 4 hours to toughen the skin.
3. Keep the heels off the mattress or frame when in bed.

k. Encourage the child to perform breathing exercises.

l. Institute range of motion activities.

m. Provide age-appropriate stimulation. See *Stimulation.*

1. Supply prism glasses for reading.
2. Provide activities that allow release of aggressive feelings.
3. Encourage peer interaction.

n. Modify a wheelchair (Stagnara's traction) so the child can be upright and mobile (Moe et al., 1978).

7. Meet the needs of the child who requires instrumentation and spinal fusion.

a. Explain to the child and parents how the cast applied preoperatively will be bivalved or windowed to allow for surgery.

b. Introduce the child to incentive spirometry, IPPB, or blow bottles to be used postoperatively.

c. Prepare the child and parents for surgery. See *Preoperative Care* and *Preparation for Surgery.*

d. Keep the bed flat postoperatively.

e. Log roll the child every 2 hours.

f. Irrigate the nasogastric tube as ordered.

g. Provide mouth care every 2 hours.

h. Assess neurological status every 2 hours.
   1. Color.
   2. Temperature.
   3. Capillary filling.
   4. Presence or absence of edema.
   5. Sensation.
   6. Motion.

i. Provide Foley catheter care twice a day or as ordered.

j. Observe, record, and report the child's response to respiratory therapy.

k. Observe, record, and report the child's response to pain medication. See *Pain*.

l. Observe, record, and report bleeding or drainage from the donor site on the iliac crest if bone grafts were used during the fusion.

m. Monitor the central venous pressure (CVP) line as ordered.

n. Prepare the child for suture removal 10 days postoperatively.

o. Prepare the child for application of a Risser cast or molded plastic cast 10 to 14 days postoperatively.
   1. A new cast will be applied after suture removal.
   2. An initial cast will be applied if one was not applied immediately postoperatively.

p. Teach the child and parents home management.
   1. Review the surgeon's recommendations for ambulation or bed rest.
   2. Review cast care. See *Cast Care*.
   3. Encourage the child to exercise at home to promote muscle tone and circulation.
   4. Have parents demonstrate application of antiembolism stockings, if appropriate.
   5. Arrange for a tutor, home-bound teacher, or communication link-up so the child can continue schoolwork.
   6. Encourage peer activities.
   7. Review need for safe environment, e.g., handrails on stairs, no scatter rugs, firm, solid shoes, etc.
   8. Encourage cosmetics, clothing, hairstyle, etc. to improve the adolescent's self-esteem.

8. Help the child adjust to cast removal.
   a. Reassure the child that treatment accomplished correction, although total improvement is not possible.
   b. Encourage the child to verbalize feelings about altered appearance and prolonged dependence on others.
   c. Support the child who falls frequently after the brace or cast is removed and explain that normal balance will be regained.
   d. Review the surgeon's recommendations for resuming activity.

Seborrhea. See *Dermatitis, Seborrheic*.

Seizures (epilepsy). Recurrence of periodic, excessive, and sudden outbursts of electrical activity from abnormal brain neurons which interfere with normal behavior (Swift, 1978).

A. **General Considerations.**
   1. Seizures are a symptom and not a disease.
   2. Seizures are categorized with subcategories as follows (Norman and Browne, 1981):
      a. Partial (seizures begin locally).
         1. Elementary partial (simple partial, focal) seizures.
         2. Complex partial (psychomotor, temporal lobe) seizures.
      b. Generalized seizures.
         1. Absence seizures (petit mal).
         2. Myoclonic seizures.
         3. Infantile spasms.
         4. Clonic seizures.
         5. Tonic seizures.
         6. Tonic-clonic seizures (grand mal).
         7. Atonic seizures.
         8. Akinetic seizures.
      c. Unilateral (involving one hemisphere).
      d. Unclassified.
   3. Epilepsy may be classified as:
      a. Primary (idiopathic)—without a known cause.
      b. Secondary—with a known cause such a tumor, meningitis, encephalitis, head trauma, etc.
   4. Activity seen during a seizure is dependent upon the cells affected, and a child may exhibit different types of seizures at different times.
   5. Auras (warnings) which are less common in children:
      a. May be broadly classified as:
         1. Motor—confused behavior.
         2. Sensory—flashing lights, blurred vision, G.I. upset, unusual smell.
         3. Psychic—change in mood.
      b. Are actually a part of the seizure.
      c. May or may not occur, e.g., characteristically absent with grand mal seizures.
      d. Can occur by themselves as small seizures.
   6. Elementary partial (simple partial, focal) seizures:

a. Result from local cortical discharge.
b. Are not accompanied by loss of consciousness.
c. Have symptoms related to the area of the brain that is discharging and include motor, sensory, and/or autonomic symptoms.

7. Complex partial (psychomotor, temporal lobe) seizures:
   a. May be preceded by an aura.
   b. May be accompanied by alterations in, or loss of, consciousness because discharge spreads to both hemispheres.
   c. Have symptomatology which may be:
      1. Cognitive—deja vu.
      2. Affective—fear, anxiety.
      3. Psychosensory—hallucinations, illusions.
      4. Psychomotor—automatisms such as lip smacking, purposeless movements.
   d. Are followed by a period of drowsiness or confusion.

8. Tonic–clonic (grand-mal) seizures:
   a. Are characterized by:
      1. Loss of consciousness at the onset.
      2. Tonic movements—stiffening of the body followed by:
      3. Clonic movements—alternating periods of tension and relaxation.
      4. A "cry" produced by forced expiration of air over the vocal cords in the tonic phase.
      5. Cyanosis in the tonic phase.
      6. Frothing at the mouth due to increased secretions from autonomic nervous system stimulation.
      7. Loss of bowel and bladder control.
   b. Are followed by a postictal state that may be characterized by:
      1. Confusion.
      2. Sleepiness.
      3. Poor coordination.
      4. Difficulty with speech and vision.

9. Absence seizures (petit mal):
   a. Are characterized by:
      1. Sudden brief loss of contact without falling.
      2. A "day dreaming" appearance.
      3. Resumption of activity where the child stopped.
      4. Slight jerking of arms and legs in some children.
      5. No aura.
      6. No memory for the event.
   b. Are not usually associated with organic disorders but may show hereditary factors.
   c. May cease in adolescence although a child may go on to develop grand mal seizures.
   d. May be precipitated by:
      1. Hypoglycemia.
      2. Emotional and/or physical stress.
      3. Hyperventilation.

10. Myoclonic seizures are characterized by:
    a. Sudden brief jerking movements of a muscle or group of muscles.
    b. No loss of consciousness.
    c. No postictal state.

11. Infantile spasms ("salaam" attack):
    a. Are characterized by:
       1. Sudden, brief, symmetrical contractions of muscles.
       2. Rolling of the eyes.
       3. A cry that precedes or follows the seizure.
       4. Absence of postictal drowsiness or sleep.
    b. May or may not be accompanied by a loss of consciousness.
    c. Most seizures stop by age 5, but a high percentage of children with infantile spasms have severe retardation.

12. Akinetic seizures:
    a. Are characterized by:
       1. Sudden, momentary loss of muscle control which results in falls in the older child and in a dropping forward of the head and neck and extension of the arms in the infant who does not stand.
       2. Momentary loss of consciousness.
    b. May occur frequently during the day.
    c. May result in serious injury, since the older child cannot extend his arms to break the fall.

13. Diagnosis is made on the basis of:
    a. History.
    b. Physical and neurological exams.
    c. Diagnostic tests.
       1. EEG—measures the electrical impulses of the brain.
       2. Lumbar puncture—to rule out meningitis.
       3. Skull films—to rule out trauma.
       4. CAT or CT scan, brain scan, and/or pneumoencephalogram—to rule out a space-occupying lesion.
       5. Arteriogram—to rule out vascular malformations.
       6. CBC and urinalysis—to rule out the presence of other illnesses.
       7. EKG—to rule out underlying cardiac arrhythmias.

14. Treatment for recurrent seizures is aimed at reduction or elimination of seizure activity by the use of:
    a. Anticonvulsant drugs which decrease the:
       1. Excitability of abnormal cells.
       2. Responsiveness of normal cells to the increased stimulus.
    b. Ketogenic diet which:

S

1. Uses a high fat, low carbohydrate diet to maintain a mild ketosis that inhibits seizure activity.
2. Is used with antiepileptic drugs for optimal effectiveness.
  c. Surgery if:
    1. A definite focal lesion is found.
    2. The seizures are causing progressive brain damage.
    3. There is no response to drugs.
  d. Implantation of a cerebellar stimulator in the cerebellum in the child with intractable seizures (Muehl, 1979).
15. Anticonvulsant drugs:
  a. Are numerous, but the major drugs are:
    1. Phenobarbital (Luminal).
    2. Phenytoin (Dilantin).
    3. Primidone (Mysoline).
    4. Ethosuximide (Zarontin).
    5. Carbamazepine (Tegretol).
    6. Valproic acid (Depakene).
    7. Cloazepam (Clonopin).
  b. May be more effective against one type of seizure than another, and several drugs, or combinations of drugs, may be tried.
  c. Are more rapidly metabolized and not as well absorbed in children as in adults which contributes to poor seizure control.
  d. Are not habit forming and do not cause brain damage.
  e. Can be given with medications for the other illnesses, and do not interfere with their actions.
  f. Will be monitored by periodic blood level determinations, since certain blood levels must be maintained to prevent seizure activity.
  g. Frequently produce mild side effects, e.g., rash.
  h. May produce blood dyscrasias, and the blood should be checked every 6 months.
  i. All have dose-related toxic effects.
16. Status epilepticus is a medical emergency which:
  a. Exists when seizures occur at such frequent intervals that the child does not regain consciousness between them.
  b. Must be stopped in order to prevent brain damage or death from hypoxia.
17. People with seizures, contrary to the myths that surround them:
  a. Do not pass their disorder directly to their children: hereditary factors are present but genetic counseling should be based on many factors.
  b. Show the same variation in intellectual ability as seen in the general population.
  c. Are not violent, insane, or contagious.

18. The frequency of seizures may be increased if the child/adolescent:
  a. Does not take medication on a regular basis (most common).
  b. Is ill, and especially if he runs a fever.
  c. Is under emotional stress.
  d. Has had too little or too much activity.
  e. Has a fluid and electrolyte imbalance.
  f. Consumes excessive amounts of alcohol and/or takes drugs.
  g. Is premenstrual.
  h. Is hypoglycemic.
  i. Hyperventilates.
  j. Has not had enough sleep.
19. The child with seizures should lead as normal a life as possible.
20. Seizure precautions include:
  a. Pad the crib, playpen, and side rails.
  b. Supervise the young child in the bathtub and on the toilet.
  c. Do not use pillows with infants and young children, since they may suffocate.
  d. Place gates across the top and bottom of stairs (for the toddler).
  e. Keep the child away from high and dangerous places.
  f. Supervise the child during swimming.
  g. Consider safety when selecting toys.
  h. Have the child who experiences frequent seizures wear a helmet.
  i. Have the child/adolescent avoid, when possible, those events known to trigger seizures.

B. Nursing Management.
1. Support the child and parents during hospitalization. See *Hospitalization, Support During*.
2. Initiate discharge planning. See *Discharge Planning*.
3. Obtain a nursing history to assist in the diagnosis and/or treatment of the disorder. See *History Taking*.
4. Prepare the child and parents for the tests which will be performed. See *Preparation for Procedures*.
5. Meet the needs of the child having a seizure (Norman and Browne, 1981).
  a. Remain calm so that you can function effectively.
  b. Stay with the child until the seizure is over.
  c. Prevent injury.
    1. Help the child who is out of bed to lie down, if this is possible.
    2. Pad side rails of bed with blankets. Keep side rails up and the bed in low position if the child has grand mal seizures.

3. Do not place anything in the child's mouth.

4. Remove any pillows and loose bedding if the child is in bed.

5. Cushion child's head if on a hard surface.

6. Do not restrain the extremities, since this may result in fractures.

7. Do not move the patient unless he or she may injure himself on an object which cannot be moved.

8. Move dangerous objects away from the child.

d. Prevent aspiration or suffocation.

1. Turn the child on the side, head back, and face downward so saliva and vomitus, if present, can drain.

2. Loosen tight clothing, especially around the neck.

3. Suction the child as needed.

e. Do not let people gather to watch the child.

f. Reorient and reassure the child after a seizure.

g. Provide for rest as needed.

h. Provide hygienic care for the incontinent child and reassure the child that you understand that he or she cannot stop this from happening during a seizure.

6. Observe, record, and report the following about the seizure:

a. Where it started.

b. Progression of seizure activity.

c. Length of time the seizure lasted.

d. Types of movements noted, e.g., tonic, clonic.

e. Pupillary changes.

f. Incontinence of bowel or bladder.

g. Appearance of the skin, e.g., flushed, pale, cyanotic.

h. Behavior after the seizure, e.g., alert, confused, sleepy.

i. Ask the child about any aura related to the start of the seizure.

7. Meet the needs of the child with status epilepticus.

a. Establish and maintain an airway.

b. Suction as needed.

c. Administer medications as ordered.

1. Diazepam (Valium).

2. Phenobarbital (Luminal).

3. Phenytoin (Dilantin).

d. Have resuscitative equipment on hand, since I.V. administration of drugs to stop seizures may cause cardiac and/or respiratory arrest, or arrest may occur from the prolonged seizure activity.

8. Teach the child and parents home management.

a. Tell the child and parents that adherence to the medication regimen is the best method of seizure prevention.

b. Teach the parents care of the child during a seizure.

c. Review seizure precautions with the child and parents.

d. Teach the child or parents to administer anticonvulsants and foster compliance with the medication for maximum effectiveness. See *Administration of Medications, Parental.*

1. Explain that the drug must be taken on schedule to keep a certain drug level.

2. Tell the child and parents that the drug dosage must not be altered except as directed by the physician.

3. Explain that failure to take the right dose at the right time will increase the chance of seizures.

4. Tell them that drug dosages will need to be adjusted to the child's individual needs.

5. Help the child and parents to remember to give drug(s) by scheduling them with meals and/or putting each day's supply in a container so the number taken can be checked.

6. Help the schoolchild/adolescent by planning a dosage schedule which does not require medications at school so the child does not feel "different."

7. Teach child and parents to renew the prescription before the last pill.

e. Tell parents to record their observations of all seizures.

f. Tell parents to call the physician about:

1. Any drug reaction so the dosage and/or drug can be adjusted.

2. A sore throat or easy bruising which may indicate adverse drug reaction.

g. Discuss the need to avoid situations which increase the frequency of seizures.

h. Explain that the child should lead as normal a life as possible.

1. Attend school.

2. Participate in normal activities with peers.

3. Eat a regular diet unless otherwise instructed.

i. Discuss with parents the fact that the child with seizures requires consistent limit-setting as other children do and that discipline will not provoke seizures. See *Discipline.*

j. Discuss the importance of:

1. Long-term care for the child.

2. Periodic blood studies.

3. Having the child wear a Medic-Alert bracelet or necklace and carry a wallet card stating that the child has seizures and what medications are taken.
   k. Refer to Epilepsy Foundation. (See page 321).
9. Meet the special needs of the adolescent.
   a. Recognize the fact that the adolescent may have difficulty complying with a medication schedule due to the need for independence.
   b. Support the adolescent in seeing the nurse/physician without a parent.
   c. Encourage the adolescent to participate in making decisions about care.
   d. Encourage responsibility in taking own medication.
   e. Tell the adolescent girl that:
      1. Seizures may be more likely at the time of her menstrual period.
      2. Participation in sexual activity and/or childbirth does not cure seizures.
      3. Pregnancy while on antiepileptic drugs can result in abnormalities in the infant.
   f. Discuss the state regulations for obtaining a driver's license for individuals with seizure disorders.
   g. Provide opportunities for the adolescent to verbalize feelings about restrictions imposed by the disorder.

Seizures, febrile. Transient seizure disorder occurring only in the presence of fever.

A. General Considerations.

1. Diagnostic criteria include:
   a. The first convulsion experienced by the child is associated with a temperature greater than 100.4°F (38°C).
   b. Child is less than 6 years of age.
   c. There is no evidence of infection, inflammation, or abnormal structure of the central nervous system and no fluid and electrolyte disturbance.
2. Febrile seizures may be classified as (Fishman, 1982):
   a. Benign febrile seizures which:
      1. Last less than 15 minutes.
      2. Have no significant focal features.
      3. Do not occur in a series having a duration greater than 30 minutes.
   b. Complex febrile seizures which are longer in duration, have focal features, and total duration greater than 30 minutes.
3. Febrile seizures usually:
   a. Accompany benign illness such as upper respiratory, gastrointestinal, or urinary tract infections.
   b. Occur during the first 24 hours of a fever.
   c. Occur when the temperature is rising.
   d. Occur only once during the course of the illness.
4. Signs and symptoms include:
   a. Tonic-clonic movements.
   b. General body stiffness.
   c. Eye rolling.
   d. Loss of muscle tone.
5. Predisposing factors include:
   a. Cerebral trauma at birth.
   b. Family history of febrile seizures.
   c. Allergies.
6. Febrile seizures resemble grand mal seizures except that they usually do not:
   a. Last as long.
   b. Produce as much postseizure lethargy.
7. Laboratory studies and diagnostic tests which will be done to rule out other causes of seizure include:
   a. Lumbar puncture—to rule out meningitis.
   b. Serum electrolytes, glucose, and calcium—to rule out metabolic causes.
   c. CAT scan or other radiological studies of the brain—to rule out trauma or structural abnormalities.
   d. Blood serum studies—to detect hypoglycemia or hypocalcemia which can cause seizures.
   e. Skull x-rays—may be done to rule out head trauma.
8. The EEG is of limited value in evaluation and management of children with febrile seizures because:
   a. The majority of children show some abnormality initially.
   b. It does not predict children who will experience repeated seizures or develop epilepsy.
9. Treatment of children who have experienced a febrile seizure is controversial, however the use of phenobarbital is generally accepted when treatment is used.
10. Treatment is recommended for those children at greatest risk for developing recurrent febrile seizures, neurological sequelae, and epilepsy.
    a. The child under 18 months of age.
    b. The child with complex seizures.
    c. Neurological and/or developmental abnormalities are present.
    d. There is a family history of afebrile seizures.
11. Most children who are going to have a recurrent febrile seizure will do so within 30 months (Fishman, 1982).
12. Febrile seizures may be treated by one of three approaches (Bindler and Howry, 1978).
    a. Initial therapy.

1. Diazepam (Valium) and phenobarbital are used to control the initial seizure.
2. Phenobarbital is continued for 2 to 4 years as a prophylactic measure.
3. Fever reduction measures are used when fevers develop.
  b. Intermittent therapy.
    1. Diazepam and phenobarbital are used with the initial seizure.
    2. Phenobarbital is tapered off immediately.
    3. Parents are instructed to give phenobarbital at the first sign of a febrile illness. (This is not very effective, since a seizure often heralds a febrile illness and therapeutic levels of phenobarbital take 2 days to develop.)
  c. No therapy other than fever reduction is used.
13. Recurrence of febrile seizures.
  a. 50 to 60 percent will have a second seizure.
  b. 10 to 20 percent will have three or more febrile seizures.

B. Nursing Management.
1. Support the child and parents during hospitalization. See *Hospitalization, Support During.*
2. Initiate discharge planning. See *Discharge Planning.*
3. Administer anticonvulsant drugs as ordered.
4. Initiate fever reduction measures. See *Fever Reduction.*
5. Initiate seizure precautions. See *Seizures.*
6. Observe, record, and report:
  a. Signs that may indicate a rising temperature.
    1. Behavioral changes, e.g., irritability, lethargy.
    2. Anorexia.
    3. Vomiting and/or diarrhea.
    4. Flushed face.
  b. Seizure activity.
    1. Duration of seizure.
    2. Behavior before, during, and after seizure.
    3. Body parts involved.
    4. Types of movements.
7. Teach the parents home management.
  a. Teach parents how to assess and manage a fever.
    1. Signs that may indicate fever.
    2. How to read a thermometer.
    3. Fever reduction measures.
  b. Review with parents how to care for the child during and after a seizure.
  c. Explain the rationale for giving phenobarbital if this is planned.

  d. Teach parents whose child will be taking phenobarbital.
    1. The child may experience sedation or drowsiness at the beginning of therapy but tolerance usually develops.
    2. The child may experience a paradoxical reaction and show excitement.
    3. How to administer the drug. See *Administration of Medications, Parental.*

Sepsis (septicemia). A generalized bacterial infection of the bloodstream.

A. General Considerations.
1. Infants are particularly prone to developing sepsis because of their inability to localize infection and their immature immune response.
2. Signs and symptoms, which tend to be nonspecific, include:
  a. Temperature instability, often subnormal.
  b. Poor feeding.
  c. Failure to gain weight.
  d. Vomiting.
  e. Diarrhea.
  f. Poor skin color—cyanosis, jaundice, mottling.
  g. Irritability.
  h. Lethargy.
  i. Respiratory distress.
3. Laboratory studies to identify the specific organism will be done and include cultures of the:
  a. Blood.
  b. Urine.
  c. Cerebrospinal fluid.
  d. Nasopharynx.
  e. Ear canal.
  f. Stool.
  g. Skin, if lesions are present.
4. A CBC will be done to detect:
  a. Anemia.
  b. Leukocytosis.
  c. Leukopenia.
5. Treatment measures include:
  a. Intravenous administration of antibiotics.
  b. Electronic monitoring of vital signs, including blood pressure.
  c. Supportive therapy, e.g., oxygen for respiratory distress, heat shield for temperature regulation.
6. Treatment using broad-spectrum antibiotics is often started as soon as cultures are taken and the antibiotic changed, if necessary, when culture and sensitivity reports are available.
7. Long-term antibiotic therapy predisposes the infant to:

a. Bleeding due to interference with vitamin K synthesis.

b. Growth of resistant organisms and/or fungal infections.

8. Complications include:
   a. Meningitis.
   b. Joint infection (pyarthrosis).
   c. Endotoxic shock.

9. The prognosis is generally good with early and intensive use of antibiotic therapy.

B. **Nursing Management.**
1. Support the infant and parents during hospitalization. See *Hospitalization, Support During.*
2. Initiate discharge planning as the infant's condition stabilizes. See *Discharge Planning.*
3. Administer antibiotics as ordered.
   a. Infuse within 1 hour.
   b. Give only one antibiotic at a time via a pediatric infusion set.
4. Assist with or collect cultures as ordered.
5. Isolate the infant as ordered.
6. Maintain a stable environmental temperature.
7. Observe, record, and report.
   a. The infant's response to antibiotic therapy.
   b. Alterations in vital signs.
   c. How the infant is eating, sleeping, eliminating, and responding to stimuli.
      1. Amount taken at each feeding.
      2. I.V. fluid intake.
      3. Output—urine, feces, vomitus.
      4. Hours slept.
      5. Level of consciousness—alert, drowsy, etc.
   d. Daily weight.
      1. Weigh at the same time each day, preferably before feeding.
      2. Use the same scale.
      3. Weigh infant nude.
8. Observe, record, and report signs of complications.
   a. Meningitis—bulging anterior fontanel, increasing irritability, seizures. See *Meningitis.*
   b. Joint involvement—limited movement, possible inflammation.
   c. Shock—fall in blood pressure, rapid pulse.
9. Meet the ongoing daily needs of the infant. See *Infant.*
10. Support the development of parenting skills which may be affected by early separation of infant and parents. See *Parenting.*
11. Teach parents home management.
    a. Provide a stable environmental temperature for the infant.

b. Protect the infant from individuals with infections.

c. Give medications as instructed. See *Administration of Medications, Parental.*

d. Develop a routine that meets the infant's daily needs.

Septic arthritis. See *Arthritis, Septic.*

Serous otitis media. See *Otitis Media, Serous.*

Serum hepatitis. See *Hepatitis, Viral.*

Serum sickness. A delayed hypersensitive body response to a foreign serum antigen or drug.

A. **General Considerations.**
1. Foreign substances that may create an allergic response in susceptible child include: See *Immunizations*
   a. Antibiotics, particularly penicillin.
   b. Sera.
   c. Vaccines.
   d. Toxoids.
2. Sensitization may occur within 7 to 10 days of the first exposure to the antigen and within 1 to 4 days of reexposure.
3. Signs and symptoms include:
   a. Low grade fever.
   b. Malaise.
   c. Erythematous or urticarial skin rash.
   d. Pruritis.
   e. Lymphadenopathy, local or generalized.
   f. Joint pain.
   g. Peripheral neuritis.
4. Treatment includes:
   a. Discontinuing the drug.
   b. Antihistamines.
   c. Corticosteroids in severe cases.
   d. Epinephrine and theophylline in cases of anaphylaxis.
   e. Aspirin to relieve joint pain, pruritis, and fever.
5. Serum sickness usually lasts less than a week.

B. **Nursing Management.** See ALLERGY.
1. Prevent serum sickness.
   a. Obtain a history of previous reactions and allergic responses before administering drugs, sera, vaccines, or toxoids.
   b. Perform a skin test with the sera if the history is positive for reactions or allergies.
      1. Administer a scratch test followed by intradermal testing.

S

2. Have epinephrine and emergency equipment available.
2. Explain to the child and parents why the anaphylactic or serum sickness response occurred.
   a. The child has a susceptibility to that substance.
   b. There was no error involved. (If this is true.)
3. Discuss the proper administration of medications to relieve the symptoms. See *Administration of Medications, Parental.*
4. Suggest measures to relieve itching.
   a. Cold compresses.
   b. Starch or soda baths.
   c. Antipruritic lotions.
5. Encourage the child to wear a Medic-Alert identification tag.

Sex education. Providing information about human sexuality and reproduction.

A. General Considerations.

1. Health professionals and parents need to accept that sex education should be an ongoing process through all stages of development and should include information about and discussion of the child's total sexuality.
   a. Feelings about being male or female.
   b. Development of trust and love.
   c. Attitudes toward self and others which serve as a basis for relationships.
   d. Sexual reproduction.
2. A gradual, sequential approach should be used to provide information and should take into consideration the child's level of development.
3. Factors that must be considered by the nurse before engaging in sex education include:
   a. Beliefs and values the nurse holds about sex and sexuality.
   b. Attitudes, beliefs, and relationships of the parents and other family members.
   c. Developmental level of the child.
   d. Societal norms which vary according to:
      1. Social class.
      2. Area of the country.
      3. Ethnic group and other subgroup membership.
4. The usual primary source of sex education is the peer group and there is often organized transfer of misinformation.
5. Sex education is most effective when:
   a. Parents and professionals work together to meet the needs of the child.
   b. Information is given openly and casually.
   c. Information is provided using correct terms.
   d. It is included as a part of total life education so that the child sees sex as an integral part of life.

e. Both parents are involved in giving information so the child learns to communicate sexual feelings to someone of the opposite sex.
6. Discussion of sexual morality should be avoided with the young child, but should be included before puberty (Rybicki, 1976).
7. Parents themselves may need a great deal of specific information about sex and sexuality before they are able to teach their children.
8. Questions related to sexual intercourse may be the most difficult questions for parents to answer.
9. Children learn from actions as well as words, and parents who show consideration and affection for each other tell the child a great deal about sex, love, and life.

B. Nursing Management.

1. Assess your own beliefs and values about sex and sexuality and your comfort in providing sex education before you undertake any teaching.
2. Assess the cultural and religious beliefs and values of the family as a basis for providing sex education. See *Cultural Aspects of Health Care* and *Religous Aspects of Health Care.*
3. Provide information appropriately.
   a. Be nonjudgmental about sexual beliefs and practices, since norms vary widely.
   b. Listen for the real question being asked, since the child and parents may be unable to ask direct questions, e.g., the adolescent girl who asks how big her breasts will get may be asking if her development is normal.
   c. Do not leap in with an answer; help the child or parents to develop their own answers.
4. Provide information about sexuality for parents, e.g., provide literature, refer to community classes if available, provide information yourself if possible.
5. Serve as a role model for parents by:
   a. Using correct anatomic terms for body parts and functions.
   b. Being open and casual in your discussion of sex.
   c. Answering questions as they are raised by the child.
   d. Being nonmoralistic about sexual activity.
6. Use principles of growth and development as a basis for teaching parents about the child's sexual interests and concerns.
   a. The young child is interested in his or her own body and the bodies of others and how they work.
      1. Handles own genitals when clothes are off.

2. Notices and then talks about anatomic differences.
3. May wish to touch body parts of others.
4. Asks about how baby gets in and out of mother.

b. The schoolchild becomes more interested in body functions and reproduction.
1. May ask many questions and becomes more interested in conception, pregnancy, birth, menstruation, etc.
2. Often engages in sex play, exploration, and experimentation as a means of verifying and incorporating information.
3. Becomes more aware of and interested in father's role in reproduction.
4. Engages in discussions about sex with peers and tells "sex jokes."

c. The adolescent is seeking to incorporate sexuality into a total self-identity and may become sexually active.
1. Requires assurance that sexual development is "normal."
2. Needs factual information about masturbation, homosexual experiences, contraception, pregnancy, and sexually transmitted diseases.
3. Should be seen apart from parents and helped to assume responsibility for his or her own sexuality.
4. Needs opportunities to discuss feelings about own and others' sexuality.

7. Help parents understand common areas of concern by explaining that:
a. Gender identity is firmly established by 3 to 4 years of age.
b. Masturbation (self-stimulation leading to sexual arousal or orgasm) is:
1. A normal activity.
2. Widely practiced by both boys and girls.
3. A way in which the child learns about his or her body.
4. Not a cause of emotional or physical illness.
5. Frequently seen in children who are not receiving age-appropriate stimulation or who are anxious.
6. Occasionally viewed by the adolescent as the cause of a perceived deviation in genital development.

c. Sex play and experimentation (hetero- and homosexual activity with more than one person before the onset of puberty) is:
1. A normal activity.
2. A reflection of the child's desire, through play, to learn more about how the body is made and how it functions.
3. Usually at its peak in the schoolchild.

d. Homosexual activity (sexual activity with a person of the same sex after the age of puberty) is (Wood, 1975):
1. A major source of concern to adolescents and parents.
2. Found in both males and females.
3. Usually a transitional phase in sexual development.
4. Not inconsistent with the development of mature heterosexuality.

8. Suggest ways parents can handle masturbatory behavior in the young child.
a. Do not punish the child.
b. Provide age-appropriate stimulation for the child.
c. Tell the child that this is a private activity.

9. Suggest ways in which sex play may be handled.
a. Do not condone or condemn the activity.
b. Tell the child to ask the parents if he or she has questions.
c. Suggest other activities.

10. Tell parents that the act of intercourse should be explained to the child as are other sexual activities without going into all the adult feelings about intercourse which the child does not have the developmental ability to understand.

11. Support the parents who are not comfortable in discussing sex with their child.
a. Explain that the child who sees a caring, affectionate relationship between the parents is learning a positive lesson about sexuality.
b. Suggest that the parents and child read the same sex education literature and discuss it, since this is often a more comfortable approach.
c. Discuss the parents' willingness to have a health care professional provide sex education.
d. Reassure parents that they should not do anything they are uncomfortable with, since the child senses their discomfort and will be influenced by it more than by their words.

12. Teach parents activities or discussions related to sex education which can be used with the child (Quinn, 1976).
a. Child age 4 to 8 years.
1. Grow plants from seeds.
2. Raise small male and female animals.
3. Take trips to a farm or zoo.
b. Child age 8 to 10 years.
1. Discuss different types of fertilization.
2. Discuss prenatal development.
3. Study growth patterns.
c. Child age 10 to 12 years.
1. Discuss the emotional and physical changes of puberty.

S

2. Study human growth and reproduction.
3. Discuss interpersonal relationships and responsibilities.
13. Support the adolescent in dealing with sexual concerns and needs.
  a. See the adolescent apart from parents and provide opportunities to discuss sexual needs and concerns.
  b. Provide information about:
    1. Normal sexual development.
    2. Masturbation.
    3. Homosexual experiences.
    4. Sexually transmitted disease. See *Sexually Transmitted Disease.*
    5. Contraception, whether sexually active or not.
    6. Pregnancy.
    7. Abortion.
14. Provide anticipatory guidance on sex education at each well-child visit even though the parent may not bring up the topic.

Sexual abuse. A form of child abuse in which there is exploitation of a child for the sexual gratification of an adult.

A. General Considerations.
1. Sexual abuse can be divided into (Jones, 1982):
  a. Nonfamilial abuse which:
    1. Usually occurs as a single event.
    2. Includes sexual behavior which ranges from nonviolent activities such as fondling, genital touching, and orogenital contact to violent acts of rape.
    3. Is perpetrated by someone known to the child/adolescent in the majority of cases.
    4. Is likely to be brought to the attention of health care providers and authorities for care and legal action.
    5. Has a generally good prognosis for normal psychological development of the child, especially if the family is supportive.
  b. Familial abuse (incest) which:
    1. Is defined as sexual intercourse between persons too closely related to be legally married.
    2. Occurs much more frequently than nonfamilial abuse.
    3. May occur as a single episode or occur over a number of years.
    4. May involve any combination of family members, but is most often reported between father/stepfather and daughter.
    5. May not be brought to outside attention or may be made known when mother and/or daughter retaliate

against the father or the adolescent seeks to end the relationship and tells someone.
    6. Has profound effect on the psychological adjustment of the child/adolescent.
2. Signs and symptoms which may indicate a child/adolescent is being/has been abused include:
  a. Physical.
    1. Unexplained genital trauma or explanation inconsistent with physical findings.
    2. Sexually transmitted disease present in child/young adolescent.
    3. Pregnancy in young adolescent.
    4. Vaginal or penile discharge.
    5. Physical abuse.
  b. Behavioral.
    1. Depression, somatic complaints, withdrawal from societal contacts.
    2. Behavior disturbances, suicidal gestures/attempts.
    3. Running away from home, school truancy.
    4. Use of alcohol and/or drugs.
    5. Aggressive and/or sexual acting out, e.g., stealing, prostitution.
    6. Comments suggesting sexual abuse, e.g., "He fooled around with me," "I don't like to be alone with my father."
    7. Young child acts out situation or draws picture of sexual activity.
3. The child is often unable to disclose the abusive situation and/or the offender because of:
  a. Guilt feelings.
  b. Fear that they will not be believed.
  c. Threats by the offender.
  d. Fear of loss of love.
  e. A limited vocabulary which prevents describing the situation.
  f. Failure to recognize the situation as abuse.
4. Immediate treatment measures for sexually abused children include:
  a. Interview to collect pertinent information (should be carried out, tactfully, by a trained individual and the child and parents should be seen separately).
  b. Physical examination to determine need for further care and to collect evidence for legal use.
  c. Medication: gonorrhea, pregnancy, and/or tetanus prophylaxis as indicated.
  d. Laboratory studies: semen and sperm analysis, VDRL, pregnancy test, and gonococcal cultures of vagina, rectum, and mouth.
  e. Notification of appropriate authorities: all 50 states have laws against sexual abuse which require reporting of the event.
  f. Protection of the child from further harm;

may require placement of the child out of the home.

g. Counseling for the child and parents, carried out by professionals skilled in crisis intervention.

5. Short-term follow-up includes:
   a. VDRL, repeated in 1 to 2 months.
   b. Gonococcal cultures, repeated in 7 to 10 days, if prophylaxis was administered, or in 4 days, if it was not.
   c. Assessment of how the family and child are coping, with referrals made as needed for further assistance.

6. Long-term follow-up therapy is necessary in rape and incestuous situations of sexual abuse.
   a. Rape victims may experience symptoms of grief, anger, and fear which constitute the Rape Trauma syndrome.
   b. Families which experience incest require a multidisciplinary approach in order to reach the goal of a nonincestuous, stable, appropriately functioning family.

7. Parents of children who have experienced nonfamilial sexual abuse need to know that:
   a. The way that they respond to the event will play a major part in how the child responds.
   b. The child may demonstrate regressive behavior for a period of time after the event.
   c. The child is rarely scarred for life, if the parents can support the child.
   d. The goal of care is as rapid a return to normal as possible.

8. Male children and adolescents are at significant risk for being sexually abused (DeJong, Emmett, and Hervada, 1982).

9. Proper collection, labeling, and handling of specimens is imperative since they may be needed as evidence in the event of legal prosecution.

10. Sexual abuse occurrences initially reported by the child/adolescent as being nonfamilial may later be found to be incestuous in origin.

11. It is helpful to have a trained child counselor who can work with the child/adolescent and family and coordinate the many facets of care.

12. A complete history of the event should be obtained only once in order to avoid creating additional stress for the child/adolescent and family.

B. Nursing Management.
1. Support the child/adolescent and family who have experienced nonfamilial sexual abuse.
   a. Obtain a history which includes the following information if not already gathered:
      1. Areas of physical injury.

2. Date, time, and type of sexual assault.
3. Whether the child/adolescent has urinated, defecated, bathed, douched, or been cleaned in any way since the assault.
4. Date of the last menstrual period; if adolescent is menstruating.

b. Provide detailed explanations to the parents and age-appropriate ones to the child/adolescent about the medical procedures which will be done. See *Preparation for Procedures.*
   1. Complete physical examination.
   2. Pelvic examination if rape has occurred, under analgesia or anesthesia in the young child.
   3. Visual assessment of the genital area without pelvic examination in nonrape cases.
   4. Collection of specimens for medical and legal purposes, e.g., swabs for seminal fluid and gonorrhea, blood for type and group.

c. Assist with the examination and collection of specimens.

d. Administer medications as ordered for treatment and/or prophylaxis.

e. See that the parents are informed about the results of the examination.

2. Provide care for the child/adolescent and family experiencing nonfamilial abuse if hospitalization is required. See *Hospitalization, Support During.*
   a. Administer medications and carry out procedures as ordered.
   b. Observe, record, and report aspects of the adolescent's behavior without drawing conclusions or making judgments.
      1. Coping mechanisms. See *Coping.*
      2. Response to treatment.
      3. Play activities of the younger child, e.g., is the child acting out the assault situation?
      4. Comments made by adolescents.
   c. Observe, record, and report parenting behaviors that will affect their ability to support the child/adolescent, e.g., calm reassuring manner or anger at the child.
   d. Observe, record, and report signs that may indicate that incest, rather than nonfamilial abuse, has taken place.
      1. Acting out of the situation in play.
      2. Desire of the child/adolescent to remain in the hospital.
      3. Fear of a parent.
      4. Low self-esteem and expressions of guilt, or sexually provocative behavior in the adolescent.
   e. Provide additional preparation for and

support during traumatic procedures which may remind the child of the sexual assault or be seen as punishment.

f. Protect the right of the child/adolescent and parents to privacy and confidentiality.

g. Help the child/adolescent work through the situation.

   1. Provide play situations for the younger child. See *Play, Therapeutic.*

   2. Encourage the older child to draw and/ or verbalize concerns to parents or primary caretaker, but not to peers since they may not understand.

h. Support the child/adolescent and parents in transition from care by the nurse in the immediate situation to long-term follow-up care by the social worker.

i. Prepare the child/adolescent for discharge.

   1. Prepare parents for possible regressive behavior.

   2. Encourage a rapid return to a regular routine.

   3. Tell parents to permit verbalization of feelings about the incident but to avoid questioning.

   4. Encourage the parents to express affection for the child/adolescent, if this has been missing.

   5. Inform parent of community agencies and support groups which they might find helpful.

   6. Initiate referral to a nurse clinician, social worker, or public health nurse as indicated.

3. Support the child/adolescent and family who have experienced familial sexual abuse.

a. Maintain a relaxed, reassuring, tactful manner when talking with the family.

b. Interview the child/adolescent without the parents present.

c. Provide treatment as indicated for any acute physical needs.

d. Assist the family in dealing with their reactions to this crisis situation.

e. Work with a multidisciplinary team to develop a plan for treatment services.

f. Prepare the family for the process of reporting the situation to the authorities and the involvement of legal and child welfare agencies which will occur.

Sexually transmitted diseases. Diseases spread by intimate sexual contact.

  A. General Considerations.

    1. The term sexually transmitted disease (STD) is now used in place of the earlier term venereal disease (VD) because:

a. It encompasses all diseases which may be spread during sexual contact whereas VD did not.

b. It has a less negative connotation than VD.

2. Multiple factors have contributed to the increase in STD among adolescents including:

a. Increasing rate of sexual intercourse.

b. Multiple sexual partners.

c. The presence of asymptomatic carrier states.

d. Limited screening of adolescents for STD during routine health care.

e. Delay in seeking treatment.

f. Stopping of treatment when symptoms subside but while the adolescent is still infective.

3. Adolescents may avoid seeking treatment because syphilis and gonorrhea must be reported to the health department so they can follow up on sexual contacts.

4. Most states have laws which permit the treatment of adolescents having a sexually transmitted disease without parental consent, and it is important to know your local laws.

5. An adolescent may use sexual activity as a way of reaching out for closeness to another individual and seeking a personal identity.

6. The diagnosis of a sexually transmitted disease may have an adverse effect on the adolescent's:

a. Self-image.

b. Reputation.

c. Family and peer relationships.

d. Sexual relationship.

7. Treatment of sexually transmitted diseases should involve:

a. Medical care of the specific STD.

b. Counseling of the adolescent.

c. Education about STDs.

8. There are many possible complications of gonorrhea including:

   1. Epididymitis.

   2. Meningitis.

   3. Septicemia.

   4. Pelvic inflammatory disease.

   5. Arthritis.

   6. Sterility from scarring.

   7. Blindness in an infected infant.

9. Herpes genitalis.

a. The causative organism may be either Type I or Type II herpes simplex virus.

b. Infection is acquired through direct physical contact and an infant may acquire herpes at birth if the mother has herpes.

c. Primary infections are followed by milder, but repeated recurrences.

d. Signs and symptoms appear after an incubation period which may be a few days or a year or more and include:

1. Multiple shallow, yellowish vesicles, lesions, or crusts on the genitals, buttocks, and inner thighs.
2. Inguinal adenopathy.
3. Pain.
4. Fever.
5. Pain on urination.
6. Urinary retention.
7. Thick, foul smelling vaginal discharge.
8. Malaise.

e. Diagnosis is usually made on the appearance of the lesions and a tissue culture provides definitive diagnosis.

f. Treatment is symptomatic and measures include:

1. Application of acyclovir (Zovirax) to lesions during an initial infection to control the disease.
2. Cold compresses, topical solutions (Burow's), topical anesthetics, low dry heat from hair dryer.
3. Analgesics and bed rest.
4. Catheterization for urinary retention.
5. Avoidance of sexual contact.
6. Avoidance of sitz baths and ointments as these may lead to spread of the disease.

g. Complications include:

1. Nervous system infections, e.g., neuralgia.
2. Neonatal herpes.

h. If herpes is cultured from the cervix in the last prenatal week, a cesarian section should be performed before the membranes rupture or within 4 hours of rupture to prevent neonatal herpes.

i. A higher incidence of cervical cancer is seen in women who have had herpes infections.

10. Nongonococcal urethritis (nonspecific urethritis, NGU, NSU).

a. Causative organisms include:

1. *Chlamydia trachomatis.*
2. *Ureaplasma urealyticum.*
3. Other organisms include *Trichomonas vaginalis, Candida albicans.*

b. Diagnosis is made by clinical findings and tissue cultures.

c. Symptoms include:

1. For males—mild dysuria, penile discharge (watery or thick), prostatitis.
2. For females—often asymptomatic but may have mild cervicitis and endocervical discharge.
3. For both—proctitis and pharyngitis.

d. Treatment includes the use of antibiotics.

e. Complications include epididymitis and sterility.

f. All pregnant women should be screened for chlamydia since it can cause neonatal conjunctivitis or interstitial pneumonitis.

11. Syphilis (Lues):

a. Causative organism is the *Treponema pallidum.*

b. Syphilis may be acquired through direct sexual contact with an open, active lesion or occur in a congenital form in an infant born to a mother with untreated syphilis.

c. Syphilis occurs in several stages: primary, secondary, latent, and tertiary.

d. Signs and symptoms of primary syphilis include:

1. A lesion (chancre) at the point of entry which is hard, red, painless, indurated, and has some yellow, serous discharge.
2. Lymph node enlargement in a lymph chain adjacent to the chancre.

e. Signs and symptoms of secondary syphilis appear 1 to 3 months after the initial lesion and include:

1. Skin rash that may mimic other rashes.
2. Flu-like symptoms such as headache, sore throat, achiness, and slight fever.
3. Lymph node enlargement.

f. Signs and symptoms are absent from the latent period which may last from 1 to 20 years, but a blood test would be positive.

g. Signs and symptoms associated with tertiary syphilis do not usually occur in the pediatric age group but include severe neurological and cardiac involvement.

h. Congenital syphilis occurs via placental transfer after the 18th week of gestation and causes the following signs and symptoms:

1. Rhinitis (severe and may be blood tinged)
2. Maculopapular rash after 1 to 2 weeks in some infants.
3. Fissures around the lips, nares, and anus may occur.
4. Generalized symptoms, e.g., fever, hepatosplenomegaly, anemia, and jaundice.
5. Notched teeth (Hutchinson's teeth), fractures due to epiphyseal separation, frontal bulging of the head, and painless swelling of the knee from fluid accumulation occur in the older child with congenital syphilis.

i. Screening for syphilis may be done by the use of serological reagin tests (VDRL, RPR card, and ART tests).

j. Diagnosis is made by:

1. Identification of the causative organism by microscopic dark-field examination.
2. Performing a FDRL test on the cerebrospinal fluid and checking cell count and protein concentration.
3. The use of the *Treponema pallidum* immobilization (TPI) and fluorescent treponemal antibody-absorption (FTS-ABS) tests.

k. Treatment includes the use of:
1. Penicillin (if not allergic).
2. Tetracycline or erythromycin (if allergic to penicillin).

l. Adolescents may experience the Jarisch-Herxheimer reaction following treatment for syphilis, especially secondary (Evans and Graf, 1979).
1. Chills.
2. Fever.
3. Headache.
4. Muscle aches.
5. Reappearance of old syphilitic lesions.

m. Sexually transmitted diseases can usually be treated on an outpatient basis except in the case of complication, e.g., intravenous antibiotic therapy for gonococcal arthritis, or infected infants.

B. Nursing Management.
1. Employ a straightforward, nonjudgmental approach in caring for the adolescent with a sexually transmitted disease.
2. Obtain a history of the adolescent's sexual contacts for reporting to the health department.
    a. Reassure the adolescent that the information will be kept confidential.
    b. Explain why it is necessary to report the infection and to follow up on sexual contacts, e.g., provide prophylactic treatment, prevent further spread.
3. Administer medications as ordered.
    a. Explain that reinfection is possible after treatment.
    b. Teach the adolescent with syphilis to observe for signs of the Jarisch-Herxheimer reaction following treatment and to call the clinic or physician (see above).
    c. Explain the importance of taking all the medication to eradicate the disease if more than just one injection is required.
4. Assess the adolescent's knowledge about sexually transmitted diseases.
    a. Make sure the adolescent understands the symptoms to report and treatment available (see above).
    b. Dispel myths—these diseases are not con-

tracted from drinking glasses, toilet seats, towels, etc.
    c. Provide education about prevention of sexually transmitted diseases.
    1. Teach the adolescent to wash the genitalia with soap and water before and after intercourse, urinate before and after intercourse, and to use a condom to decrease the chance of infection.
    2. Explain that douching will not prevent a sexually transmitted disease and may drive the organisms up into the uterus.
    3. Explain the relationship of the use of "the pill" to contracting a sexually transmitted disease.
    4. Discuss alternative forms of birth control for the adolescent taking "the pill."
    d. Discuss with the adolescent ways to meet the need for belonging and personal identity other than sexual activity, e.g., participation in clubs, school sports.
    e. Support the adolescent who would like to talk with his parents but is afraid of their reaction, e.g., be willing to meet and talk with parents.
    f. Explain the need for follow-up evaluation to make sure the disease is eradicated.
5. Meet the needs of the infant or child hospitalized with a sexually transmitted disease.
    a. Practice meticulous handwashing to prevent cross-contamination.
    b. Isolate the infected infant or child as ordered.
    c. Wear gloves when handling infected secretions and/or areas which may harbor the organism.
    d. Administer medications as ordered.
    e. Observe, record, and report the response to medication.
    f. Refer family members and sexual partners to the health department for follow-up.

Shingles. See *Herpes zoster.*

Shoes. See *Clothing.*

Shunt. See *Hydrocephalus.*

Sibling. A brother or sister.

A. General Considerations.
1. The birth of a sibling can be a traumatic event, particularly for the toddler.
    a. The child may feel displaced by the new arrival.

b. The child may regress to demanding a bottle, bedwetting, thumbsucking, etc.

2. Preparation for the birth of the new sibling will help the child cope with the feelings of displacement, but will not eliminate sibling rivalry.

3. Young siblings who are similar in age can serve as playmates.

4. Older siblings can serve the younger child as role models for sex-appropriate and age-appropriate behavior.

5. Older siblings in large families may have considerable responsibility for the care and discipline of younger siblings.

6. The extent of influence that siblings have on each other is affected by factors such as sex of the siblings and age differences between them.

7. Sibling rivalry continues to be a problem throughout childhood.
   a. The older sibling envies the attention received by the younger child.
   b. The younger sibling envies the older sibling's freedom and skills.

8. Interaction patterns with siblings will influence how the child interacts in school, with peers, and with the community.

9. Siblings who have been prepared for the birth of a new brother or sister have difficulty understanding the concept of an anomaly or life-threatening illness which prevents the newborn from coming home with mother.

10. Siblings of a child hospitalized for even a minor illness experience disturbing changes.
    a. Separation from parent(s).
    b. Change in routines, caregivers, or environment.
    c. Separation from the sibling.
    d. Feelings of guilt for having caused the illness.

11. Siblings of the hospitalized child may have behavioral responses to the stress.
    a. Regression.
    b. Demand for parents' attention.
    c. School problems.
    d. Social withdrawal
    e. Psychosomatic complaints.

12. Chronic illness, handicaps, and/or mental retardation of a child can have serious effects on siblings.
    a. Parents may not give enough attention to the siblings.
    b. Parents may set high aspirations for the sibling(s) to compensate for the affected child's lack of accomplishment.
    c. Siblings may experience depression, envy, and bitterness.
    d. Siblings may be given increased responsibility for the care of the child.

e. Older siblings may be concerned about bringing peers home.
   f. Adolescent siblings may have fears about genetic transmission of the disease.

13. Children who have experienced the death of a sibling may feel responsible for the death.

14. Siblings of the ill child are more vulnerable if they are experiencing concurrent stress such as entering school, moving, etc. or if they have few coping strategies (Whaley and Wong, 1983).

B. Nursing Management.
1. Prepare the child for the birth of a sibling.
   a. Tell the preschooler when the mother's pregnancy becomes obvious.
   b. Tell the older child when the news is being shared with friends and relatives.
   c. Move the young child out of the crib to be used for the new baby well in advance.
   d. Enroll the preschool child in nursery school several months before or after the new baby is born to minimize feelings of displacement.
   e. Have the child participate in an orientation to the maternity unit and/or special classes about the birth of a new baby.
   f. Prepare the child for separation from mother.
      1. Tell the child who will care for him or her.
      2. Show the child the hospital where mother will be, then go directly home so the child is reassured that mother can find her way back to him or her.

2. Support the acceptance of the new sibling.
   a. Have the mother call the child from the hospital and/or visit with the child whenever hospital policy permits.
   b. Explain when the mother and baby will be home in terms the child can understand, e.g., "The day cartoons are on TV."
   c. Have the father carry the new baby into the house so mother can greet the sibling.
   d. Plan some special time for the sibling when the newborn is brought home and continue these special times.
   e. Let the sibling open gifts brought for the new baby.
   f. Let the preschool child bathe, change, and feed a doll while mother cares for the infant.
   g. Provide quiet play activities which the young child can do in the room when mother is caring for the new baby.

3. Support the child whose newborn sibling is unable to come home with the mother because of an anomaly or life-threatening illness.

a. Show the siblings pictures of the baby, if appropriate.

b. Describe the baby in appropriate terms. "The baby is very small and needs a special crib to keep warm."

c. Tell the child it is no one's fault the baby is sick.

d. Use written material such as a special coloring book to give information to the sibling (Oehler, 1981).

4. Support the siblings of the child who is hospitalized.

a. Explain the ill sibling's disease or medical problem in appropriate developmental terms. See *Preparation for Hospitalization* and *Preparation for Procedures*.

b. Plan for consistency in child care with someone the child knows and trusts if the parents will stay at the hospital with the ill child.

c. Have the substitute caregiver stay at the child's home and maintain the normal routine, if possible.

d. Telephone the child frequently.

e. Show the child pictures of the hospitalized sibling.

f. Drive by the hospital and point out the sick child's room.

g. Alter visiting restrictions if either the sibling or the hospitalized child is severely affected by the separation or if the hospitalization will be lengthy.

h. Have the sibling draw pictures or make a gift for the sick child.

i. Explain the sick child's illness in terms the sibling can understand.

j. Reassure the sibling about his or her own good health.

k. Encourage the older sibling to verbalize feelings about assuming added home responsibilities during the sick child's hospitalization.

l. Help parents identify ways to spend time exclusively with the well sibling(s).

m. Encourage participation in sibling support groups if available.

5. Support the child whose sibling has a chronic illness, handicap, and/or mental retardation.

a. Encourage parents to spend specific periods of time with the normal child.

b. Discuss the need for parents to see the normal child as an individual with personal goals which may or may not meet parental aspirations.

c. Encourage the parents to involve the normal child in the care of the affected sibling, but do not assign responsibility beyond the normal child's ability to cope.

d. Discuss with parents that the normal sibling needs an opportunity to verbalize his or her feelings about the affected child.

e. Explain to parents that the sibling needs verbal praise, as well as tangible evidence of how the parents appreciate involvement in the affected child's care.

f. Provide genetic counseling for the normal sibling when appropriate. See *Genetic Counseling.*

6. Support the child who has experienced the death of a sibling.

a. Find out what the child believes has happened.

b. Explain the death in terms based on the child's concept of death. See *Death, Concept Development.*

c. Clarify any misconceptions and answer the child's questions honestly.

d. Allow the child to express the feelings of anger, sadness, anxiety, and resentment which are common responses.

Sickle cell disease. See *Anemia, Sickle Cell.*

SIDS. See Sudden Infant Death Syndrome.

Single parent family. A family unit headed by one parent.

A. **General Considerations.**

1. The single parent family should be considered as an alternative rather than deviant, disorganized, or disintegrated family type.

2. The single parent family may occur because of death of a spouse, abandonment, separation and/or divorce, single parent adoption, or out-of-wedlock birth.

3. The sudden burden of 24-hour responsibility for child care with no relief is overwhelming for some parents.

4. The aspect of parenting most difficult for the male custodial parent is handling the child's emotional upsets.

5. The child in the single parent family must cope with stresses different from the child in the two-parent family.

6. The child may be negatively affected by the parents' separation and/or divorce.

a. The child may feel responsible for the divorce and suffer guilt and expect retribution from the remaining parent.

b. The child may fear that the remaining parent will abandon him or her.

c. The child will have to go through the grief process.

S

d. The child will have to cope with additional losses if the family moves to a new home.

e. The child may develop physical illnesses as a manifestation of his inability to cope (Jackson and Runyon, 1983).

7. The child whose parents have separated and/or divorced will make efforts to reunite the parents.

a. The child wants to return to the previous family state.

b. The child will no longer have to feel guilty about causing the split.

8. The custodial parent may have difficulty facilitating the child's grief over loss of the noncustodial parent because of negative feelings toward the former spouse.

9. The widowed single parent needs to help the child cope with death of the parent.

a. The young child may feel responsible for the parent's death.

b. The child may have concern about whether the surviving parent will die or abandon him or her.

c. The schoolchild may express anger at the surviving parent and feel that the death was not "fair."

d. The adolescent may be unwilling to give up the lost parent.

10. The majority of single-parent families are headed by females, but the number of males who are custodial parents is increasing, particularly in the middle and upper classes.

11. The female single parent endures greater social stigma and discrimination than the male.

a. Adequate pay for work.

b. Opportunity to establish credit.

c. Expectation of assuming family roles.

d. Less community support.

e. Blame for not keeping the family together.

12. The homosexual parent must cope with the additional societal disapproval for his or her sexual orientation.

13. The adult's ability to cope with single parenthood will be affected by:

a. The sexual stereotyping within marriage, if a marriage previously existed, e.g., domestic roles.

b. The adequacy of current living arrangements.

c. The knowledge of available resources.

d. Financial status.

e. Available support systems.

f. Past success at solving problems.

g. Ability to differentiate own individuality from being part of a "couple."

14. The single parent may overcompensate for guilt feelings by constantly providing new toys or activities for the child.

15. The single parent may also spend so much time and energy in being "super" parent and "super" housekeeper, cook, etc., that there is nothing left for the parent's personal needs for companionship, career goals, etc.

16. The single parent may unconsciously begin to rely on the child for support and sharing of decisions which were part of the former spouse's role.

B. **Nursing Management.** See CRISIS INTERVENTION and WORKING MOTHER.

1. Assist the child whose parents have separated and/or divorced.

a. Find out the child's understanding of what has happened and why.

b. Encourage the parents to clarify any misconceptions the child has about the situation.

c. Reassure the child about his parents' love if this is true.

d. Facilitate the child's expression of grief.

1. Provide creative materials for the young child, e.g., crayons, paint, playdough, clay, blocks.

2. Encourage verbalization of feelings by the older child, e.g., "I would be sort of sad and sort of mad if that happened to me."

e. Help the child identify positive goals which will increase self-esteem when they are accomplished, e.g., obtaining a special rank in scouting, learning to bake a cake.

f. Identify the support system for the adolescent and encourage the teenager to seek their help.

g. Encourage the older child or adolescent to tell the parents to make their own decisions if each parent is trying to get the child on his or her side in disagreements.

h. Suggest that the parent and/or older child obtain books on divorce. See *References and Resources, section on Books for Children.*

2. Assist the child who has lost a parent through death. See *Death, Concept Development.*

a. Find out what the child understands of what has happened and why.

b. Encourage the parent to clarify any misconceptions the child has.

c. Facilitate the child's expression of grief.

1. Provide creative materials for the young child, e.g., crayons, paint, playdough, clay, blocks.

2. Encourage verbalization of feelings by the older child, e.g., "I would be sort of sad and sort of mad if that happened to me."

d. Allow the child to regress, but support a

return to independence as the child copes effectively with the mourning process.

3. Assess how the parent is coping with the single-parent situation.
   a. What resources are available to the family?
      1. Support system.
      2. Financial assets.
   b. What does the parent view as family problems?
   c. What does the parent view as family strengths?
   d. What has the separated or divorced parent worked out with the noncustodial parent about visiting, financial responsibility, discipline, etc.?
4. Provide information about resources available.
   a. Family service agency.
   b. Consumer credit counseling.
   c. *Parents Without Partners.*
   d. Fathers United for Equal Justice. (Support group for custodial fathers.)
   e. Adult single groups through religious organizations, YWCA, YMCA, etc.
5. Help the parent plan ways to be an individual.
   a. Analyze daily activities and decide what can be reduced or eliminated to allow the parent a private time every day.
   b. Designate a private space and have the child respect it.
   c. Continue membership in adult organizations.
   d. Ask a relative or friend to take the child for a weekend or exchange child care responsibilities with a friend to have some time alone.
   e. Acknowledge basic sexual needs and decide how to deal with them in a way which does not cause trauma for the child.
6. Make practical suggestions to help the parent adjust to single parenthood.
   a. Seek help from others when it is needed; it makes others feel good to help.
   b. Make contingency child-care plans for emergency situations.
   c. Expose the child to more than one baby sitter so the child does not have to adjust to a new caretaker in a tense situation.
   d. Keep a card with all pertinent information on the parent and child in a wallet or purse for reference in case of an emergency.
   e. Install protective devices to make the parent feel safe.
7. Help the parent adjust to the need for professional counseling (if needed) by explaining that referral to a specialist is not uncommon for complex problems.

Sinusitis. Inflammation of the ethmoid, maxillary, or frontal sinuses.

A. **General Considerations.**
   1. Sinusitis is uncommon in infants and children and common in adolescents because of the progressive development of the sinuses; development of the sinuses to the point where they can harbor infection occurs as follows:
      a. Maxillary and ethmoid—birth.
      b. Sphenoid—3 to 4 years.
      c. Frontal—6 to 7 years.
   2. Bacteria are the usual causative agent but the rhinoviruses have also been implicated in causation.
   3. The condition may be acute or chronic in nature.
   4. Signs and symptoms of acute sinusitis include:
      a. Pain: may be throbbing in nature.
      b. Tenderness over the affected sinus.
      c. Periorbital or facial edema.
      d. Purulent nasal discharge.
      e. Postnasal drip.
   5. Signs and symptoms of chronic sinusitis include:
      a. Chronic cough.
      b. Persistent, purulent drainage.
      c. Recurrent headache.
      d. Mouth breathing.
   6. Diagnosis is made by:
      a. Clinical findings.
      b. X-ray studies; an air-fluid level in the sinuses is diagnostic (DeAngelis, 1979).
   7. Cultures of secretions may be done to identify pathogenic organisms.
   8. Treatment of acute sinusitis can usually be managed at home with:
      a. Antibiotics for infection.
      b. Oral and topical decongestants to promote sinus drainage.
      c. Antipyretics for fever.
      d. Analgesics.
      e. Supportive measures, e.g., local heat, hydration, air humidification, rest.
   9. Treatment of chronic sinusitis includes treatment as outlined above plus eradication of the underlying cause:
      a. Treatment of allergies; most common cause of chronic sinusitis.
      b. Removal of adenoids; they impede sinus drainage.
      c. Correction of any nasal deformities, e.g., deviated septum.
   10. Vasoconstrictive nose drops or sprays should not be used longer than 3 to 4 days to prevent rebound swelling and phenylephrine products should not be used with infants to avoid tachycardia.

S

11. Complications include:
    a. Development of subacute or chronic sinusitis following an acute episode.
    b. Meningitis.
    c. Orbital or facial cellulitis.
    d. Osteomyelitis.

B. **Nursing Management.**
1. Teach parents.
    a. Use nasal spray as instructed for no longer than 4 days, since rebound swelling may occur.
    b. Force fluids to liquify secretions. See *Forcing Fluids.*
    c. Give antibiotics, decongestants, antipyretics, and analgesics as instructed. See *Administration of Medications, Parental.*
    d. Apply warm, moist compresses over affected area.
    e. Run cool steam vaporizer.
2. Tell parents that the child may swim after the acute stage but that diving should be avoided or the child should wear nose plugs.
3. Tell parents to call the physician if the child develops:
    a. A high fever.
    b. Earache.
    c. Increased redness or swelling over the affected sinus.
    d. Marked irritability.

Sleep. A period of slumber.

A. **General Considerations.**
1. The infant/child needs a routine for sleep as a part of general body and psychosocial health.
2. Individual differences in sleep patterns begin in the newborn period even though the baby may sleep up to 20 hours a day.
3. The sleep-awake cycles of newborns are shorter than adults. Newborns wake up every 3 to 4 hours.
4. The amount of sleep the infant requires decreases very little between 2 and 12 months of age.
5. A definite sleep routine is established by most infants by 4 months of age, and the baby should sleep through the night by 5 months.
6. The toddler's need for sleep gradually decreases from 12 hours at night plus two naps to 9 or 10 hours at night plus an afternoon nap.
7. The preschooler needs 10 to 12 hours of sleep which may or may not include an afternoon nap.
8. The schoolchild needs about 10 hours of sleep per night.

9. The adolescent usually requires around 8 hours of sleep per night.
10. Nightmares are common in the preschool period when the child's imagination is active.
11. The young schoolchild may also have nightmares when other children discuss ghosts and monsters or when he or she begins to fear death.
12. The adolescent's sleep may be restless because of environmental stress.
13. The adolescent may consider staying up late as a mark of adulthood.
14. Sleep problems are most common in the toddler and preschool age groups.
    a. The child enjoys the interactions with parents and does not want to be separated from them.
    b. The child is mastering a new task, such as walking, and wants to continue to practice.
    c. The child has acquired poor sleep habits.
15. Night waking often begins around 8 months of age when the infant demonstrates separation anxiety and is rewarded by the mother's presence when he cries.
16. If conservative measures fail, the parents must endure several difficult nights by not going to the infant/child even after prolonged crying.

B. **Nursing Management.**
1. Discuss with parents general measures to facilitate sleep.
    a. Explain to parents that a general routine for sleep that is compatible with family life style is important for the infant/child's health.
    b. Encourage parents to tell the child in advance that it is almost nap time or bed time.
    c. Plan quiet activities for 20 to 30 minutes to help the child "wind down" before sleep.
    d. Offer milk to induce sleep, if the child needs a bedtime snack.
    e. Dress the child in pajamas of appropriate warmth.
    f. Obtain a firm mattress to support the child's back.
2. Teach parents how to meet the specific needs of the infant.
    a. Observe the infant's sleep-awake pattern and do not awaken for feeding when the child is in deep sleep.
    b. Place the baby on the abdomen for sleep if feeding has just been completed.
    c. Do not put a pillow in bed for the infant since suffocation could occur.
    d. Give the older infant time to adjust to separation by placing him in bed while you

straighten the next room or prepare clothing for the next day so the child knows you are near.

3. Teach the parents how to meet the specific needs of the toddler.
   a. Follow a bed time ritual, but do not allow it to become so long and complex that the child is able to manipulate bedtime.
   b. Provide a chair or stool so the toddler can get out of bed safely once he or she has learned to climb out of the bed or crib.
   c. Offer only one toy to take to bed for nap time, since a variety of toys will distract the toddler from sleep.
   d. Do not allow a choice if the toddler does not have one, e.g., "What toy to you want to take to bed?" rather than "Are you ready to go to bed?"
   e. Move the child to a single bed several months before a new sibling is born, to prevent the toddler from feeling displaced.

4. Teach the parents ways they can meet the specific needs of the preschooler.
   a. Provide the child a private space for sleeping, if possible.
   b. Provide a night light if the child expresses fear of the dark.
   c. Explain the causes of shadows in the room and night noises.
   d. Do not insist on an afternoon nap if the nursery school includes a rest period after lunch as most of them do.
   e. Arrange a quiet time for reading a story or singing a song when the child is in his or her bed.

5. Teach parents how to meet the specific needs of the schoolchild.
   a. Plan a few minutes of quiet talk before bed time to discuss the day's activities, future plans, or things in general.
   b. Recognize that the child may resist sleep as he or she becomes aware of the finality of death.
   c. Provide opportunities for the child to talk about school pressures if nightmares occur.

6. Teach parents to meet the specific needs of the adolescent.
   a. Set a good example by obtaining adequate sleep.
   b. Help the teenager make realistic plans for the number of outside activities which can be balanced with good health habits.

7. Meet the needs of parents who complain that the child has sleep problems.
   a. Ask the parents to describe the sleep patterns of the child and of other family members.
   b. Explore if the parents are able to set limits about other aspects of the child's behavior.
   c. Involve the parents in planning approaches to the problem.
      1. Tell the parents it will not be easy, but they can do it.
      2. Write down the plan.
      3. Record the effects of the approaches.
      4. Do not use putting the child to bed as punishment.
      5. Establish a specific, time-limited ritual which is repeated at nap time and at bed time (Younger, 1982).
      6. Tell the child what the new sleep routine will be.
      7. Break the habit of a nighttime bottle by adding water to the milk in increasing proportions until the bottle contains water only. See *Nursing Bottle Syndrome.*
      8. Stay with the child who awakens during the night, but do not take the child from the crib or bed.
      9. Do not allow the child to sleep more than is age-appropriate during the day.
      10. Reinforce the child for appropriate sleep behavior.
      11. Ignore behavior such as crying, since giving attention will encourage the child to continue this behavior.
      12. Obtain a chain lock for the parent's bedroom door if the child's getting into the parent's bed is one of the problems.
      13. Introduce neurorelaxation methods to induce sleep in the young child (Schumann, 1981).
         a. Select one word such as heavy, slow, easy, and use this word to convey a relaxed state.
         b. Have the child hyperextend body to stretch from head to toes with back arched.
         c. Have the child take several deep breaths.
         d. Instruct the child to relax each part of his body from toe to head while parent tells the child that the body part is heavy or other word selected as above.
         e. Repeat instructions for each part 6 to 8 times in a monotone while firmly stroking that part.

8. Meet the needs of the child who has nightmares.
   a. Go to the child's room quickly.
   b. Turn on a light.
   c. Soothe the child.

d. Tell the child he or she had a bad dream and help return to sleep.

e. Talk to the child in the morning to determine if there are environmental factors or stress related to the nightmares if they recur.

Slipped femoral epiphysis (coxa vara). Downward and backward displacement of the femoral head.

A. General Considerations.
1. The cause is unknown.
2. Most slipped epiphyses occur during adolescence when the growth plate is weaker.
3. Symptoms are frequently referred to the groin, lower third of the thigh or to the knee.
   a. Mild pain or discomfort is usually gradual.
   b. Knee pain secondary to favoring the hip.
   c. Fatigue after walking or standing.
   d. Slight limp.
   e. Progressive external rotation deformity of the hip resulting in a "Charlie Chaplin" walk.
   f. Knees hit the handlebars when cycling since the knee moves away from the midline.
   g. Affected leg shortened with a severe slip.
4. The diagnosis is confirmed by x-ray.
5. Treatment varies with the degree of slipping and with the individual surgeon.
   a. Strict bed rest with the leg in internal rotation is enforced as soon as diagnosis is made.
   b. Manipulation and traction may be used preoperatively.
   c. Minimal slips may be treated with a hip spica cast interrupted by periods of traction to maintain hip motion.
   d. Insertion of nails or pins to align the epiphysis and femoral head is the most common surgical procedure.
   e. A corrective osteotomy may be necessary in severe cases.
   f. A pinning procedure may be performed initially followed by a corrective osteotomy when the growth plate closes.
6. Complications include:
   a. Avascular necrosis secondary to damage to the blood supply to the femoral head during surgery or closed manipulation.
   b. Cartilage necrosis if severe synovitis of the hip is associated with the slip.
7. Strenuous sports and games are not permitted after a pinning procedure until the growth plate has closed and the pins have been removed.
8. Early and adequate treatment results in a good hip function if the displacement is not severe.
9. Severe displacement or late treatment may result in permanent damage regardless of the type of treatment.
10. A slip of the opposite hip occurs in about one-third of the children.

B. Nursing Management.
1. Support the child and parents during hospitalization. See *Hospitalization, Support During*.
2. Initiate discharge planning. See *Discharge Planning*.
3. Meet the needs of the child in traction if used preoperatively or postoperatively. See *Traction, Care of Child*.
4. Find out what the child and parents have been told about casting or traction postoperatively and record on the Kardex.
5. Provide the child an opportunity to discuss feelings about the immobilization and activity restrictions which will be necessary postoperatively. See *Immobilized Child*.
6. Prepare the child and parents for surgery. See *Preoperative Care* and *Preparation for Surgery*.
7. Meet the needs of the child postoperatively. See *Postoperative Care*.
   a. Provide care for the child who is in traction to minimize discomfort and muscle spasm after an osteotomy.
   b. Provide care for the child in a cast. See *Cast Care*.
8. Teach the child and parents home management.
   a. Have the child demonstrate proper crutch-walking if appropriate.
   b. Discuss ways to meet the child's need for schooling and peer relationships if no weight bearing is allowed for a prolonged period.
   c. Explain to the child and parents why follow-up care to examine the opposite hip is necessary.
   d. Review symptoms of involvement of the opposite hip which should be reported to the orthopedist.

Smoking, cigarette. Use of tobacco.

A. General Considerations.
1. Tobacco is an addicting, legal drug containing nicotine which is:
   a. Habit forming.
   b. Capable of producing both stimulation and relaxation depending on the amount smoked.

c. Able to reduce hunger contractions of the stomach.

2. Cigarette smoking:
   a. Increases the risk of:
      1. Coronary artery disease.
      2. Emphysema.
      3. Lung cancer.
   b. During pregnancy is believed to contribute to:
      1. Lowered birth weights.
      2. Early deliveries.
      3. Irritability in the infant.
   c. By a breast-feeding mother may produce the following in the infant if more than a pack per day is consumed:
      1. Vomiting.
      2. Diarrhea.
      3. Restlessness.
3. Smoking is on the increase in the teenage population, especially among girls.
4. Social use of cigarettes is all pervasive in our society and children model adult behavior.
5. The older schoolchild and adolescent may experience a great deal of pressure from their peer group to engage in smoking.
6. Smoking is a source of oral gratification.
7. No single approach to the problem has been shown to be more effective than another in preventing or stopping people from smoking.

B. **Nursing Management.** See ADOLESCENT.
1. Approach all discussions related to smoking in a nonjudgmental manner.
2. Talk with the child about why he or she smokes.
   a. Peer group smokes.
   b. Thinks it makes him or her seem older.
   c. Parents smoke.
   d. Relieves tension or boredom.
   e. Something to do while studying.
   f. Keeps him or her from eating.
3. Remember that an individual must be motivated to change behavior before change can take place.
4. Seek to motivate the child to stop smoking.
   a. Emphasize being an adult, independent thinker rather than someone controlled by a group.
   b. Give concrete information about the relationship of smoking to the development of health problems but avoid preaching.
   c. Stress positive benefits of not smoking, e.g., increased endurance in sports due to improved respiratory function, decreased staining of teeth and fingers, etc.
   d. Have child/adolescent calculate the cost of smoking for a month and consider what could be purchased with the money.
5. Support the child who wishes to stop smoking.

a. Explain that you understand how difficult it is to give up smoking since nicotine is addicting.
b. Encourage the child to avoid those places, groups, situations etc. which prompt him to smoke, especially in the early stages of withdrawal.
c. Suggest changing the place where the child studies if this is when he smokes.
d. Discuss substitutes for oral gratification if needed.
   1. Keep low calorie snacks on hand, e.g., carrot or celery sticks, plain popcorn.
   2. Chew sugarless gum.
   3. Drink water or sugarless beverages.
e. Explore age-appropriate activities to meet the child's need for relief of boredom and/or tension, e.g., school sports teams.
f. Refer older adolescent to local groups for people trying to stop smoking.
6. Provide good role modeling.
   a. Do not smoke yourself.
   b. Encourage parents who smoke to quit.
   c. Find out if the school permits smoking in student lounges and encourage the discontinuance of this practice.
7. Praise all positive efforts that the child makes to stop smoking and ignore smoking that occurs.
8. Serve as an advocate for nonsmoking; be willing to meet and talk with students, parents, teachers, and youth groups.

Snellen test. See *Vision Screening.*

Speech screening. Assessment of the child's oral language production.

A. **General Considerations.**
1. Speech screening should include assessment of:
   a. Articulation—correct and appropriate sound production.
   b. Voice production—pitch, loudness, and quality.
   c. Fluency—smooth, flowing sound production.
2. The child with delayed speech may have difficulty with:
   a. Vocabulary—number of words to express needs, feelings, and thoughts.
   b. Syntax—putting words together according to the rules of grammar.
3. Delayed speech is common in children with:
   a. Limited intelligence.
   b. Hearing deficit.
   c. Poor motor development who cannot con-

trol their tongues and facial muscles to form words.

4. The health professional who is responsible for assessing the child's speech must know normal speech development and that the child should master (Van Hattum, 1975):
   a. Vowels by 3 years.
   b. P, b, m, w, and h by 3½ years.
   c. T, d, n, k, g, ng, and y by 4½ years.
   d. F, s, z (s and z are usually lost when incisors are lost), by 5½ years.
   e. Sh, r, v, th (as in that), and l by 6½ years.
   f. S, z, th (as in think), ch, and j by 7½ years.
   g. Consonant blends, e.g., pl, bl, sp by 8 years.

5. More than one-half of the child's speech should be intelligible by 2 years, and almost all of the child's speech should be intelligible by 4 years.

6. Repetitions in words or hesitations are common in the 2- to 4-year-old, but speech should be fluent without repetitions or hesitations by 7 years.

7. Causes of articulation disorders include:
   a. Limited intellectual growth.
   b. Frequent respiratory infections.
   c. Lack of or poor role models.
   d. Poor motivation.
   e. Faulty dentition.

8. Voice disorders may be caused by:
   a. Organic or structural defects such as cleft palate, hearing loss, or cerebral palsy.
   b. Shyness.
   c. Poor role models.

9. The most common fluency disorder is stuttering.
   a. The specific cause is unknown.
   b. Stuttering is common in 3- and 4-year-olds.
   c. Telling the child to stop and talk slowly or to repeat the words or statements is ineffective.
   d. Take time to listen to what the child has to say and ask easy questions to help the child express his thoughts.

B. Nursing Management. See HEARING SCREENING.

1. Obtain a history from the parents about the young child's speech.
   a. Does the child over 15 months produce some sound combination which is identifiable?
   b. Does the child of 16 to 18 months use words to make things happen? (e.g., Shout "up" to be picked up?)
   c. Does the child over 18 months make two-word sentences?
   d. Does the child comprehend questions or instructions even though he lacks language to express his thoughts?

2. Observe the spontaneous communications between the child and the parents or initiate conversation with the child.

   a. Is the child's speech intelligible?
   b. Has the child mastered vowels and/or consonant sounds appropriate to chronological age?
   c. Are repetitions or hesitations noted?
   d. Is voice production of pleasant quality and sufficiently loud for the environment?

3. Administer a language/speech test such as the Denver Articulation Screening Examination (DASE) if appropriate.

4. Record the child's speech on tape for validation by a speech pathologist if abnormalities are noted.

5. Assess the child's overall development by use of a screening tool such as the Denver Developmental Screening Test (DDST) to decide whether the developmental lag is general or limited to speech.

6. Initiate a referral for specialized speech evaluation.
   a. If the screening test continues to be abnormal when repeated 2 weeks after the initial testing.
   b. If the child has a lag of more than 6 months in the young child or 12 months in the older child in expected articulation mastery.
   c. If the child or the parents are overly concerned about the child's speech.

7. Refer for specialized hearing evaluation if speech and/or hearing screening tests suggest hearing deficit.

Spider bites. See *Home Management of Minor Emergencies.*

Spina bifida. Defective closure of the vertebral column.

A. General Considerations.
1. There are two types of spina bifida.
2. Spina bifida occulta:
   a. Occurs when the posterior laminae of the vertebrae do not fuse.
   b. Is rarely symptomatic.
   c. May be diagnosed when an x-ray is done for another purpose.
   d. May have physical manifestations such as dimpling of the skin or abnormal tufts of hair over the defect.
3. Spina bifida cystica includes two anomalies.
   a. Meningocele—midline lesion which contains meninges only or meninges and nerve roots.
      1. The defect is covered by dura, meninges, or skin that undergoes rapid epithelization.
      2. Neurological deficit is absent.

3. Secondary hydrocephalus may develop and require surgery before the sac is closed.
4. Sac closure may be delayed until the infant is 3 months of age and a better candidate for elective surgery.

b. Meningomyelocele (myelomeningocele)—midline lesion which contains CSF, incompletely formed meninges, and malformed spinal cord.

1. The sac may leak in utero or rupture at birth.
2. A thin membrane covers the sac.
3. Closure of the sac is performed immediately because of the threat of ascending meningitis or further motor impairment.
4. Some sensory-motor deficit will be present in the limbs and cutaneous areas below the lesion.
5. Secondary hydrocephalus frequently occurs because of the Arnold–Chiari malformation with partial or complete occlusion of the Aqueduct of Sylvius.

4. Spina bifida cystica can be diagnosed prenatally.
a. The concentration of alpha-fetoprotein (AFP) is high in amniotic fluid.
b. The maternal serum level of AFP may be elevated.
c. Ultrasound scanning of the uterus.

5. Repair of the defect may not always be possible and/or recommended.
6. Some surgeons prefer to shunt the hydrocephalus first, then repair the defect.
7. Not all nerve roots are involved in the sac so the child may have some movement and/or sensation in the lower extremities.
8. Bowel and bladder dysfunction occur if a defect is located below the third sacral vertebra, even if motor development is normal.
9. The true impact of the neurogenic bladder and bowel may not be realized by parents until the child cannot be toilet trained.
10. Orthopedic problems that may occur in the child with meningomyelocele include:
a. Scoliosis.
b. Kyphosis.
c. Lordosis.
d. Congenital hip dysplasia.
e. Hip contractures.
f. Clubfeet.
g. Fractures due to osteoporosis.
11. The child and the parents may need to cope with numerous procedures and operations if the child has associated anomalies.
a. Closure of the sac.
b. Shunting for hydrocephalus.
c. Shunt revision(s).

d. Casting for clubfeet.
e. Long-leg or Milwaukee braces for spinal deformity.
f. Correction of hip dysplasia.
g. Scoliosis repair.
12. Urinary incontinence may be managed by one or more of the following:
a. Urinary tract antiseptic drugs.
b. Clean, intermittent catheterization.
c. Manual expression of urine (Credé maneuver).
d. Artificial urinary sphincters.
e. Behavior modification program.
f. Biofeedback.
13. Bowel incontinence may be managed by behavior modification and/or bowel training programs.
14. Education of the child and family about the defect and its treatment should be consistent and continuous.
a. The child's adjustment to the defect is primarily dependent on the parents' attitudes toward and investment in the child.
b. The focus of the child's and parents' concerns will change as the child becomes older, e.g., from physical care to educational needs and concern about peer relationships.
c. The child and family can get "lost in the system" of numerous specialty clinics if a nurse or other health team member does not assume responsibility for coordination of services.
15. Habilitation of the child with meningomyelocele involves a team composed of a neurosurgeon, plastic surgeon, pediatrician, urologist, orthopedic surgeon, orthotist, physical therapist, nurse coordinator, public health nurse, social worker, occupational therapist, psychiatrist, and play therapist.
16. Parents need assistance with allowing the child to be as independent as possible, e.g., encouraging the child to walk with braces and crutches rather than using a wheelchair.
17. Decisions about regular versus special school should be made according to the child's best opportunity for a normal life style as well as quality education. (Public Law 94-142 mandates education for all handicapped children.)
18. Death in early infancy is usually due to CNS infection or hydrocephalus.
19. The life span of the older child is determined by the severity of the renal disease or pulmonary disease caused by kyphoscoliosis.

B. **Nursing Management.** See CRISIS INTERVENTION.
1. Support the child and parents during hospitalization. See *Hospitalization, Support During.*

2. Initiate discharge planning as soon as it is clear what home management will be appropriate. See *Discharge Planning*.
3. Help the parents cope with their feelings about the child. See *Exceptional Child*.
4. Meet the needs of the infant whose defect has not been repaired.
   a. Maintain the infant's temperature. See *Neonate*.
   b. Observe, record, and report indications of nerve supply.
      1. Dribbling of urine and feces.
      2. Absence or presence of leg movement.
   c. Keep the dressings over the sac moistened with antibiotic solution or ointment as ordered.
   d. Observe, record, and report:
      1. Leaks of the sac.
      2. Irritation of the sac.
      3. Signs of infection.
   e. Apply a protective shield over the sac if ordered.
   f. Protect the sac from contamination by urine and feces by taping a sterile plastic sheet just below the defect.
   g. Keep the perineal area clean and dry.
      1. Apply a protective ointment after cleansing.
      2. Air dry the perineum several times a day.
   h. Use a Bradford frame if ordered to prevent contamination of the sac.
   i. Place the infant on sheepskin or foam to reduce pressure on the knees and ankles.
   j. Position the infant prone, hips slightly flexed, legs abducted with a pad between the knees, and small roll under the ankles.
      1. Turn prone to side.
      2. Turn side to side.
   k. Provide passive range of motion to the foot, ankle, and knee joints as ordered.
   l. Measure the head circumference daily.
   m. Observe, record, and report the signs and symptoms of increased intracranial pressure. See *Increased Intracranial Pressure*.
   n. Observe, record, and report signs and symptoms of infection.
      1. Fever.
      2. Irritability.
      3. Lethargy.
      4. Nuchal rigidity.
   o. Observe, record, and report the infant's response to antibiotics.
   p. Hold the infant for feedings or feed in a prone position with the head held in the nurse's hand and turned to one side.
      1. The baby may be turned slightly to the side if approved by the surgeon.

   2. Burp the baby by gently rubbing or patting the infant's back.
   q. Prevent urinary stasis by manual emptying of the bladder (Credé maneuver).
   r. Provide age-appropriate auditory and visual stimulation. See *Stimulation*.
5. Meet the needs of the infant after the repair. See *Postoperative Care*.
   a. Maintain normal temperature.
   b. Continue preoperative nursing measures as appropriate.
   c. Position the infant prone and lower the head 8 to 10 degrees, if ordered, to prevent leakage of CSF from the operative site and to prevent pressure on the operative site.
   d. Hold the infant for feedings as soon after surgery as the surgeon will allow (usually 7 to 10 days).
6. Involve the parents in the child's care when they are able to participate and progress slowly in giving them responsibility.
   a. Demonstrate the care and explain what you are doing and why.
   b. Ask the parent to hand you things or otherwise assist.
   c. Have the parent perform the care while you assist.
   d. Support the parent who performs the care independently.
7. Teach the parents home management. See *Handicapped Child*.
   a. Discuss the infant's stimulation needs with the parent so they can help the child reach the ultimate potential.
   b. Encourage the parents to introduce new foods, finger foods, etc. as the child is ready, but discourage excess caloric intake, since the child is less active and therefore more likely to be overweight (Killam et al., 1983). See *Nutrition* and *Obesity*.
   c. Discuss with the parents precautions necessary due to paralysis and insensitivity of the lower extremities.
      1. Maintain proper body alignment.
      2. Make sure shoes and socks fit properly.
      3. Do not purchase shoes with rough seams.
      4. Pad the playpen or infant seat.
      5. Protect the child from contact with a radiator or heater.
      6. Observe the skin twice daily for pressure areas.
      7. Give the older child a mirror to use when examining the skin for pressure areas.
      8. Check the temperature of bath water.

9. Protect the child with adequate clothing.
10. Remove all toys from the crib for sleep.
d. Explain the care of the unrepaired sac.
　1. Keep the baby in a prone position.
　2. Protect the sac from fecal and urine contamination.
　3. Wash the sac gently with wet cotton balls if it does become soiled.
　4. Hold the infant by supporting the back above the sac.
　5. Cut a foam rubber doughnut to fit the sac so the infant can be placed in an infant seat.
　6. Notify the physician if the sac leaks or becomes larger.
e. Explain the care of the repaired sac.
　1. Keep the incision line clean and dry.
　2. Cleanse the incision with an antiseptic solution if instructed.
　3. Protect the incision from fecal and urine contamination.
　4. Keep the infant on his abdomen or side except for diaper changes and sponge baths until the incision is healed.
f. Review the signs of increased intracranial pressure.
g. Review teaching about the shunt if appropriate. See *Hydrocephalus*.
h. Discuss bladder management with parents.
　1. Emphasize that frequent follow-up and long-term administration of medications as ordered is essential to the child's survival. See *Administration of Medications, Parental*.
　2. Encourage a fluid intake for the child of 2 ounces/pound/day (Hill et al., 1969).
　3. Encourage a diet high in acid-ash foods, e.g., meat, eggs, cheese, breads, cranberries, plums, prunes, etc., which acidify the urine and decrease bacterial growth.
　4. Discuss measures of good perineal skin care.
　5. Teach the parents those symptoms of urinary tract infections which the child might manifest, e.g., unexplained fever, lethargy, and foul-smelling urine. See *Urinary Tract Infection*.
　6. Teach the parents the use of nonsurgical management as appropriate, e.g., nonsterile intermittent catheterization, external collecting devices, or Credé maneuver.

7. Discourage parents from continuing to use diapers to manage incontinence once the child has reached the age of 3 years.
i. Discuss bowel management with parents.
　1. Avoid constipating foods. See *Constipation*.
　2. Encourage physical activity.
　3. Administer a laxative or fecal modifier if dietary management is ineffective.
　4. Maintain a routine of placing the child on a potty chair. See *Toilet Training*.
　5. Have the child blow up a balloon to increase intra-abdominal pressure when on the potty chair. (Supervise the child for safety.)
　6. Administer a glycerin suppository just prior to toileting if the child needs it.
　7. Discuss behavior modification techniques for the older child (Jeffries, Killam, and Varni, 1982).
j. Discuss the child's need for mobility.
　1. Use an infant seat to help the baby see the world.
　2. Pursue the use of sitting braces, standing braces, or a parapodium which allow the child to have hands free for exploration even though the child cannot walk.
　3. Obtain or build a creeper (similar to a large skateboard) to allow the toddler to move independently by propelling the creeper with hands and arms.
k. Discuss the child's need for a positive body image. See *Body Image*.
　1. Provide the child with physical contact such as touching and hugging.
　2. Provide the child with as many age-appropriate activities as possible, e.g., pajama parties, group outings.
8. Meet the needs of the child who requires treatment for congenital hip dysplasia, clubfoot, or scoliosis. See *Clubfoot, Congenital Hip Dysplasia*, and *Scoliosis*.
9. Provide the family with information on community resources for long-term support and assistance, e.g., local or state Spina Bifida Association, public health nurse, local or state association for retarded persons (if appropriate), Easter Seal Society, March of Dimes, etc.

Splints. See Cast Care.

Squint. See *Strabismus*.

St. Vitus' dance. See *Rheumatic Fever.*

Still's disease. See *Arthritis, Juvenile Rheumatoid.*

Stimulation. The introduction of stimuli to enrich the child's environment and to promote development.

A. General Considerations.
1. Tactile, visual, and auditory stimuli should be provided as part of care beginning in the newborn period.
2. Teaching mothers to provide tactile–kinesthetic stimulation to their premature infants has resulted in gains in neurological development, weight gain, and mental development.
3. The nurse and/or parent planning stimulation activities must be familiar with normal growth and development. See *Appendix v.*
4. Programs involving intensive sensory–motor stimulation and behavior shaping can be very successful even with profoundly retarded children.
5. Stimulation of language development, personal–social development, fine motor skills, and gross motor skills should be discussed with every parent.
6. Stimulation activities may promote development in more than one area.
7. Infants can be stimulated by minor changes in their environment.
   a. Turning room lights on and off.
   b. Moving the crib from one place in the room to another.
   c. Hanging wind chimes outside the window.
   d. Making sounds such as "click-click," puffing, kissing, etc.
8. The items on the Denver Developmental Screening Test (DDST) can be used to help the parents learn which activities should be stimulated. See Appendix.
9. Activities and toys selected for stimulation should be free of sex bias, since male and female children need to experience a variety of stimuli.
10. Play space which is safe and large enough for the child to practice gross motor skills is important beginning with the latter half of the first year of life.
11. Children who are not provided with appropriate stimulation by adults will resort to self-stimulation activities such as masturbating, head-banging, and rocking.

B. **Nursing Management.** See LANGUAGE DEVELOPMENT.
1. Provide stimulation for the infant.
   a. Personal–social development.
      1. Meet the infant's physical needs consistently.
      2. Hold and comfort the infant when he is distressed.
      3. Talk to the baby in gentle, reassuring tones.
      4. Stroke the infant's body using fingers and palms.
      5. Rock the baby.
      6. Put an unbreakable mirror on the crib side.
      7. Provide a change in environment, e.g., put the infant in a playpen in the room where the parent is working; take for a walk outside.
      8. Provide toys that make sounds and have bright colors.
      9. Play interactive games such as pat-a-cake, this little piggy, and peek-a-boo.
      10. Provide toys for water play during the bath.
   b. Fine-motor development.
      1. Crib mobiles.
      2. Toys of different textures.
      3. Toys suitable for grasping and mouthing.
      4. Nesting and stacking toys.
      5. Large plastic beads to snap together.
      6. Music boxes with moving figures.
      7. Crib dangle bells.
      8. Cracker or cookie for self-feeding (around 6 to 8 months).
      9. Cloth books to turn pages.
      10. Shape and color matching toys.
   c. Gross-motor development.
      1. Rattles.
      2. Squeeze toys.
      3. Grip balls.
      4. Crib exerciser and cradle gym to encourage reaching.
      5. Blocks.
      6. Object strung across crib for kicking.
      7. Jumpers or walkers (around 6 months).
      8. Blocks or cups to bang together.
2. Provide stimulation for the toddler.
   a. Personal–social development.
      1. Toy telephone.
      2. Interactive games such as ring-around-the-rosy.
      3. Songs which involve touching body parts.
      4. Little chores to perform around the house.
      5. Shelves so the child can put away toys.
      6. Books to be read aloud by the parents.
      7. Exposure to people and places in the neighborhood.
   b. Fine-motor development.

1. Shape and color matching toys.
2. Large piece puzzles.
3. Large crayons.
4. Milk carton and clothespins to drop into it.
5. Sandbox.
6. Toys which fit together and come apart.
7. Hammering toys.
8. Water and pouring toys.
   c. Gross-motor development.
   1. Pots and pans to stack and bang together.
   2. Push and pull toys.
   3. Pedal toys such as tricycle.
   4. Big, soft toys.
   5. Large toys to carry around.
   6. Materials to build forts and hideaways.
3. Provide stimulation for the preschooler.
   a. Personal–social development.
   1. Field trips to the zoo, farm, etc.
   2. Supervised play with peers in the neighborhood or nursery school.
   3. Books to be read aloud by parents.
   4. Clothes for dramatic play.
   5. Educational television programs (*Mister Roger's Neighborhood, Sesame Street*).
   6. Household chores.
   7. Record player.
   8. Puppets.
   9. Interactive games such as tag, drop the handkerchief.
   b. Fine-motor development.
   1. Puzzles.
   2. Construction sets, blocks.
   3. Sand and water play.
   4. Playdough, clay, fingerpaints, chalkboard.
   5. Simple musical instruments.
   6. Printing of letters and numbers.
   7. Cutting and pasting.
   c. Gross-motor development.
   1. Tricycle, scooter, wagon, etc.
   2. Outdoor swing set.
   3. Balls of all kinds.
   4. Roller skates.
   5. Trees, logs, etc. to climb.
   6. Swimming.
   7. Exercises such as elephant walk, leap frog, wheelbarrow, etc.
   8. Jump rope.
   9. Hopscotch.
4. Provide stimulation for the schoolchild.
   a. Personal–social development.
   1. Organized peer activities such as scouting, clubs.

2. Having friends over for meals, sleepovers, etc.
3. Specific household chores.
4. Helping with family activities such as holiday baking.
5. Field trips to museums, manufacturing plants, historical sites, etc.
6. Letters to relatives or pen pals.
7. Books about the larger world around him.
   b. Fine-motor development.
   1. Model-building kits.
   2. Sewing or needle work.
   3. Puzzles.
   4. Arts and craft activities.
   5. Tools and mechanical equipment.
   6. Musical instruments.
   7. Collections, e.g., stamps, coins, baseball cards.
   c. Gross-motor development.
   1. Organized sports activities.
   2. Bicycles.
   3. Balls of all kinds.
   4. Kites.
   5. Gymnastics.
   6. Running.
   7. Hiking.
   8. Skating.
5. Provide stimulation for the adolescent.
   a. Personal–social development—organized clubs and activities and informal social get-togethers.
   b. Fine-motor development—hobbies and handicrafts.
   c. Gross-motor development—competitive athletics and informal sports activities.
6. Provide stimulation for the hospitalized infant/child.
   a. Assess the development and identify specific lags.
   b. Plan appropriate activities to stimulate the development and record on the Kardex.
   c. Share the plan with family members and encourage their participation.
   d. Integrate the activities into the child's daily care on a routine basis.
   e. Provide consistency by assigning a minimal number of caregivers.
   f. Adjust the plan as the child's condition changes and as his development progresses.
   g. Include observations of developmental progress in the nurses' notes.
   h. Consider ways to stimulate gross-motor development, since this is usually the area of greatest delay in the long-term patient.
   1. Playpen or blanket on the floor for the infant.

S

277

2. Small slide or stairs in the playroom for the toddler.
3. Walks outside with physician's permission for all age groups.

   i. Use a planned guide, e.g., the Washington guide or the Porter guide, for stimulating development if the hospitalization will be lengthy.

Strabismus (squint, "crossed-eyes").

Incoordination of extraocular muscles resulting from an imbalance of tone among the muscles or from a paralysis of one or more muscles.

A. **General Considerations.**
   1. Strabismus may be caused by:
      a. Refractive errors.
      b. Corneal scarring.
      c. Cataracts.
      d. Optic atrophy.
      e. Amblyopia: a visually impaired eye does not participate in fusion and may deviate.
      f. Anisometropia.
   2. Abnormal deviations may be either:
      a. Tropias—observable deviations.
      b. Phorias—latent deviations that are observed when binocular vision is disturbed.
   3. Direction of the deviations are described as follows:
      a. Esotropia, esophoria—actual or latent inward deviation.
      b. Exotropia, exophoria—actual or latent outward deviation.
      c. Hypertropia, hyperphoria—actual or latent upward deviation.
      d. Hypotropia, hypophoria—actual or latent downward deviation.
   4. If the deviation remains the same as the child looks in all directions, the strabismus is called *comitant*, and if it varies, the strabismus is called *noncomitant*.
   5. Infants under the age of 4 months may have periods of uncoordinated eye movement but it should not be persistent or continue after this age.
   6. Amblyopia results from suppression of vision in the deviating eye if the strabismus is not diagnosed and treated before age 7. See *Amblyopia*.
   7. Diagnosis is made by the use of:
      a. Direct visualization of an obvious deviation.
      b. The cover test. See *Vision Screening*.
      c. The Hirschberg test. See *Vision Screening*.
      d. Vision evaluation by an ophthalmologist.
   8. Pseudostrabismus may be apparent in the infant and/or very young child due to a flat nasal bridge, wide epicanthal folds, and deep set eyes.
   9. The degree of amblyopia is not related to the degree of deviation; small deviations can cause pronounced amblyopia and vice versa.
   10. Many children can alternate the seeing eye and therefore do not develop amblyopia.
   11. Treatment measures to promote binocular vision and improved cosmetic appearance include the use of one or more of the following:
       a. Glasses or contact lenses.
       b. Medications that control eye muscle action.
       c. Occlusion of the good eye for periods of time to prevent or treat amblyopia.
       d. Surgery to restore the balance between the two eyes by adjusting one or more of the ocular muscles.
       e. Orthoptic exercises as adjunctive therapy to reinforce binocular single vision.
   12. Surgery will not correct visual loss due to amblyopia and may need to be repeated to bring eyes into alignment.
   13. Results of treatment vary but are usually better if treatment is done before age 2 (Ellis, 1976).

B. **Nursing Management.**
   1. Support the child and parents during hospitalization. See *Hospitalization, Support During*.
   2. Initiate discharge planning. See *Discharge Planning*.
   3. Meet the needs of the child requiring surgery.
      a. Meet the child's needs preoperatively. See *Preoperative Care, Preparation for Procedures*, and *Preparation for Surgery*.
         1. Tell the child the eye will be "fixed" but do not say "cut."
         2. Demonstrate eye patches and arm restraints on doll or puppet.
         3. Let the child play out the situation. See *Play, Therapeutic*.
         4. Have the child try patches over both eyes and arm restraints.
         5. Let the child express his or her fears and/or concerns about not seeing and being restrained.
         6. Tell the child when the patches will come off and that he will be able to see.
      b. Meet the child's needs postoperatively. See *Postoperative Care*.
         1. Encourage parents to stay with the child to provide security.
         2. Provide verbal support and stimulation while the child cannot see and move about freely.
         3. Increase fluid intake slowly, since the child may experience vomiting.

4. Give the child his security object, since he cannot see to find it, e.g., toy, blanket.
5. Restrain the child only as necessary for his safety.
6. Speak to the child before touching him.
7. Change eye patches as ordered.
4. Teach the child and parents eye muscle exercises as ordered.
5. Teach the older child who will wear glasses.
   a. Keep glasses in case when not wearing or fold and place with lenses facing upward.
   b. Use a hand on each side piece when putting on and taking off to avoid bending or breaking.
   c. Wash daily and dry with soft tissue.
   d. Clean lenses with special lens cleaners or soft tissue, not paper towels or clothing.
6. Teach parents of child who will wear glasses.
   a. Plastic lenses are lighter and safer but scratch more easily than do safety glass.
   b. Scratch filler is available for plastic lenses.
   c. Plastic frames are more durable than metal.
   d. Permit the child to have a choice in selecting frames to encourage wearing of glasses.
   e. Safety straps are available to keep glasses in place on active children.
   f. Inspect area on top of ears and at bridge of nose for redness, pressure, or irritation which indicates glasses need adjustment.
   g. Buy two pairs if possible in case of accidental breakage.
   h. Take a positive attitude about child's appearance in glasses.
7. Teach the child and parents about eye patching.
   a. Explain that the "good" eye is patched in order to force the deviated eye to work and therefore improve the amblyopia.
   b. Tell them that the patches must be worn at all times for a 6- to 8-week period.
   c. Advise the parents of the schoolchild to contact the teacher and explain that schoolwork may suffer in quality when the eye is first patched.
8. Teach the child and parents about the use of anticholinesterase ophthalmic drops to promote accommodation.
   a. Use drops as instructed.
   b. Report signs of side effects.
      1. Visual blurring.
      2. Headaches.
      3. Obstruction to tear drainage.
      4. Irritation of the external eye structure.
      5. Systemic symptoms, e.g., sweating, flushing, diarrhea, enuresis, or precipitation of an asthmatic attack.
9. Support the child and parents in accepting:

a. Loss of visual acuity that may have occurred.
b. Repeated surgical procedures which may be required to straighten the eyes.
c. Altered body image.

Strep throat. See *Pharyngitis, Streptococcal.*

Stye (hordeolum). Staphylococcal infection of the sebaceous glands of the lid margin.

A. **General Considerations.**
1. Symptoms include localized tenderness, redness, and swelling.
2. The following contribute to the development of styes:
   a. Adolescent hormonal changes.
   b. Incomplete removal of eye makeup.
   c. Rubbing of the eyes as a result of itching due to allergens or strain due to visual problems.
   d. Chronic debilitating illnesses.
   e. Carrying staphylococcus in the nose or throat without symptoms of infection.
3. Treatment consists of:
   a. Warm moist compresses to the affected eye.
   b. Application of antibiotic or sulfonamide ophthalmic ointment.
   c. Incision and drainage when the lesion becomes pointed, if spontaneous rupture does not occur.

B. **Nursing Management.**
1. Teach the child and parents.
   a. Apply warm, wet dressings every 4 hours.
   b. Use ophthalmic ointment as ordered. See *Administration of Medications, Parenteral.*
   c. Do not attempt to rupture stye.
   d. Care for eye after rupture of the stye occurs.
      1. Remove drainage with clean cloth or dressing.
      2. Do not apply pressure.
      3. Continue soaks until drainage stops.
2. Stress to adolescent girl.
   a. Remove eye makeup once a day with soap and water.
   b. Discard eye makeup used prior to infection.
   c. Discard mascara after 3 months, since bacterial growth may occur in the cosmetic.
3. Evaluate vision. See *Vision Screening.*
4. Initiate further evaluation if history reveals allergic symptoms.

Subdural hematoma. Venous bleeding into the subdural space as a result of tearing of the bridging veins that run from the cerebral surface to the major dural sinuses.

S

A. **General Considerations.**
1. Subdural hematomas in infants and children are usually associated with contusion and hemorrhage in the brain as a result of accidental or inflicted head injury.
2. Injury at birth may be the cause in some cases.
3. Signs and symptoms include:
   a. Seizures.
   b. Vomiting.
   c. Irritability and other behavioral changes.
   d. Enlarged head.
   e. Bulging fontanels.
   f. Retinal hemorrhage.
   g. Symptoms of increased intracranial pressure. See *Increased Intracranial Pressure*.
   h. Anemia.
   i. Developmental delay.
4. The older child with chronic subdural hematoma may be admitted with a probable diagnosis of brain tumor.
5. Diagnostic tests include computerized axial tomography (CAT scan), EEG, and subdural taps.
6. Subdural hematomas may be classified according to the age of the lesion.
   a. Acute—3 days or less.
   b. Subacute—3 days to 3 weeks.
   c. Chronic—older than 3 weeks.
7. Treatment varies with the type of lesion.
   a. Acute and subacute—evacuation of the clots through burr holes or craniotomy is usually sufficient. Placement of a subdural drain for 24 hours or craniectomy may be necessary in some cases.
   b. Chronic (in the infant)—daily subdural taps may be performed for 2 to 3 weeks or longer. A subdural shunt to the peritoneal cavity or pleural space may be necessary. The shunt will be removed in 2 to 3 months.
   c. Chronic (in the older child)—evacuation of the clot is done through a burr hole or subtemporal craniectomy. Placement of a subdural drain or subdural shunt to the pleural or peritoneal cavity may be necessary.
8. Acute subdural hematoma carries a high mortality rate.
9. The survival rate with chronic subdural hematoma is good, but the following sequelae are serious:
   a. Seizures.
   b. Mental retardation.
   c. Spasticity.

B. **Nursing Management.**
1. Support the child and parent during hospitalization. See *Hospitalization, Support During*.
2. Initiate discharge planning. See *Discharge Planning*.
3. Observe, record, and report signs and symptoms of subdural hematoma.
4. Provide good skin care, particularly if the head is enlarged.
   a. Place a sheepskin under the child's head.
   b. Reposition the child every 2 hours.
5. Prepare the child and parents for the diagnostic procedures. See *Preparation for Procedures*.
6. Restrain the child securely during the subdural tap.
7. Observe, record, and report drainage on the dressing after the tap.
   a. Reinforce the dressing if serous drainage occurs.
   b. Notify the physician and reinforce the dressing if frank bleeding occurs.
8. Observe, record, and report signs and symptoms of increased intracranial pressure.
9. Use mitts or elbow restraints to prevent the child from dislodging the dressing when the parents or nurse are not present to supervise the child. See *Restraints*.
10. Prepare the child and parents if burr hole(s) or craniectomy is/are necessary. See *Preoperative Care* and *Preparation for Surgery*.
11. Meet the needs of the child postoperatively. See *Postoperative Care*.
    a. Position the child with the head of the bed flat or slightly elevated as ordered.
    b. Reposition the child every hour in the immediate postoperative period.
    c. Observe, record, and report:
       1. Rapid increase in drainage or bright red blood on the dressing.
       2. Urinary incontinence (in the toilet-trained child) or retention.
       3. Signs and symptoms of increased intracranial pressure.
    d. Reinforce the dressing with a sterile towel or pads as needed.
       1. Use a ballpoint pen to outline drainage, since fluid from a felt tip pen may penetrate the dressing.
       2. Clarify with the surgeon how much drainage should be expected.
12. Meet the postoperative needs of the child who had a shunt inserted.
    a. Observe, record, and report signs and symptoms of increased ICP.
    b. Position the child flat or with head and shoulders elevated as ordered.
    c. Provide good skin care.
       1. Clarify with the surgeon to which side and how often the child should be turned.

S

2. Place cotton behind the ears and over the ears under the head dressing if needed to prevent skin breakdown.
   3. Place sheepskin under the head.
   d. Offer oral feeding in small amounts, since vomiting increases intracranial pressure.
   1. Record successful approaches on the Kardex.
   2. Offer feedings on demand rather than on a schedule.
   e. Provide age-appropriate stimulation as the child's condition improves. See *Stimulation.*
13. Teach the parents home management.
   a. Assess the parents' ability to meet the child's physical needs and reinforce as appropriate, e.g., skin care, nutrition.
   b. Teach the signs and symptoms of increased ICP.
   c. Encourage the parents to provide appropriate stimulation.
   d. Encourage the parents to maintain medical follow-up to evaluate for sequelae.
   e. Discuss accident prevention if appropriate. See *Accident Prevention.*

Sudden infant death syndrome (SIDS). Unexpected death, during sleep, usually in the infant of 1 to 6 months of age.

A. **General Considerations.**
1. The cause of the syndrome is unknown, but several theories have been partially substantiated.
   a. Functional abnormality of the autonomic nervous system.
   b. Delayed maturation of the cardiorespiratory system.
   c. Periodic apnea of unknown cause during sleep.
2. It is likely that there is more than one cause, since no one factor has been found in all sudden infant deaths.
3. There have been some instances, called "near misses" where parents have resuscitated the limp, cyanotic, and apneic infant.
4. Some physicians recommend that the parents of the "near miss" infant use an apnea monitor at home when the infant sleeps.
   a. Health professionals frequently criticize the psychological demands on parents who use home monitors.
   b. In spite of difficulties, parents generally prefer home monitoring to prolonged hospitalization or no monitoring (Dimaggio and Sheetz, 1983).

1. Mothers express concerns about the monitor functioning and false alarms.
   2. Isolation and social deprivation of the mother is common.
   3. Normal concerns of new infant and maternal physiological restoration.
5. There are monitors sold in retail stores, but parents of healthy infants should be discouraged from purchasing them unless the physician feels this is necessary.
6. The infant victim of SIDS is usually found by the parent in a disheveled bed with blood-tinged secretions in the mouth and nose.
7. Parental attempts at resuscitation may discolor the body in such a way that emergency personnel, e.g., policemen and firemen, may misinterpret the appearance as evidence of child abuse.
8. An autopsy should always be performed and the parents notified of the results immediately.
9. Accusations of abuse or neglect by emergency personnel, neighbors, or relatives may cause serious emotional problems for the family.
10. Parents often need assistance in handling their grief from public health nurses or other professionals.
   a. Parents have guilt feelings as well as shock and numbness.
   b. Somatic expressions of feelings may occur after a few days.
      1. Sleeplessness.
      2. Anorexia.
      3. Fatigue.
   c. Continued questioning by neighbors, police, etc. may interfere with the parents' grieving.
   d. Parents may experience anger at health professionals who were unable to prevent the infant's death.
11. Some communities have SIDS organizations which help the parents with counseling services.
12. Intervention by the public health nurse or SIDS nurse–counselor will need to extend over time according to the ability of the parents to resolve their grief.

B. **Nursing Management.** See CRISIS INTERVENTION.
1. Assist the parents of the "near miss" infant if home monitoring is used.
   a. Teach the parents to attach the monitor with the belt.
   b. Have the parents perform a return demonstration of monitor operation during hospitalization or provide a home visit.
   c. Provide written instructions.
   d. Teach the parents to assess the infant dur-

ing the alarm situation and to document their observations and interventions (Duncan and Webb, 1983).

   e. Notify family's electric company and nearest emergency unit that the equipment is in the home (Bakke and Dougherty, 1981).

2. Offer support to the parents if the infant is brought to the emergency room.

   a. Provide privacy for the parents and stay with them.

   b. Avoid asking questions that may increase the parents' guilt, e.g., "Did you burp him well?" or "How long was he sick before you took him to the doctor?"

   c. Accompany the parents to the examining room when they see the infant.

   d. Answer the parents' questions about SIDS.

   e. Allow the parents to express their anger without personalizing their statements and becoming defensive.

   f. Reinforce the physician's explanations about the diagnosis.

   g. Help the parents plan how to help the siblings.

      1. Tell the children that the infant was sick even though he did not appear sick.

      2. The parents and others tried to help the baby.

      3. It is not the parents' fault, the siblings' fault, or anyone else's.

   h. Refer the parents to the public health nurse and the local SIDS chapter, if one exists.

3. Provide support for the family during the process of grief resolution, keeping in mind that the resolution may take considerable time.

   a. Listen to whatever feelings or experiences the parents want to share.

   b. Assess what they understand about what happened to the infant.

   c. Correct any misconceptions they have about the diagnosis.

   d. Provide assurances about the parents' ability to care for a child.

   e. Explain the concept of death held by the siblings. See *Death, Concept Development.*

   f. Help the parents plan for a relationship with their children which is supportive, but does not lead to overprotectiveness.

   g. Help the parents identify the effectiveness of their usual coping mechanisms and what approaches might be more applicable in this situation.

   h. Encourage the parents, particularly the mother, to verbalize reactions to suggestions from others that they have a "replacement" child.

      1. Each being is individual and one infant can never truly replace another.

      2. Parents often find it difficult to allow the new baby to establish individuality.

      3. Parents find it difficult to attach successfully with a new infant within a year of loss.

   i. Encourage the parents to share their feelings of grief so they can support, rather than "spare" each other.

4. Support the parents during a subsequent pregnancy.

   a. Provide opportunities for expression of fears and concerns.

   b. Provide assurances about their parenting abilities by focusing on their knowledge and positive feelings toward children.

   c. Discuss the possibility that the parents will want to be very protective of the infant during the first year of life.

5. Meet the needs of the parents who lost an infant with SIDS and now have an ill or hospitalized infant or child.

   a. Record the information on the Kardex.

   b. Keep the parents well informed about the child's progress and encourage the physicians to do so.

   c. Comment positively on those child care activities the parents provide.

   d. Provide opportunities for the parents to express their fears and concerns and assure them that this is natural.

6. Serve as an advocate in the community. See *Advocate.*

   a. Support and/or participate in education of policemen and firemen who have initial contact with the family of the SIDS infant.

   b. Participate in staff development programs for emergency room personnel.

   c. Support legislation which will assist families of SIDS victims.

   d. Assist with the establishment and/or participate in the local SIDS chapter.

Suicide. Taking one's own life.

  A. General Considerations.

    1. Many "accidents" in childhood and adolescence are, in reality, suicide attempts.

    2. Motives for suicide include:

      a. Separation from or loss of a loved one.

      b. Aggression.

      c. Attempts to manipulate others.

      d. Attempts to escape or call attention to an unbearable life situation.

      e. School difficulties.

      f. Sexual difficulties in the adolescent.

g. A developmental crisis.

3. Suicidal children and adolescents manifest symptoms of depression different from those seen in adults.
    a. Isolation from peers.
    b. Eating and sleep disturbances.
    c. Alcohol or drug abuse.
    d. Irritability.
    e. Hyperactivity.
    f. Frequent accidents.
    g. Lack of outside interests.
    h. Truancy or school problems.
    i. Running away from home.
    j. Boredom.
    k. Sexual promiscuity.

4. Feelings of hopelessness usually occur before the child/adolescent plans suicide.

5. Suicide attempts and completions increase in adolescence when the teenager is faced with the developmental task of forming a clear identity.

6. The suicidal child or adolescent has a limited variety of coping behaviors and views suicide as the only solution to his problems.

7. The adolescent who contemplates suicide is most often an isolated teenager who comes from a disorganized family background.

8. The risk of suicide increases when the child/ adolescent has no adequate social network (Valente, 1983).
    a. No one to talk with when feeling bad.
    b. No one to ask for help.
    c. No clear idea of where to get help.
    d. No supportive relationship.

9. A precipitating event can be identified in most suicide attempts or completions, e.g., parental death or divorce, pregnancy, broken love affair.

10. The child who has attempted suicide or who has a family member who attempted or completed suicide is at risk.

11. Statements such as "It won't matter after Friday," giving away prized possessions, or a sudden mood elevation should be considered signals of an imminent suicide attempt.

B. **Nursing Management.**
    1. Observe, record, and report symptoms of depression which are obtained in the nursing history.
    2. Assume that the child who verbalizes suicide intentions is serious.
    3. Ascertain whether the depressed child has a supportive adult, e.g., health professional, counselor, teacher, etc. with whom to talk.
    4. Share information about community resources that can help the child.
        a. Family service agency.
        b. Crisis intervention or suicide hot line, etc.
        c. School counselor.
        d. Religious leader.
    5. Support the child and family if referral is made for professional counseling or therapy.
    6. Provide accurate sex education or refer if appropriate, since sexual difficulties can be a suicide motive. See *Sex Education*.
    7. Discuss outlets for aggressive feelings, e.g., organized sports, jogging, etc.
    8. Meet the needs of the hospitalized child/adolescent who has attempted suicide.
        a. Confront your own attitudes toward the child and ask for reassignment if you have angry or resentful feelings.
        b. Support the child and parents during hospitalization. See *Hospitalization, Support During*.
        c. Initiate discharge planning as soon as decisions about treatment are made. See *Discharge Planning*.
        d. Orient the child to reality as needed.
        e. Let the child know that you care.
        f. Evaluate the safety of the environment if a significant risk for a repeated suicidal attempt is present.
        g. Observe, record, and report the patient's:
            1. Sensory perception.
            2. Mood.
            3. Self-image.
            4. Relationships with others.
            5. Anxiety level.
            6. Response to hospitalization.
            7. Attention span.
            8. Mental status.
            9. Suicidal statements.
            10. Response to medications.
        h. Earn the child's trust by being honest at all times.
        i. Provide personal attention to decrease the child's feelings of isolation and hopelessness.
            1. Leave the door to the room open except when privacy needs for physical care are met.
            2. Allow reasonable choices about routine care activities such as bathing, etc.
            3. Avoid an approach of extreme cheerfulness or solemnity.
            4. Help the child identify his own strengths as a way of improving his self-image.
            5. Initiate involvement in peer activities when the physical condition permits.
            6. Provide the young or less verbal child with play or art materials to facilitate expression of feelings.

S

j. Provide opportunities for the parents to discuss their ambivalent feelings toward the child.
  1. Anger toward the child for doing this to them.
  2. Concern for the child's welfare.
k. Observe, record, and report actions which indicate the return of destructive impulses.
  1. Increased tension.
  2. Anxiety.
  3. Rapid mood swings.
  4. Withdrawal.
  5. Secretive behavior.
l. Involve the child in setting limits and enforce them consistently.
m. Support the child and parents' need for professional counseling or therapy.

Surgery, outpatient. Minor surgery performed in a short-stay unit without overnight hospitalization.

A. **General Considerations.**
  1. Advantages of admitting the child as an outpatient include:
    a. The child is separated from home and normal routine for less than a day.
    b. Exposure to infectious children is minimized.
    c. Costs are decreased for the family or third-party payer.
    d. Better utilization of inpatient facilities occurs.
  2. Several factors must be considered when the use of a short-term unit is contemplated.
    a. The child under 1 year may need observation by professional staff even if the procedure is minor.
    b. The child with heart disease or chronic respiratory disease may require overnight hospitalization for a thorough preoperative evaluation and/or postoperative observation.
    c. The parents must be comfortable and competent in assuming responsibility for postoperative observations and care.
    d. The risk of complications following the surgical procedure must be minimal.
  3. Preoperative screening tests are usually completed the day before admission at the clinic, hospital, or physician's office.

  4. Parents should be provided with written instructions about:
    a. When and where to have preoperative screening tests completed.
    b. How to prepare the child for the procedure.
    c. The routines and procedures they should expect, e.g., preoperative sedation, NPO period, I.V.s, etc.
    d. Postoperative observation and care.
  5. Preoperative medication may not be required for all surgical procedures.

B. **Nursing Management.**
  1. Provide an orientation to the unit for the child and his parents individually or as part of a group. See *Preparation for Hospitalization.*
  2. Give the parents written instruction for preparation and care appropriate to the child's age and surgical procedure. See *Preparation for Surgery.*
  3. Help the child and parents adjust to the unit. See *Admission to Hospital, Elective.*
  4. Meet the needs of the child preoperatively. See *Preoperative Care.*
  5. Meet the needs of the child postoperatively. See *Postoperative Care.*
    a. Encourage parental participation, since they will be assuming responsibility for the care after discharge.
    b. Demonstrate any special procedures which parents should know.
    c. Give the parents written instructions for home care.
    d. Supply the parents with equipment to care for the child at home.
      1. Disposable pads or emesis basin to use in the car for the trip home.
      2. Disposable hospital gown if the child has a surgical incision which would be irritated by clothing.
    e. Tell the parents what signs and symptoms to report to the physician.
    f. Give the parents the name and number of whom to call if there are questions or concerns.

Sydenham's chorea. See *Rheumatic Fever.*

Syphilis. See *Sexually Transmitted Diseases.*

S

Talipes equinovarus. See *Clubfoot.*

Teeth. See *Dental Care.*

Teething. The eruption of the deciduous teeth.

A. **General Considerations.**
1. The eruption of the deciduous teeth occurs as follows.
   a. Maxillary.
      1. Central incisors—6 to 8 months.
      2. Lateral incisors—8 to 11 months.
      3. Cuspids—16 to 20 months.
      4. First molars—10 to 16 months.
      5. Second molars—20 to 30 months.
   b. Mandibular.
      1. Central incisors—5 to 7 months.
      2. Lateral incisors—7 to 10 months.
      3. Cuspids—16 to 20 months.
      4. First molars—10 to 16 months.
      5. Second molars—20 to 30 months.
2. Signs and symptoms associated with teething include irritability, drooling, and swelling where the tooth will erupt.
3. The child should be provided with safe, firm objects to chew, but otherwise the gums should be left alone.
4. Teething does not cause systemic illness or fever.
5. Sucking may increase gum discomfort during teething.
6. Dental care should start when the teeth begin to erupt.
7. Normal dentition can be affected by nutritional or hormonal disturbances.
8. Ethnic and cultural groups may hold firm beliefs about teething and practice home remedies. See *Cultural Aspects of Health Care.*

B. **Nursing Management.**
1. Explain the normal sequence of dentition to parents.
2. Point out that there will be a space between the lateral incisor and first molar until the cuspid erupts.
3. Teach parents what they can do to relieve discomfort.
   a. Provide teething rings which have been chilled.
   b. Give Zwieback or hard bagel to chew on.
   c. Offer milk and cool fluids by cup if sucking is painful.
   d. Let toddler chew on cool fruit slices.
4. Teach parents not to:
   a. Rub or break gum over erupting tooth since secondary infection may occur.
   b. Place aspirin against gum since gingival erosion and/or aspiration may occur.
5. Advise parents to call physician if signs of systemic illness develop while child is teething.
6. Encourage parents to provide extra cuddling when irritability, due to discomfort, is present.
7. Stress the importance of maintaining a safe environment, since the teething child puts everything in his mouth.
8. Do not discourage home remedies, unless careful nursing assessment indicates they are harmful.

Temper tantrums. Negativistic behavior characterized by kicking, screaming, foot stomping, and repeated yelling of "no, no."

A. **General Considerations.**
1. Temper tantrums frequently develop between the ages of 1 to 3 years because the child is:
   a. Egocentric.
   b. Seeking to establish autonomy.
   c. Capable of doing more things and thinking more thoughts than he has language to describe and frustration results.
2. Factors which precipitate temper tantrums include:
   a. Hunger.
   b. Tiredness.
   c. Illness/hospitalization.
   d. The child's inability to make a decision which causes frustration.
   e. Unrealistic behavior expectations by parents.
   f. Too frequent use of the word "no" in response to the child's behavior.
   g. Situational stressors, e.g., toilet training.
   h. Inconsistent limit-setting.
   i. Overindulgence or overprotectiveness by the parents.
   j. The need to gain attention from parents who may be ignoring the child.
3. Temper tantrums may be accompanied by breath holding spells in which the child may become apneic, lose consciousness, and have a convulsion.

4. Breath holding spells must be differentiated from seizure activity.
5. The active, assertive, energetic child is more likely to have temper tantrums than is the quieter, more passive child.
6. The most effective treatment includes (Scipien, 1979):
   a. Ignoring the behavior.
   b. Reducing environmental stimuli.
   c. Removing objects on which the child might hurt himself.
   d. Supporting the child as control is regained.
7. If tantrums persist after consistent use of the above measures, careful evaluation of the child's physical and emotional environment should be done and underlying causes eliminated.

B. **Nursing Management.** See *Behavior Problems.*
   1. Obtain a nursing history to determine factors in the child's environment which may precipitate temper tantrums. See *History Taking* and *Appendix iv.*
   2. Use the data from the nursing history to help the parents identify ways in which the number of tantrums may be reduced such as:
      a. Seeing that the child gets adequate rest. See *Sleep.*
      b. Feeding the child on a schedule which meets his needs.
      c. Limiting the number of decisions the child is asked to make.
      d. Setting realistic limits on behavior and enforcing them in a consistent manner. See *Discipline.*
      e. Distracting the child with an alternative activity rather than saying "no" or "do not do that."
      f. Expecting the child to master one, rather than several, developmental tasks at a time.
      g. Giving the child some undivided attention at different times during the day.
   3. Provide anticipatory guidance about growth and development so parents understand what behaviors can be expected at different ages. See *Appendix v.*
   4. Ask the parent to describe breath holding spells so they can be differentiated from seizure activity (Pillitteri, 1977).
      a. Temper tantrums are usually provoked by some factor whereas seizures occur without provocation.
      b. Cyanosis occurs before the child falls to the ground during a temper tantrum whereas it occurs after the child falls in a seizure.
      c. Alert, responsive behavior follows a breath holding spell whereas the child is usually sleepy following a seizure.

5. Teach parents how to manage temper tantrums.
   a. Explain the treatment as outlined above.
   b. Tell parents that they should neither give in to nor punish the child for throwing a temper tantrum, since this encourages repetition of the behavior.
   c. Teach parents not to respond to the child's behavior by screaming, smacking, etc., since this reinforces the child's behavior.
6. Support the parents in appropriate management of temper tantrums.
   a. Tell them that you recognize that it is difficult to change behavior patterns.
   b. Praise parents for setting consistent limits.
   c. Explain that as the child matures and learns to handle frustration, temper tantrums decrease.
7. Meet the needs of the hospitalized child who has temper tantrums.
   a. Remember that illness and/or separation from home may cause regression. See *Regression.*
   b. Handle temper tantrums as outlined above.
   c. Decide on a consistent approach to the child and record it on the Kardex.

Terminal illness. See *Dying Child.*

Testes, undescended. See *Cryptorchidism.*

Tetralogy of Fallot. See *Congenital Heart Disease.*

Therapeutic play. See *Play, Therapeutic.*

Thrush. See *Candida albicans.*

Thumb sucking. See *Behavior Problems.*

Tinea (ringworm). Superficial fungus infection of the skin.

A. **General Considerations.**
   1. Classification of tinea is based primarily on the area of the body affected.
   2. Tinea capitis is ringworm of the scalp.
      a. May be caused by a fungus from a human or animal host.
      b. Infection begins around a single hair, but spreads in a circular fashion.
      c. Symptoms include:

1. Scaly patches of broken-off hair.
2. Partial alopecia.
3. Erythema and weeping of the scalp.
4. Pustule formation.
  d. The use of a Wood's lamp will demonstrate yellow-green fluorescence of affected hairs in some fungal types.
3. Tinea pedis (athlete's foot) is ringworm of the feet.
  a. Symptoms affect spaces between the toes or on the instep.
    1. Macerated superficial epithelium.
    2. Fissures.
    3. Intense itching.
  b. Similar symptoms in the young child are usually caused by atopic or contact dermatitis.
  c. Wearing occlusive shoes, such as sneakers, facilitates fungal growth.
4. Tinea cruris (jock itch) is ringworm of the groin in the male or female.
  a. Symptoms include:
    1. Inflammation.
    2. Itching.
  b. The infection tends to recur.
  c. Infection of preadolescent children is rare.
5. Tinea corporis is ringworm of the skin.
  a. Often transmitted by infected pets to the child.
  b. Symptoms include:
    1. Rounded or slightly irregular, reddish-pink small patches with scaling borders.
    2. Mild itching.
  c. Body areas affected are the neck, face, forearms, and hands.
6. Diagnosis of all tinea infections is confirmed by dissolving the scales in potassium hydroxide and examining them under a microscope or by culturing the scraped scales.
7. Treatment for these fungal infections may include the oral antifungal agent, griseofulvin, and/or local application of antifungal powders, creams or lotions, e.g., Desenex, Tinactin, Micatin, Lotrimin.

B. Nursing Management.
1. Teach the child and parents home management of tinea capitis.
  a. Administer griseofulvin with milk or ice cream, since fat increases the absorption of the medication.
  b. Continue administration of the medication until it is discontinued in 4 to 6 weeks.
  c. Cover the head with a cloth or stockinette cap or scarf.
  d. Boil the cap or scarf daily to prevent spread of the infection.
  e. Keep the nails clean and clipped.

2. Teach the child and parents home management of tinea pedis.
  a. Administer the topical powder or ointment as instructed.
  b. Sterilize or discard socks and shoes contaminated by the fungus.
  c. Purchase cotton or cotton/nylon socks; avoid stretch or all nylon socks.
  d. Have the child wear well-ventilated shoes.
  e. Restrict the child from going barefoot in public places until the infection clears.
3. Teach the child and parents home management of tinea cruris.
  a. Administer the topical powder or ointment as instructed.
  b. Use warm compresses or sitz baths as instructed.
  c. Keep the groin area clean and dry.
  d. Bathe frequently, particularly in warm weather.
  e. Rinse well to remove soap.
  f. Dress the child in loose-fitting, absorbent underwear.
4. Teach the child and parents home management of tinea corporis.
  a. Administer the topical powder or ointment as instructed.
  b. Keep the skin clean and dry.
  c. Rinse well to remove soap.
  d. Keep the nails clean and clipped.

Toddler. Child in the period of development between 1 and 3 years of age.

A. General Considerations.
1. The toddler is faced with a number of developmental tasks which include (Duvall, 1977):
  a. Adjusting to healthy daily routines.
  b. Mastering good eating habits.
  c. Mastering toilet training.
  d. Developing age-appropriate physical skills.
  e. Becoming a member of the family.
  f. Learning to communicate effectively.
2. The rate at which each child masters these tasks will vary.
3. The rate of growth slows dramatically during the toddler period.
4. Physiological responses are similar to those of the older child, but fluid and electrolyte balance must still be monitored carefully.
5. The family is the most important social group for the toddler, and separation anxiety remains strong.
6. Play is important to the toddler's optimal development.
7. Ritualism is common in the toddler period.
8. Accidents are common during this period, since the toddler asserts autonomy, becomes more

mobile, and overestimates physical capabilities.

9. The toddler's favorite word is "no" and represents attempts to become autonomous.

B. Nursing Management.

1. Support the parents in meeting the child's needs. See *Parenting.*
2. Support the toddler's adjustment to hospitalization. See *Hospitalization, Support During.*
   a. Find out what the daily home routine has been, record it on the Kardex, and follow it as much as possible.
   b. Find out about the toddler's usual means of coping and any known fears. See *Coping* and *Fears.*
   c. Use knowledge of the toddler's response to hospitalization as a basis for care. See *Hospitalization, Response to.*
3. Meet daily physical needs.
   a. Bathe:
      1. In a tub if possible.
      2. Plan bath for after breakfast and before linen change to avoid having to repeat the task.
      3. Let parents bathe the toddler in the evening, especially if this is the home routine.
      4. Permit the toddler to assist with the bath, e.g., get the towels and soap ready, put soap on the washcloth.
      5. Wash hair as needed.
      6. Clean outer ears with a washcloth.
      7. Do not use cotton applicators to clean ear canal, since cerumen may become impacted.
   b. Administer mouth care.
      1. Provide a small tooth brush.
      2. Allow the older toddler to brush his or her own teeth, assist the younger toddler, and help both as needed to reach all teeth.
   c. Provide adequate nutrition. See *Nutrition.*
   d. Provide for rest and sleep routines. See *Sleep.*
      1. Plan naps on basis of home schedule.
      2. Give the toddler security object to take to bed, e.g., blanket, toy.
      3. Schedule procedures, tests, etc. around the nap schedule if possible.
      4. Plan a "slowdown" period prior to naps and bedtime so the toddler begins to relax, e.g., read a story, hold and sing to the child.
      5. Provide a pillow if the toddler is used to having one.
      6. Place top covers in the crib during nap and bedtimes.

   e. Meet the needs of the toddler who is not toilet trained or who regresses.
      1. Change diapers as soon as wet or soiled.
      2. Wash and dry the area.
      3. Provide care for diaper rash if needed. See *Dermatitis, Diaper.*
      4. Use double diapers, especially for sleeping, since urine volume increases.
   f. Meet the needs of the toddler who is being trained or is trained. See *Toilet Training.*
      1. Follow home schedule.
      2. Keep potty chair available, since the toddler often cannot wait to go to the bathroom.
      3. Do not use diapers.
      4. Praise all successes and ignore all accidents.
   g. Protect from injury.
      1. Know where the toddler is at all times!
      2. Keep the side rails all the way up when no one is with the child.
      3. Obtain a "climber crib" for the toddler who attempts to get out of the crib.
      4. Keep the crib away from equipment hung on the walls and electrical outlets.
      5. Keep any gooseneck or moveable overbed lights up out of the way to avoid burns.
      6. Do not leave safety pins on the bedside table.
      7. Supervise the toddler who is out of bed.
      8. Remove equipment and electrical cords from activity areas.
      9. Make sure that toys have no sharp points or edges.
   h. Prevent infection.
      1. Do not care for the toddler if you have an infectious illness.
      2. Prevent contact with other children on the unit who have infectious illnesses.
      3. Practice good handwashing technique.
   i. Provide for exercise. See *Exercise.*
4. Consider the toddler's developmental level when:
   a. Taking vital signs. See *Preparation for Procedures.*
      1. Count respirations when the toddler is quiet.
      2. Let the toddler become used to the stethoscope before you take an apical pulse, e.g., let him handle it, listen to his own heartbeat, etc.
      3. Take a rectal temperature last, since this is an intrusive procedure, and the toddler may need to be restrained for safety during the procedure.
   b. Administering medications. See *Administration of Medications* and *Appendix iii.*
5. Meet the emotional needs of the toddler.

T

a. Involve the parents in the care of the toddler.
b. Provide for rooming-in of a parent if possible.
c. Follow home rituals and routines as recorded on the Kardex.
d. Support the toddler in his efforts to master developmental tasks by encouraging to do what he can for himself, e.g., feed self finger foods, put on socks and shirt, use the potty chair, etc.
e. Support the toddler when he or she needs to be dependent, e.g., hold and comfort when parents must leave, feed when the child wishes you to, etc.
f. Do not reinforce normal developmental negativism.
   1. Approach the toddler with a positive attitude.
   2. Limit the number of choices the toddler must make and present them in an either/or manner, e.g., "Do you want a hot dog or a hamburger for lunch?"
   3. Do not offer a choice where none is present, e.g., if you plan to put the toddler down for a nap, say, "It's time for a nap" not "Would you like to take a nap?"
   4. Handle temper tantrums appropriately. See *Temper Tantrums.*
g. Plan for play activities which promote fine and gross-motor development and allow an outlet for the toddler's normal aggressive behavior. See *Play.*
h. Limit the number of caregivers to whom the child must adjust.
i. Spend time with the toddler when you are not giving direct physical care.
6. Provide anticipatory guidance to parents related to the following areas as indicated on the basis of assessment:
   a. Growth and development norms. See *Appendix v.*
   b. Common problems, e.g., negativism, temper tantrums.
   c. Nutritional needs and eating habits. See *Nutrition.*
   d. Safety. See *Accident Prevention.*
   e. Ways to stimulate development. See *Stimulation.*
   f. Provision for ongoing health care, e.g., seeing a dentist. See *Well-Child Care.*

Toilet training. The process by which the child learns to control bowels and bladder.

   A. General Considerations.
   1. Toilet training should be started when the child demonstrates signs of physical and psychological readiness which include:
      a. The ability to stand and walk well, and to voluntarily let go of an object, indicating physiological capability of sphincter control.
      b. Some regularity in bowel movements, e.g., usually has a bowel movement after breakfast.
      c. The ability to hold urine for at least 2 hours.
      d. The ability to recognize and to indicate the need to eliminate.
      e. A willingness to cooperate in order to please the caregiver.
      f. The ability to sit still for 5 to 10 minutes.
   2. Toilet training should not be started during a time of family stress, e.g., moving, illness.
   3. Training for bowel and bladder control can be done at the same time if the child is over 2 years of age, bowel training may precede bladder training, and the child achieves daytime bladder control before night control.
   4. Parents are most likely to be successful in toilet training if their teaching style is (Erikson, 1981):
      a. Positive.
      b. Consistent.
      c. Geared to the particular child.
      d. Nonpunitive.
      e. Nonpressured
   5. The child may be proud of what he or she produces to please the mother and:
      a. May not want the toilet flushed or the potty chair emptied.
      b. May want to examine what he produces.
   6. Negative responses to this normal exploratory behavior may cause the child to think he or she is "bad."
   7. The child may fear the flushing of the toilet, since the child thinks he or she too may be flushed away.
   8. Occasional "accidents" may occur for some time when the child is:
      a. Busy with play.
      b. Excited.
      c. Tired.
      d. Ill.
      e. Stressed, e.g., birth of sibling, hospitalization.
      f. Trying to convey a message that he or she is being pressed to learn or to do too much at a time.
   9. The use of a potty chair and clothing which is easy to get off and on facilitates the training process.
   10. The child who balks at toilet training should not be pushed; it is better to wait a few weeks and reintroduce the subject.

B. **Nursing Management.**
1. Assess parental attitudes toward toilet training and discuss parental behaviors which are known to facilitate toilet training.
   a. Readiness of parents to become involved in teaching the child.
   b. Willingness to reward toileting behavior when it occurs.
   c. Time available each day to spend with the child in learning control.
   d. Knowledge of child's usual daily patterns of bowel and bladder elimination.
   e. Preparations for training underway or complete, e.g., toilet seat or potty chair available, easily removable clothes, and training pants ready.
   f. Ability to accept child's lapses in training without anger, guilt, or punitive behavior.
2. Explain to parents that toilet training should be individualized to their child.
3. Teach parents the signs of physical and psychological readiness which the child should exhibit before training is started.
4. Discuss methods of preparing the child for toilet training.
   a. Explain the need for a regular schedule to help the child develop regular elimination habits.
   b. Plan the training for a time when the parent will be able to devote time to the process.
   c. Purchase training pants.
   d. Decide on what type of toilet to use.
      1. Potty chair—allows child to place feet on floor for support and is easy to use but requires emptying and cleaning.
      2. Regular toilet—does not require care that potty chair does but child will need a step stool and smaller toilet seat in order to feel secure.
5. Provide parents with guidelines for the actual training process.
   a. Introduce the concept of using the bathroom and wearing training pants.
      1. Let the child see the toilet being used by a parent or sibling so he can learn by imitation.
      2. Show underpants to the child and explain that people who use the bathroom wear these and not diapers.
      3. Buy training pants for the child and present them as a sign that he or she is getting bigger and can be more like an adult.
   b. Take the child to the bathroom on a regular schedule such as:
      1. When the child wakes up.
      2. After breakfast.
      3. Midmorning.
      4. Before lunch.
      5. After lunch/before nap.
      6. After nap.
      7. Before and after dinner.
      8. Before bedtime.
   c. Place the child on the potty chair or toilet.
      1. Help with clothing.
      2. Do not keep on the toilet for longer than 10 minutes (less if the child objects).
      3. Do not make this a play time.
      4. Remove the child from the toilet at the end of the time; praise the child for cooperating in the process whether or not he or she goes to the bathroom.
      5. Do not use the potty chair as a seat at other times, since this confuses the child about its purpose.
   d. Respond to the child's cues that he or she needs to use the bathroom on a consistent basis even though in the beginning the cue and actual elimination may occur together.
   e. Tell parents not to use laxatives, suppositories, or enemas in an attempt to "regulate" the child.
   f. Explain the need to praise all success and disregard any accidents, since this helps the child develop self-confidence and a desire to master other developmental tasks.
6. Tell parents that the child may fear the flushing of the toilet and to wait until the child is off the toilet to flush.
7. Help parents cope with the child who wishes to save and/or play with what is produced.
   a. Explain the child's inability to understand why the parent wants to get rid of something the parent was so proud of the child for producing.
   b. Tell them to wait until the child leaves the bathroom to dispose of waste products.
   c. Discuss the fact that the child does not share the parents' distaste for this behavior and that they should avoid telling the child "bad," "dirty," etc., lest the child feel these terms apply to him as a person.
   d. Tell parents of the child who engages in playing with feces to:
      1. Give the child clay or play dough which have the same texture.
      2. Change the child as soon as he defecates.

Tongue tie. Inability to elevate or protrude the tongue due to a short lingual frenulum.

A. **General Considerations.**
1. The frenulum is short and near the end of the tongue in the newborn.

2. As the anterior portion of the tongue grows the frenulum is further back.
3. Tongue tie does not interfere with nursing or speech development.
4. Clipping of the frenulum in the older child may be done if the child cannot extend the tongue beyond the teeth.

B. Nursing Management.
1. Reassure parents regarding normal development of the lingual frenulum.
2. Teach the child and parents home management of the child who has the frenulum clipped.
   a. Change gauze packing as needed until oozing stops.
   b. Start with clear liquids and progress diet as tolerated.
   c. Rinse mouth after eating.
   d. Call the physician if frank bleeding occurs or signs of infection develop.
   e. Use analgesic as ordered for discomfort. See *Administration of Medications, Parental.*
   f. Return to physician for removal of suture.

Tonsillectomy and adenoidectomy.
Removal of the palatine tonsils and the pharyngeal tonsils (adenoids).

A. General Considerations.
1. Tonsillectomy and adenoidectomy is the most frequently performed pediatric surgical procedure, although new research suggests indications for the combined procedure are rare.
2. Indications for tonsillectomy include:
   a. Cor pulmonale secondary to severe chronic upper airway obstruction.
   b. Swallowing difficulty caused by enlarged tonsils.
   c. Chronic tonsillitis.
   d. Peritonsillar abscess.
   e. Chronic anterior cervical lymphadenitis.
   f. Voice changes secondary to enlarged tonsils.
3. Indications for adenoidectomy include:
   a. Nasal obstruction resulting in breathing discomfort and speech distortion.
   b. Chronic or recurrent otitis media associated with:
      1. Sensorineural hearing loss.
      2. Conductive hearing loss.
      3. Chronic mastoiditis.
      4. Cholesteatoma.
   c. Chronic sinusitis or nasopharyngitis.
4. Tonsillectomy and adenoidectomy is performed only when indications for both are present.
5. Since surgery is delayed until infection is no longer present it is difficult for the child to un-

derstand why an operation is necessary if his throat is not sore.
6. Bleeding and clotting time should be obtained as well as routine CBC.
7. Surgery may be done in a short-stay surgical unit and overnight hospitalization will not be required.
8. Postoperative complications include:
   a. Hemorrhage.
   b. Pneumonia.
   c. Lung abscess.
   d. Septicemia.
9. Hemorrhage may occur:
   a. In the operating room.
   b. When the anesthetic wears off.
   c. 5 to 8 days postoperatively.

B. Nursing Management.
1. Support the child and parents during hospitalization. See *Hospitalization, Support During.*
2. Initiate discharge planning. See *Discharge Planning.*
3. Meet the preoperative needs of the child. See *Preoperative Care* and *Preparation for Surgery.*
   a. Check the results of bleeding and clotting time.
   b. Observe, record, and report any loose teeth.
   c. Show the child an ice collar and let him try it on if this is an expected postoperative order.
   d. Tell the child his throat will be sore, but he will be able to talk.
4. Meet the needs of the child postoperatively. See *Postoperative Care.*
   a. Facilitate drainage by positioning the child prone with a pillow under the chest or semi-prone with one knee flexed.
   b. Observe, record, and report signs and symptoms of hemorrhage.
      1. A pulse rate of 120 per minute, if the child is quiet.
      2. Pallor.
      3. Frequent swallowing.
      4. Trickling of bright blood from the mouth or nose.
      5. Emesis of bright red blood.
      6. Frequent throat clearing.
   c. Be familiar with the location of suction apparatus and equipment for control of hemorrhage.
   d. Explain to the child and parents that vomiting old, dark blood and mucus is not unusual.
   e. Encourage noncitric clear liquids when the child is alert.
   f. Apply an ice collar if ordered.
   g. Keep the child on bed rest as ordered.
   h. Observe, record, and report the child's response to pain medication.

      i. Observe, record, and report cyanosis, stridor, or rapid respirations which indicate obstruction.

        1. Notify the surgeon.

        2. Clear the airway by raising the child's hips or pulling the head and shoulders over the bedside and then slap the child between the shoulder blades.

        3. Support the jaw to keep the tongue forward.

        4. Suction the accumulated secretions.

      j. Offer mouth care frequently.

      k. Progress the child to a soft, bland diet as ordered since eating increases the blood supply to the throat which hastens healing.

    5. Teach the child and parent home management.

      a. Review activity restrictions for the next week as instructed by the surgeon.

      b. Give appropriate information about pain medication to be given at home. See *Administration of Medications, Parental.*

      c. Describe examples of appropriate diet.

        1. Soft bread, but not toast.

        2. Mashed potatoes, but not french fries.

        3. Soft eggs, but not bacon.

      d. Review observations that should be reported to the surgeon.

        1. Transient earache.

        2. Frequent swallowing.

        3. Vomiting of blood.

        4. Fever.

      e. Provide the phone number of the private physician or emergency department.

Tonsillitis/adenoiditis.

Infection and inflammation of the palatine tonsils/Infection and inflammation of the pharyngeal tonsils.

  A. General Considerations.

    1. Tonsillitis and adenoiditis are sometimes included under the broader diagnostic category of acute pharyngitis which describes any throat infection.

    2. Tonsillar tissue increases during the preschool years when the child is exposed to many new organisms.

    3. The tonsils are believed to act in the formation of antibodies and to filter pathogenic organisms from the head and neck area.

    4. Signs and symptoms of infection of the palatine tonsils include:

      a. Drooling as a result of painful swallowing.

      b. High fever.

      c. Lethargy.

      d. Pus on the tonsillar crypts.

      e. Bright red enlarged tonsils.

    5. Signs and symptoms of infection of the pharyngeal tonsils include:

      a. Nasal speech.

      b. Mouth breathing.

      c. Hearing difficulty.

      d. Fever.

      e. Lethargy.

      f. Pharyngeal pain.

      g. Edema of the involved tissue.

    6. The causative agent may be viral or bacterial.

    7. Treatment is based on the child's symptoms and the identification of the causative organism by throat culture.

      a. Oral penicillin if group A beta hemolytic streptococcus is identified.

      b. Antipyretics.

      c. Analgesics.

    8. Intramuscular penicillin may be administered if the parent is presumed to be noncompliant in returning for culture report or in administering the oral antibiotic accurately.

    9. Tonsils may hypertrophy or atrophy after an infection.

    10. Chronic tonsillitis occurs when the tonsils are chronically hypertrophied and infected.

    11. Signs and symptoms of chronic tonsillitis include:

      a. Persistent or repeated sore throat.

      b. Swallowing difficulty.

      c. Breathing difficulty.

      d. Enlarged cervical lymph nodes.

    12. Signs and symptoms of chronic adenoiditis include:

      a. Constant mouth breathing.

      b. Persistent rhinitis.

      c. Nasal speech.

      d. Chronic cough.

      e. Halitosis.

      f. Decrease in the sense of taste, smell, and hearing.

    13. Tonsillectomy and/or adenoidectomy may be necessary in cases of chronic infection. See *Tonsillectomy and Adenoidectomy.*

  B. Nursing Management.

    1. Explain the purpose of and procedure for a throat culture to the child and parents. See *Preparation for Procedures.*

    2. Review the administration of antibiotic therapy. See *Administration of Medications, Parental.*

    3. Discuss comfort measures for the child.

      a. Keep the child on bed rest during the febrile period. See *Home Management of Minor Illnesses.*

      b. Initiate fever reduction measures. See *Fever Reduction.*

      c. Apply hot or cold throat compresses depending on which is more soothing to the child.

    d. Provide cool mist vaporizer during periods of mouth breathing.

    e. Have the older child gargle with warm salt water. One tsp. of salt per 8 ounce glass of water.

    f. Administer analgesics as instructed.

    g. Provide cool, bland fluids frequently. See *Forcing Fluids.*

4. Teach the child and parents to report symptoms of abscess formation.

    a. Dyspnea.

    b. Respiratory obstruction.

      1. Cyanosis.

      2. Stridor.

      3. Rapid respirations.

Total parenteral nutrition (TPN, intravenous alimentation, hyperalimentation).

Intravenous administration of all nutrients in amounts sufficient to promote overtly normal growth (Winters, 1982).

A. General Considerations.

1. The solution for parenteral nutrition contains:

    a. Amino acids.

    b. Glucose (10 to 25 percent).

    c. Electrolytes.

    d. Minerals.

    e. Trace metals.

    f. Vitamins.

2. Solutions may be administered by two routes.

    a. Central venous via superior vena cava, innominate or intrathoracic subclavian veins, or inferior vena cava.

    b. Peripheral veins via dorsal aspect of hand or foot or superficial veins of the scalp.

3. Advantages and disadvantages associated with each route include:

    a. Central.

      1. Advantages: no limit to the amount of nutrients which can be given and the lines may remain in place for a long period of time.

      2. Disadvantages: complications may occur at insertion site, greater risk of mechanical and metabolic complications, greater difficulty in care of the lines and administration of fluids.

    b. Peripheral.

      1. Advantages: care is similar to that of other I.V.s, no special technique must be used for placement, and there are fewer technical and metabolic complications.

      2. Disadvantages: site must be changed at least every 48 hours, there is a potential for thrombophlebitis and/or sloughing

of skin, there is a limit to the amount of nutrients which can be given and a false assumption may be made that nutrient needs are being met.

4. Total parenteral solutions may cause allergic reactions.

    a. Rash.

    b. Tachycardia.

    c. Nausea and vomiting.

5. The solutions is administered through regular I.V. tubing with a millipore filter attached to remove organisms or particles in the solution.

6. Central venous alimentation:

    a. Is required for use with glucose solutions greater than 10 percent because they are hyperosmolar and require a high blood flow for dilution.

    b. Will be used for long-term therapy because it enhances growth.

    c. Will be started in the OR.

    d. Are usually administered using a constant infusion pump.

7. Peripheral venous alimentation.

    a. Solutions contain dilute glucose-protein hydrolysates.

    b. Are used for shorter-term therapy because they maintain or promote only slight gain in weight.

    c. Can be started on the pediatric unit.

8. Complications associated with parenteral nutrition are more common with the central venous route and may be:

    a. Metabolic: related to the child's capacity to handle the solution.

      1. Hyperglycemia.

      2. Azotemia.

      3. Acid-base imbalance.

      4. Electrolyte imbalance.

      5. Fluid overload.

      6. Hyperosmotic dehydration.

    b. Catheter: related to the I.V. line and its placement; all of the following are related to central lines except for infection:

      1. Infection (major complication encountered).

      2. Pneumothorax.

      3. Perforation.

      4. Hemothorax.

      5. Thrombosis formation at the catheter tip.

      6. Air embolism.

      7. Phlebitis.

      8. Tissue damage if the line dislodges and solution leaks into surrounding tissues.

9. The volume of fluid ordered will depend on the child's:

    a. Age.

    b. General condition.

    c. Response to therapy.

d. Oral nutritional intake, if not NPO.

10. The TPN solution must be changed every 24 hours and the dressings and tubing changed on a regular basis according to agency policy.

11. Intravenous fat emulsions:

   a. May be Intralipid®, a soybean emulsion, or Liposyn®, a safflower oil emulsion.

   b. Supply essential fatty acids and are the major source of calories in peripheral alimentation.

   c. Are isotonic and may be given via a central or peripheral vein.

   d. Are used by the body in the same way as food fats.

   e. Must be run through a separate I.V. line without a filter and mixed with other solutions close to the site of insertion in order to maintain stability of the emulsion.

   f. Promote the growth of organisms and are more likely to support growth of pathogens than the glucose/amino acid solution.

   g. May produce hyperlipemia and need to be discontinued.

   h. Are started at a slow rate and gradually increased to rate ordered.

   i. May produce the following reactions (close monitoring is necessary and the infusion should be stopped and the physician notified if a reaction occurs):

      1. Dyspnea.
      2. Cyanosis.
      3. Pain in the chest or back.
      4. Sweating.
      5. Drowsiness.
      6. Temperature elevation.

   j. Administration may be followed by the development of a fat-overload syndrome which can occur days or weeks later and presents with the following:

      1. Fever.
      2. Jaundice.
      3. Easy bruising.
      4. Abnormal clotting studies.
      5. Focal seizures.
      6. Leukocytosis.
      7. Shock.

   k. Should be used with caution or not at all when any of the following are present:

      1. Infection.
      2. Pulmonary disease.
      3. Hyperbilirubinemia.
      4. Lipemia.
      5. Thrombocytopenia.

12. Growth and metabolic parameters will need to be evaluated and the child constantly monitored for infection.

13. The infant or young child receiving TPN may fail to develop an association between food intake and the relief of hunger because the gastrointestinal tract is not stimulated.

14. The feeding situation plays an integral part in the psychosocial development of the child and therefore the child who is receiving long-term total parenteral nutrition has special psychosocial needs.

15. Selected children on long-term total parenteral nutrition can be managed at home with administration of solutions via a Broviac catheter.

B. Nursing Management.

1. Explain the therapy to the child and parents. See *Preparation for Procedures*.

2. Assist with catheter insertion as ordered if the procedure is done on the unit.

3. Meet the needs of the child preoperatively if insertion in the OR is planned. See *Preoperative Care* and *Preparation for Surgery*.

4. Meet the needs of the child postoperatively. See *Postoperative Care*.

5. Record on Kardex where catheter is placed.

6. Observe, record, and report signs and symptoms of complications of catheter insertion.

7. Observe, record, and report signs and symptoms of an allergic reaction to the solution.

8. Prevent infection.

   a. Do not open the TPN line to:
      1. Withdraw blood.
      2. Measure central venous pressure.
      3. Administer I.V. bolus drugs.
      4. Piggyback other infusions.

   b. Use aseptic technique in all catheter care.

   c. Do not hang a bag or bottle which has precipitate or any holes or cracks.

   d. Change the following every 24 hours:
      1. I.V. tubing.
      2. Filter.
      3. Solution.

   e. Follow hospital procedure for catheter care and dressing change procedure.

9. Observe, record, and report signs of sepsis due to infection.

   a. Poor feeding.
   b. Fever.
   c. Lethargy.
   d. Irritability.
   e. Vomiting.

10. Observe, record, and report the following when the dressing is changed:

    a. Loose sutures at the cutdown site.
    b. Kinking of the line.
    c. Redness.
    d. Edema.
    e. Sediment around the insertion site.
    f. Leaking of fluid which will cause tissue damage.

11. Prevent dislodging of catheter.
    a. Restrain the child as needed. See *Restraints*.
    b. Do not put pressure on or pull on tubing.
12. Prevent air embolus.
    a. Do not disconnect the tubing.
    b. Use a padded hemostat to clamp the central venous line during a change.
13. Maintain a constant infusion rate, since:
    a. Increasing the rate of the hypertonic solution can cause:
       1. Hyperglycemia.
       2. Osmotic diuresis.
       3. Brain toxicity.
    b. Decreasing the rate may cause hypoglycemia.
14. Monitor the following (Winters, 1982):
    a. Growth variables (obtain and record).
       1. Daily weight.
       2. Weekly length.
       3. Weekly head circumference.
    b. Metabolic variables (obtain and/or review laboratory values as they are ordered and report abnormal results).
       1. Plasma electrolytes.
       2. Blood urea nitrogen.
       3. Plasma calcium, magnesium, and phosphorus.
       4. Acid-base status.
       5. Serum protein.
       6. Liver function studies.
       7. Urine glucose.
15. Observe, record, and report signs of phlebitis at the peripheral catheter site.
16. Maintain stability of the Intralipid®.
    a. Refrigerate until time of infusion.
    b. Do not add anything to the emulsion.
    c. Do not hang if solution is "frothy."
    d. Infuse through a separate line.
17. Observe, record, and report signs of fatty acid deficiency.
    a. Dry, scaly skin.
    b. Eczematous lesions.
18. Provide frequent mouth care.
19. Meet the psychosocial needs of the infant. See *Infant* and *Neonate*.
    a. Provide simulated feedings (Conway and Williams, 1976).
       1. Give the infant a pacifier to suck for 15 to 20 minutes at a feeding time.
       2. Hold and cuddle the infant while he sucks.
       3. Maintain eye contact.
       4. Remove pacifier and return the infant to bed.
    b. Provide age-appropriate stimulation. See *Stimulation*.

20. Meet the psychosocial needs of the toddler. See *Toddler*.
    a. Minimize the amount of restraint needed. See *Immobilized Child*.
    b. Provide for play. See *Play* and *Play, Therapeutic*.
    c. Provide substitute activities for the child at mealtime, e.g., take for a walk, read a story.
21. Meet the psychosocial needs of the preschooler. See *Preschooler*.
    a. Minimize restraints.
    b. Provide substitutes for active play, e.g., racing a car on a table, building and demolishing block towers.
    c. Decrease fears by providing consistent, age-appropriate explanations.
    d. Tell the child that you know it is hard to give up favorite foods and let her or him talk about the situation.
22. Meet the psychosocial needs of the schoolchild and adolescent. See *Adolescent* and *Schoolchild*.
    a. Support the child in coping with an altered body image due to nutritional changes. See *Body Image*.
    b. Let the child select the time for treatment to provide some control.
    c. Supply information about TPN.
23. Support the older child and parents during termination of parenteral nutrition to increase caloric intake.
    a. Offer small, frequent feedings of high caloric foods, e.g., milk, ice cream, custards, peanut butter, cheese cubes.
    b. Give the child a choice when possible.
    c. Find out favorite foods and record on Kardex.
    d. Encourage family to bring in favorite foods.
24. Develop a plan of care for the child who will receive total parenteral nutrition at home (Whaley and Wong, 1983).
    a. Assess the parents for their readiness and ability to provide care in the home.
    b. Assess availability of support systems required to provide home administration, e.g., pharmacy to prepare the solution, physician availability, insurance coverage.
    c. Involve the hospital social services department and community health nurse in developing and implementing the plan.
    d. Instruct the child and parents in administration of the solution(s) via the Broviac catheter.
    e. Provide a period of time during which the parent(s) assume total care of the child with professional assistance readily available.

T

f. Provide, and review with parents, a complete written set of instructions.

Toys.
Articles used for amusement primarily by the child from 1 to 8 years of age.

A. **General Considerations.**
1. Toys should be selected with several considerations in mind.
   a. Is it safe?
   b. Is it appropriate to the child's developmental level?
   c. Can the child become involved with it?
   d. How much creativity will it permit?
   e. How much supervision or instruction is required for its use?
   f. Will it hold the child's interest?
   g. Will it last?
2. Children do not need a large number of toys, but they do need a variety, since what they want to learn, practice, and explore changes quickly.
3. Children can be taught early to take care of their toys.
4. Toys can serve an educational value for the child.
   a. A large ball can facilitate gross-motor skills such as balance, throwing, and kicking.
   b. Dolls with removable clothing can facilitate fine motor skills.
   c. Musical toys that repeat phrases can encourage speech.
5. Items available in the home, e.g., wooden spoons, pots and pans, empty boxes, can provide many happy play hours for the child.
6. Many toys can be made from materials in the home.
   a. Encourage parents to save milk cartons, empty spools, juice containers, etc. for special projects.
   b. The child and/or the parent may create new toys.
   c. Many books are available to help the child and/or parent who needs assistance.
7. Children need toys for indoor and outdoor play.
8. Children should have the opportunity to play with a variety of toys without regard for sexual stereotyping.
   a. Play with dolls can teach the child of either sex about loving and caring.
   b. Playing with trucks or baseballs will not guarantee masculinity or destroy femininity.
9. The older child may have definite ideas about what toy(s) he or she wants.
10. Children will usually enjoy receiving a new toy once a month or so, rather than being overwhelmed on holidays or birthdays.
11. Selection of toys for the hospitalized child must be selected with awareness that:
    a. Regression usually occurs.
    b. The child's energy level may be decreased.
    c. The immobilized child needs an outlet for aggression.
    d. Washable toys may be necessary for the child in isolation.

B. **Nursing Management.**
1. Select appropriate toys for the hospitalized child.
   a. Infant.
      1. Soft toys such as stuffed animals or rag dolls.
      2. Mobiles (change frequently).
      3. Musical toys.
      4. Rubber or plastic toys which can be chewed on, but are too large to be swallowed.
      5. Large, colorful plastic or wooden beads which can be hooked together.
      6. Large blocks.
      7. Rattles.
      8. Balls.
      9. Mirrors.
   b. Toddler.
      1. Soft toys such as stuffed animals or rag dolls.
      2. Pull or push toys.
      3. Toys which can be ridden.
      4. Blocks.
      5. Balls and beanbags.
      6. Crayons and paper.
      7. Musical toys.
      8. Playdough and clay.
      9. Empty and fill toys such as a milk container and clothespins.
      10. Hammer and pegs.
      11. Water and water toys.
      12. Large piece puzzles.
      13. Books.
   c. Preschooler.
      1. Riding toys.
      2. Large beads to string.
      3. Blocks and other materials to construct things.
      4. Crayons and finger paints.
      5. Scissors.
      6. Hammer and pegs.
      7. Jump rope.
      8. Clothing and equipment for dramatic play.
      9. Small slides and stairs to climb.
      10. Puzzles.
      11. Books.
      12. Balls and beanbags.

T

13. Card games for older preschoolers.
14. Playdough and clay.
15. Dolls.
2. The schoolchild may not be interested in toys but will enjoy:
   a. Puzzles.
   b. Model kits.
   c. Board games.
   d. Card games.
   e. Construction sets such as logs or small plastic blocks that fit together.
   f. Small electronic games.
   g. Craft activities.
3. Discuss the selection of toys with parents using the above list as a resource.
   a. Review some basic safety considerations.
      1. Can the child take the toy apart and be injured by what is inside?
      2. Are the parts small enough to be swallowed?
      3. Could the toy shatter and cut (e.g., glass or brittle plastic toys)?
      4. Are there any sharp edges?
      5. Is the noise made by the toy too loud?
      6. Is the paint safe?
      7. Is the wiring of electrical toy safe?
      8. Is the toy safe for any child in the family who might decide to play with it?
      9. Can the child's finger get caught in the trigger mechanism?
      10. Is there a possibility of an explosion?
   b. Discuss with parents that many products state that a particular toy is suitable for children of a large age range and they must consider their child's development.
   c. Discourage parents from purchasing a toy that is too sophisticated because they feel their child is brighter than average or that the child will grow into it.
   d. Discuss with parents that children should not be influenced by parents to prefer "boy" or "girl" toys.

Tracheobronchitis. See *Laryngotracheobronchitis*.

Tracheoesophageal fistula (TEF). A congenital anomaly in which the upper esophagus ends in a blind pouch below the level of the trachea and the lower esophageal segment communicates with the trachea.

A. General Considerations.
1. There are other types of esophageal atresia, but the type described above is the most common.
2. Signs and symptoms of TEF are frequently observed by the alert nurse in the newborn nursery.
   a. Constant bubbling of oral secretions.
   b. Coughing, cyanosis, or coughing with feeding.
   c. Gradually increasing respiratory distress.
   d. Abdominal distention.
3. The first feeding of the newborn should be sterile water to avoid problems if the feeding is aspirated.
4. An unsuccessful attempt to pass a nasogastric catheter during a newborn examination will suggest the diagnosis.
5. X-ray examination with a radiopaque catheter will confirm the diagnosis.
6. Pneumonia may occur as an early complication due to:
   a. Aspiration of oral feedings.
   b. Reflux of stomach contents through the fistula between the lower esophageal segment and the trachea.
7. Surgical treatment varies with the infant's condition and the extent of the defect.
   a. A gastrostomy under local anesthesia may be performed on the infant to empty the stomach of gastric secretions and to prevent reflux into the lungs.
   b. A primary repair with ligation of the fistula and anastomosis of the esophageal segments will be performed if:
      1. The infant is full-term.
      2. There is minimal pulmonary contamination.
      3. The distance between the esophageal segments is minimal.
   c. Repeated operations over time (staging) will be necessary if:
      1. The infant is premature.
      2. The baby has pneumonia or sepsis.
      3. The distance between the esophageal segment or the difference in size of the ends of the segments is significant.
8. Staged repair often includes:
   a. Gastrostomy.
   b. Constant suction of the upper pouch or externalization of the upper esophageal segment (cervical esophagostomy).
   c. Anastomosis of the esophageal segments.
   d. Esophageal reconstruction using a segment of the colon (colon transplant or colon interposition) when the child is 18 to 24 months of age.
9. Associated defects may include:
   a. Congenital heart disease.
   b. Genitourinary anomalies.
   c. Anorectal malformations.
10. Supportive measures which are used preoperatively include:

T

a. I.V. therapy.
b. Warm, high humidity environment.
c. Constant suction of the upper pouch via double lumen catheter.
d. Positioning the baby at a 30 degree elevation to prevent reflux and aspiration.
e. Oxygen if necessary.
f. Temperature and EKG monitoring.
g. Broad-spectrum antibiotic therapy if aspiration occurs.

11. Hyperalimentation may be used for the infant whose repair will be staged. See *Total Parenteral Nutrition.*

12. Introduction of oral feedings will be difficult if the sucking reflex is not stimulated in simulated feedings in the infant with long-term gastrostomy or hyperalimentation therapy.

13. It is possible to introduce the child who will need a colon transplant to age-appropriate feeding habits if the surgeon and parents agree.
    a. A small portion of the gastrostomy tube feeding or age-appropriate pureed or junior food can be fed the child, since it will exit through the cervical esophagostomy.
    b. If the parents can deal with this approach aesthetically, the major concern is good skin care around the esophagostomy.

14. Complications of the esophageal reconstruction are ischemia of the transplanted segment and stricture.

15. Dilatations may be performed routinely after anastomosis or colon transplant or only when stricture is evident.

B. Nursing Management.

1. Support the infant and parents during hospitalization. See *Hospitalization, Support During.*

2. Initiate discharge planning as soon as it is apparent what the parents will need to know. See *Discharge Planning.*

3. Meet the needs of the infant preoperatively. See *Preoperative Care* and *Preparation for Surgery.*
   a. Maintain the temperature and humidity as ordered.
   b. Elevate the infant 30 degrees or as ordered.
   c. Observe, record, and report signs and symptoms of respiratory distress:
      1. Retractions.
      2. Circumoral cyanosis.
      3. Nasal flaring.
   d. Suction the mouth frequently.
   e. Aspirate secretions from the esophageal pouch frequently if continuous suction is not used.
   f. Provide care of the esophagostomy and gastrostomy sites.
      1. Use gauze pads as dressings.
      2. Apply a protective ointment such as zinc oxide or silicone.
      3. Apply a colostomy bag if the infant's skin tolerates this.
   g. Monitor I.V. or hyperalimentation accurately.
   h. Leave the gastrostomy to straight drainage.
   i. Monitor the oxygen level every hour or as indicated in hospital policy.
   j. Change the infant's position every 2 hours.
   k. Observe, record, and report the infant's response to antibiotic therapy.

4. Meet the needs of the infant after anastomosis.
   a. Continue to monitor temperature, humidity, and oxygen as ordered.
   b. Use a marked catheter for nasopharyngeal suctioning to prevent damage to the anastomosis.
   c. Leave the gastrostomy tube to straight drainage until feedings are begun.
   d. Measure and record gastrostomy drainage.
   e. Weigh daily.
   f. Monitor intake and record.
   g. Monitor urine specific gravity.
   h. Observe, record, and report the amount of drainage from the chest tube.
   i. Provide mouth care frequently.
   j. Change the infant's position every 2 hours.
   k. Observe, record, and report the infant's response to antibiotic therapy.
   l. Institute gastrostomy feeding when ordered.
      1. Aspirate stomach contents before feeding and subtract this volume from the amount of formula to be fed.
      2. Return aspirated stomach contents, then feed formula.
      3. Feed slowly.
      4. Hold the infant during the gastrostomy feeding as soon as his condition permits.
      5. Elevate the tubing and leave open by suspending the tubing through the top of the incubator or suspend from an I.V. pole.
      6. Attach a syringe to the tubing to allow for reflux of formula.
   m. Provide appropriate stimulation as the baby's condition improves.
   n. Progress to oral feedings as ordered.
      1. Elevate the infant slightly for feedings.
      2. Feed the infant slowly and observe his response.

T

3. Maintain consistency by recording the most effective feeding technique on the Kardex for all caregivers to follow.
4. Complete the feeding by gastrostomy, if ordered, to prevent tiring the infant.
5. Teach the parents home management of the infant following anastomosis.
  a. Discuss the feeding techniques that have been most effective.
    1. Give the child food that is cut into appropriate size when the diet has progressed to table food.
    2. Encourage the child to chew food thoroughly.
  b. Review signs of respiratory distress.
  c. Teach the parents the signs and symptoms of stricture.
    1. Refusal to eat.
    2. Pronounced coughing.
    3. Dysphagia.
  d. Teach the parent emergency measures to use if the child becomes obstructed, e.g., syringe suctioning, CPR.
  e. Discuss basic infant care, particularly if this is the first-born child. See *Infant.*
6. Teach the parents home management of the infant who will require colon transplant.
  a. Have parents demonstrate gastrostomy feeding procedure.
    1. Encourage parents to hold the infant during the feeding and offer a pacifier to stimulate the sucking reflex.
    2. Teach the parents to clamp the tube securely after feeding.
  b. Teach the parents to prepare the feedings in a blender.
  c. Arrange for the dietician to explain when to add different foods to the feedings as the child grows.
  d. Review skin care of the esophagostomy and gastrostomy sites.
  e. Discuss with parents how offering a small portion of the feeding orally or offering a lollipop or sucker will help meet the child's oral needs.
7. Meet the needs of the infant undergoing colon transplant.
  a. Provide preoperative care. See *Preoperative Care* and *Preparation for Surgery.*
  b. Provide postoperative care. See *Postoperative Care.*
    1. Observe, record, and report chest tube drainage.
    2. Position the child to facilitate adequate respiration.
    3. Elevate the gastrostomy tube and do not clamp in the immediate postoperative period.
    4. Clamp the tube 30 to 45 minutes after

feeding once gastrostomy feedings have been resumed.
  c. Initiate oral feedings gradually, particularly if the child has never been fed orally.
    1. Dip a nipple or pacifier in formula or milk to allow the child to adjust to the taste.
    2. Try cup feedings if the child's sucking need has disappeared through lack of stimulation.
    3. Use patience and gentle reassurance when attempting feedings.
    4. Maintain consistency by recording the most effective approach on the Kardex for all caregivers to follow.
  d. Reassure parents that frequent burping and a strong stool odor to the breath are common, but will disappear in time.
  e. Teach parents home management.
    1. Discuss the feeding techniques that have been most effective.
    2. Teach the signs and symptoms of stricture, e.g., refusal to eat, pronounced coughing, and dysphagia.
    3. Discuss how to progress the diet according to the child's developmental level.
    4. Discuss the need to provide age-appropriate care. See *Toddler.*

Traction, care of child. Measures to meet the needs of the child treated by application of a pulling force to an extremity or other part of the body.

  A. General Considerations.
    1. Traction may be used to:
      a. Correct displacement of fracture fragments.
      b. Immobilize a fracture.
      c. Decrease spinal curvature.
      d. Reduce muscle spasm (rare).
      e. Reduce a dislocation.
      f. Rest an extremity.
    2. There are two general categories of traction.
      a. Skin traction that is applied to skin and soft tissue and results in an indirect pull on the skeletal system.
      b. Skeletal traction that is applied directly to the bone via a pin, wire, tongs, etc.
    3. The pulling force is accomplished by the use of ropes, pulleys, and weights.
    4. Countertraction to balance the applied traction is provided by the child's own weight.
    5. The foot of the bed may need to be elevated on shock blocks to maintain countertraction if the child's weight is light in relation to the weights.
    6. A solid Bradford frame may be used with a

T

young child in traction to obtain additional countertraction or to assist with immobilization.

7. The young child will need to be restrained so that proper body alignment can be maintained.

8. Possible complications of the traction and immobilization include:
   a. Impairment of neurovascular status.
   b. Pressure areas.
   c. Infected pin sites.
   d. Contractures.
   e. Foot drop.
   f. Constipation.
   g. Renal calculi.

B. **Nursing Management.** See *Fractures* and *Immobilized Child.*
   1. Support the child and parents during hospitalization. See *Hospitalization, Support During.*
   2. Initiate discharge planning. See *Discharge Planning.*
   3. Observe the traction setup and follow the course of each weight and pulley.
      a. Do not release the traction unless there is a specific order to do so.
      b. Do not remove a weight or lay it on the bed.
      c. Be sure that all ropes are in the grooves of the pulley.
      d. Be sure all weights are hanging free and are not caught on the bed frame or in the linen.
      e. Be sure the ordered amount of weight is applied.
      f. Do not allow the footplate or the knot in the rope to come in contact with the pulley or the foot of the bed.
      g. Check the rope for fraying.
      h. Keep the child's foot from resting on the mattress.
      i. Check skin traction bandages every 4 hours to assure they are positioned correctly.
   4. Observe, record, and report the child's neurovascular status.
      a. Obtain baseline data before traction is applied if possible.
      b. Assess the following factors:
         1. Color.
         2. Capillary filling.
         3. Temperature.
         4. Presence or absence of edema.
         5. Sensation.
         6. Motion.
      c. Assess status every hour for 24 hours after application, then every 4 hours unless ordered otherwise.
      d. Assess status 30 minutes after skin traction is reapplied.

5. Assess the child's need for pain medication. See *Pain.*
6. Clarify with the orthopedist or follow agency procedure for how the child should be positioned, e.g., degree of elevation of head of bed, prone or supine, etc.
7. Be sure the child is in proper alignment.
   a. Place a diagram of the desired alignment on the traction apparatus.
   b. Draw lines with a crayon on the sheet to remind the child where to lie.
   c. Use a sling, jacket, or diaper restraint to keep the young child from sitting up.
      1. Explain the reason for the restraint to the child, if old enough, and to the parents.
      2. Apply the restraint as soon as the child is placed in traction.
      3. Use the restraint consistently on all shifts.
      4. Remove the restraint every 4 hours for skin care and observation.
8. Promote skin integrity.
   a. Keep the linen wrinkle-free.
   b. Provide sheepskin, egg crate, or alternating pressure mattress.
   c. Provide a trapeze bar for the older child to lift his back and shoulders off the bed for skin care.
   d. Use alcohol for skin care, since this toughens the skin and lotions or oils soften the skin and predispose to breakdown.
   e. Massage the back, sacral area, and bony prominences three times a day.
   f. Skin care should be given to the extremity in skin traction every 4 hours when the extremity is unwrapped.
   g. Observe for signs and symptoms of an allergic reaction to adhesive traction straps.
      1. Severe itching.
      2. Rash.
      3. Blister formation.
   h. Obtain a written order for the type of pin care to be given, if any, to the child in skeletal traction.
9. Prevent constipation which may occur because of immobilization. See *Constipation.*
   a. Offer natural fruit juices, particularly prune juice.
   b. Encourage raw fruits and vegetables.
   c. Maintain an adequate fluid intake.
   d. Obtain an order for a stool softener if needed.
10. Prevent formation of renal calculi by forcing fluids and by limiting the child's milk intake to two glasses per day. See *Forcing Fluids.*
11. Meet the child's need for stimulation and diversion. See *Stimulation.*
    a. Move the child's bed to the playroom or

hall unless the child's bed is on shock blocks.

b. Provide crafts and activities the child can do while maintaining proper alignment.

c. Provide activities to help the immobilized child release aggression.

d. Provide foot puppets which provide diversion and improve circulation.

e. Suspend mobiles, greeting cards, drawings, etc. over the traction bars.

12. Teach the parent management of the traction if it will be used at home (Villalon and Smith, 1982).

a. Have the parents do a return demonstration of traction application.

b. Give the parents written instructions.

c. Help the child understand the traction is to help him get better and is not a form of punishment.

d. Make a home visit or refer the family to the community health nurse.

e. Give the parents a contact number if they need assistance.

f. Provide the young child with opportunities to work through the trauma of hospitalization. See *Play, Therapeutic.*

Transposition of the great vessels. See *Congenital Heart Disease.*

Truncus arteriosus. See *Congenital Heart Disease.*

Trust. See *Appendix v.*

Tumor, bone. See *Osteosarcoma* and *Ewing's Sarcoma.*

Tumor, brain. See *Brain Tumor.*

Tumor, Wilms'. See *Wilms' Tumor.*

Umbilical hernia. See *Hernia, Umbilical.*

Undescended testes. See *Cryptorchidism.*

Urinary tract infection. Bacterial infection of any portion of the urinary tract.

A. **General Considerations.**

1. Urinary tract infections may be classified as follows (Carvajal and Travis, 1980):

a. Symptomatic or asymptomatic.

b. Initial infection or recurrent infection.

c. Simple (no anatomic or functional abnormalities present) or complex (anatomic or functional abnormalities present).

d. Lower (urethra, bladder) or upper (ureters, kidneys).

2. Classification serves as a basis for the treatment plan, e.g., an initial, symptomatic, simple infection of the bladder will be treated differently than a recurrent, symptomatic, complex infection of the kidneys.

3. Signs and symptoms vary and are influenced by the age of the child and the location of the infection.

a. Neonates and infants may exhibit such nonspecific signs and symptoms as:

1. Poor feeding.
2. Diarrhea.
3. Vomiting.
4. Irritability.
5. Convulsions.
6. Failure to thrive.

b. Older children with lower urinary tract infections may exhibit:

1. Dysuria.
2. Frequency of urination.
3. Urgency when urinating.
4. Lower abdominal pain.
5. Foul smelling urine.
6. Enuresis.
7. Hematuria.

c. Older children with upper urinary tract infections may exhibit:

1. Fever.
2. Chills.
3. Costovertebral angle tenderness.
4. Back pain.

4. The child may also be entirely asymptomatic or exhibit only fever.

5. Diagnosis is made by the finding of 100,000

or more organisms per milliliter in a fresh, clean voided, promptly cultured midstream urine or the presence of any bacteria in a specimen obtained by a suprapubic urine tap.

6. Differentiation between upper and lower urinary tract infections is important and laboratory studies which contribute to localization of the infection include examination of the urine for:
   a. Glitter cells and leukocyte casts.
   b. Increased leukocytes—counts greater than 1,000,000 strongly suggest pyelonephritis.
   c. Urine concentration—decreased in upper urinary tract infections.
   d. Serum antibodies—increased in upper urinary tract infections.

7. Treatment of all infections is aimed at:
   a. Eradication of the infectious organism by:
      1. Systemic antibiotics for 10 to 14 days.
      2. Urinary tract antiseptics for long-term use to maintain urine sterility.
   b. Elimination, if possible, of underlying contributing factors.
      1. Neurological factors affecting the voiding mechanism.
      2. Obstruction.
      3. Renal calculi.
      4. Gross vesicoureteral reflux.
      5. Constipation which produces functional obstruction of the bladder neck and urethra.
   c. Follow-up to ensure eradication of infection and detection of recurrent infection, e.g., repeat urine cultures.

8. The use of an antibiotic which does not alter the intestinal flora is important because those that do predispose the child to recurrent infection.

9. Renal damage rarely occurs from infection unless there is an underlying contributing factor.

10. All children with a first infection should have an intravenous pyelogram and a voiding cystourethrogram.

11. Cystoscopy is not indicated unless significant problems are revealed by the urethrogram (Kunin, 1979).

12. A variety of kits are available for use at home to screen children for urinary tract infections.

13. The intrusive nature of the intravenous pyelogram makes this a stressful procedure for the child.

14. Factors which predispose the child/adolescent to urinary tract infections include:
   a. Short female urethra.
   b. Close proximity of the urethra to the anus in the female.
   c. Incomplete emptying of the bladder.
   d. Concentrated and alkaline urine.
   e. Poor personal hygiene and tight, nonabsorbent underwear.

15. Home management is usually possible for the older child and x-ray studies can be done on an outpatient basis, but the infant or acutely ill child will be hospitalized.

B. Nursing Management.
1. Support the child and parents during hospitalization. See *Hospitalization, Support During.*
2. Initiate discharge planning. See *Discharge Planning.*
3. Observe, record, and report signs and symptoms.
4. Observe, record, and report the child's response to antibiotic therapy.
5. Promote hydration. See *Forcing Fluids.*
6. Reduce fever as ordered. See *Fever Reduction.*
7. Collect a clean catch midstream urine specimen in the toilet trained child as ordered, making sure that the:
   a. Labia or penis and meatus are washed and rinsed.
   b. Container does not touch the body.
   c. Urine is collected in midstream.
   e. Specimen goes directly to the lab or is refrigerated, since bacteria double in number every 20 to 30 minutes at room temperature.
8. Assist with the collection of a suprapubic bladder tap in the untrained child as ordered making sure that the:
   a. Child has not voided within the last hour.
   b. Child is restrained so the needle can be safely introduced into the bladder.
   c. Skin has been prepared with iodine and alcohol.
   d. Specimen goes to the lab or is refrigerated.
9. Observe, record, and report hematuria following a suprapubic tap.
10. Prepare the child/adolescent and parents for an intravenous pyelogram. See *Preparation for Procedures.*
   a. Review history for presence of any allergy to shellfish or prior allergic response to radiopaque dye (renograms can be done with radionuclides in children with these allergies).
   b. Tell younger child what he will feel, e.g., small stick when needle put in, warm all over when pictures are taken.
   c. Tell older child what he will feel and why procedure is done, e.g., to see if there are any problems with his kidneys which need to be fixed.
   d. Do not use the term "dye" since child may interpret this as "die."
   e. Draw diagrams of urinary tract for school-

age child/adolescent to show what will be done.

11. Prepare the child and parents for a voiding cystourethrogram.
    a. Explain that the procedure will detect problems.
    b. Tell the child that it will not hurt.
    c. Explain the need for urinary catheter insertion.
    d. Insert the catheter carefully since any edema may distort the films.
    e. Tell the child that he will be asked to urinate while on the x-ray table and that everybody understands.

12. Explain the importance of follow-up care since the recurrence rate tends to be high.
    a. Administer all medications as ordered. See *Administration of Medications, Parental.*
    b. Return to the office or clinic as instructed for repeat urine studies to detect bacteria.

13. Teach measures which help prevent infection:
    a. Wipe from front to back.
    b. Take showers rather than tub baths to prevent bacteria entrance into the short female urethra.
    c. Avoid tight clothing.
    d. Wear absorbent cotton crotch underwear.
    e. Check for vaginitis or pinworms if the child is scratching the genitalia. See *Worms.*
    f. Have the child void frequently and completely empty the bladder.
    g. Avoid constipation, since retained stool acts as a functional obstruction. See *Constipation.*
    h. Encourage fluid intake, especially cranberry juice that promotes urine acidification.

14. Assess sexual activity in the adolescent who develops a urinary tract infection and determine need for sex education and contraceptive counseling.

15. Prepare the child and parents for surgery, if planned, to correct an abnormality known to be contributing to infection.

Vaccination. See *Immunization.*

Vaginitis, gonorrheal. See *Sexually Transmitted Diseases.*

Vaginitis, monilial. See *Candida albicans.*

Varicella. See *Chickenpox.*

Venereal disease. See *Sexually Transmitted Diseases.*

Ventricular septal defect. See *Congenital Heart Disease.*

Viral hepatitis. See *Hepatitis, Viral.*

Vision screening. The use of testing procedures to identify deficits in the child's vision.

A. **General Considerations.**
1. Good vision is vital to the child's:
   a. Perceptual development.
   b. Cognitive development.
   c. Development of hand–eye coordination.
   d. Safety.
2. Signs and symptoms that may indicate a visual deficit include:
   a. Failure of infant to fixate on mother's face.
   b. Inattention or overattention to visual stimuli.
   c. Squinting.
   d. Covering or closing an eye when reading, working, and/or playing.
   e. Crossing of the eyes on an occasional or regular basis after the age of 6 months.
   f. Complaints of headache, dizziness, or nausea following use of the eyes.
   g. Rubbing of the eyes and/or consistent blinking.
   h. Poor school performance.
   i. Consistent tilting of head in same direction.
   j. Nystagmus.

3. Vision screening should be part of well-child care and should include evaluation of (See *Well-child Care*):
   a. Visual acuity.
   b. Muscle balance.
   c. Peripheral vision.
   d. Color vision in males. (Color blindness is a sex-linked recessive characteristic.)
4. The Snellen E Chart can be used to screen visual acuity in most children by age 4.
5. The Snellen alphabet can be used to screen visual acuity when the child knows the alphabet.
6. The cover and Hirschberg tests are reliable screening methods to detect muscle imbalance.
7. Visual acuity improves as the child grows.
   a. Birth—20/300.
   b. 1 year—20/100.
   c. 2 years—20/40.
   d. 3 years—20/30.
   e. 4 to 5 years—20/20 (normal adult level).
8. The child with a visual deficit should be referred to an ophthalmologist for a thorough examination.
9. Vision screening is very difficult in the infant, but all infants should be checked to see that they have some vision.
10. Vision screening should be carried out in the schools, since many schoolage children are not seen by a physician on a regular basis.
11. The Titmus Vision Testor:
    a. Is a closed vision tester into which the child looks to read either the Snellen E or Snellen Alphabet Chart.
    b. Eliminates distractions.
    c. Prevents memorization of letters on the lines that is possible with wall charts.
12. Vision screening techniques must be modified for the child with mental or emotional retardation (Holland, 1979).

B. Nursing Management.
1. Explain to the parents the importance of having the child's vision screened on a regular basis.
2. Screen the infant.
   a. Assess red reflex.
   b. Move a penlight or bright object in different directions and observe whether the infant follows.
   c. Assess ability to fixate on mother's face.
   d. Assess ocular movements by having infant follow an object through various positions of gaze.
   e. Any infant who does not appear to see should be evaluated further.
3. Prepare the older child for the screening test(s) to be performed. See *Preparation for Procedures.*
4. Screen visual acuity in child over 3 years of age.
   a. Screen the child who wears glasses with his glasses on.
   b. Screen the older child who does not know the alphabet by using the Snellen E (illiterate E) chart.
      1. Ask the child to point in the direction that the E points.
      2. Help the child cooperate in the test by comparing the E to a table and asking which way the "legs" point or by pasting colorful pictures of objects above, below, and on either side of the chart and asking the child toward which picture the "legs" are pointed.
   c. Screen the visual acuity of the older child who knows the alphabet by using the Snellen Alphabet Chart.
   d. Assist a trained individual in doing the screening or make sure you have been taught how to set up and administer the tests to increase the accuracy of the screening procedure.
   e. Refer the child for further evaluation if you observe:
      1. An obvious disorder such as strabismus no matter what the child's visual acuity.
      2. Visual acuity difference of one line or more.
      3. Visual acuity in either eye less than 20/40 in child over age 4.
      4. Visual acuity in either eye less than 20/50 in child under age 4.
5. Help parents to prepare their child for the test by asking them to practice with the child at home using an E drawn on a piece of paper.
6. Screen the child for muscle imbalance. See *Strabismus.*
   a. Perform a Hirschberg test.
      1. Hold a flashlight in a horizontal position 14 inches away from the child's eyes.
      2. Have the child look at a spot on your forehead.
      3. Move the light to eye level and direct it into the child's eyes.
      4. Observe whether the light is reflected from the same location in both eyes.
      5. Refer the child whose eyes reflect light from different spots.
   b. Perform a cover test.
      1. Hold flashlight 14 inches from child's eyes.
      2. Cover one eye (do not touch it) with an occluder held across the nose and forehead.
      3. Have the child keep both eyes open and look at the light.

4. Remove the occluder and watch for any movement in the eye as it is uncovered.
5. Repeat with the other eye.
6. Refer any child in whom eye movement was noted when the occluder was removed.
7. Screen for amblyopia. See *Amblyopia.*
   a. Hold an object for the child to focus on.
   b. Cover one eye and observe whether the child continues to focus on the object.
   c. Repeat with the other eye.
   d. Refer a child for further evaluation if he objects to having an eye covered.
8. Screen peripheral vision.
   a. Stand behind the child.
   b. Have the child look straight ahead.
   c. Wiggle a finger from behind the right side of the child's head until he sees your finger.
   d. Repeat on left side.
   e. Refer the child for further evaluation if he or she does not see the figure as it approaches a 90 degree angle with direct line of vision.

Vital signs. See *Appendix i.*

Volkmann's contracture. See *Fracture.*

Volvulus. Twisting of the intestine resulting in obstruction.

A. **General Considerations.**
   1. Malrotation of the colon, midgut volvulus, and adhesive bands usually occur together.
   2. The abnormalities occur during fetal life.
      a. The cecum remains in the upper right quadrant.
      b. The duodenum is pulled out of position resulting in partial obstruction.
      c. Duodenal bands fix the cecum to the abnormal site.
      d. The mesentery is not attached normally and the small intestine twists around the base of the mesentery.
   3. Signs and symptoms of the intestinal obstruction occur when the intestine twists.
      a. Intense crying.
      b. Pain.
      c. Drawing up the legs.
      d. Abdominal distention.
      e. Bile stained vomitus.
      f. Absence of stools.
      g. Abdominal mass.
   4. Necrosis of the intestine may result from lack of blood supply.

5. The obstruction is diagnosed by a barium enema and upper gastrointestinal series.
6. Fluid and electrolyte imbalance secondary to the vomiting will be corrected preoperatively with I.V. fluid therapy. See *Fluid and Electrolyte Imbalance.*
7. Surgery is necessary to relieve the volvulus, dissect the duodenal bands, and mobilize the cecum.

B. **Nursing Management.**
   1. Support the child and parents during hospitalization. See *Hospitalization, Support During.*
   2. Initiate discharge planning. See *Discharge Planning.*
   3. Meet the needs of the infant/child preoperatively. See *Preoperative Care* and *Preparation for Surgery.*
      a. Maintain NPO status.
      b. Monitor I.V. accurately.
      c. Irrigate nasogastric tube as ordered.
      d. Provide mouth care frequently.
      e. Provide a pacifier to meet sucking needs.
      f. Help the parents to feel at ease while comforting the child by rocking, touching, etc.
      g. Explain to parents that their feeding technique did not cause the problem.
      h. Reassure parents that this problem will not recur.
   4. Meet the needs of the child postoperatively. See *Postoperative Care.*
   5. Teach the parents home management.
      a. Teach parents to protect the wound site.
         1. Pin the diaper low.
         2. Give a sponge bath until the incision is healed.
      b. Review measures to prevent infection.
         1. Frequent handwashing.
         2. Adequate rest.
         3. Adequate nutrition.

Vomiting. Forceful evacuation of the contents of the stomach often accompanied by nausea.

A. **General Considerations.**
   1. True vomiting must be differentiated from:
      a. "Wet burp"—formula brought back up with a burp during feeding and which is not sour, since it was not in contact with gastric secretions.
      b. Regurgitation or "spitting up"—formula returned from the stomach, usually associated with feeding and burping.
   2. Vomiting is a symptom that may accompany a variety of conditions but is most commonly associated with:
      a. Gastrointestinal problems.
      b. Central nervous system disorders.

c. Urinary tract infections.
d. Upper respiratory infections.
e. Feeding problems.
f. Gastroenteritis (less common).
3. Projectile vomiting, vomitus raised so forcefully that it is projected 3 to 4 feet from the child, is often associated with pyloric stenosis or increased intracranial pressure and is usually not accompanied by nausea.
4. Persistent vomiting is associated with an anomaly of the gastrointestinal tract.
5. The child with vomiting may also have:
   a. Nausea.
   b. Diarrhea. See *Diarrhea.*
   c. Abdominal cramps.
   d. Headache.
   e. Signs and symptoms of dehydration.
6. Treatment will be based on the underlying etiology.
7. Antiemetics are generally not indicated in the treatment of gastroenteritis, since they are potentially toxic.
8. Metabolic alkalosis and dehydration may develop with severe or prolonged vomiting, and the use of I.V. fluids may be necessary.
9. The child with vomiting due to a neurological condition or pyloric stenosis is usually refed, since there is no accompanying nausea or gastric irritation.
10. Home management of short-term episodes of vomiting is usually possible, but hospitalization may be required if any one of the following are present:
    a. Forceful vomiting in an infant under 3 months.
    b. Severe abdominal pain.
    c. Vomiting without improvement for more than a day.
    d. Signs of dehydration.
    e. Blood in the vomitus.

B. Nursing Management.
1. Support the child and parents during hospitalization. See *Hospitalization, Support During.*
2. Initiate discharge planning. See *Discharge Planning.*
3. Isolate the child whose vomiting is due to an infectious process. See *Isolated Child.*
4. Progress the diet as ordered or in the following way in children with vomiting due to infection.
5. Explain the rationale for the slow progression of the diet.
   a. Keep NPO for 2 to 4 hours (the younger the child the shorter the period of NPO).
   b. Offer clear liquids.
      1. One tbs. every 15 to 20 minutes for 2 hours.
      2. Two tbs. every ½ hour for 4 times in the older child and every 2 hours for the next 12 to 18 hours in the infant.
      3. Increase amounts slowly.
      4. Use such fluids as flat coke, ginger ale, weak tea, Gatorade, or a commercial pediatric electrolyte solution.
   c. Offer a soft diet the second day and progress to a regular diet as tolerated.
   d. Give liquids at room temperature to avoid further gastric irritation.
   e. Do not boil milk, since this increases the renal solute load and may cause hypernatremia.
6. Observe, record, and report:
   a. Response to dietary management.
   b. Response to antiemetic medications if these are given.
   c. Forceful vomiting.
   d. Signs and symptoms of dehydration. See *Fluid and Electrolyte Imbalance.*
   e. Development or presence of severe abdominal pain.
   f. Blood in the vomitus.
7. Observe, record, and report the following about the vomiting:
   a. Amount.
   b. Number of times.
   c. Color.
   d. Consistency.
   e. Associated factors, e.g., vomited after crying or coughing, complained of headache just before vomiting.
8. Meet the needs of the infant with regurgitation.
   a. Feed slowly.
   b. Thicken feedings with infant's cereal.
   c. Place in infant seat for ½ to 1 hour after feeding.
   d. Elevate the head of the bed.
9. Teach parents to:
   a. Manage vomiting at home by progressing the diet.
   b. Manage regurgitation.
   c. Call the physician if the child has:
      1. Forceful vomiting.
      2. Signs of dehydration.
      3. Blood in vomitus.
      4. Abdominal pain.

V

Warts. Flesh-colored papules caused by a virus.

A. General Considerations.
1. There are several morphological types of warts.
   a. Plantar and palmar-elevated or flat lesions that may have punctate dots on the surface and that occur on the soles of the feet or palms of the hands.
   b. Flat-discrete, multiple flesh-colored brown papules on the face or extensor arm surfaces.
   c. *Verrucae vulgaris* (common warts)—grey-, brown-, or flesh-colored elevations of the dorsal hand surfaces or around the nails.
   d. *Verrucae accuminata* (venereal warts)—flesh-colored, wet, cauliflower papules on the genital regions.
2. Therapy for warts is avoided if possible, since many of the lesions will resolve in 6 to 9 months if the viral infection is mild.
3. Facial warts may be removed for cosmetic reasons.
4. Plantar warts appear on the soles of the feet and require removal if they cause pain when the child walks.
5. Treatment of plantar warts is usually with 40 percent salicylic acid plasters which cause painless atrophy of the lesions.
6. Venereal warts are treated with one or more applications of 25 percent podophyllin in alcohol.
7. Other treatment methods include surgical removal, electrocautery, curettage, cryotherapy (liquid nitrogen), caustic solutions, and x-ray therapy.
8. The recurrence rate for warts is 20 to 30 percent.

B. Nursing Management. See BODY IMAGE and COPING.
1. Explain to the child and parents that warts are caused by a virus, not contact with toads or frogs.
2. Discuss with the child and parents how to explain to teachers and peers that warts are not very contagious and the child is not a threat to others.
3. Explain to the child and parents that the child should not "pick at" the wart(s).
4. Review the specific therapy prescribed with the child and parents.

Wax, ear. See *Cerumen.*

Weaning. See *Nutrition.*

Well-child care. Routine health supervision and health promotion.

A. General Considerations. See AMBULATORY CARE.
1. The focus of well-child care is the promotion and maintenance of health. See *Health Promotion and Maintenance.*
2. The American Academy of Pediatrics has established Guidelines for Health Supervision which serve as a guide for health care services for children in different age groups. See *Appendix vi.*
3. Parents must be helped to value the concept of keeping the well-child well, since many parents bring the child for health care only when he is ill.
4. The role of the nurse in well-child care includes:
   a. Supporting the child and parents during the visit.
   b. Obtaining a nursing history.
   c. Preparing the child and parents for, and carrying out procedures.
   d. Assisting with the physical exam.
   e. Administering screening tests.
   f. Providing anticipatory guidance.
   g. Assisting children in becoming more responsible for their own health care.
5. The waiting time in clinics and offices provides an excellent opportunity for health teaching of the child and parents.

B. Nursing Management. See *Preparation for Well-child Visit.*
1. Welcome the child and parents to the doctor's office or clinic.
2. Help the child and parents feel comfortable in the waiting area.
   a. Provide safe, age-appropriate toys for the younger child. See *Toys.*
   b. Have appropriate reading materials available for the older child and parents.
   c. Provide some small chairs for the younger child if possible.
3. Obtain a nursing history. See *History Taking* and *Appendix iv.*
4. Use a questionnaire to determine informational needs and interests which can be filled out and kept with the chart for later reference.

5. Use the waiting time as teaching time.
    a. Provide anticipatory guidance about:
        1. Growth and development. See *Appendix v*.
        2. Establishing a sound parent–child relationship. See *Parenting*.
        3. Safety needs. See *Accident Prevention*.
        4. Nutrition. See *Nutrition*.
        5. Screening procedures to be done during the visit. See *Hearing Screening, Speech Screening,* and *Vision Screening*.
        6. Dental care. See *Dental Care*.
        7. Sex education. See *Sex Education*.
    b. Discuss the importance of and schedule for immunizations. See *Immunizations*.
    c. Offer guidance and support to the parents in coping with common childhood problems.
        1. Colic. See *Colic*.
        2. Behavior problems. See *Behavior Problems* and *Discipline*.
        3. Feeding problems. See *Feeding Problems*.
        4. Minor illnesses. See *Home Management of Minor Illnesses*.
        5. Accidents. See *Home Management of Minor Emergencies*.
        6. Toilet training. See *Toilet Training*.
        7. Temper tantrums. See *Temper Tantrums*.
    d. Use wall hung posters and distribute pamphlets.
    e. Assist the child in becoming more responsible for his/her own health care.
        1. Teach/review habits which promote/maintain health, e.g., handwashing, tooth brushing, eating foods from the four basic food groups.
        2. Teach the five basic rules of PACT (Participatory and Assertive Consumer Training) (Motivating Children to Become Assertive Health Consumers, 1982).
            a. Talk to health professionals.
            b. Listen and learn from health professionals.
            c. Ask questions of the health professional.
            d. Decide with the health professional what to do about a health problem or how to meet health related goals.
            e. Do what was decided.
        3. Provide a small personalized record book for children which they can bring to each visit and use to record information about their health, e.g., blood pressure measurements, weight, and height.
        4. Provide adolescents with a written record of their health care and encourage them to assume responsibility for scheduling their own appointments.
6. Prepare the child and parents for the examination and procedures to be done. See *Preparation for Procedures* and *Appendix vi*.
    a. State what is planned for the visit.
    b. Provide privacy, especially for the older child.
    c. Let the parent undress the child who experiences stranger anxiety.
    d. Allow the preschooler to keep on underpants.
    e. Arrange for the adolescent to be seen alone.
7. Obtain and record the child's temperature.
    a. Take a rectal temperature until the child is able to hold the thermometer under his tongue with his mouth closed (approximately 4 years of age).
    b. Have the parent hold the infant and young child across the knees to take temperature.
    c. When taking a rectal temperature:
        1. Insert the thermometer just past the internal anal sphincter in the infant and no more than 1 inch in the older child.
        2. Place a hand on the buttocks of the infant and young child and hold the thermometer firmly in place.
8. Obtain and record height.
    a. Measure child under 2 years of age lying down.
    b. Measure child from 2 to 3 years of age lying down or standing up, but record on appropriate growth chart.
        1. Zero to 36 months chart if lying down.
        2. Two to 18 years chart if standing up.
    c. Measure child over 3 years of age standing up.
    d. Measure the supine child accurately.
        1. Use two people.
        2. Have one person hold the child's head in alignment with the child looking up and the top of the head in contact with the headboard.
        3. Have the second person hold the child's feet with the toes straight up and press down gently on the knees while bringing the footboard in contact with the sole of the foot.
    e. Measure the standing child accurately.
        1. Have the child stand straight with eyes looking directly ahead.
        2. Measure the child without shoes.
        3. Have the child keep his heels down.
9. Obtain and record weight.
    a. Make sure the scale is balanced.
    b. Weigh the infant nude and weigh the older child wearing only underpants or a light cotton gown.

c. Obtain weight to the nearest half ounce for infants and nearest quarter pound for older children.

10. Obtain and record head circumference.
    a. Use a flexible, nonstretchable tape or use disposable paper tape.
    b. Pass the tape just above the ridges of the eyebrows and around the fullest part of the occiput; pull the tape tight.
    c. Record measurement to the nearst ⅛".

11. Obtain and record blood pressure measurement on all children over 2 years of age.
    a. Explain the procedure. See *Preparation for Procedures*.
    b. Have the child in a quiet state while obtaining blood pressure in order to avoid high readings.
    c. Fully expose the upper arm.
    d. Use a cuff whose inner rubber bladder covers at least two-thirds of the length of the upper arm and encircles the extremity without overlapping.
    e. Wrap the cuff snugly with the lower edge above the antecubital space.
    f. Inflate the cuff rapidly to 30 mm Hg above the point where the radial pulse disappears.
    g. Lower the pressure in the inflated cuff at the rate of 3 to 5 mm Hg per second in order to prevent a false low reading.
    h. Use the fourth Korotkoff sound, when muffling occurs, as the diastolic reading.
    i. Do not use heavy pressure on the stethoscope, since this distorts Korotkoff sounds.

12. Collect urine for screening.
    a. Wash the external genitalia according to agency policy.
    b. Apply pediatric urine collector to child who is not trained.
    c. Have the older child urinate in a small collecting cup; provide privacy.
    d. Do not offer water if the child is unable to urinate, since this dilutes the urine thus altering the result, e.g., collect the specimen later in the visit or have the parent collect at home and bring in.

13. Perform screening tests as ordered.
    a. Obtain hemoglobin, hematocrit or other laboratory screening tests according to office or clinic procedure and record the results.
    b. Screen vision, hearing, and speech. See *Vision Screening, Hearing Screening*, and *Speech Screening*.
    c. Administer or assist with the administration of developmental screening tests.
       1. Become proficient in the administration of any developmental screening test used.

2. Establish rapport with the child and parents before starting.
3. Explain the test to parents and provide age-appropriate explanations to the child.
4. Administer the test using correct procedure.
5. Evaluate the results of the test.
6. Follow agency policy for providing feedback to the parents and arranging for any follow-up evaluation which may be necessary.
    d. Perform gross evaluation of development, if formal evaluation is not possible, by asking about specific developmental milestones and use results to determine if further evaluation is needed. See *Appendix v*.

14. Support the child during the physical exam. See *Preparation for Procedures*.

15. Administer immunizations as ordered. See *Immunizations*.

16. Provide time after the visit to:
    a. Reinforce or clarify the physician's comments or instructions; write out specific instructions.
    b. Discuss questions that may have arisen during the examination.
    c. Initiate referrals which may be needed, e.g., visit to ophthalmologist for further vision evaluation.
       1. Make sure the child and parents understand why further evaluation is needed.
       2. Explain to the older child that "failure" of a screening test does not mean he is a failure.

17. Teach the adolescent girl how to examine her breasts and the adolescent boy how to examine his testes. See *Appendix viii*.

"Wet dreams." See *Nocturnal Emissions*.

Wilms' tumor (nephroblastoma). Embryonal, encapsulated tumor of the kidney.

A. **General Considerations.**
   1. Wilms' tumor may be unilateral or bilateral.
   2. The child with Wilms' tumor may have an associated congenital abnormality.
      a. Genitourinary malformations.
      b. Hemihypertrophy.
      c. Absence of the iris.
   3. The child may manifest few signs and symptoms.
      a. Asymptomatic abdominal mass noted by parents during physical care or by a health professional during well-baby examination.

    b. Hematuria, fever, and abdominal pain are infrequent.

    c. Rupture of the tumor capsule during a fall may cause symptoms of an acute abdomen.

4. Diagnostic tests may include:

    a. IVP.

    b. CAT scan.

    c. Aortic arteriogram of the opposite kidney.

    d. Vena-cavagram.

    e. Organ and skeletal x-ray surveys, tomograms, and bone scans to rule out metastasis.

    f. Liver function tests to detect metastasis and abnormalities which may alter chemotherapeutic agent metabolism.

    g. Renal function tests to evaluate kidney function.

5. Metastasis may occur by:

    a. Local extension into perirenal connective tissues and the renal vein to the inferior vena cava.

    b. Lymphatics to regional lymph nodes.

    c. Bloodstream to lungs and occasionally the liver and bones.

6. Wilms' tumor is usually classified into stages based on the extent of tumor involvement.

7. Tumor cells may be classified histologically as favorable or unfavorable and more aggressive therapy is required when the cell type is unfavorable.

8. Surgical excision usually begins the treatment.

    a. Radical nephrectomy is performed if the tumor is unilateral.

    b. Exploration of the abdominal cavity and opposite kidney is done for staging.

    c. A radical nephrectomy of the more involved kidney and partial removal of the opposite kidney may be done if bilateral masses are present.

    d. Pulmonary nodules resulting from metastatis may be excised.

9. Radiation therapy is used when the tumor has extended through the renal capsule.

10. All children will be treated with chemotherapy, usually dactinomycin and vincristine.

11. The prognosis for the child with Wilms' tumor is very good, particularly if metastasis has not occurred at diagnosis.

B. **Nursing Management.** See CRISIS INTERVENTION and LIFE-THREATENING ILLNESS.

1. Support the child and parents during hospitalization. See *Hospitalization, Support During.*

2. Initiate discharge planning. See *Discharge Planning.*

3. Place a sign on the bed which advises others not to palpate the abdomen, since rupture of the capsule will spread the malignant cells.

4. Provide consistency and continuity of care, since the child must endure so many painful diagnostic and therapeutic procedures. See *Preparation for Procedures.*

5. Accompany the physician, if possible, when explanations are given to the child and parents so that consistent, accurate information is communicated.

    a. Anxiety interferes with the ability of the child and parents to comprehend information.

    b. The information should be recorded on the Kardex so that the same explanation can be given each time the child or parent asks.

      1. Answer all questions honestly.

      2. Use terminology the child understands.

    c. Arrange for uninterrupted periods of contact with the child and parents so that supportive discussions can be held.

6. Meet the needs of the child and parents preoperatively. See *Preoperative Care* and *Preparation for Surgery.*

    a. Anticipate that the child and parents will be very anxious since surgery will be scheduled 24 to 48 hours after diagnosis.

    b. Inform the child and parents that the incision will be long since both kidneys must be examined during surgery.

    c. Monitor blood pressure accurately since hypertension may occur secondary to excess renin production.

    d. Verify that parents understand that radiation therapy and chemotherapy will begin in the immediate postoperative period.

7. Meet the needs of the child and parents postoperatively. See *Postoperative Care.*

    a. Monitor intake and output to assess kidney functioning.

    b. Institute or monitor pulmonary hygiene therapy which is ordered to prevent pulmonary complications.

    c. Monitor blood pressure for decrease after tumor removal.

8. Meet the needs of the child receiving radiation therapy and chemotherapy. See *Chemotherapy* and *Radiation Therapy.*

9. Teach the child and parents home management.

    a. Encourage the parents to make the home life as normal as possible.

      1. Have the child resume normal activities such as play groups or school.

      2. Encourage normal peer relationships.

      3. Maintain normal discipline. See *Discipline.*

      4. Encourage normal rest and nutrition for all family members.

b. Encourage therapeutic play to help the child to work through feelings about intrusive procedures since radiation and chemotherapy will continue on an outpatient basis. See *Play, Therapeutic*.

10. Meet the needs of the child who does not respond to therapy. See *Dying Child*.

Working mother. Mother employed outside the home.

A. General Considerations.

1. The number of working mothers is increasing each year.
2. Mothers work because of:
   a. Economic necessity.
   b. A desire to increase the family's standard of living.
   c. Boredom with the day to day home routine.
   d. A desire to meet their own personal developmental needs.
   e. A desire to pursue a career in a special field.
3. It is the quality of the mother–child interaction rather than the quantity of time that the mother spends with the child that influences the parent–child relationship most directly.
4. Children of working mothers tend to:
   a. Show few ill effects from the separation.
   b. Be self-reliant.
   c. Do well in school.
5. The child between the ages of 6 months and 4 years reacts to separation from the mother more strongly than the young infant or older child.
6. A working mother will be better able to cope with the stresses that working produces if she:
   a. Has the support of her family.
   b. Does not feel guilty about working.
   c. Has adequate child care.
7. Stresses include those related to:
   a. Meeting the ongoing day to day needs and activities related to running a home.
   b. Finding time to pursue personal activities and have some time for herself.
   c. Meeting the child's needs for well-child care or care when he is ill or hospitalized.
      1. Physician's offices and clinics may not have hours when she can bring the child.
      2. Day care centers will not accept an ill child.
      3. The mother often cannot stay with the ill child at home or in the hospital for any length of time for fear she may lose her job.
      4. When both parents work, it is usually the mother who is absent from the job to stay with the hospitalized child (Knafl, Deatrick, and Kodadek, 1982).

8. The working mother may feel she needs to be "Supermom" and handle her family, home, and job without help.

B. Nursing Management.

1. Assess those factors known to affect how well the mother copes with the stresses related to working (see above).
2. Provide support as indicated.
   a. Give the mother an opportunity to talk about her work, since this may help her work out her feelings.
   b. Be nonjudgmental about the mother's attitude toward working.
   c. Tell her that children of working mothers need not have any more problems than children whose mothers stay home.
   d. Explain that she should not attempt to deal with guilt feelings by indulging the child, since this may lead to insecurity in the child and increased demands.
   e. Discuss ways to evaluate a day care center if she has concerns about child care. See *Day Care Center*.
   f. Encourage her to discuss sharing of housework, chores, etc., so that she does not feel that she must handle everything.
3. Discuss specific ways in which the mother can promote the child's adjustment to her working.
   a. Plan some time each day that is spent just with the child, e.g., reading a story, having the child tell you about his or her day.
   b. Develop a routine for daily activities.
      1. Lay out clothes for the next day to avoid a morning rush.
      2. Make and refrigerate lunches the night before for easy packing in the morning.
      3. Plan meals ahead and cook in quantity and freeze some for another meal.
      4. Make sure the older child knows what the schedule will be for the day, e.g., "The day care bus will pick you up after school and I will come for you at the day care center at 5 o'clock."
   c. Give the older child responsibility for some daily activity, e.g., making bed, putting away the wash.
   d. Take the child to see where she works and to meet some of her co-workers if possible.
   e. Discuss with the older child why she works and how she feels about her job.
   f. Set consistent limits.
4. Assist the mother in planning for well-child care.
   a. Give her the last appointment in the day if it is possible for her to bring the child after work.
   b. Discuss whether the child could be brought by someone else (grandparent, neighbor) and

schedule a telephone conference to discuss the results of the visit.

5. Help the mother identify ways of coping if the child is ill at home and she must continue to work, locate a neighbor who stays at home who would be willing to watch the child; the adolescent can stay by himself, if not too ill, and can be checked on by phone.

6. Support the working mother who is unable to stay with her hospitalized child.
   a. Recognize the fact that the mother may feel very guilty about having to leave the child.
   b. Make sure you have her office number and know how to reach her.
   c. Arrange a time when she can call and talk to her child and/or talk with the nurse assigned to the child.
   d. Discuss what is planned for the child's care, since the mother might be able to plan to be present for specific tests or procedures if she has a schedule.

Worms (helminths). Parasitic infection of the intestinal tract.

A. General Considerations.
1. Hookworm (Ancylostomiasis).
   a. Fecal contamination of soil is the source of the infection.
   b. Infection occurs when the larvae penetrate the skin and enter the bloodstream.
   c. The larvae:
      1. Reach the lungs via the bloodstream.
      2. Exit into the alveoli from the lungs.
      3. Migrate from the alveoli to the pharynx and are swallowed.
   d. The larvae develop into adults in the upper intestine where they feed on blood and reproduce.
   e. Signs and symptoms are variable.
      1. Weakness.
      2. Anemia.
      3. Pallor.
      4. Weight loss.
      5. Occult blood in the stools.
      6. Abdominal discomfort.
      7. Intense itching at the spot where the larvae entered.
   f. Diagnosis is made by detecting the presence of ova in fecal smears.
   g. Treatment includes the use of an anthelmintic and iron therapy for the anemia.
   h. Severe cardiac decompensation may occur if the iron deficiency anemia becomes severe.
   i. The prognosis is good except for severely anemic children.

2. Roundworm (Ascariasis).
   a. Fecal contamination of the ground leads to wide disbursement of the ova in the soil.
   b. Infection occurs when contaminated soil is carried to the mouth via fingers, toys, etc. and is swallowed.
   c. The larvae reach the intestines in the same manner that the hookworm does.
   d. Signs and symptoms associated with larvae invasion and migration to the lungs include:
      1. Cough.
      2. Dyspnea.
      3. Fever.
      4. Rales.
   e. Signs and symptoms associated with intestinal infestation by adult worms are often absent but may include:
      1. Anorexia.
      2. Nausea.
      3. Vomiting.
      4. Epigastric pain.
   f. Diagnosis is made when ova are detected in fecal smears.
   g. Complications include:
      1. Pneumonia caused by large numbers of larvae in the lungs.
      2. Intestinal obstruction due to large masses of worms.
      3. Acute appendicitis due to blockage of the appendiceal lumen by worms.
   h. Treatment involves the use of an anthelmintic drug.

3. Pinworms (Enterobiasis).
   a. Pinworm ova are (Wittner, 1982):
      1. Released in the environment when the adult female migrates externally and lays her eggs in the anal skin folds.
      2. Able to survive at room temperature for 2 to 3 weeks.
      3. Resistant to most household disinfectants.
      4. Often airborne since they are light and will float when pajamas or bedlinens are removed.
   b. Infection occurs when the ova are inhaled or swallowed.
   c. Signs and symptoms include:
      1. Intense anal itching, especially at night, when the eggs are deposited.
      2. Vaginitis and pruritus vulvae in young girls.
      3. Observation of the creamy, white worms in the perianal area.
   d. Diagnosis is made from the microscopic detection of ova on an anal swab which can be done at home.
   e. Treatment:
      1. Consists of the use of an anthelmintic drug.

2. May be repeated in 2 to 3 weeks (Wittner, 1982).
3. Is often recommended for the entire family, since crosscontamination is common.

   f. Acute infection often occurs if the infected child scratches and then brings his fingers to the mouth.

   g. Complications are rare but may include secondary bacterial infection of scratched areas of acute appendicitis from filling of the appendiceal lumen with worms.

4. The prognosis is good and home management is possible except in cases involving severe complications.

B. Nursing Management.

1. Be nonjudgmental in your care of the child with worms.

2. Assess the general hygienic practices of the child and parents in relation to:
   a. Handwashing.
   b. Disposal of feces.
   c. Food preparation.

3. Provide health education as needed in relation to:
   a. Washing of hands.
   b. Keeping fingernails short and clean.
   c. Cleaning toys that may be contaminated.
   d. Disposing of feces.

4. Administer, or teach parents to administer, the anthelmintic drugs as ordered. See *Administration of Medications, Parental.*

5. Teach the child and parents signs and symptoms of complications, as above, which are to be reported to the physician.

6. Meet the additional needs of the child with hookworms.
   a. Collect a stool specimen for examination.
   b. Teach parents to manage the anemia. See *Anemia, Iron Deficiency.*

     1. Administer iron supplement as instructed.
     2. Schedule the anemic child's activities so he does not become overfatigued.
     3. Bring the child in for periodic evaluation of his anemia.

   c. Explain that reinfection can be prevented by:
     1. Wearing shoes.
     2. Avoiding the handling of soil contaminated with feces.
     3. Preventing fecal contamination of soil in which vegetables are grown.

7. Meet the additional needs of the child with pinworms.
   a. Teach parents to collect an anal swab.
     1. Provide a tongue blade with one end covered with cellophane tape, sticky side out, and a microscope slide.
     2. Have the parent press the tongue blade against the child's anus in the morning before the child bathes or defecates.
     3. Tell the parent to press the swab to the microscope slide and bring it to the office or clinic for examination.

   b. Explain that the use of pyrivium pamoate (Povan) will turn the stools red.

   c. Prevent autoinfection.
     1. Have the child wear underpants under pajamas to prevent scratching.
     2. Teach child to wash hands carefully after using the bathroom and before eating.
     3. Change and launder underwear, pajamas, and bedlinens daily.

   d. Prevent crossinfection.
     1. Have child sleep by himself.
     2. Do not shake the child's clothes or bedlinens.
     3. Have all family members treated simultaneously.

REFERENCES AND RESOURCES

Adams, RM, & Roeser, R: The ultimate hearing test: Evoked response audiometry. The Journal of School Health 49: 536, 1979

Aguilera, DC & Messick, JM: Crisis Intervention. 4th Ed. St. Louis: Mosby, 1982

Alexander, MM, Brown, MS: Pediatric History Taking and Physical Diagnosis for Nurses. New York: McGraw-Hill, 1979

Altemer, WA, O'Connor, S, Vietze, PM, Sandler, HM, Sherrod, KB: Antecedents of child abuse. The Journal of Pediatrics 100: 823–829, 1982

Ament, ME, Barclay, GN: Chronic diarrhea. Pediatric Annals 11: 124–131, 1982

American Academy of Pediatrics: Report of the Committee on Infectious Diseases 17th Ed. Evanston, IL.

Anderson, DJ, Thibault, J: Nursing management of the pediatric patient with Kawasaki's disease. Issues in Comprehensive Pediatric Nursing 5: 1–10, 1981

Babington, MA, Spadero, DC: Cariogenic medications. Pediatric Nursing 8: 165–170, 1982

Bakke, K & Dougherty, J: Sudden infant death syndrome and infant apnea: current questions, clinical management, and research directions. Issues in Comprehensive Pediatric Nursing 5: 77–88, 1981

Barnard, B, Creswell, J, Erickson, V, Ivey, J, Johnston B, Alexander, LS: Exercise for children with physical disabilities. Issues in Comprehensive Pediatric Nursing 5: 99–108, 1981

Barnard, KE, Erickson, ML: Teaching Children with Developmental Problems 2nd Ed. St. Louis: Mosby, 1976

Bass, LW, & Cohen, RL: Ostensible versus actual reasons for seeking pediatric attention. Another look at the parental ticket of admission. Pediatrics 70: 870–874, 1982

Benoliel, JQ: Nursing care for the terminal patient: a psychosocial approach. In B. Schoenberg (Ed.). Psychosocial Aspects of Terminal Care. New York: Columbia University Press, 1972

Benoliel, JQ: Terminal illness in childhood. In Scipien, G. M., Comprehensive Pediatric Nursing 2nd Ed. New York: McGraw-Hill.

Bettoli, EJ: Herpes: Facts and fallacies. The American Journal of Nursing 82: 924–929, 1982

Bindler, RMcG: Home care for a child with a cardiac defect. Issues in Comprehensive Pediatric Nursing 3: 48–60, 1979

Boffman, JH, & Boffman, RT: Early detection of hearing impairment. Issues in Comprehensive Pediatric Nursing 5: 11–20, 1981

Boyd, CW: A bed for infants with gastroesophageal reflux. Pediatric Nursing 7: 53–55, 1981

Boyd, CW: Postural therapy at home for infants with gastroesophageal reflux. Pediatric Nursing 8: 395–398, 1982

Bradshaw, TW: Teething. The American Journal of Maternal Child Nursing 7: 41–42, 1981

Braff, A: Telling children about their adoption: new alternatives. The American Journal of Maternal Child Nursing 2: 254–259, 1977

Branch, MF, Paxton, PP: Providing Safe Nursing Care for Ethnic People of Color. Norwalk, CT: Appleton, 1976

Brazelton, TB: Infants and Mothers: Differences in Development. New York: Delta, 1969

Brockhaus, JPD, Brockhaus, RH: Adopting an older child: The emotional process. The American Journal of Nursing 82: 288–291, 1982

Brodoff, AS: Think rocky mountain spotted fever! Patient Care, 16: 21–39, 1982

Brown, MH, Kiss, ME: Standards of clinical nursing practice: The side effects of chemotherapy in the treatment of leukemia. Cancer Nursing 5: 317–323, 1982

Buntain, WL, & Cain, WC: Caustic injuries to the esophagus: A pediatric overview. Southern Medical Journal 74: 590–593, 1981

Burgess, AW: Nursing Levels of Health Intervention Englewood Cliffs, NJ: Prentice-Hall, 1978

Burgess, AW, Baldwin, B: Crisis Intervention Englewood Cliffs, NJ: Prentice-Hall, 1981

Burnett, JW: Infections of the skin. In A.M. Rudolph (Ed.), Pediatrics 17th Ed., Norwalk, CT: Appleton, 1982

Cadden, V: Crisis in the family. In G. Caplan (Ed.). Principles of Preventive Psychiatry New York: Basic Books, 1964

Campbell, CE, Herten, RJ: Vd to std: Redefining venereal disease. The American Journal of Nursing 81, 1629–1635, 1981

Capano, K & Brindle, S: Bridging the gaps in discharge planning. Pediatric Nursing 4: 245–249, 1978

Carvajal, HF, & Travis, LB: Infections of the urinary tract. In AM Rudolph (Ed.), Pediatrics pp. 1209–1214. Norwalk, CT: Appleton, 1980

Cestaro-Seifer, DJ: Developing an instructional unit on toxic shock syndrome for adolescent girls. Issues in Comprehensive Pediatric Nursing 6: 107–126, 1983

Chambers, T: Nocturnal enuresis: Fears and tears. Nursing Mirror, 153: 52–53, 1981

Chameides, L: Congenital heart disease: Its effect on the schoolage child. The Journal of School Health 49: 205–209, 1979

Chiappa, KH, & Ropper, AH: Evoked potentials in clinical medicine. New England Journal of Medicine 306: 1140-1209, 1982

Chinn, PL, & Leitch, CJ: Child Health Maintenance: A Guide to Clinical Assessment 2nd Ed. St. Louis: Mosby, 1979

Chung, JHT, & Lilly, JR: Congenital intestinal malformations and obstructions. In AM Rudolph (Ed.), Pediatrics 17th Ed. Norwalk, CT: Appleton, 1982

Clark, JB, Queener, SF, Karb, VB: Pharmacological Basis of Nursing Practice St. Louis: Mosby, 1982

Cleaveland, MJ: Nursing care in childhood cancer—brain tumor. American Journal of Nursing 82: 422-424, 1982

Clore, ER: Lice: Ancient pest with new resistance. Pediatric Nursing 9: 347-350, 1983

Coughlin, MK: Teaching children about their seizures and medications. The American Journal of Maternal Child Nursing 4: 161-162, 1979

Cox, BP, Edelin, P: Hearing deficits. In PR Magrab (Ed.). Psychological Management of Pediatric Problems: Vol. II. Sensorineural Conditions and Social Concerns pp. 173-215. Baltimore: University Park Press, 1978

Crumette, B, Munton, MT: Mothers' decisions about infant nutrition. Pediatric Nursing 6: 16-19, 1980

Curole, DN: Managing genital herpesvirus infection: The state of the art. Consultant 21: 47-53, 1981

Dalgas, P: Reye's syndrome update. Pediatric Nursing 9: 345-349, 1983

Damon, J, & Taylor, LF: Brain tumors in children. Nursing Clinics in North America 15: 99-113, 1980

Daniel, WA: Nutrition: Judging the adolescent's true needs. Consultant 22: 42-44, 1982

Davidson, M: Diarrhea. In AM Rudolph (Ed.), Pediatrics 17th Ed. pp. 924-925. Norwalk, CT: Appleton, 1982.

Davis, AJ: When parents disagree on treatment. The American Journal of Nursing 80: 2080-2082, 1980

Davis, GT, Hill, PM: Cerebral palsy. Nursing Clinics of North America 15: 35-49, 1980

Davis, M: Getting to the root of the problem: Hair grooming techniques for black patients. Nursing 77 7: 60-65, 1977

De Angelis, C: Pediatrics for the Primary Health Care Provider 2nd Ed. Boston: Little-Brown, 1979

deChesnay, M: Incest: A family triangle. Nursing Times 79: 64-65, 1983

De Jong, AR, Emmett, GA, Hervada, AA: Epidemilogic factors in sexual abuse of boys. The American Journal of Diseases of Children 136: 990-993, 1982

De Jong, AR, Emmett, GA, Hervada, AA: Sexual abuse of children. The American Journal of Diseases of Children 136: 129-134, 1982

Denny, FW: Viral pneumonia. In EL Kendig & Chernick (Eds.). Disorders of the Respiratory Tract in Children Chap. 22. Philadelphia: Saunders, 1983

DePanfilis, D: Clients who refer themselves to child protective services. Children Today 11: 21-25, 1982

Diagram Group: Child's Body. New York: Paddington, 1977

Dimaggio, GT, Sheetz, AH: The concerns of mothers caring for an infant on an apnea monitor. MCN 8: 294-297, 1983

Downes, M, Orr, DP: Adolescent sexual abuse: How to recognize and deal with a delicate problem. Consultant 21: 37-47, 1981

Duncan, JA & Webb, LZ: Teaching families home apnea monitoring. Pediatric Nursing 9: 171-175, 1983

Duvall, E: Marriage and Family Development, 5th Ed. Philadelphia: Lippincott, 1977

Eland, J: Pain and Crayons. Nursing 13: 94, 1983

Fireman, P., Friday, GA, Gira, C, Vierthaler, WA, Michaels, L: Teaching self-management skills to asthmatic children and their parents in an ambulatory care setting. Pediatrics 68: 341-347, 1981

Fishman, MA: Understanding convulsions in children. Consultant 22: 82-85, 1982

Fletcher, GH: Textbook of Radiotherapy 2nd Ed. Philadelphia: Lea and Feiberger, 1980

Fraiberg, S: Insights from the Blind. New York: Basic Books, 1977

Friedman, SB, & Hoekelman, RA: Behavioral Pediatrics: Psychosocial Aspects of Child Health Care. New York: McGraw-Hill, 1980

Gaddy, DS: Nursing care in childhood cancer-update. The American Journal of Nursing 416-421, 1982

Glen, SA: Hospital admission through the parents eyes. Nursing Times 78: 1321-1323, 1982

Graf, CM: Sexually transmitted disease: A new look at an old problem. Issues in Comprehensive Pediatric Nursing, 2: 12-20, 1978

Gray, A: Genital herpes. Nursing Mirror 156: 58-59, 1983

Glass, LB, Verkins, CA: The ups and downs of serum pH. Nursing 83, 13: 34-41, 1983

Gorline, LL, & Stegbauer, CC: What every nurse should know about vaginitis. The American Journal of Nursing 82: 1851-1855, 1982

Green, M, Haggerty, RJ: Ambulatory Pediatrics II. Philadelphia: Saunders, 1977

Griffiths, SS: Changes in body image caused by antineoplastic drugs. Issues in Comprehensive Pediatric Nursing 4: 17-27, 1980

Grosso, C, Barden, M, Henry, C: The Vietnamese American family. . . and grandma makes 3. The American Journal of Maternal Child Nursing 6: 177-180, 1981

Gyulay, JE: The Dying Child. New York: McGraw-Hill, 1978

Hall, M, DeLaCruz, A, Russell, P: Working with neglecting families. Children Today 11: 6-9+, 1982

Hausman, KA: Critical care of the child with increased intracranial pressure. Nursing Clinics of North America 16: 647-655, 1981

Hazinski, MF: Critical care of the pediatric cardiovascular patient. Nursing Clinics of North America, 16: 671-697, 1981

Helberg, JLaM: Documentation in child abuse. The American Journal of Nursing 83: 234-239, 1983

Heller, P: Sickle cell anemia: Questions most often asked. Consultant 22: 249-265, 1982

Henneman, A, Koziol, J: Preschool feeding problems: It's not nutritious unless they eat it. Issues in Comprehensive Pediatric Nursing 4: 7-12, 1980

Hoffmann, AD (Ed.): Adolescent medicine. Reading, MA: Addison-Wesley, 1983

Holland, SH: Vision testing for special children. Nursing 9: 74-79, 1979

Honig, PJ, Charney, EB: Children with brain tumor headaches. American Journal of Diseases of Childhood 136: 121-123, 1982

Horner, MME, McClennan, MA: Toilet training: Ready or not? Pediatric Nursing 7: 15-18, 1981

Horowitz, JA, Hughes, CB, & Perdue, BJ: Parenting Reassessed. A Nursing Perspective. Englewood-Cliffs, NJ: Prentice-Hall, 1982

Howard, RB, Herbold, NH: Nutrition in Clinical Care 2nd Ed. New York: McGraw-Hill, 1982

Howry, LB, Bindler, R McG & Tso, Y: Pediatric Medications. Philadelphia: Lippincott, 1981

Huber, HL: Draining the "fluid ear" with myringotomy and tube insertion. Nursing 8: 28–31, 1978

Hutchinson, MM: Administration of fat emulsions. The American Journal of Nursing 82: 275–277, 1982

Irwin, CE, Jr, Shafer, M: Suicide in children and adolescents. In AM Rudolph (Ed.), Pediatrics 17th Ed., Norwalk, CT: Appleton, 1982

Jackson, PL, Runyon, N: Caring for children from divorced families. The American Journal of Maternal Child Nursing 8: 126–130, 1983

Jeffries, JS, Killam, PE, Varni, JW: Behavioral management of fecal incontinence in a child with myelomeningocele. Pediatric Nursing 8: 267–270, 1982

Johnson, MP: Support groups for parents of chronically ill children. Pediatric Nursing 9: 160–163, 1982

Jonas, M & Cunha, BA: The ticks of summer. Emergency Medicine 14: 146–159, 1982

Jones, JG: Sexual abuse of children. The American Journal of Diseases of Children 136: 142–146, 1982

Jones, R, Shearin, R: Communicating with adolescents and young adults about sexuality. Pediatric Nursing 11: 733–738, 1982

Jonides, L: Childhood obesity: A treatment approach for private practices. Pediatric Nursing 8: 320–322, 1982

Joseph, K, MacEwen, GD, Boos, ML: Home traction in the management of congenital dislocation of the hip. Clinical Orthopedics and Related Research, 1982

Kee, JL: Fluids and Electrolytes with Clinical Applications 3rd Ed. New York: Wiley, 1982

Kelly, M & Parson, E: The Mother's Almanac. Garden City, NY: Doubleday, 1975

Kempe, CH, Silver, HK, O'Brien, D (Eds.): Current Pediatric Diagnosis and Treatment. Los Altos, CA: Lange, 1982

Killam, PE, Apodaca, L., Manella, KJ, Varni, JW: Behavioral pediatric weight rehabilitation for children with myelomeningocele. The American Journal of Maternal Child Nursing, 8: 280–286, 1983

Killim, SW, McCarthy, SM: Hospitalization of the autistic child. The American Journal of Maternal Child Nursing 5: 413–423, 1980

Kilmon, C & Helpin, ML: Update on dentistry for children. Pediatric Nursing 7: 41–44, 1981

Kirilloff, LH & Tibbals, SC: Drugs for asthma. The American Journal of Nursing 83: 55–61, 1983

Knafl, KA, Destrick, JA, & Kodadek, S: How parents manage jobs and a child's hospitalization. The American Journal of Maternal Child Nursing 7: 125–127, 1982

Knight, RW: A Practical Approach to Fluid, Electrolyte and Acid-base Balance. Madison, NC: Total Health Information Company, 1982

Koren, ME, Herrmann, CS: Cancer immunotherapy: What why, when, how. Nursing 81 11: 34–41, 1981

Kurfiss, DD: Positioning as treatment for infant gastroesophageal reflux. The American Journal of Nursing 82: 1535–1537, 1982

Labson, LH: Giving acute care in childhood cancer. Patient Care 16: 151–8, 1982

Lane, PL, Lee, MM: Special care for special casts. Nursing 13: 50–51, 1983

Langford, RW: Teenagers and obesity. The American Journal of Nursing 81: 556–559, 1981

Lanzkowsky, P: Iron deficiency and resultant anemia in adolescents. Consultant, 21: 164–172, 1981

Lappin, MA: Preparation for menarche: Maturational event vs. hygienic crisis. Pediatric Annals 11: 751–760, 1982

Lasky, PA, Gulbrandson, M, Scoblic, M: Health education translated into health behavior. Issues in Comprehensive Pediatric Nursing 5: 167–175, 1981

Laughlin, JJ, Brady, MJ, Eigen, H: Changing feeding trends as a cause of electrolyte depletion in infants with cystic fibrosis. Pediatrics, 68: 203–207, 1981

Leininger, M: Transcultural Nursing New York: Masson, 1979

Leininger, M: Transcultural Nursing: Concepts, theories, practices. New York: Wiley, 1978

Leitch, CJ & Tinker, RV (Eds.): Primary Care, Philadelphia: Davis, 1978

Lillo, R, Masteller, D: Outpatient management of children in diabetic ketoacidosis. Pediatric Nursing. 8: 383–385, 1982

Litt, IF, Cuskey, WR, Rosenberg, A: Role of self-esteem and autonomy in determining medication compliance among adolescents with juvenile rheumatoid arthritis. Pediatrics, 64: 15–17, 1982

Loggie, JMH: Pediatric hypertension: Pharmacologic alternatives amid therapy controversy. Consultant 21: 245–259, 1981

Loughlin, GM: Bronchitis. In E. L. Kenodig & V. Chernick (Eds.). Disorders of the respiratory tract in children. (Chap. 16). Philadelphia: Saunders, 1983

Lushbaugh, MA: Critical care of the child with burns. Nursing Clinics of North America, 16: 635–646, 1981

Lynch, JM: Helping patients through the recurrent nightmare of herpes. Nursing 82 12: 40–41, 1982

Lynch, MH, Gray, JL: Kawasaki disease. Pediatric Nursing 8, 96–101, 1982

Marvin, JA: Planning home care for burn patients. Nursing 83 13: 65–67, 1983

McCaffry, M: Pain relief for the child. Pediatric Nursing 3: 11–16, 1977

McCarthy, AM, Mehegan, J: Migraine headaches in children: treatment. Pediatric Nursing 8: 173–176, 1982

McCrory, WW: Essential hypertension in childhood. Pediatric Annals 11: 585–590, 1982

McCrory, WW: Finding an elevated blood pressure—what does it mean? Pediatric Annals 11: 581–584, 1982

McEnery, PT, Strife, F: Nephrotic syndrome in childhood. Pediatric Clinics of North America 29: 875–894, 1982

McGuire, L, Dizard, S: Managing pain in the young patient. Nursing 82: 52–55, 1982

McKeever, PT: Fathering the chronically ill child. The American Journal of Maternal Child Nursing 6: 124–128, 1981

McLaughlin, C: The Black Parents Handbook. New York: Harcourt, 1979

McLaury, P: Head lice: Pediatric social disease. The American Journal of Nursing 83: 1300–1303, 1983

Mayfield, JK, Riseborough, EJ, Jaffe, N, Nehma, AM: Spinal deformity in children treated for neuroblastoma. The Journal of Bone and Joint Surgery 63-A: 183-193, 1981

Megzitt, BF, Juett, DA, Smith, JD: Cast-bracing for fractures of the femoral shaft. The Journal of Bone and Joint Surgery 63-B: 12-23, 1981

Meyer, TM: TENS relieving pain through electricity. Nursing 82: 57-59, 1982

Miller, J, Arsenault, L: Reye's syndrome. Journal of Neurosurgical Nursing 15: 155-163, 1983

Miller, KA: Child abuse and neglect. The Journal of Family Practice 14: 571-575, 1982

Misik, IM: When the anorectic patient challenges you. Nursing 11: 46-49, 1981

Modcrin, MA, Schott, J: An update of congestive heart failure in infants. Issues in Comprehensive Pediatric Nursing 3: 5-22, 1979

Moe, JH, Winter, RB, Bradford, DS, Lonstein, JE: Scoliosis and other spinal deformities. Philadelphia: Saunders, 1978

Moore, ML: Realities in Childbearing (2nd Ed.). Philadelphia: Saunders, 1983

Motivating children to become assertive health care consumers. Nursing 82 12: 94-95, 1982

Murray, R, Zentner, J: Nursing Concepts for Health Promotion 2nd Ed. Englewood, NJ: Prentice-Hall, 1979

National Committee for Prevention of Child Abuse: Basic Facts About Sexual Child Abuse. Chicago: National Committee for Prevention of Child Abuse, 1982

National Heart, Lung, and Blood Pressure Institute: Report of the task force on blood pressure control in children. Pediatrics 59: 798-803, 1977

Nelms, BC: What is a normal adolescent? The American Journal of Maternal Child Nursing 6: 402-406, 1981

Nopshitz, J: On masturbation. Pediatric Annals 11: 747-749, 1982

Norman, SE, Browne, TR: Seizure disorders. The American Journal of Nursing 81: 984-989, 1981

Oehler, J: The frog family books: color the pictures "sad" or "glad." The American Journal of Maternal Child Nursing 6: 281-283, 1981

Ormond, EAR & Caulfield, C: A practical guide to giving oral medications to young children. The American Journal of Maternal Child Nursing 1: 320-325, 1976

Ostchega, Y: Preventing . . . and treating . . . cancer chemotherapy's oral complications. Nursing 80 10: 47-52, 1980

Pantell, RH, Fries, JF & Vickery, PM: Taking Care of Your Child. Reading, MA: Addison-Wesley, 1977

Papin, D: Long-term care for children who have ingested corrosive substances. Issues in Comprehensive Pediatric Nursing, 4: 55-68, 1980

Pedley, TA, DeVivo, DC: Seizure disorders in infants and children. In AM Rudolph (Ed.), Pediatrics 17th Ed. pp. 1654-1671. Norwalk, CT: Appleton, 1982

Peralta, G: Workbook: Home hyperalimentation and intravenous therapy. The Coordinator 2: 20-27, 1983

Petrillo, M, Sanger, S: Emotional Care of Hospitalized Children 2nd Ed. Philadelphia: Lippincott, 1980

Pidgeon, V: Characteristics of children's thinking and implications for health teaching. Maternal Child Nursing Journal 6: 1-7, 1977

Pierce, PM, Giovinco, G: Reach: self-care for the chronically ill child. Pediatric Nursing 9: 37-39, 1983

Pillitteri, A: Nursing Care of the Growing Family: A Child Health Text. Boston: Little, Brown, 1977

Pinney, M: Pneumonia. The American Journal of Nursing 81: 517-518, 1981

Pinyerd, BJ: Siblings of child with myelomeningocele: examining their perceptions. Maternal Child Nursing Journal 12: 61-69, 1983

Pipes, P: Nutrition in Infancy and Childhood. St. Louis: Mosby, 1983

Pless, IB: Practical problems and their management. In A Scheiner and I Abrams (Eds.) Practical Management of the Developmentally Disabled Child. St. Louis: Mosby: 416, 1980

Poole, SR, Morrison, JD: Adolescent health care in family practice. The Journal of Family Practice 16: 103-109, 1983

Powell, ML: Assessment and Management of Developmental Changes and Problems in Children 2nd Ed. St. Louis: Mosby, 1981

Pridham, KF, Hansen, MF, Bradley, ME, Heighway, SM: Issues of concern to mothers of new babies. The Journal of Family Practice 14: 1079-1085, 1982

Pringle, SM, Ramsey, BE: Promoting the Health of Children: A Guide for Caretakers and Health Care Professionals. St. Louis: Mosby, 1982

Pritchard, DJ: Indications for surgical treatment of localized Ewing's sarcoma of bone. Clinical Orthopedics and Related Research 153: 39-43, 1980

Powers, RJ, Andrassy, RJ, Brennan, LP, Weitzmann, JJ: Alternate approach to the management of acute perforating appendicitis in children. Surgery, Gynecology and Obstetrics 152: 473-475, 1981

Raab, EL & Leopold, IH: Strabismus. In H. C. Shirkey (Ed.). Pediatric Therapy 6th Ed. (Chap. 28). St. Louis: Mosby, 1980

Rapoff, MA, Christophersen, ER: Improving compliance in pediatric practice. The Pediatric Clinics of North America 29: 339-355, 1982

Reeder, S, Mastroiani, L: Maternity Nursing. Philadelphia: Lippincott, 1983

Redman, BK: The Process of Patient Teaching in Nursing. St. Louis: Mosby, 1980

Rice, BL: Nutritional problems of developmentally disabled children. Pediatric Nursing 7: 15-18, 1981

Rice, MA, Kibbee, PE: Review: identifying the adolescent substance abuser. The American Journal of Maternal Child Nursing, 8: 139-142, 1983

Riggs, RS: Incest: The school's role. The Journal of School Health, 52: 365-369, 1982

Ritchie, JA: Nursing the child undergoing limb amputation. The American Journal of Maternal Child Nursing 5: 114-120, 1980

Rodgers, BM, Hillemeier, MM, O'Neill, E, Slonim, MB: Depression in the chronically ill or handicapped child. The American Journal of Maternal Child Nursing 6: 266-273, 1981

Romney, MC: Incest in adolescence. Pediatric Annals 11: 813-817, 1982

Rooks, Y, Pack, B: A profile of sickle cell disease. Nursing Clinics of North America 18: 131-138, 1983

Rose-Williamson, K, Rathbun, SB: Planning discharge for a patient with osteogenic sarcoma. Oncology Nursing Forum 8: 38-40, 1981

Rosenberg, AJ, Vela, AR: A new simplified technique for

pediatric anorectal manometry. Pediatrics 71: 240–244, 1983

Rozzell, MS, Hijazi, M, Pack, B: The painful episode. Nursing Clinics of North America 18: 185–199, 1983

Rudolph, AM (Ed.): Pediatrics 17th Ed. Norwalk, CT: Appleton, 1982

Rutter, M, Bartak, L: Special education treatment of autistic children: a comparative study. II Follow-up findings and implications for service. Journal of Child Psychology and Psychiatry 14: 241–270, 1973

Sasso, SC: Prostaglandin E-1 for the infant with congenital heart disease. The American Journal of Maternal Child Nursing 1: 29, 1983

Sataloff, RT: Pediatric hearing loss. Pediatric Nursing 6: 16–18, 1980

Sataloff, RT, Colton, CM: Otitis media: A common childhood infection. The American Journal of Nursing 81: 1480–1483, 1981

Schumann, MJ: Neuromuscular relaxation—a method for inducing sleep in young children. Pediatric Nursing 7: 9–13, 1981

Scipien, GM, Barnard, MU, Chard, MA, Howe, J, Phillips, PJ: Issues in Comprehensive Pediatric Nursing 2nd Ed. New York: McGraw-Hill, 1979

Scott, E, Jan, J, Freeman, R: Can't Your Child See? Baltimore: University Park Press, 1977

Seashore, JH: Esophageal malformations. In A. M. Rudolph (Ed.), Pediatrics 17th ed., Norwalk, CT: Appleton, 1982

Seleckman, J: Immunization: What's it all about? The American Journal of Nursing 80: 1440–1445, 1980

Sergis-Deavenport, E, Varni, JW: Behavioral techniques in teaching hemophilia factor replacement procedures to families. Pediatric Nursing 8: 416–419

Shubin, S: Nursing patients from different cultures. Nursing 80 10: 79–81, 1980

Simkins, R: The crises of bronchiolitis. The American Journal of Nursing 81: 514–516, 1981

Simone, J: Leukemia. In AM Rudolph (Ed.), Pediatrics 17th ed. pp. 1097–1102. Norwalk, CT: Appleton, 1982

Sloane, PD: Sore throats: They're common, but full of surprises. Consultant, 22: 110–127, 1982

Smith, KM: Recognizing cardiac failure in neonates. The American Journal of Maternal Child Nursing 4: 98–100, 1979

Smith, ML: When a child dies at home. Nursing 82 12: 66–67, 1982

Spadaro, DC: Factors involved with patient compliance. Pediatric Nursing 6: 27–29, 1980

Spinetta, JJ, Deasy-Spinetta, P: (Eds.). Living with Childhood Cancer. St. Louis: Mosby.

Steele, SM: Health Promotion of the Child with Long-Term Illness 3rd ed. Norwalk, CT: Appleton, 1983

Stone, AC: Facing up to acne. Pediatric Nursing 8: 229–234, 1982

Tauer, KM: Promoting effective decision-making in sexually active adolescents. The Nursing Clinics of North America 18: 275–292, 1983

Tealey, AR: Getting children to keep still during radiotherapy. The American Journal of Maternal Child Nursing 2: 178–181, 1977

Tennant, FS, LaCour, J: Children at high risk for addiction and alcoholism. Pediatric Nursing 6:26–27, 1980

Teung, AG: Growth and Development. Norwalk, CT: Appleton, 1982

Tesler, M, Savedra, M: Coping with hospitalization: A study of school-age children. Pediatric Nursing 7: 35–38, 1981

Toguri, AG: Urologic Abnormalities. In AM Rudolph(Ed.). Pediatrics 17th Ed. Norwalk, CT: Appleton, 1982

Travis, LB: The nephrotic syndrome. In AM Rudolph (Ed.), Pediatrics pp. 1188–1192 Norwalk, CT: Appleton, 1982

Valent, S: Suicide in school aged children: theory and assessment. Pediatric Nursing 9: 25–29, 1983

Vestal, KW (Ed.): Pediatric Critical Care Nursing. New York: Wiley, 1982

Villalon, D, Smith, MN: At home with traction. Pediatric Nursing 8: 15–16, 1982

Voyles, JB: Bronchopulmonary dysplasia. The American Journal of Nursing 81: 510–514, 1981

Wachtel, D: Preventing scabies outbreaks. Nursing 79 9: 68–71.

Waechter, E: The adolescent with a handicapping, chronic, or life threatening illness. In R. Mercer (Ed.), Perspective on Adolescent Health Care pp. 186–209. Philadelphia: Lippincott, 1979

Walsh, S: Parents of asthmatic kids (PAK): A successful parent support group. Pediatric Nursing 7: 28–29, 1981

Watson, KW: Adoptive and foster parents. In LE Arnold (Ed.). Helping Parents Help Their Children. New York: Brunner-Mazel, 1978

Weaver, BM, Vines, DW: Case recognition and assessment of father-daughter incest. Issues in Comprehensive Pediatric Nursing 4: 67–76, 1980

Webster-Stratton, C: Recognizing and assessing conduct disorders in children. The American Journal of Maternal Child Nursing 8: 336–339, 1983

Wenger, DR: Selective surgical containment for Legg-Perthes disease: recognition and management of complications. Journal of Pediatric Orthopedics 1: 153–160, 1981

Whaley, LF, Wong, DL: Nursing Care of Infants and Children 2nd ed. St. Louis: Mosby, 1983

Wilken, B, Brown, RD, Urwin, R, Brown, DA: Cystic fibrosis screening by dried blood spot trypsin assay: results in 75,000 newborn infants. The Journal of Pediatrics 102: 383–387, 1983

Williams HA: Screening for testicular cancer. Pediatric Nursing 7: 38–40, 1981

Williams, L: Childhood immunizations. Pediatric Nursing 8: 18–21, 53, 1982

Wittner, M: Diseases caused by arthropods. In AM Rudolph (Ed.), Pediatrics pp. 709–710, Norwalk, CT: Appleton.

Wittner, M: Parasitic diseases. In AM Rudolph (Ed.), Pediatrics, 17th ed. Norwalk, CT: Appleton, 1982

Wong, D, Dornan, LR: Nursing care in childhood cancer-retinoblastoma. The American Journal of Nursing 82: 425–431, 1982

Wood, SP: School aged children's perceptions of the causes of illness. Pediatric Nursing 9: 101–104, 1983

Wooldridge, M, Surveyer, JA: Skin grafting full-thickness burn injury. The American Journal of Nursing, 80: 2000–2004, 1980

Younger, JB: The management of night waking in older infants. Pediatric Nursing 8: 155–158, 1982

Zamerowski, ST: Helping families cope with handicapped children. Topics in Clinical Nursing 4: 41–56, 1982

Selected Books for Children

Death and Dying

Bernstein JE, Gullo SV: When People Die. New York, Dutton, 1977 (Grades K–3)

Byars, B: The Night Swimmer. New York, Delacorte, 1980 (Grades 5 and up)

Grollman EA: Talking About Death. New York, Beacon, 1976 (3–10 years)

Krementz J: How It Feels When a Parent Dies. New York, Knopf, 1981 (Grades 4 and up)

Peavy A: Grandfather. New York, Scribner, 1981 (Grades K–2)

Pevaner S: And You Give Me a Pain, Elaine. New York, Seabury, 1978 (Grades 5–7)

White EB: Charlotte's Web. New York, Harper, 1952 (Grades 1–4)

Divorce

Blume J: It's Not the End of the World. New York, Bantam, 1977 (Grades 3–8)

Boeckman C: Surviving Your Parent's Divorce. New York, Watts, 1980 (Grades 6 and up)

Hyde MO: My Friend Has Four Parents. New York, McGraw, 1981 (Grades 4 and up)

Koningsburg EL: Journey to an 800 Number. New York, Atheneum, 1982 (Grades 4 and up)

LeShan J: What's Going to Happen to Me—When Parents Separate or Divorce. New York, Four Winds, 1978 (Grades 6 and up)

List JA: The Day the Loving Stopped. New York, Fawcett Juniper, 1981 (Grades 7 and up)

Williams B: Mitzi and the Terrible Tyrannosaurus Rex. New York, Dutton, 1982 (Grades 2–5)

Williams VB: A Chair For My Mother. New York, Greenwillow, 1982 (Grades K–2)

Wolkoff J: Happily Ever After . . . Almost. Scarsdale, NY, Bradbury, 1982 (Grades 5 and up)

Family Life and Relationships

Aliki: We Are Best Friends. New York, Greenwillow, 1982 (Grades K–2)

MacLachlen P: Cassie Binegar. New York, Harper, 1982 (Grades 3–6)

McCaffrey M: My Brother Ange. New York, Crowell, 1982 (Grades 3–6)

Miles B: I Would If I Could. New York, Knopf, 1982 (Grades 3–5)

Rodgers, M: Summer Switch. New York, Harper, 1982 (Grades 5 and up)

Schwartz A: Bea and Mr. Jones. Scarsdale, NY, Bradbury, 1982 (Grades K–2)

Sebastyen O: IOU's Boston, Little, 1982 (Grades 5 and up)

Hospitalization and health care

Chase F: A Visit to the Hospital. New York, Gross, 1977 (Grades K–3)

Ciliotta, C, Livingston C: Why Am I Going to the Hospital? Secaucus, NJ, Stuart, 1983 (Grades K–3)

Clark B, Coleman LL: Pop-up Going to the Hospital. New York, Random, 1971 (Grades K–3)

Froman R: Let's Find Out About the Clinic. New York, Watts, 1968 (Grades K–3)

Howe J: The Hospital Book. New York, Crown, 1981 (Grades 2–4)

Kay, E: The Clinic. New York, Watts, 1971 (Grades 5–7)

Kay, E: First Book of the Emergency Room. New York, Watts, 1970 (Grades 5–7)

Rey M, & Rey HA: Curious George Goes to the Hospital. Boston, Houghton, 1966 (3–8 years)

Rockwell A, Rockwell H: Sick in Bed. New York, Macmillian, 1982 (Grades K–2)

Scarry R: Nicky Goes to See the Doctor. New York, Western, 1971 (3–7 years)

Singer M: It Can't Hurt Forever. New York, Harper, 1978 (Grades 4–6)

Sex education

Bell R: Changing Bodies, Changing Lives; A Book for Teens on Sex and Relationships. New York, Random, 1981 (Grades 7 and up)

Blume J: Are You There, God? It's Me Margaret. Scarsdale, NY, Bradbury, 1972 (Grades 4–9)

Blume J: Deenie. Scarsdale, NY, Bradbury, 1973 (Grades 4–9)

Blume J: Then Again, Maybe I Won't. Scarsdale, NY, Bradbury, 1971 (Grades 4–9)

Caveney S: Inside Mom: An illustrated Account of Conception, Pregnancy, and Childbirth. New York, St. Martin's, 1977 (Grades 4–6)

Eyerly J: He's My Baby Now. Philadelphia, Lippincott, 1977 (Grades 7–10) (deals with illegitimate child)

Godon S: Facts About Sex For Today's Youth. New York, Ed-U-Press, 1973 (Grades 6–10)

Gordon S: Girls Are Girls and Boys Are Boys—So What's the Difference? New York, Ed-U-Press, 1974 (Grades K–3)

Gordon S, Gordon J: Did the Sun Shine Before You Were Born? New York, Ed-U-Press, 1974 (3–7 years)

Hautzig D: Hey Dollface. New York, Greenwillow, 1978 (Grades 7–9) (deals with homosexuality)

Hettlinger RF: (1971). Growing Up With Sex. New York, Seabury, 1971 (Grades 6–10)

Johnson EW: Love and Sex in Plain Language. New York, Bantam, 1977 (Grades 6–10).

Mandara L: What's Happening To My Body?: A Growing Up Guide For Mothers and Daughters. New York, Newmarket, 1983 (Grades 4–8)

Mayle P: Where Did I Come From? Secaucus, NJ, Stuart, 1973 (Grades K–3)

Nourse AE: Menstruation: Just Plain Talk. New York, Watts, 1980 (Grades 3 and up)

Wibblesman C, McCoy K: The Teenage Body Book. New York, Simon, 1978 (Grades 7–10)

Miscellaneous

Betancourt J: Smile! How to Cope With Braces. New York, Knopf, 1982 (Grades 4 and up)

Brown M: Arthur Goes to Camp. Boston, Little, 1982 (Grades K–2)

Brown M: Dinosaurs Beware! A Safety Guide. Boston, Little, 1982 (Grades K–2)

Cohen M: Jim Meets the Thing. New York, Greenwillow, 1981 (Grades K–2) (dealing with fears)

Gilson J: Do Bananas Chew Gum? New York, Lothrop, 1980 (Grades 4–6) (learning disabled child)

Greenfield E, Revis A: Alesia. New York, Philomel, 1981 (Grades 5 and up) (diary of a child handicapped after car accident)

Hyman J: Deafness. New York, Watts, 1980 (Grades 4–6)

Jonas A: When You Were a Baby. New York, Greenwillow, 1981 (Grades K–2)

Keller H: Cromwell's Glasses. New York, Greenwillow, 1981 (Grades K–2)

Lasker J: The Do-Something Day. New York, Viking, 1982 (Grades K–2) (runaway children)

Linburg P: The Story of Your Heart. New York, Coward, 1979 (Grades 5 and up)

MacLachen P: Mama One, Mama Two. New York, Harper, 1982 (Grades K–2) (foster home care)

Marcus RB: Being Blind. New York, Hastings, 1981 (Grades 5 and up)

Risking M: Apple Is My Sign. New York, Houghton, 1981 (Grades 5 and up) (deaf child)

Riedman SR: Diabetes. New York, Watts, 1980 (Grades 4 and up)

Robinet HG: Ride the Red Cycle. New York, Houghton, 1980 (Grades 3–5) (physically handicapped child)

Schlee A: Ask Me No Questions. New York, Holt, 1982 (Grades 5 and up) (child abuse)

Schott E: Adoption. New York, Watts, 1980 (Grades 4 and up)

Seixas JS: Tobacco—What It Is, What It Does. New York, Greenwillow, 1981 (Grades 1–4)

Silverstein A, Silverstein V: Runaway Sugar; All About Diabetes. Philadelphia, Lippincott, 1981 (Grades 3–5)

Smith DB: Last Was Lloyd. New York, Viking, 1981 (Grades 4–6) (overprotected child)

Trier CS: Exercise: What It Is, What It Does. New York, Greenwillow, 1982 (Grades 1–3)

Voight C: Dicey's Song. New York, Atheneum, 1982 (Grades 5 and up) (sibling's response to mentally ill mother)

Wolf B: Michael and the Dentist. New York, Four Winds, 1980 (Grades K–3)

Community and National Resources

American Academy of Pediatrics
P.O. Box 1034
Evanston, Ill. 60204

American Cancer Society
77 Third Avenue
New York, N.Y. 10017

American Diabetes Association, Inc.
1 East 45th Street
New York, N.Y. 10020

American Foundation for the Blind
15 West 16th Street
New York, N.Y. 10011

American Heart Association
44 East 23rd Street
New York, N.Y. 10011

American Lung Assocation
1740 Broadway
New York, N.Y. 10019

Anorexia Nervosa and Associated Diseases (ANAD)
550 Frontage Road
Department N79
Northfield, Ill. 60093

Association for the Aid of Crippled Children
345 East 46th Street
New York, N.Y. 10017

Association for Children with Learning Disabilities
4156 Library Road
Pittsburgh, Pa. 15234

Epilepsy Foundation of America
1828 L Street, N.W.
Washington, D.C. 20036

National Association for Retarded Children, Inc.
386 Park Avenue South
New York, N.Y. 10016

National Association for Sickle Cell Disease, Inc.
945 South Western Avenue
Suite 206
Los Angles, Ca.

National Association for the Deaf, Inc.
2495 Shattuck Avenue
Berkeley, Ca. 94720

National Association for Visually Handicapped
305 East 24th Street
New York, N.Y. 10010

National Cystic Fibrosis Research Foundation
3379 Peachtree Rd., N.E.
Atlanta, Ga. 30326

National Institute of Mental Health
5600 Fishers Lane
Rockville, Md. 20852

The Arthritis Foundation
1212 Avenue of the Americas
New York, N.Y. 10036

The National Foundation for Sudden Infant Death
1501 Broadway
New York, N.Y. 10036

The National Hospice Organization
Tower Suite 506
301 Maple Avenue West
Vienna, Va. 22180

National Hemophilia Foundation
25 West 39th Street
New York, N.Y. 10018

United Cerebral Palsy Association, Inc.
66 East 34th Street
New York, N.Y. 10066

APPENDIXES

Normal Respiration, Pulse, and Blood Pressure Values

TABLE 1
NORMAL RESPIRATION AND PULSE VALUES FOR CHILDREN

	Age	Approximate rate/min
Normal respiratory rates at rest	0–12 mo	30–50
	1–5 yr	20–30
	5–12 yr	15–25
	12–18 yr	12–20
Normal heart rate at rest	0–1 mo	120–160
	1–6 mo	110–140
	6–12 mo	100–120
	1–2 yr	85–125
	2–6 yr	70–110
	6–10 yr	65–100
	10–16 yr	75–90

TABLE 2
NORMAL RANGE OF BLOOD PRESSURE VALUES FOR CHILDREN

Age	Systolic / Diastolic
Infant (1–12 mo)	65–120
	40–80
Toddler (1–3 yr)	69–123
	38–90
Preschooler (3–6 yr)	76–120
	46–80
Schoolchild (6–12 yr)	85–128
	48–68
Adolescent (12–18 yr)	85–140
	45–85

Wide variations in normal blood pressure range are common in children and serial readings should be done when it is necessary to determine an upward or downward trend.

Blood and Laboratory Test Values

TABLE 1
AVERAGE RANGE OF BLOOD VALUES AT DIFFERENT AGES

	Birth	3 mo	6 mo	1 yr	2 yr	4 yr	8–12 yr	Adult *male*	Adult *female*
Hemoglobin (g/dl)	13–20	9.5–14	10.5–14	11–15	12–15	12.5–15	12–16	13–18	11–16
Hematocrit (g/dl)	44–64	23–41	33–42	32–40	34–40	36–44	39–47	42–52	37–47
WBC/mm³(thousands)	9–38	6–18	1–15	4.5–13.5	9–12	8–10	8	5–10	5–10
Monocytes (%)	6–12	7	5	5	5–8	5–8	5–8	5–8	5–8
Lymphocytes (%)	30–31	55–63	48–60	48–53	48–50	40–48	30–38	30–35	30–35
Neutrophils (%)	40–80	30–35	30–45	40–50	40–50	50–55	55–60	35–70	35–70
Eosinophils (%)	2–3	—	—	—	—	—	—	—	2–3
Platelets (per mm³)	350,000	250,000	—	—	—	—	—	(250,000–350,000)	
Reticulocytes	2–8	0.5–1.6	—	—	—	—	—	—	0.5–1.6

Compiled from a variety of sources.

TABLE 2
HEMATOLOGICAL DATA IN SICKLE CELL DISEASE

	Normal *Average*	Sickle Cell *Average*	Sickle Cell *Range*
Hemoglobin	12	7.5	5.5–9.5
Hematocrit	36	22	17–29
Reticulocytes	1.5	12	5–30
Nucleated RBC	0	3	1–20
WBC	7500	20,000	12–35,000

From Rudolph AM, Barnett HL, Einhorn AH (eds): Pediatrics, 16th ed. New York, Appleton, p 1153, 1977, used with permission.

TABLE 3
LABORATORY TEST VALUES

Hematology	*Values*

Erythrocyte sedimentation rate	Newborn: 0–2 mm/hr
	4–14 year old: 3–13 mm/hr
	>14 years (Westergren):
	    male: 0–15 mm/hr
	    female: 0–20 mm/hr

Factor assay	
Factor VIII: Antihemophilic factor	Minimum hemostatic level: 30–35% concentration
Factor IX: Plasma thromboplastin component (PTC, Christmas factor)	Minimum hemostatic level: 30% concentration
Hematocrit	Newborn: 42–54% 1–3 years: 29–40% 4–10 years: 36–38% >age 10: male: 40–54% female: 36–46%
Hemoglobin (Hb or Hgb)	Newborn: 14–24 g/dl Infant: 10–15 g/dl Child: 11–16 g/dl >age 12: male: 13.5–18 g/dl female: 12–16 g/dl
Platelet count (thrombocytes)	Premature: 100,000–300,000 mm Newborn: 150,000–300,000 mm Infant: 200,000–475,000 mm >1 year: 150,000–450,000 mm

Reticulocytes	Newborn: 2.5–6.5% of all RBC
	Infant: 0.5–3.5% of all RBC
	Child: 0.5–2.0% of all RBC
White blood cell differential	Child: 2 weeks to 12 years
Neutrophils	29–47%
Segments	50–65%
Bands	0–5%
Eosinophils	0–3%
Basophils	1–3%
Lymphocytes	38–63%
Monocytes	4–9%

Chemistry	*Values*
Alkaline phosphatase	Infant: 40–300 U/L
	Child: 60–270 U/L
Bilirubin	Newborn: total = 12 mg/dl
	Child: total = 0.2–0.8 mg/dl
Blood urea nitrogen (BUN)	Infant: 5–15 mg/dl
	Child: 5–20 mg/dl
	Thereafter: male: 10–25 mg/dl
	female: 8–20 mg/dl
Calcium (Ca)	Newborn: 3.7–7 mEq/L
	Infant: 5–6 mEq/L
	Child: 4.5–5.8 mEq/L
	Thereafter: 4.5–5.5 mEq/L
Carbon dioxide combining power	20–28 mEq/L
Chloride (Cl)	Newborn: 94–112 mEq/L
	Infant: 95–110 mEq/L
	Child: 98–105 mEq/L
	Thereafter: 95–105 mEq/L
Creatinine	Infant to 6 years: 0.3–0.6 mg/dl
	6–18 years: 0.4–1.22 mg/dl
	Thereafter: 0.6–1.2 mg/dl
Fasting blood sugar (FBS)	Newborn: 30–80 mg/dl
	Child: 60–100 mg/dl
	Thereafter: 70–110 mg/dl

Glucose tolerance test

>6 years	Serum(mg/dl)	Blood (mg/dl)
Fasting	70–110	60–100
0.5 Hr	<160	<150
1 Hr	<170	<160
2 Hr	<125	<115
3 Hr	fasting level	fasting level

Magnesium	Newborn: 1.4–2.9 mEq/L
	Child: 1.6–2.6 mEq/L
	Thereafter: 1.5–2.5 mEq/L
Osmolality	270–290 mOsm/Kg/H_2O
Phosphorus	Newborn: 3.5–8.6 mg/dl
	Infant: 4.5–6.7 mg/dl
	Child: 4.5–5.5 mg/dl
	Thereafter: 2.5–4.8 mg/dl
Potassium	Infant: 3.6–5.8 mEq/L
	Child: 3.5–5.5 mEq/L
	Thereafter: 3.5–5.0 mEq/L
Sodium	Infant: 134–150 mEq/L
	Child: 135–145 mEq/L
	Thereafter: 135–145 mEq/L

Serology	*Values*
Antistreptolysin O (ASO)	Newborn: similar to mother's
	Infant: <160 U/dl
	Preschool: <150 U/dl
	Schoolage: <200 U/dl
C-Reactive protein (CRP)	0
RPR (rapid plasma reagin)	Negative
Rubella antibody detection (HAI or HI)	<1:8 titer = susceptible
	1:8–1:32 past exposure
	1:32–1:64 immunity
	>1:64 definite immunity
VDRL (venereal disease research laboratory)	Negative

Urine Chemistry	*Values*
Osmolality	Newborn: 100–600 mOsm/Kg/H_2O
	Child: 50–1200 mOsm/Kg/H_2O
	Average: 200–800 mOsm/Kg/H_2O
Urinalysis	
pH	Newborn: 5–7
	Child: 4.5–8
	Thereafter: same as child
Specific gravity	Newborn: 1.001–1.020
	Child: 1.005–1.030
	Thereafter: same as child
Protein	Negative
Glucose	Negative
Ketones	Negative
RBC	Rare
WBC	0–4
Casts	Rare
Vanillylmandelic acid (VMA)	1.5–7.5 mg/24 hours

Other	*Values*
Cerebrospinal fluid (CSF)	
Pressure	50–100 mm H_2O
Cell count	0–8 mm
Protein	15–45 mg/dl
Chloride	120–128 mEq/L
Glucose	35–75 mg/dl
Culture	No organisms
Sweat chloride	<50 mEq/L

Note: These are reference values only. Each laboratory must report its own normal range for the technique it uses and the population it serves. Consult the agency laboratory for specific values.

Kee J LeF: Laboratory Tests and Diagnostic Tests with Nursing Implications. Norwalk, CT: Appleton, 1983, used with permission.

TABLE 4
NORMAL AND ABNORMAL BLOOD GAS MEASUREMENTS

Normal Values	pH	pCO_2	HCO_3 (mEq/L)	CO_2
Child	7.35–7.45	35–45	24–26	25–28
Term Infant - birth	7.26–7.29	54.5		
- 1 hr	7.30	38.8		20.6
- 3 hr	7.34	38.3		21.9
- 1 to 3 d	7.38–7.41	34–35		21.4
Premature >1250 g - 1 to 3 d	7.38–7.39	38–39		
<1250 g - 1 to 3 d	7.35–7.36	37–44		

Abnormal Values	pH	pCO_2	HCO_3 (mEq/L)	CO_2
Metabolic acidosis	↓	↓	↓	↓
Acute respiratory acidosis	↓	↑	← →	Sl. ↑
Compensated resp. acidosis	← → or Sl. ↓	↑	↑	↑
Metabolic alkalosis	↑	Sl. ↑	↑	↑
Acute respiratory alkalosis	↑	↓	← →	Sl. ↓
Compensated resp. alkalosis	← → or Sl. ↑	↓	↓	↓

Reproduced with permission from Johns Hopkins Hospital: The Harriet Lane Handbook, 9th ed., edited by Jeffrey A. Biller and Andrew Yeager. Copyright 1981 by Year Book Medical Publishers, Inc., Chicago.

Drug Administration

TABLE 1
CALCULATING SAFE DRUG DOSAGE

	Unit of Measurement	Formula for Safe Dosage	Examples
Surface area rule	Total body surface area	$\dfrac{\text{Surface area of child (square meters)}}{1.7}$	
Clark's rule	Child's weight	$\dfrac{\text{Adult dose} \times \text{weight of child (in pounds)}}{150}$	Adult dose is 3 grains Child weighs 50 pounds *Solution:* $\dfrac{3 \times 50}{150} = \dfrac{150}{150} = 1$ grain
Fried's rule (under age 2)	Child's age	$\dfrac{\text{Adult dose} \times \text{age of child (in months)}}{150}$	Adult dose is 30 ml Child is 10 months old *Solution:* $\dfrac{30 \times 10}{150} = \dfrac{300}{150} = 2$ ml
Young's rule (over age 2)	Child's age	$\dfrac{\text{Adult dose} \times \text{age of child (in years)}}{\text{Age of child (in years)} + 12}$	Adult dose is 350 mg. Child's age is 6 years *Solution:* $\dfrac{350 \times 6}{6 + 12} = \dfrac{2100}{18} = 117$ mg.

TABLE 2
CALCULATING I.V. FLOW RATES

Situation	Formula	Example
When using a micro- or mini-drip administration set which yields 60 drops per ml	Prescribed number of ml/hr = flow rate in drops/minute	Order is 15 ml/hr $\dfrac{60 \times 15}{60} = 15$
When using a macro-drip administration set	Drops/ml set yields × prescribed ml/hr divided by 60 = flow rate in drops/minute	Set yields 10 drops/ml and the prescribed rate is 18 ml/hr $\dfrac{10 \times 18}{60} = \dfrac{180}{60} = 3$ drops/minute

TABLE 3
PEDIATRIC ORAL MEDICATION GUIDELINES

Developmental Tasks and Behaviors		Nursing Implications
1 to 3 mo		
Motor	Reaches randomly toward mouth; shows strong palmar grasp reflex.	Infant's hands should be monitored or controlled to prevent spilling of medications.
	Head drops or exhibits bobbing control.	Head must be well supported.
Feeding	Sucks reflexively in response to tactile stimulation.	Medication should be administered using this natural behavior: medication should be given via nipple.
	Corners of the mouth may not seal effectively and the tongue may be reflexively forced against the palate.	Correct position of the nipple, if used, must be assured for adequate sucking.
	Tongue movement may project food out of mouth.	A syringe or dropper, if used, should be placed in the center back portion of the mouth. If placed along the gums, it must be toward the back of the mouth.
	Sucking strength increases (3 mo).	Amount of medication presented must be controlled. Infant may choke or drool because he can take in more medication than he can control.
	Stops taking fluids when full; progresses to fading of sucking reflex (3 mo).	Medication more easily given in small volumes and when infant is hungry.
Interactive	Basic trust vs. mistrust stage.	
	Infant becomes socially responsive.	Medication administration requires feeding behavior that establishes an easy, comfortable situation. This is part of the child's learning to form a trust relationship.
3 to 12 mo		
Motor	Advances from sitting well with support (3–4 mo) to crawling (10 mo).	Safety precautions regarding where medications are placed and kept become extremely important.
	Begins to develop fine motor hand control.	
	Advances from lying as placed (3 mo) to standing with support (12 mo).	Child who does not want to cooperate has ability to resist with his whole body.
Feeding	Starting at 12-month-old level:	
	Smacks and pouts lips in act of shifting food in mouth and in swallowing. Lower lip active in eating.	Child may spit out food and medicine he does not want.
	Tongue may protrude during swallowing.	Eating is inefficient, so medications may need to be retrieved and refed.
	Learns to drink from cup. Generally has poor approximation of corners of the mouth when drinking.	A small medicine cup may be more effective than a spoon.
	Feeding behaviors become individualized.	Feeding patterns and routines at home need to be considered.
	Learns to finger-feed self.	
Interactive	Basic trust vs. mistrust and oral sensory stages:	
	Communication skills develop from random social responses (3 mo) to making simple requests by gesturing (12 mo).	One must be alert for child's indicating his own needs (12 mo).
	Is sensitive and responsive to tactile stimulation. Begins developing responsiveness to other stimuli.	Physical comforting will be most effective with child. Verbal comforting secondary.
	Recognizes immediate family and, very important, may exhibit intense separation anxiety.	Exhibits early memory. May recall negative experiences, precipitating negative response in another similar situation.
12 to 18 mo		
Motor	Advances from standing with support to independent walking.	Have the child choose a position for taking medication or hold him to provide control and comfort. Forcing the child to take medicine when he is lying down takes away his sense of independence and will frequently result in very resistive behavior.
Feeding	Begins independent self-feeding, but is still messy.	Home feeding habits should be considered.
	Develops voluntary tongue and lip control.	Spits out disagreeable tastes effectively. Disguise crushed tablets and contents of capsules in a small amount of familiar solid. Be prepared to refeed.
	Spits deliberately.	
Interactive	Autonomy vs. shame and doubt.	
	Indicates needs and wants by pointing.	
	Speaks 4 to 6 words. Uses individual jargon.	Find out what words child uses for drinking, swallowing, and how oral medicines have been given at home.
	Responds to familiar commands.	

TABLE 3
PEDIATRIC ORAL MEDICATION GUIDELINES (Con't.)

		Developmental Tasks and Behaviors	Nursing Implications
		Responds to and participates in the routines of daily living.	Let child explore an empty medication cup. He will likely be more cooperative if familiar items are used.
			When possible, involve the parents. They are familiar and trusted persons, which is an important factor during an unfamiliar experience.
			Tell parents and staff the approach used for medication. Report its effectiveness.
		Exhibits notable independence, resistance, self-assertiveness, and ambivalence.	Allow the child as much freedom as possible.
			Allow the child to assert himself by choosing a drink to wash down the medicine.
		Begins to have temper tantrums.	Use games to gain cooperation.
			Tell the child what you expect and then follow through. A consistent, firm approach is essential.
18 to 30 mo	Motor	Walks, climbs into chair (18 mo).	Child is able to run away and kick.
		Advances to running without falling (24 mo).	
		Advances to obtaining and throwing small objects.	Child may throw materials placed within his reach. Never leave medications sitting on the bedside stand.
	Feeding	Generally feeds self. Advances to proficiency with minimal spilling.	Allow child opportunity to drink liquids from a medicine cup by himself.
		Second molars erupted (20–30 mo).	Permits greater flexibility in choosing form of medication.
		Exhibits increased rotary chewing, manages solid food particles.	
		Controls mouth and jaw proficiently.	Child is effective in spitting out unwanted medications and in clamping mouth tightly closed in resistance.
	Interactive	Autonomy vs. shame and doubt.	
		Has some sense of time, but no words for time (18 mo). Then responds to "just a minute" (21 mo). Advances to understanding, "play after you drink this" (24 mo).	Tell the child getting medicine that any bad taste will only last "a minute."
			Learn child's level of time awareness from nursing history.
		Carries out two to three directions given one at a time.	Give simplified directions: "Open your mouth, drink, and then swallow."
		Shows ability to respond to and participate in routines of daily living.	Include child in establishing medicine-taking routine.
		Helps put things away; carries breakable objects.	
		Exhibits independence, resistance, self-assertiveness, and ambivalence.	Use a firm, consistent approach.
		Throws temper tantrums frequently.	Resistive behaviors are at a peak.
		Shows pride in accomplished skills.	Give immediate, positive tactile and verbal response to cooperative taking of medicine. Ignore resistive behavior.
		Does not know right from wrong.	
		Shows conflict between holding on and letting go.	Give choices when possible: "Do you want to sit in the chair or on my lap to take your medicine?"
2½ to 3½ yr	Motor	Continues to develop proficiency. Basic skills have all been initiated.	Child may be quite adept in resistive behavior.
	Feeding	Becoming more proficient in skills.	
		Eating likes and dislikes are definite but changeable.	Medication tastes can be disguised with variable effectiveness.
		May be influenced by others' reactions in responding to new food experiences.	A calm, positive approach is needed to gain a cooperative response from the child, quick tense approach is likely to produce similar behavior in the child.
	Interactive	Initiative vs. guilt.	
		Gives full name.	Begin asking for verbal identification of patient before giving medications.
		Is ritualistic.	Communicate administration methods.
		Has little understanding of past, present, or future.	Use concrete and immediate rewards.
		Shows concrete thinking, egocentricity.	Tolerates frustration poorly.
			Child's initial response to reason appears positive, but without consistent effect.

TABLE 3
PEDIATRIC ORAL MEDICATION GUIDELINES (Con't.)

Developmental Tasks and Behaviors	Nursing Implications
	Prolonged bargaining is frustrating and frightening to the child because no one is in control of the situation.
Exhibits early aggressiveness; coercive, manipulative behavior.	Give a choice when possible. Do not give a choice if the child does not have one.
Has many fantasies.	Begin giving simple, honest explanations of why the medication is given (not because the child was bad).
May be frightened by his "power."	Child's sense of security is dependent upon the nurses' consistent expectations of his behavior.

3½ to 6 yr

Motor	Develops proficiency of coordination.	Child can attempt and master pill taking.
	Can identify the parts of a complete movement or task.	
Feeding	Exhibits olfactory, gustatory, and kinesthetic refinement.	Disguising tastes is generally less effective than it is at younger ages. Child can distinguish medicine tastes and smells.
	Begins to lose temporary teeth (5 yr).	Loose teeth may need to be considered when selecting form of medication.
Interactive	Initiative vs. guilt.	
	Makes decisions.	Child should be active in making decisions that affect him.
	Sense of time allows enjoyment of delayed gratification.	Rewards which are not immediately received and social interaction can be used as effective motivators.
	Is able to tolerate frustration.	Child is able to understand the purpose of medications in simple terms.
	Seeks companionship.	
	Shows pride in accomplishments.	
	Has ability to follow directions and remember several instructions for a period of minutes to hours.	Teaching can have long-term benefits.
	Exhibits developing conscience. Needs limits set to help control his frightening sense of "power."	Prolonged reasoning or arguing may frighten the child; a simple command by a trusted adult may be more effective.
	Exhibits genital interest, general mutilation fears.	Explain the relationship between cause, illness, and treatment. Use simple terms.
	Illness often seen as punishment.	Give control when possible—child needs to make choices.
	Shows changeable response to parents.	Child may be more cooperative in medicine taking for the nurse than for the parent.

From Ormond EAR, Caulfield C: Am J Matern Child Nurs 1:321–325, September/October 1976, used with permission.

TABLE 4
PEDIATRIC INTRAMUSCULAR MEDICATION GUIDELINES

	Developmental Tasks and Behaviors	Nursing Management
Birth to 12 mo		
Physical development	Immature nervous system produces diffuse reflexive movement.	Restrain as necessary even though infant is small. Use two people (not mother): one to restrain, the other to give injection in older infant.
	Progressive maturation: roll over, sit, stand, walk, constant movement.	
	Gluteal muscle small and not developed.	Give injection in vastus lateralis muscle. Alternate right and left legs.
	Sciatic nerve close to area.	
Cognitive development	Unable to understand explanations.	State what you are going to do and then proceed with injection.
	Stranger anxiety develops in second half of first year. May associate syringe and needle with painful stimuli.	Spend time with child prior to giving injection. Prepare injection out of visual range of child.
Emotional/social development	Trust vs. mistrust.	
	Responds to tactile stimulation.	Hold and cuddle after injection. Physical comfort is more effective than verbal.
	Infant is distractible.	Offer toy to hold or something to look at during procedure.
1 to 3 yr		
Physical development	Locates injection site easily and works to push syringe away.	Use two people for procedure if needed for safe care.
	Highly mobile, runs.	
	Gluteal area not well developed until child has been walking for a year.	Give injection in vastus lateralis muscle. Rotate injection sites.
Cognitive development	Preoperational thought processes. Egocentric, short attention span. Obeys simple commands.	State what you are going to do and then proceed with injection. Use simple words and short phrases.
	Sense of time is developing from about 18 months.	Tell child "This will just take a minute and then you can play or get up."
	Distractible.	Give child something to look at, hold, or play with during procedure.
	Limited concept of body boundaries.	Apply band-aid.
Emotional/social development	Autonomy vs. shame and doubt. Rituals and consistency very important to child. Child sees minor changes as new experiences.	Use consistent approach. Record approach on Kardex.
	Self-assertive behavior; "me do."	Let child hold alcohol swab or band-aid.
	Resistant to restriction of freedom.	Restrain only as needed and for as brief a period as possible.
	Negativism and temper tantrums present.	Ignore negative behavior. Use firm, consistent approach.
	Many fears, especially fear of separation from parents.	Encourage parents to hold child and comfort child.
	Cannot use play to decrease fears.	Use tactile and verbal comfort measures.
	Fantasies are prominent at this age.	Give simple, honest reason for injection.
	Takes pride in own accomplishments.	Reward positive behaviors immediately.
3 to 6 yr		
Physical development	Increasing coordination.	Restrain as necessary.
	Gluteus muscle usually well developed.	Use only if absolutely necessary as vastus lateralis is still site of choice.
	Deltoid muscle developed.	Administer maximum of 1 ml.
Cognitive development	Remains egocentric; is a concrete thinker.	Tell child what he will feel.
	Concept of body boundaries incomplete; believes skin holds in body contents.	Explain body contents will not leak out of injection site.
		Apply band-aid.
	Learns by seeing and handling things.	Encourage child to handle alcohol swab, syringe, and band-aid prior to experience.
	Developing a conscience.	Tell child injections are never used as punishment.
	Can follow directions.	Teach child what he can do to help himself, e.g., lie still.
	Understands simple explanations.	

TABLE 4
PEDIATRIC INTRAMUSCULAR MEDICATION GUIDELINES (Con't.)

	Developmental Tasks and Behaviors	Nursing Management
Emotional/social development	Initiative vs. guilt.	State relationship of medication to child's situation.
	Genital phase; concerns about mutilation.	Give simple explanations. Provide privacy during injection.
	Seeks to master situations; takes pride in accomplishments.	Permit choice when possible, e.g., which leg? Foster development of coping mechanisms, e.g., let child hold someone's hand, say "ouch" when stuck, or count seconds it takes to give injection.
	Play is useful as a means of dealing with fears and fantasies.	Provide child with equipment and opportunity necessary to play "giving injection." Permit use of needle under nursing supervision. Observe for cues that child needs to play.
	Fears intrusive procedures. Injection seen as an aggressive act.	Give medication by injection only when necessary. Use vastus lateralis which is less threatening site than gluteus.
6 to 12 yr		
Physical development	Gluteal muscle well developed.	Permit child to select site if possible. Rotate sites.
Cognitive development	Understands concept of causality.	State injection not given because of any wrong doing.
	Capable of logical thinking and deduction; greater comprehension of relationships.	Give simple explanation of why medication is being given by injection.
	Understands time concept.	May be able to accept present discomfort for future gains.
Emotional/social development	Industry vs. Inferiority.	
	Wants to take part in situations.	Provide choice when possible, e.g., right or left leg for injection?
	Thrives on praise.	Praise child for positive contribution to procedure, e.g., you hold still very well.
	Decreased dependence on family; increased involvement with peer group.	Give verbal support.
	Fears the unknown.	Provide clear explanations. Repeat explanations as needed, since anxiety may be high.
	Verbalization replaces play as an effective means of dealing with anxiety.	Plan nursing care to allow for opportunities just to talk with the child.
Adolescent		
Physical development	Same sites as used for adults are appropriate to adolescent.	Assess muscle mass development. Provide choice when possible. Rotate sites.
Cognitive development	Capable of dealing with both reality and abstract thought.	Give as much information as adolescent desires about medication.
	Occasionally demonstrates some egocentrism.	Tell him how medication will feel.
Emotional/social development	Identity vs. role confusion.	
	Fears regression. Desire to be like others.	Support coping mechanisms. Tell him his reactions are like others.
	Concerns over body image.	Provide privacy. Permit choice of site if possible. Refrain from comments about adolescent's physical development.

Sample Nursing History

TABLE 1
SAMPLE NURSING HISTORY

Child
Name (nickname preferred). _____
Age. _____
Grade in school. _____

Chief Complaint
Why is _____ (fill in child's name) being hospitalized/seen in the clinic/doctor's office?

Present Illness
What signs and symptoms of illness does _____ have? (include child's name as you collect data.)
Has _____ received any treatment? If so what type?
Does _____ have any allergies?
What was _____ told about coming here?
What have you been told about the illness/hospitalization/visit?
What have you been told will be done for _____ ?
What have you told other family members?
Will someone be able to visit? (hospitalized child)
Is there anything else you would like to tell us?

Family
Who are the family members and where do they live?
What is a usual day like at home?
Who do you go to when you need help?
Does your family have beliefs or practices which may affect health care?
Do any family members have a current illness?
Has anyone been hospitalized? How do you feel about the care they received?
Is there anything else you would like to tell us about your family?

Child
Tell me what _____ is like?
How do you think _____ is growing? or What new things has _____ learned to do lately.
What is _____ day usually like?
Does _____ have any special fears?
How does _____ like day care/school? (if applicable)
How does _____ get along with others?
How is _____ disciplined?
What has _____ health been like?
What immunizations has _____ received?
When was _____ last seen by the dentist?

Review of Systems
Eyes, Ears, Nose and Throat
Are there frequent: nosebleeds, sore throats, colds, earaches? Do the eyes ever appear to be crossed? Does the older child ever report that he/she has difficulty seeing things?

Cardiorespiratory
Does the infant/child have trouble: breathing, finishing a 3- to 4-ounce bottle without tiring? Does running cause problems for the child? Does the infant/child ever turn blue?

Gastrointestinal
Does the child have problems with: vomiting, diarrhea, constipation, blood in the stools? Has the child complained of gastrointestinal pain?

Genitourinary
Is the child's urinary stream straight and strong? Is there any history of frequency, urgency, or pain related to urination? If the patient/client is an older girl, does she menstruate?

Neurological
Has the child had: febrile seizures, nonfebrile seizures, headaches, or dizzy spells? Have unusual behaviors been noted?

TABLE 1
SAMPLE NURSING HISTORY (Con't.)

Musculoskeletal

Have there been any: sprains or broken bones, swelling and/or redness of joints?

Senses

Does the child: see and hear as well as the parent feels he/she should? Can he/she see the blackboard in school?

Habits (young child)

Eating

Does _____ feed him/herself?

What types of food does _____ like?

What food does _____ dislike? Food allergies?

Does _____ take a bottle? Is the milk warmed?

Sleeping

Does _____ take a special toy or blanket to bed?

What does _____ call it?

Does _____ take a nap? When? How long?

What is _____ usual bedtime?

How many hours does _____ sleep at night?

What are _____ special bedtime routines?

Hygiene

What help does _____ need with bathing, dressing, toothbrushing, going to the bathroom?

Play

What are _____ favorite toys and activities?

Is there anything else about _____ you would like us to know?

Play/Exercise

What are _____ favorite toys and activities?

What kinds of exercise does _____ engage in?

Is (for older child) _____ engaged in any team sports?

Is there anything else about _____ that you would like us to know?

TABLE 2
ADOLESCENT—MODIFIED HISTORY

Personal history
    Name (nickname).
    Age.
    Grade in school.
    Employment.

Chief complaint
    Why have you been admitted to the hospital/come to the doctor or clinic?

Present illness
    What signs and symptoms do you have?
    Are you taking or doing anything for them?
    Do you have any allergies?
    What have you been told about your hospitalization/clinic visit?

Adolescent
    How would you describe yourself?
    How do you think you are growing?
    What is a usual day like for you?
    How do you spend your leisure time?
    Is there anything you would like to ask us or tell us?

Review of Systems (as above)

Habits
    Do you smoke?
    Do you drink alcohol or beer?
    Do you take drugs?
    Are you sexually active?

Growth and Development

Theories of Development

TABLE 1
PIAGET'S PERIODS OF COGNITIVE DEVELOPMENT IN CHILDHOOD

Cognitive Period	Description of Period	Behaviors to Observe
Sensory to motor phase (0–24 mo)	The child's thought derives from sensation and movement and is therefore linked to, and limited by, motor and sensory experiences.	Progression of behaviors: Reflexes (0–1 mo). Reaches for object. Manipulates object. Experiments with manipulation. Imitates actions.
Concrete operations: Preoperational thought (2–4 yr)	The child uses symbols and figures to stand for objects, and performs mental combinations by trial and error. Child becomes increasingly able to think (internally represent events) and less dependent on his physical activities for direction of behavior.	Egocentric: thinks everyone thinks and feels as he does. Attributes life to inanimate objects. Confuses inner and outer. Judges events by their outward appearance. Cannot perform a completed process in reverse (irreversibility).
Intuitive subperiod (4–7/8 yr)	The child bases his conclusions on his perceptions. Thought is intuitive and prelogical.	Identifies only one quality of an object at a time (centering). Remains egocentric. Correctly identifies things as having life or motion. Develops a sense of past, present, future.
Operational thought (7/8–11 yr)	The child develops logical operations that can be applied to concrete problems but is unable to apply logic to abstract problems.	Can consider more than one characteristic or relationship at a time (decentering). Can see another person's viewpoint. Able to perform or imagine a process in reverse (reversibility). Develops detailed classification systems. Makes deductions from simple experiences. Understands that something is essentially the same even when shape and texture change (conservation).
Formal operations: (11–15 yr)	Hypothetical and theoretical thinking develop. Uses experimentation and logical analysis to determine relationships between and among things. Can apply logic to problems regardless of content.	Able to think in the abstract. Engages in experimentation. Seeks relationships on an adult level.

TABLE 2
FREUD'S PERIODS OF DEVELOPMENT IN CHILDHOOD

Period	Description of Period	Behaviors to Observe
Oral	The child receives stimulation and pleasure through his mouth.	The child attempts to put everything into his mouth. Receives pleasure from sucking. Tension is reduced by sucking.
Anal (1½–3½ yr)	The child's interest is focused on the anal region and he finds pleasure in holding on and letting go. Muscles are used for expression of control and inhibition.	Engages in play which includes putting things "into" and taking things "out of." Toilet training is mastered by the end of this period.
Genital (phallic) (4–7 yr)	The child exhibits a great deal of intrusive behavior. The Oedipal phase occurs in which the child turns toward the parent of the opposite sex and fears castration by the same sex parent. The Oedipal phase is usually resolved toward the end of this period.	Engages in exhibitionism. States plans to "marry" parent of opposite sex. Exhibits interest in sex differences. Exhibits preoccupation with loss of body parts and bodily injury. Asks many questions related to sexuality. Identification with same sex parent.
Latency (7–11 yr)	The sexual drive (libido) is controlled and repressed during period. Emphasis during this period is on the development of skills and talents.	Devotes energies to the accomplishment of concrete tasks and the acquisition of skills.
Adult sexuality	Resurgence of sexual drives occurs along with a recapitulation of the Oedipal phase. Mastery of this period results in the development of the ability to love and to work.	Separates from parents. Develops relationships with members of the opposite sex. Seeks a role model to replace the parent of the same sex.

TABLE 3
ERIKSON'S DEVELOPMENTAL TASKS FOR CHILDHOOD

Developmental Task	Description of Task	Behaviors to Observe
Trust vs. Mistrust (0–12 mo)	Trust develops when an infant's needs are met consistently and effectively. Mistrust develops when care is inconsistent and inadequate.	Enjoys eating and sucking. Attends to environment. Mother relates to child in a positive manner. Infant reaches out for objects in the environment.
Autonomy vs. Shame/Doubt (1–3 yr)	Autonomy develops when the child is permitted to assert himself. Shame and doubt develop if the child did not develop a sense of trust and/or learns his assertiveness is not acceptable or his actions are ineffective.	Shows a sense of will; "me." Seeks and receives parental reassurance. Explores the environment.
Initiative vs. Guilt (3–6 yr)	Initiative develops if the child is allowed the freedom to initiate motor play, to ask questions, and to engage in fantasy play. Guilt develops if the child is made to feel that his activity is bad, that he is asking too many questions, or that his play is silly.	Starts many tasks; completes few. Interacts more with parents and peers. Exhibits intrusive behavior. Initiates motor activities. Engages in fantasy play. Asks many questions.
Industry vs. Inferiority (6–13 yr)	Industry develops if the child is encouraged in efforts to make things, permitted to do it by himself, and praised for the results. Inferiority develops if the child is not encouraged to do things, and if activities are seen as a nuisance.	Wants to learn to do things well and completes tasks. Participates in a variety of activities. Takes pride in accomplishments. Relives real life situations in play activities.
Identity vs. Role Confusion (13–18 yr)	Identity develops when the adolescent is able to bring together life experiences into a whole and integrate them into an acceptable self image. Role confusion develops when the adolescent is not able to integrate life experiences into a whole and is not sure who he or she is or what he or she can do.	Picture of self held by the adolescent is similar to that held by significant others. Makes long range plans for occupation. Tests social norms. Tries out different life styles. Develops some basic philosophy.

TABLE 4
GROWTH AND DEVELOPMENT NORMS

Gross Motor	Fine Motor-Adaptive	Language	Personal-Social
Newborn to 3 mo			
Lifts head when in prone position momentarily. Lies with head to one side (tonic neck reflex). Head lag when pulled from supine to sitting. Makes swimming movements when in prone position. Head erect with bobbing in vertical position. Sits with back rounded when supported. Raises chest when in prone position—usually supported on forearm.	Sucking, rooting, and Moro reflexes present. Palmar and plantar grasp reflexes present. Does not reach for object but holds object when placed in hand for a moment. Random movement of arms. Follows moving object to midline. Holds hands in front of himself, plays with hands. Reaches for or bats at shiny objects. Brings hands to mouth. Holds rattle for brief time. Movements are symmetrical.	Cries when hungry and uncomfortable. Responds to moderate sound by ceasing activity or widening eyes. Makes small throaty sounds. Pays attention to speaking voice.	Stares at surroundings. Notices faces or bright objects in line of vision. Smiles responsively. Makes no distinction between himself and his environment. Crying differentiated between pain and hunger. Longer periods of wakefulness without crying. Smiles spontaneously.
3 to 6 mo			
Symmetrical body posture. Holds head steady. Lifts head and shoulders up 90 degrees. Tries to roll from back to side. Tonic neck reflex disappears. Supports some weight on legs. No head lag when pulled to sitting. Moro reflex disappears. Sits propped. Neck righting reflex developing. Turns over both ways. May pull self to sitting. Stepping reflex disappearing.	Palmar grasp disappearing. Holds hands open. Moves arms at sight of toy. Hand to mouth movements. Reaches for objects beyond grasp. Whole hand grasp of moderate sized objects. Holds object in each hand briefly. Raking grasp.	Coos and gurgles. Very "talkative." Laughs out loud. Vocalizes displeasure. Babbles. Shows displeasure with crowing.	Initiates social play by smiling. Enjoys having people around. Recognizes familiar objects. Thrashes arms and legs in frustration. Begins to distinguish familiar from unfamiliar faces. Very self-centered. Can tolerate some delay.
6 to 9 mo			
Head precedes body when pulled to sitting. Sits alone leaning on arms. Plays with feet. Bounces when in standing position. Sits alone steadily. Hitches. Crawls. Creeps. Gets to sitting position. Parachute reflex developing.	Bangs two objects together. Transfers toys from hand to hand. Reach and grasp is direct. Beginning pincer grasp. Holds own bottle. Puts nipple in and out at will. Feeds self cracker. Rooting, sucking, and plantar grasp reflexes disappear.	Makes two syllable sounds. Says *Ma Ma* and *Da Da* without meaning. Imitates expressions. Sounds stand for things. Responds to adults' emotional tone. Cries when scolded.	Shows wariness of strangers. Prefers mother. Emotionally changeable from crying to laughing. Affection for other family members. Beginning awareness of separation from environment. Eight-month stranger anxiety.
9 to 12 mo			
Sits steadily. Does not like to lie down except when sleepy. Pulls self to standing. Creeps well. Cruises.	True pincer grasp. Picks up small objects. Can release a toy. Can hold and mark with crayon.	Says one or two words appropriately. Knows own name. Uses jargon. Communicates with self and others.	Feeds self a cookie. Drinks from cup. Likes to eat with fingers. Uses spoon with help. Plays simple games: bye, bye; pat-a-cake; peek-a-boo.

TABLE 4
GROWTH AND DEVELOPMENT NORMS (Con't.)

Gross Motor	Fine Motor-Adaptive	Language	Personal-Social
Stands erect with help of mother's hand. Walks with help. Can sit down without help. Landau reflex developing.		Recognizes *No No.* Speech development slows with onset of walking.	Cooperates with dressing. Shows variety of emotions. Cries for affection. Extends and releases toy upon request. Can follow simple commands, one at a time. Concerned mostly with self. Attachment to mother is still great. Uses mother as a safe haven from which to explore. Beginning of self-assertion.
1 yr old Walks alone—wide based gait. Walking improves, becomes form of play. Creeps up stairs. Runs—seldom falls. Pulls toy behind. Walks backward. Climbs steps or upon furniture. Seats self on small chair.	Builds tower of 2-4 blocks. Throws objects. Opens boxes. Pokes fingers in holes. Turns pages of a book. Differentiates between straight and curved lines. Throws ball. Scribbles vigorously. Grasps spoon, takes to mouth but spills food.	Uses jargon. Names familiar pictures or objects. Vocalizes wants. Points to desired objects. Knows about 10 words. Uses short phrases. Points to several body parts.	Drinks from cup. Plays pat-a-cake. Indicates wants (not by crying). Shifts attention rapidly. Gets into everything. Temper tantrums if things go wrong. Resists sleep after put to bed. May control bowel movements. Thumb sucking when sleepy. Enjoys solitary play or watching others' activity. Selects a favorite toy or object—like blanket. Beginning acceptance of real world rather than complete and immediate gratification of wishes.
2 yr old Steady gait. Walks up and down stairs—both feet on one step. Runs—fewer falls. Walks on tip toes. Can stand on one foot alone. Can ride a tricycle. Throws ball overhand. Kicks ball forward.	Builds tower of 5-8 blocks. Can make cubes into a train. Can open door by turning knob. Imitates vertical strokes. Uses spoon with little spilling. Manipulates play material. Can drink from small glass held in one hand.	Has about 300 words. Uses pronouns. Jargon disappears. Makes 3-4 word sentences. Does not readily ask for help. Enjoys hearing stories.	Obeys simple commands. Treats other children as if they were objects. Drinks well from a glass. Helps to undress himself. Can pull on simple garments. May be toilet-trained in daytime. Does not know right from wrong. Enjoys play with dolls—parallel play. Cannot share possessions. Mimics activities of adults. Takes favorite toy to bed. May begin food likes and dislikes and becomes a "picky" eater. Increasing sign of sense of identity—knows self as separate person. Begins to have a conscience when can control some areas of behavior to conform to social demands.

TABLE 4
GROWTH AND DEVELOPMENT NORMS (Con't.)

	Gross Motor	Fine Motor-Adaptive	Language	Personal-Social
3 yr old	Able to ride tricycle. Walks up stairs alternating feet. Beginning disappearance of sway back and pot belly. Increased coordination.	Begins to use scissors. Can handle beads, blocks. Can unbutton buttons if on side or front. Copies a circle.	Vocabulary about 900 words. Talks in sentences. Stuttering may occur. Can state name.	Decrease in temper tantrums. Can understand simple reasons. Learning from experience is rapid due to interest in new activities. Completely toilet trained. Aware of sexual differences. Begins to work through problems of family relations with other children in play.
4 yr old	Very active. Enjoys activities requiring balance. Can climb and jump well. Throws ball overhand with increased skill.	Uses scissors successfully. Can lace shoes. Can brush teeth. Makes detailed constructions with blocks.	Vocabulary about 1500 words. Exaggerates, boasts, tattles. Much questioning asking how, why. Likes nonsense words.	More noisy, argumentative, aggressive. Talks with and plays with imaginary playmate. Projects on imaginary companion what is bad in self. Developing strong sense of family and home. Imaginative play. May have some friends of the same sex. Beginning sense of morality and conscience.
5 yr old	Increase in muscle coordination. Can hop and jump rope. Increase in strength and coordination. Control over large muscles still greater than control over small muscles.	Dresses with assistance. May be able to tie shoes. Can form some letters correctly. Can use hammer and nails.	Vocabulary about 2100 words. Talks constantly. Asks questions which show thought. Knows names of days of week and week as unit.	Internalizes social norms. Kindergarten important in socialization. Develops personality which gives indication of what he or she will be like as an adult. Wants to accept responsibility and glories in achievements. Serious, businesslike, realistic, literal. Strong feeling for family and identification with parent of same sex. Child lives in the here and now.
6 yr old	Still using large muscles. Movements more coordinated and graceful. Balance improving. Seems to be always active. Throws and catches a ball. Able to ride a bicycle.	Deliberate eye–hand coordination. Develops manual dexterity. Able to print capital letters. Knows right hand from left. Aware of hands as tools; able to cut and paste well.	Command of every form of sentence structure. Uses language as a tool to share in experiences of others. Defines objects in terms of use. Some concept of abstract words.	Learning social role as male or female. Prefers to be with friends of same sex rather than family. Developing mental abilities in school. Learning cooperation and fair play. Gaining self-mastery and independence. Very ritualistic. Self-centered, show-off. Able to complete simple tasks. Enjoys physical activity. Beginning interest in concept of God. Rigid moralism: sees "black" and "white" no "gray" areas in ethics.

TABLE 4
GROWTH AND DEVELOPMENT NORMS (Con't.)

Gross Motor	Fine Motor-Adaptive	Language	Personal-Social
7 and 8 yr olds			
Repeats performances to master them.	Draws human figures more accurately.	Increased ability to use words as vehicles of expression.	Intense—short lived interests.
Moves between very active and passive play activities.	Drops pencil frequently when working.	Increased use of adjectives, adverbs, and conjunctions.	Does some household tasks.
Is more cautious in motor activities.	Can make capital and small letters.		More independent play.
Always on the go.	Increased speed and smoothness in fine motor activity.		Can be reasoned with.
Actions are smoother.	Uses perspective in drawings.		Interested in collecting.
Ready for organized sports.	Can do jigsaw puzzles.		Increasing concept of right and wrong.
	Enjoys building models.		Likes a reward system.
			Forms secret clubs.
			Does not like to lose at games.
			Seeks praise.
			Peer group important.
			Has same-sex best friend.
9 and 10 yr olds			
Likes to display motor skills.	Can use both hands independently.	More accurate and flexible in use of proper names.	May become concerned about health.
Timing better controlled.	Well-developed eye–hand coordination.	Increased use of prepositions and pronouns.	Peer oriented.
Apt to overdo.	Adds details to drawings.	Increased use of compound and complex sentences.	Completes tasks.
Enjoys large muscle, rough and tumble activities.	Can write for longer periods of time.		Concerned about missing school.
Increased stamina.	Builds more complex models; sews and knits.		Somatic complaints may develop when chores are to be done.
			Rebels against parental control.
			Positive feelings about self.
			Begins to think of career.
			Interested in rules.
11 and 12 yr olds			
Likes taking walks; enjoys exploring.	Increasing detail added to work.	Vocabulary of 50,000 words.	Behavior is often paradoxical.
Takes part in team sports.	Improved hand writing.	Better understanding of abstract relationships between words.	More independent and tolerant.
Enjoys constructing things.	Involved in more refined motor activities.		Interested in money.
Seems clumsy inside but is agile in outdoor sports.	Makes collections for display.		Loves conversation.
			Resists doing tasks.
			Enjoys variety and change.
			Relates well with peers.
			Develops interest in opposite sex.
			Well-developed sense of conscience.

Early Adolescence 12–14	Midadolescence 15–16	Late Adolescence 17 ⟶
Adolescent Profile		
Sports participation represents the most common form of gross-motor activity.	There is decreased play activity and talking becomes the major pasttime.	Work may serve as the "play" of earlier years.
Fine motor development involves the refinement of skills.		
Loud boisterous behavior is common.	Develops intense relationships.	Develops ability to maintain stable relationships.
Physical maturity precedes emotional maturity.	May engage in sexual experimentation with peers.	More independent.
Boys generally less concerned about appearance than girls.	Narcissistic behavior is common.	Behavior more predictable.
Vacillation between dependence and independence is common.	Engages in a rich fantasy life.	Experiences less conflict with parents and peers.
Questions traditional values.	Develops deductive reasoning.	Becomes more future oriented.
In conflict with parents.	Disengages from parents.	Develops a sense of community awareness.
	May be hypochondriacal.	Relationship with opposite sex highly valued.

TABLE 5
EVALUATING DEVELOPMENT

Age (months)	Posture and Locomotion	Manipulation	Language	Social
3 mo	Does he support himself on forearms when lying? Does he hold his head up steady while on his stomach?	Are his hands usually open at rest? Does he pull at his clothing?	Does he laugh or make happy noises? Does he turn his head to sounds?	Does he smile at you? Does he reach for familiar people or objects?
6	Does he lift his head when lying on his back? Does he roll from back to front?	Does he transfer a toy from one hand to the other? Does he pick up small objects?	Does he "babble," repeat sounds together (i.e., mum-mum-mum)? Is he frightened by angry noise?	Does he stretch his arms out to be picked up? Does he show his likes and dislikes?
9	Does he sit for long periods without support? Does he pull up on furniture?	Does he pick up objects with his thumb and one finger? Does he finger-feed any foods?	Does he understand "no-no," "bye-bye"? Will he imitate any sounds or words if you make them first?	Does he hold his own bottle? Does he play any nursery games ("peek-a-boo," "bye-bye")?
12	Is he walking (alone or with hand held)? Does he pivot when sitting?	Does he *throw* toys (objects)? Does he give you toys (let go) easily?	Does he have *at least* one meaningful word other than "mama," "dada"? Does he shake his head for "no"?	Does he cooperate in dressing? Does he come when you call him?
18	Does he walk upstairs with help? Can he throw a toy while standing without falling?	Does he turn book pages (2 or 3 at a time)? Does he fill spoon and feed self?	Does he have *at least* 6 real words besides his "jargon?" Does he point at what he wants?	Does he copy you in routine tasks (sweeping, dusting, etc.)? Does he play in the company of other children?
2 yr	Does he run well without falling? Does he walk *up* and *down* stairs alone?	Does he turn book pages one at a time? Does he remove his own shoes, pants?	Does he talk in short (2–3 words) sentences? Does he use pronouns ("me," "you," "mine")?	Does he ask to be taken to the toilet? Does he play in company of other children?
2½	Does he jump, getting both feet off the floor? Does he throw a ball overhand?	Does he unbutton any buttons? Does he hold a pencil or crayon adult fashion?	Does he use plurals or past tense? Does he use the word "I" correctly most of the time?	Does he tell his first and last name if asked? Does he get himself a drink without help?
3	Does he pedal a tricycle? Does he alternate feet (one stair per step) going upstairs?	Does he dry his hands (if reminded)? Does he dress and undress fully including front buttons?	Does he tell little stories about his experiences? Does he know his sex?	Does he share his toys? Does he play well *with* another child? Take turns?
4	Does he attempt to hop or skip? Does he alternate feet going downstairs?	Does he button clothes fully? Does he catch a ball?	Does he say a song or a poem from memory? Does he know all his colors?	Does he tell "tall tales" or "show off?" Does he play *cooperatively* with a small *group* of children?
5	Does he skip, alternating feet? Does he jump rope or jump over low obstacles?	Does he tie his own shoes? Does he spread with a knife?	Can he print his first name? Does he ever ask what a word means?	Is he a "mother's helper," likes to do things for you? Does he play competitive games and abide by the *rules*?

Capute A, Biehl R: (1973). Developmental attainment form. The Pediatric Clinics of North America 20: 8–9, Philadelphia Saunders, used by permission.

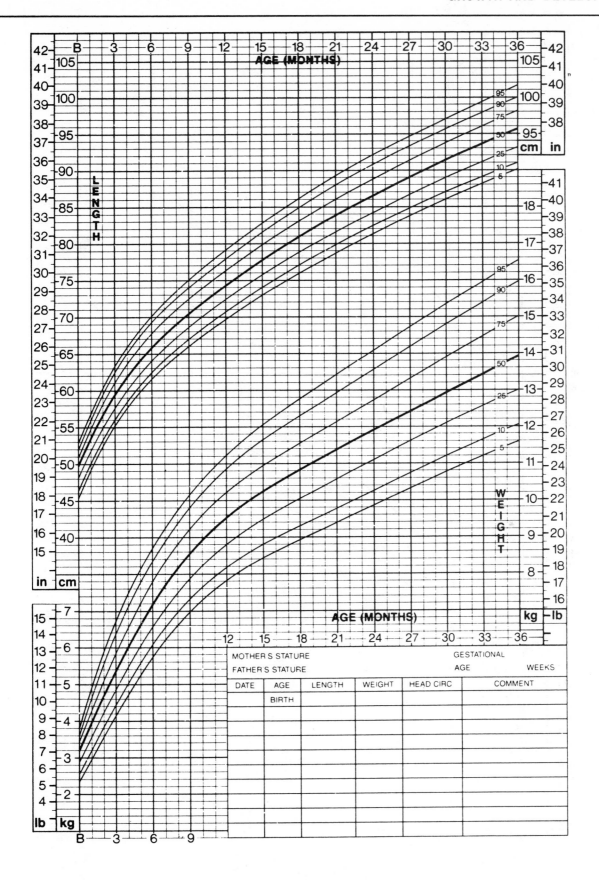

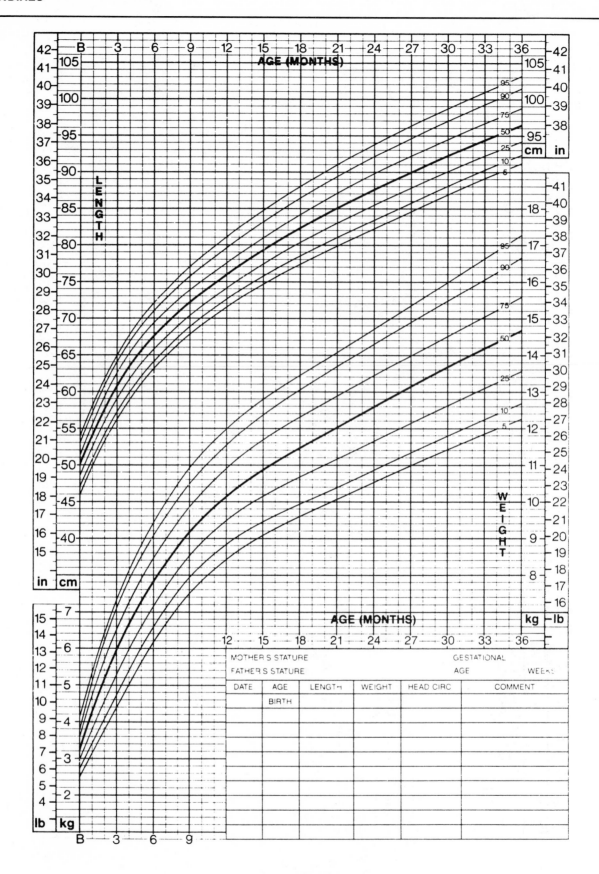

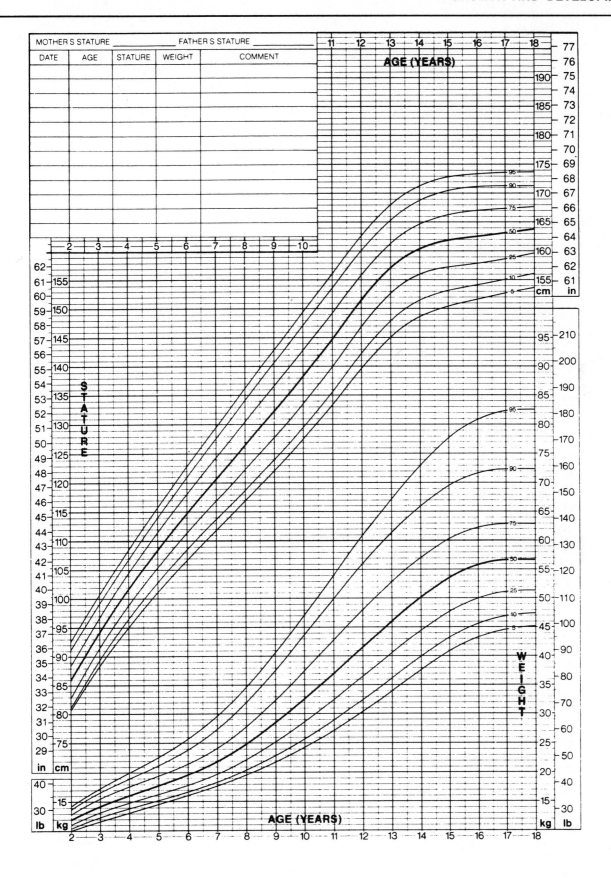

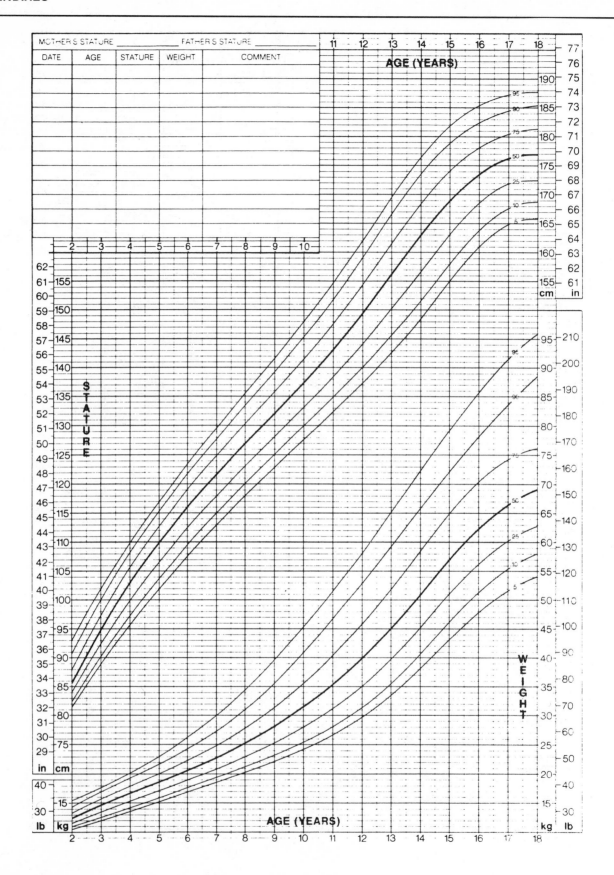

DATE	AGE	STATURE	WEIGHT	COMMENT

MOTHER'S STATURE _____ FATHER'S STATURE _____

AGE (YEARS)

STATURE

WEIGHT

AGE (YEARS)

Health Promotion

TABLE 1
GUIDELINES FOR HEALTH SUPERVISION

Each child and family is unique: therefore these **Guidelines for Health Supervision of Children and Youth**[1] are designed for the care of children who are receiving competent parenting, have no manifestations of any important health problems, and are growing and developing in satisfactory fashion. **Additional visits may become necessary** if circumstances suggest variations from normal. These guidelines represent a consensus by the Committee on Practice and Ambulatory Medicine, in consultation with the membership of the American Academy of Pediatrics through the Chapter Chairmen.

The Committee emphasizes the great importance of **continuity of care** in comprehensive health supervision[2] and the need to avoid **fragmentation of care**[3].

A **prenatal visit** by the parents for anticipatory guidance and pertinent medical history is strongly recommended.

Health supervision should begin with medical care of the newborn in the hospital.

AGE[4]	Infancy						Early Childhood					Late Childhood					Adolescence			
	By 1 mo.	2 mos.	4 mos.	6 mos.	9 mos.	12 mos.	15 mos.	18 mos.	24 mos.	3 yrs.	4 yrs.	5 yrs.	6 yrs.	8 yrs.	10 yrs.	12 yrs.	14 yrs.	16 yrs.	18 yrs.	20+ yrs.
HISTORY Initial/Interval	•	•	•	•	•	•	•	•	•	•	•	•	•	•	•	•	•	•	•	•
MEASUREMENTS Height and Weight	•	•	•	•	•	•	•	•	•	•	•	•	•	•	•	•	•	•	•	•
Head Circumference	•	•	•	•	•	•														
Blood Pressure										•	•	•	•	•	•	•	•	•	•	•
SENSORY SCREENING Vision	S	S	S	S	S	S	S	S	S	O	O	O	O	O	S	O	O	S	O	O
Hearing	S	S	S	S	S	S	S	S	S	S	O	O	S[5]	S[5]	S[5]	O	S	S	O	S
DEVEL./BEHAV. ASSESSMENT[6]	•	•	•	•	•	•	•	•	•	•	•	•	•	•	•	•	•	•	•	•
PHYSICAL EXAMINATION[7]	•	•	•	•	•	•	•	•	•	•	•	•	•	•	•	•	•	•	•	•
PROCEDURES[8] Hered./Metabolic Screening[9]	•																			
Immunization[10]		•	•	•			•	•				•					•			
Tuberculin Test						•			11 •					11 •					11 •	
Hematocrit or Hemoglobin[12]					•				•						•				•	
Urinalysis[13]				•					•						•				•	
ANTICIPATORY GUIDANCE[14]	•	•	•	•	•	•	•	•	•	•	•	•	•	•	•	•	•	•	•	•
INITIAL DENTAL REFERRAL[15]									•											

1. Committee on Practice and Ambulatory Medicine. 1981.
2. Statement on Continuity of Pediatric Care, Committee on Standards of Child Health Care, 1978.
3. Statement on Fragmentation of Pediatric Care, Committee on Standards of Child Health Care, 1978.
4. If a child comes under care for the first time at any point on the Schedule, or if any items are not accomplished at the suggested age, the Schedule should be brought up to date at the earliest possible time.
5. At these points, history may suffice; if problem suggested, a standard testing method should be employed.
6. By history and appropriate physical examination; if suspicious, by specific objective developmental testing.
7. At each visit, a complete physical examination is essential, with infant totally unclothed, older child undressed and suitably draped.
8. These may be modified, depending upon entry point into schedule and individual need.
9. PKU and thyroid testing should be done at about 2 wks. Infants initially screened before 24 hours of age should be rescreened.
10. Schedule(s) per Report of Committee on Infectious Disease, ed. 18, 1982.

11. The Committee on Infectious Diseases recommends tuberculin testing at 12 months of age and every 1-2 years thereafter. In some areas tuberculosis is of exceedingly low occurrence and the physician may elect not to retest routinely or to use longer intervals.
12. Present medical evidence suggests the need for reevaluation of the frequency and timing of hemoglobin or hematocrit tests. One determination is therefore suggested during each time period. Performance of additional tests is left to the individual practice experience.
13. Present medical evidence suggests the need for reevaluation of the frequency and timing of urinalyses. One determination is therefore suggested during each time period. Performance of additional tests is left to the individual practice experience.
14. Appropriate discussion and counseling should be an integral part of each visit for care.
15. Subsequent examinations as prescribed by dentist.

N.B.: Special chemical, immunologic, and endocrine testing are usually carried out upon specific indications. Testing other than newborn (e.g., inborn errors of metabolism, sickle disease, lead) are discretionary with the physician.

Key: • = to be performed; S = subjective, by history; O = objective, by a standard testing method.

TABLE 2
RECOMMENDED SCHEDULE FOR ACTIVE
IMMUNIZATION OF NORMAL INFANTS AND
CHILDREN

Recommended Age	Vaccine(s)	Comments
2 mo	DTP,* OPV†	Can be initiated earlier in areas of high endemicity
4 mo	DTP, OPV	2-mo interval desired for OPV to avoid interference
6 mo	DTP (OPV)	OPV optional for areas where polio might be imported (e.g., some areas of Southwest United States)
12 mo	Tuberculin Test‡	May be given simultaneously with MMR at 15 mo (see text)
15 mo	Measles, Mumps, Rubella (MMR)§	MMR preferred
18 mo	DTP, OPV	Consider as part of primary series—DTP essential
4–6 yr″	DTP, OPV	
14–16 yr	Td#	Repeat every 10 years for lifetime

*DTP—Diphtheria and tetanus toxoids with pertussis vaccine.
†OPV—Oral, attenuated poliovirus vaccine contains poliovirus types 1, 2, and 3.
‡Tuberculin test—Mantoux (intradermal PPD) preferred. Frequency of tests depends on local epidemiology. The Committee recommends annual or biennial testing unless local circumstances dictate less frequent or no testing (see *Tuberculosis* for complete discussion).
§MMR—Live measles, mumps, and rubella viruses in a combined vaccine (see text for discussion of single vaccines versus combination).
″Up to the seventh birthday.
#Td—Adult tetanus toxoid (full dose) and diphtheria toxoid (reduced dose) in combination.
For all products used, consult manufacturer's brochure for instructions for storage, handling, and administration. Biologics prepared by different manufacturers may vary, and those of the same manufacturer may change from time to time. The package insert should be followed for a specific product.
From American Academy of Pediatrics, Report on the Committee on Infectious Diseases, 19th ed. Evanston, IL; Copyright the American Academy of Pediatrics, 1983, used with permission.

TABLE 3
RECOMMENDED IMMUNIZATION SCHEDULES FOR INFANTS AND CHILDREN NOT INITIALLY IMMUNIZED AT USUAL RECOMMENDED TIMES IN EARLY INFANCY

Timing	Recommended Schedules				Comments
	Preferred Schedule	Alternatives			
		#1	#2	#3	
First visit	DTP #1, OPV #1, Tuberculin test (PPD)	MMR, PPD	DTP #1, OPV #1, PPD	DTP #1, OPV #1, MMR, PPD	MMR should be given no younger than 15 mo old.
1 mo after first visit	MMR	DTP #1, OPV #1	MMR, DTP #2	DTP #2	
2 mo after first visit	DTP #2, OPV #2	—	DTP #3, OPV #2	DTP #3, OPV #2	—
3 mo after first visit	(DTP #3)	DTP #2, OPV #2	—	—	In preferred schedule, DTP #3 can be given if OPV #3 is not to be given until 10–16 mo.
4 mo after first visit	DTP #3 (OPV #3)	—	(OPV #3)	(OPV #3)	OPV #3 optional for areas for likely importation of polio (e.g., some southwestern states).
5 mo after first visit	—	DTP #3 (OPV #3)	—	—	
10–16 mo after last dose	DTP #4, OPV #3 or OPV #4	DTP #4, OPV #3 or OPV #4	DTP #4, OPV #3 or OPV #4	DTP #4, OPV #3 or OPV #4	—
Preschool	DTP #5, OPV #4 or OPV #5	DTP #5, OPV #4 or OPV #5	DTP #5, OPV #4 or OPV #5	DTP #5, OPV #4 or OPV #5	Preschool dose not necessary if DTP #4 or #5 given after fourth birthday.
14–16 yr old	Td	Td	Td	Td	Repeat every 10 yr.

Alternative #1 can be used in those more than 15 months old if measles is occurring in the community.
Alternative #2 allows for more rapid DTP immunization.
Alternative #3 should be reserved for those whose access to medical care is compromised by poor compliance.
DTP = Diphtheria and tetanus toxoids with pertussis vaccine.
OPV = Oral, attenuated poliovirus vaccine contains types 1, 2, and 3.
Tuberculin test = Mantoux (intradermal PPD) preferred. Frequency of tests depends on local epidemiology. The Committee recommends annual or biennial testing unless local circumstances dictate less frequent or no testing (see *Tuberculosis* for complete discussion).
MMR = Live measles, mumps, and rubella viruses in a combined vaccine (see text for discussion of single vaccines).
Td = Adult tetanus toxoid (full dose) and diphtheria toxoid (reduced dose) in combination.
For all products used, consult manufacturer's brochure for instructions for storage, handling, and administration. Biologics prepared by different manufacturers may vary, and those of the same manufacturer may change from time to time. The package insert should be followed for a specific product.
From American Academy of Pediatrics, Report of the Committee on Infectious Diseases, 19th ed. Evanston, IL; Copyright the American Academy of Pediatrics, 1983, used with permission.

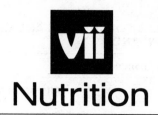

Nutrition

TABLE 1
SAMPLE NUTRITION HISTORY

Name _____

Age _____

What does _____ (name of child) usually eat for
  Breakfast
  Lunch
  Dinner
  Snacks

What did _____ eat yesterday?

How many meals does _____ eat each day and where?

Is _____ a picky or poor eater?

Do you feed _____ or does he/she feed him/herself?

How many cups of milk does _____ drink a day?

What are _____ favorite foods?

What foods does _____ dislike/not eat?

Does _____ take vitamins? Iron?

How much exercise does _____ get a day?

Is _____ allergic to any foods?

Does anyone in your family eat anything other than the usual foods (e.g., starch, clay)?

TABLE 2
GUIDE TO NUTRIENTS

Nutrient	Function
Protein Meat, poultry, fish, eggs, cheese, milk	Essential for growth and life-long body maintenance Builds resistance to disease

Minerals
  Calcium
    Milk, yogurt, cheese, collards, kale
	Forms healthy bones and teeth
	Aids in normal blood clotting
	Helps nerves and muscles react normally

Iron Liver, meat, dark greens, egg yolks, dried beans, and peas	Helps blood cells carry oxygen from the lungs to body cells Protects against some forms of nutritional anemia
Fats Shortening, oil, butter, margarine	Carry vitamins A, D, E, & K Source of energy (calories) best used in limited amounts
Carbohydrates Cereal, potatoes, dried beans, corn, bread, sugar	Inexpensive source of energy Best when consumed as fruit, sugar, or starch (bread, cereal foods, potatoes)

Vitamins
  A
    Liver, carrots, sweet potatoes, greens, butter, margarine
	Protects eyes and night vision
	Helps keep skin healthy
	Builds resistance to disease

B-complex Liver, nuts, fortified cereal products	Protects the nervous system Keeps appetite and digestion in working order Aids body cells in using fats, carbohydrates, and protein for energy
C Tomatoes, raw cabbage, broccoli, orange, strawberries	Keeps body cells and tissues strong and healthy Aids in healing wounds and broken bones
D Milk (Very important for children)	Aids in absorption and use of calcium and phosphorus by body cells Helps build strong bones and teeth

Water
  Very important for the young child with a rapid metabolic rate.
  Found in all foods, particularly fruits and vegetables
	Required to maintain homeostatis, evaporative losses, excrete renal solute load, build cells, and body fluids

Adapted from Meal Time! Happy Time! A Guide for Parents, The American Dietetic Association, used with permission.

TABLE 3
FOODS FOR EVERYDAY

	1–3 yr	4–6 yr	7–10 yr	11–Adolescence	Comment
Meat group Meat, poultry, fish, organ meats, or meat substitutes	2 servings (1 ounce each)	2 servings (1½ ounce each)	2 servings (1½–2 ounces each)	2 servings (2–3 ounces each)	Substitutes for the protein of 1 ounce meat: 1 egg, 1 ounce cheese, ¼ cup cottage cheese, ¼ cup peanuts, ⅓ cup other nuts, ½ cup cooked dry peas or beans, 2 tbsp. peanut butter
Milk group Milk (Whole, skim dry, evaporated, buttermilk) and other dairy products	2 cups	2 cups	2 cups	3–4 cups (5–6 cups for pregnant adolescents)	Substitutes for the calcium of 1 cup milk: 1 cup yogurt, 1⅓ cup cottage cheese, 1½ cup ice cream, 1¼ ounce (⅓ cup grated) natural cheese, 1¾ ounce process cheese

TABLE 3 (Con't).
FOODS FOR EVERYDAY

	1–3 yr	4–6 yr	7–10 yr	11–Adoles-cense	Comment
Vegetable-fruit group					
For vitamin A: deep yellow-orange or very dark green For vitamin C: citrus fruit, melon, strawberries, broccoli, tomatoes, raw cabbage	4 servings or more (3 tbsp each)	4 servings or more (3 tbsp each)	4 servings or more (⅓ cup each)	4 servings or more (½ cup each)	Eat one vitamin C source daily, one high vitamin A source at least every other day. Other fruits and vegetables fill out this food group.
Bread and cereal group					
Whole grain or enriched bread, cereal, rice, pasta	3 servings	4 servings	4 servings or more	4 servings or more (6 or more for boys)	Very active children, adolescents, adults, and athletes need more for energy. A serving is 1 slice bread, 1 roll, ½ cup cooked cereal products, 1 ounce dry cereal.
Calorie needs	1,300	1,800	2,400	2,400 girls, 2,800–3,000 boys	

From Meal Time! Happy Time! A Guide for Parents. The American Dietetic Association, used with permission.

TABLE 4
INFANT NUTRITION

Age (mo)	Total daily requirements	How met
0–4	20–30 ounces of milk*	Formula, breast milk
4–6	32 ounces of milk	Formula, breast milk
	4–6 tbsp. dry cereal†	Offer rice cereal first, and mixed or wheat cereal last
	3–4 tbsp. vegetables	Pureed table food or commercial baby food
	4–9 tbsp. fruit	Pureed table food or commercial baby food
	2–4 tbsp. meat	Pureed meat or commercial whole meat preparations
6–8	28 ounces of milk	Formula, breast milk, or whole milk
	½ cup cereal	Increase table foods, decrease commercial infant foods; give small finger food pieces
	4–8 tbsp. vegetables	(fruit, vegetable, cheese), provide firm foods for teething (teething biscuit)
	4–8 tbsp. fruit	
	4–8 tbsp. meat	
8–12	20–24 ounces of milk	Formula, breast milk, whole milk
	½ cup cereal	Increase table foods and eliminate commercial infant foods by end of first year. Avoid
	2 slices bread, or potato, rice, macaroni	additional salt or sugar
	4–8 tbsp. vegetable	
	4–8 tbsp. meat	
	4–8 tbsp. fruit	

*Breast milk and prepared formula purchased in the store contain 20 calories per ounce.
†Start with a teaspoon of solid food and increase the amount slowly. Divide the total amount among the meals served.

Self-Examination

How to Do Testicular Self-Examination

Cancer of the testes—the male reproductive glands—is one of the most common cancers in men 15 to 34 years of age. It accounts for 12 percent of all cancer deaths in this group.

If discovered in the early stages, testicular cancer can be treated promptly and effectively. It's important for you to take time to learn the basic facts about this type of cancer—its symptoms, treatment, and what you can do to get the help you need when it counts.

A major risk factor

Men who have an undescended or partially descended testicle are at a much higher risk of developing testicular cancer than others.

However, it is a simple procedure to correct the undescended testicle condition. See your doctor if this applies to you.

What are the symptoms?

The first sign of testicular cancer is usually a slight enlargement of one of the testes, and a change in its consistency.

Pain may be absent, but often there is a dull ache in the lower abdomen and groin, together with a sensation of dragging and heaviness.

What can I do?

Your best hope for early detection of testicular cancer is a simple three-minute monthly self-examination. The best time is after a warm bath or shower, when the scrotal skin is most relaxed.

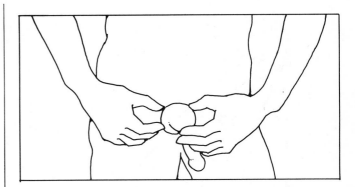

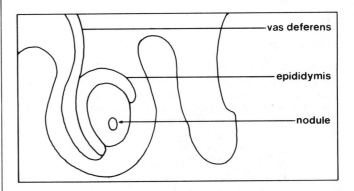

Role each testicle gently between the thumb and fingers of both hands. If you find any hard lumps or nodules, you should see your doctor promptly. They may not be malignant, but only your doctor can make the diagnosis.

Following a thorough physical examination, your doctor may perform certain x-ray studies to make the most accurate diagnosis possible.

From For Men Only: Testicular Cancer and How to do TSE. #2093-LE. The American Cancer Society, used with permission.

How to Examine Your Breasts

1

In the shower:

Examine your breasts during bath or shower; hands glide easier over wet skin. Fingers flat, move gently over every part of each breast. Use right hand to examine left breast, left hand for right breast. Check for any lump, hard knot or thickening.

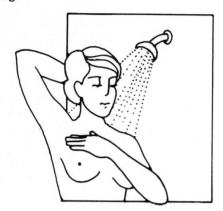

2

Before a mirror:

Inspect your breasts with arms at your sides. Next, raise your arms high overhead. Look for any changes in contour of each breast, a swelling, dimpling of skin or changes in the nipple.

Then, rest palms on hips and press down firmly to flex your chest muscles. Left and right breast will not exactly match—few women's breasts do.

Regular inspection shows what is normal for you and will give you confidence in your examination

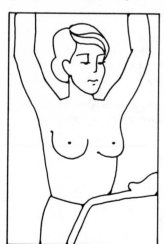 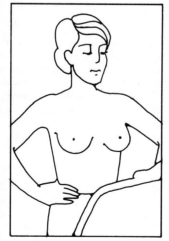

3

Lying down:

To examine your right breast, put a pillow or folded towel under your right shoulder. Place right hand behind your head—this distributes breast tissue more evenly on the chest.

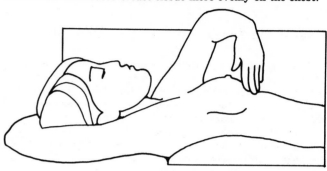

With left hand, fingers flat, press gently in small circular motions around an imaginary clock face. Begin at outermost top of your right breast for 12 o'clock, then move to 1 o'clock, and so on around the circle back to 12. A ridge of firm tissue in the lower curve of each breast is normal. Then move in an inch, toward the nipple, keep circling to examine *every part of your breast,* including nipple. This requires at least three more circles. Now slowly repeat procedure on your left breast with a pillow under your left shoulder and left hand behind head. Notice how your breast structure feels.

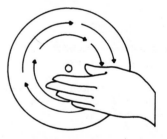

Finally, squeeze the nipple of each breast gently between thumb and index finger. Any discharge, clear or bloody, should be reported to your doctor immediately.

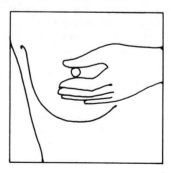

From How to Examine Your Breasts. #2088-LE. The American Cancer Society, used with permission.

Denver Developmental Screening Test

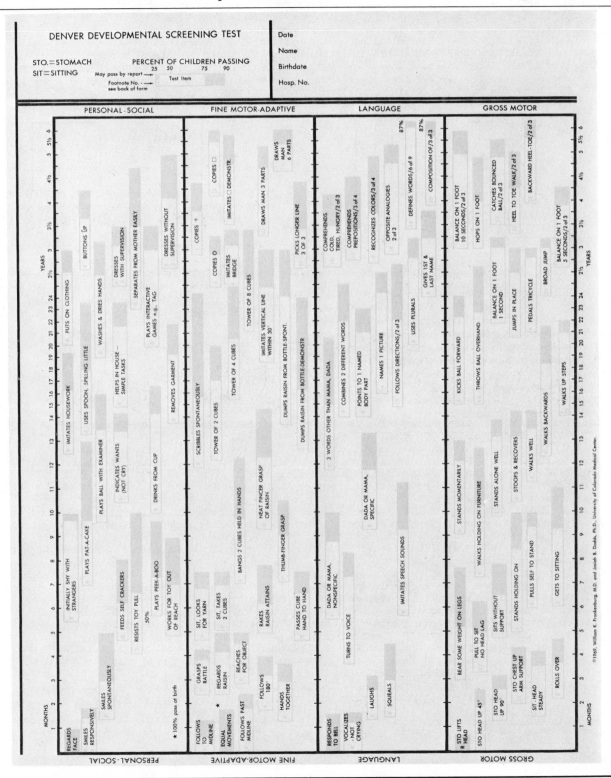

DIRECTIONS

DATE

NAME

BIRTHDATE

HOSP. NO.

1. Try to get child to smile by smiling, talking or waving to him. Do not touch him.
2. When child is playing with toy, pull it away from him. Pass if he resists.
3. Child does not have to be able to tie shoes or button in the back.
4. Move yarn slowly in an arc from one side to the other, about 6" above child's face. Pass if eyes follow 90° to midline. (Past midline; 180°)
5. Pass if child grasps rattle when it is touched to the backs or tips of fingers.
6. Pass if child continues to look where yarn disappeared or tries to see where it went. Yarn should be dropped quickly from sight from tester's hand without arm movement.
7. Pass if child picks up raisin with any part of thumb and a finger.
8. Pass if child picks up raisin with the ends of thumb and index finger using an over hand approach.

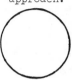 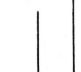 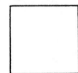

9. Pass any enclosed form. Fail continuous round motions.
10. Which line is longer? (Not bigger.) Turn paper upside down and repeat. (3/3 or 5/6)
11. Pass any crossing lines.
12. Have child copy first. If failed, demonstrate

When giving items 9, 11 and 12, do not name the forms. Do not demonstrate 9 and 11.

13. When scoring, each pair (2 arms, 2 legs, etc.) counts as one part.
14. Point to picture and have child name it. (No credit is given for sounds only.)

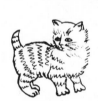 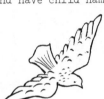 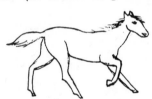 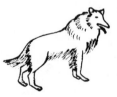 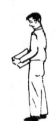

15. Tell child to: Give block to Mommie; put block on table; put block on floor. Pass 2 of 3. (Do not help child by pointing, moving head or eyes.)
16. Ask child: What do you do when you are cold? ..hungry? ..tired? Pass 2 of 3.
17. Tell child to: Put block on table; under table; in front of chair, behind chair. Pass 3 of 4. (Do not help child by pointing, moving head or eyes.)
18. Ask child: If fire is hot, ice is ?; Mother is a woman, Dad is a ?; a horse is big, a mouse is ?. Pass 2 of 3.
19. Ask child: What is a ball? ..lake? ..desk? ..house? ..banana? ..curtain? ..ceiling? ..hedge? ..pavement? Pass if defined in terms of use, shape, what it is made of or general category (such as banana is fruit, not just yellow). Pass 6 of 9.
20. Ask child: What is a spoon made of? ..a shoe made of? ..a door made of? (No other objects may be substituted.) Pass 3 of 3.
21. When placed on stomach, child lifts chest off table with support of forearms and/or hands.
22. When child is on back, grasp his hands and pull him to sitting. Pass if head does not hang back.
23. Child may use wall or rail only, not person. May not crawl.
24. Child must throw ball overhand 3 feet to within arm's reach of tester.
25. Child must perform standing broad jump over width of test sheet. (8-1/2 inches)
26. Tell child to walk forward, ⌒⌒⌒⌒⌒→ heel within 1 inch of toe. Tester may demonstrate. Child must walk 4 consecutive steps, 2 out of 3 trials.
27. Bounce ball to child who should stand 3 feet away from tester. Child must catch ball with hands, not arms, 2 out of 3 trials.
28. Tell child to walk backward, ←⌒⌒⌒⌒ toe within 1 inch of heel. Tester may demonstrate. Child must walk 4 consecutive steps, 2 out of 3 trials.

DATE AND BEHAVIORAL OBSERVATIONS (how child feels at time of test, relation to tester, attention span, verbal behavior, self-confidence, etc,):

Accepted Nursing Diagnoses*

ACTIVITY INTOLERANCE
ANXIETY
BOWEL ELIMINATION, ALTERATIONS IN:
  CONSTIPATION
BOWEL ELIMINATION, ALTERATIONS IN:
  DIARRHEA/INCONTINENCE
CARDIAC OUTPUT, ALTERATIONS IN:
  DECREASED
COMFORT, ALTERATIONS IN: PAIN
COMMUNICATION, IMPAIRED VERBAL
COPING, INEFFECTIVE INDIVIDUAL
COPING, INEFFECTIVE FAMILY:
  COMPROMISED/DISBLING
COPING, FAMILY: POTENTIAL FOR
  GROWTH
DIVERSIONAL ACTIVITY DEFICIT
FAMILY PROCESSES, ALTERATIONS IN
FEAR (SPECIFY)
FLUID VOLUME DEFICIT
FLUID VOLUME EXCESS
GRIEVING
HEALTH MAINTENANCE, ALTERA-
  TIONS IN
HOME MAINTENANCE MANAGEMENT,
  IMPAIRED
INJURY, POTENTIAL FOR (SPECIFY)
KNOWLEDGE DEFICIT (SPECIFY)
MOBILITY, IMPAIRED PHYSICAL
NONCOMPLIANCE (SPECIFY)
NUTRITION, ALTERATIONS IN:
  LESS THAN BODY REQUIREMENTS

NUTRITION, ALTERATIONS IN:
  MORE THAN BODY REQUIREMENTS
ORAL MUCOUS MEMBRANE, ALTERA-
  TIONS IN
PARENTING, ALTERATIONS IN
POWERLESSNESS
RAPE TRAUMA SYNDROME
RESPIRATORY FUNCTION, ALTERATIONS
  IN: AIRWAY CLEARANCE INEFFECTIVE
  BREATHING PATTERNS, INEFFECTIVE
  GAS EXCHANGE, IMPAIRED
SELF-CARE DEFICIT: TOTAL: FEEDING;
  BATHING/HYGIENE; DRESSING/
  GROOMING; TOILETING
SELF-CONCEPT, DISTURBANCE IN
SENSORY-PERCEPTUAL ALTERATIONS
  (SPECIFY)
SEXUAL DYSFUNCTION
SKIN INTEGRITY, IMPAIRMENT OF
SLEEP PATTERN DISTURBANCE
SOCIAL ISOLATION
SPIRITUAL DISTRESS
TISSUE PERFUSION, ALTERATIONS IN
  CEREBRAL, CARDIOPULMONARY,
  RENAL, GASTROINTESTINAL,
  PERIPHERAL
URINARY ELIMINATION, ALTERATION IN
  PATTERNS OF
VIOLENCE, POTENTIAL FOR

*This list of nursing diagnoses may be removed from the text. It is designed so that it can be folded over a 3 × 5 index card, enclosed in plastic, and used as a pocket reference.
Fifth National Congress (1982) From Carpenito, L. J. 1983 *Nursing Diagnosis:Application to Clinical Practice,* Philadelphia, Lippincott. Used with permission.